MW01038539

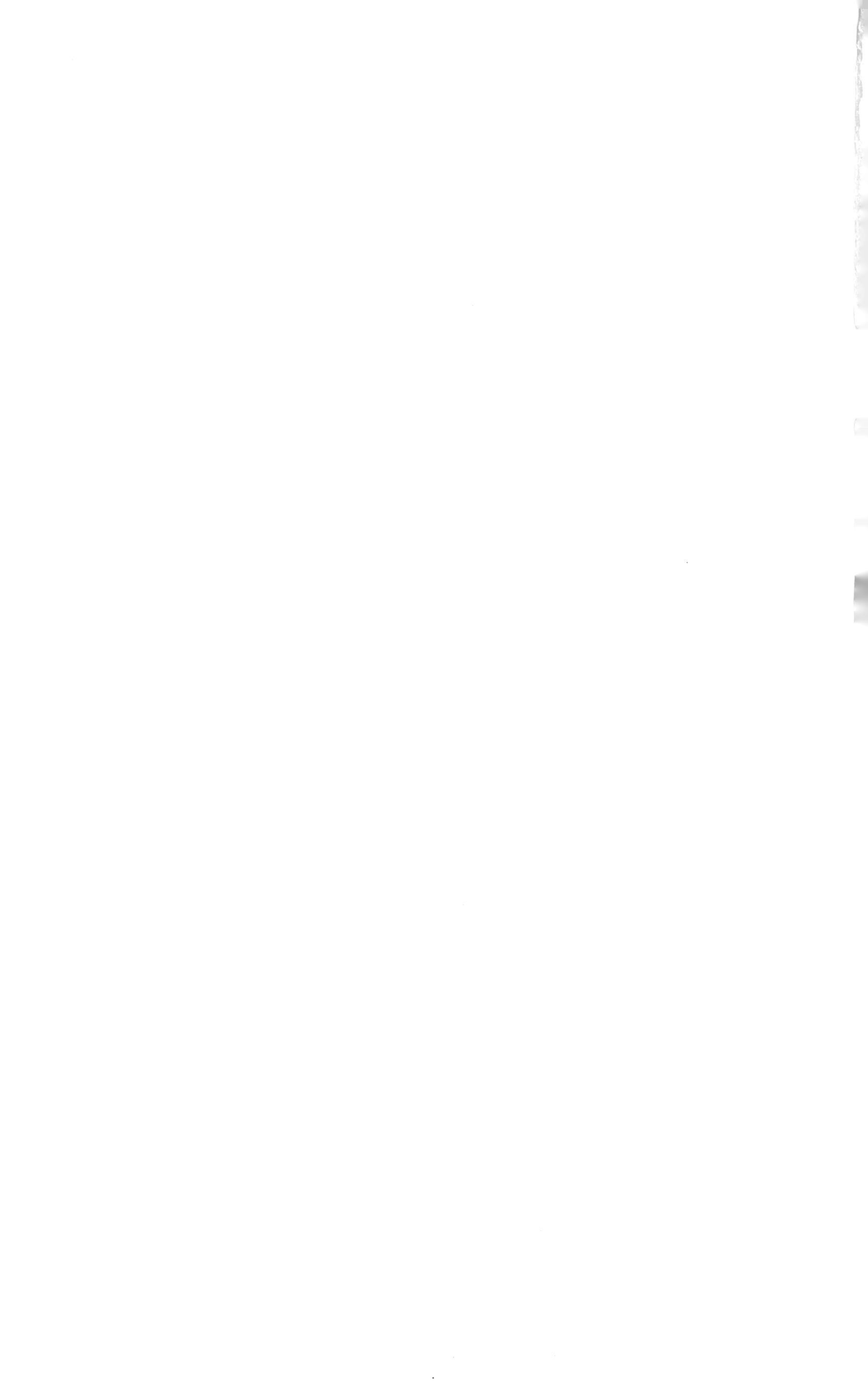

Handbook of Autism Spectrum Disorder and the Law

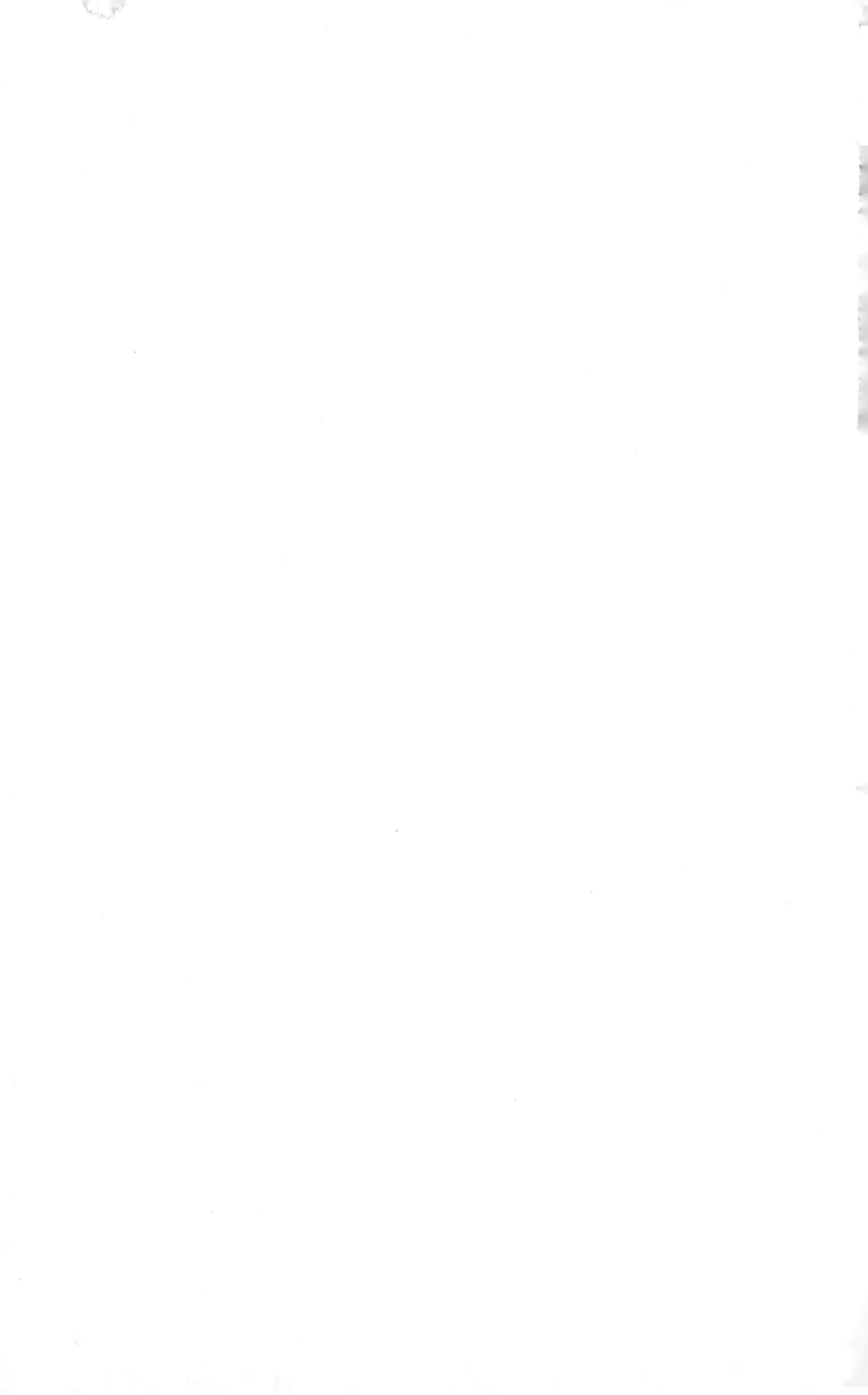

Fred R. Volkmar · Rachel Loftin ·
Alexander Westphal · Marc Woodbury-Smith
Editors

Handbook of Autism Spectrum Disorder and the Law

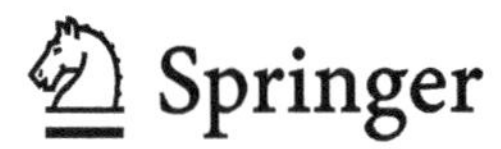

Editors
Fred R. Volkmar
Yale Child Study Center and Autism Center of Excellence
Yale University and Southern Conn. State University
New Haven, USA

Rachel Loftin
Department of Psychiatry and Behavioral Sciences
Northwestern University Feinberg School of Medicine
Chicago, USA

Alexander Westphal
Division of Law and Psychiatry
Yale School of Medicine
New Haven, USA

Marc Woodbury-Smith
Biosciences Institute
Newcastle University
Newcastle upon Tyne, UK

ISBN 978-3-030-70912-9 ISBN 978-3-030-70913-6 (eBook)
https://doi.org/10.1007/978-3-030-70913-6

This Springer imprint is published by the registered company Springer Nature Switzerland AG
The registered company address is: Gewerbestrasse 11, 6330 Cham, Switzerland

Foreword: Autism and Law

Our societal treatment of those with autism is checkered at best. For much of the twentieth century, autism has been misunderstood and misperceived as a disorder. Separated and shunned from the rest of society for much of the past century, it is only in the very recent past that integration has become de rigueur. Today, the challenge is to understand how we integrate a portion of the population that intrinsically has challenged most of us fail to comprehend and appreciate. Autism often presents itself as an invisible challenge. The casual observer may look at someone and not be able to discern whether or not the person with whom they are engaging is autistic. Yet their challenges navigating the social world can be daunting. For instance, one of the day-to-day challenges of individuals on the spectrum is comprehending and adapting to social norms—*What does that look mean? Why did he/she say that? Is someone approaching me as friend or foe?*

There is a greater understanding now of what autism is as a disorder but, more importantly, society is beginning to redefine what is possible for children, young adults and mature adults who are on the Autism Spectrum. People on the spectrum are going to college, getting jobs, integrating into the fabric of communities and, yes, even getting married. We learn that more and more people on the spectrum are not just engaging in activities previously thought to be beyond the capacity of similarly challenged persons, but excelling in ways not thought to be attainable. And there lies the rub—being encouraged, prodded and positioned to engage in society, the resultant exposure can and does lead to entanglements (some good and some bad) with the law.

Autism and the Law is a wonderful addition to the literature on autism that speaks in large measure to both scientists and laypersons. This Handbook is a treatment of the myriad instances where the law and science intersect. As is true of any substantive area of the law, no one source can cover every context in which autism intersects with legal jurisprudence. It is a fool's errand to try. What *Autism and the Law* offers the reader is a sensible and practical treatment of areas of the law that may present particular challenges to persons on the spectrum. *Autism and the Law* takes on these challenges straightforwardly, with the objective of educating and familiarizing those engaged in the law or addressing a legal situation with at least a base understanding of the challenges facing those on the spectrum and those responsible for engaging with them.

This Handbook is a true melding of science and law. The brilliance of the presentation is the contributors schooled in science and/or law present a text that is both useful and readable. The reader is made to understand how autism affects those afflicted in different instances—how does autism affect a person dealing with trauma? What effect does autism have on cognitive functioning as it relates to empathy and social ability? The varying topics effectively create a baseline of knowledge, but individually each chapter provides enough information to address many legal situations.

This Handbook is not a how to or what do I do as much as it is a desktop reference that allows one to navigate some very complicated situations where a person on the spectrum comes in contact with legal situations when a specialized understanding of autism and its effect on the person on the spectrum is critical. For example, the chapter addressing how a person's autism affects their interface with the criminal justice system, particularly, as a defendant (or a victim or witness) is fascinating. The chapter is a must-read to all involved in the criminal justice dynamic—defense attorney, prosecutor, judge and autistic witness, defendant, or victim. Based on my own background as a federal judge, a federal prosecutor, and defense attorney, I found this chapter particularly fascinating because if each player in the dynamic lacks a basic understanding of autism—justice cannot be done. An appreciation of how autism affects memory, perception, anxiety, social relationships, and language to name a few, can help maintain the delicate balance that keeps the criminal justice system on an even keel. More important, these understandings are absolutely critical to a fair adjudication for the autistic defendant or an autistic victim of a crime as well.

Those on the spectrum and those who love and care for them will surely find this Handbook insightful and useful. But this Handbook offers a farther reach. Doctors, lawyers, law enforcement personnel, medical workers, employers, and their employees will all benefit from this practical guide. The data presented in this Hand book is enormously useful in the workplace, educational settings, and the criminal justice system. As our nation faces a continuing explosion of people diagnosed on the spectrum, judges, law enforcement officers, attorneys, and employers will need source material to consult. Laws, policies, and procedures will have to continue to evolve if we are to create just and fair environments for our fellow citizens on the spectrum to be full participants in all our nation has to offer. Finally, scientists, scholars, and policymakers whose research includes autism will benefit from reading and rereading this Handbook. Advances in intervention happen when we can enhance awareness, increase understanding and reshape expectations of policy makers and practitioners about how the law impacts those on the spectrum. I suspect that the deeper and substantive treatment of the law as it relates to autism that this Handbook offers will be critical for designing more effective interventions in the future.

Twenty years ago, my daughter was diagnosed with autism. My family and I worked tirelessly to build an infrastructure around her in which she could flourish. I am honored to have the opportunity to reflect on the promise of this book as a judge, a scholar, and a father. The Handbook is just the first edition and my hope is to see it evolve over time. It will doubtless have to be updated regularly as laws, policies, views, and attitudes change. For now, it is an excellent resource that helps all who consult it.

The Honorable Joseph A. Greenaway Jr.
J.D., Judge, U.S. Court of Appeals for the Third Circuit
James A. Byrne United States Courthouse
Philadelphia, PA, USA

Contents

Chapter 1
An Introduction to Autism and the Autism Spectrum

Fred R. Volkmar, Scott Jackson, and Brian Pete

What Is Autism?

This chapter provides a brief overview of autism/autism spectrum disorder (the terms are used interchangeably)—the nature of the condition, its clinical features with an emphasis on their relevance to the legal system, and approaches to the client with autism/Autism Spectrum Disorder/Asperger's Disorder. As much as possible (and it is not always possible) we try to avoid scientific jargon and put information into terms that we hope are readily comprehensible to an educated but non-specialist reader. One of the several challenges for the novice to the field comes from the diversity of fields (medicine, psychology, education, speech pathology, occupational therapy, etc.) involved, which sometimes have their own unique nomenclature and terms of art. A glossary of terms is provided at the end of this chapter and we put terms that appear there in **Bold Face Type** each time they appear in the text. In general, we will use the terms autism and autism spectrum disorder (ASD) interchangeably. However, at times we will specify certain subtypes of autism—particularly Asperger's disorder—which may have important differences from more typical autism/ASD.

Authors also differ in their use of identity-first (i.e., "autistic people") and person-first language (i.e., "person with autism"). There is no established rule for which to

---

F. R. Volkmar (✉)
Yale Child Study Center and Autism Center of Excellence,
Yale University and Southern Conn. State University, New Haven, USA
e-mail: fred.volkmar@yale.edu

S. Jackson
Southern Connecticut States University, New Haven, CT, USA
e-mail: jacksons38@southernct.edu

B. Pete
Lewis Brisbois Bisgaard & Smith LLP, New York, NY, USA
e-mail: Brian.Pete@lewisbrisbois.com

F. R. Volkmar et al. (eds.), *Handbook of Autism Spectrum Disorder and the Law*,
https://doi.org/10.1007/978-3-030-70913-6_1

use, and decisions about identity versus person-first language can be fraught with controversy. When working directly with families and individuals, it is best to inquire about which terms are preferred.

We also give a few clinical case examples—always well disguised—to illustrate specific points. We do have some references in the text and some additional resources and websites at the end of this chapter.

Autism as a Diagnostic Concept

Put in the simplest way, autism might be thought of as a congenital social learning disability. By this we mean that those born with autism/ASD, in contrast to other infants, seem to come into the world with an inability to or difficultly in engaging the social world—this is in stark contrast to typical infants who play the "social game" from birth, if not even before. The typically developing infant thus arrives ready to engage with parents and caregivers and then learns from them about the world. These infants' learning comes both through direct interaction and learning the complexities of the social game, as well as through observation (the latter reflecting the intense social interest of the typical newborn). Thus, just watching what other people do, what they attend to, how they interact, and how they communicate makes for a tremendously rich learning environment for the typical child. In contrast, the infant with autism must learn about the world in other ways. This reflects, in large part, the considerable amount of social learning that typically developing individuals acquire very early in life without formal teaching, e.g., through their interest in watching and understanding another person. The early onset and pervasiveness of autism lead to major difficulties in efficient learning. These difficulties continue into adulthood with unusual patterns of social interactions and ways of viewing the world. These differences are exemplified in studies of eye-tracking—i.e., of where individuals with ASD look in viewing social scenes. Figure 1.1 is from one of the first of these studies and shows how the person with autism focuses on a different part of the social scene in a brief clip from the movie "Who's Afraid of Virginia Woolf?" The typical viewers focus on the top of the face, where most of the social-emotional information is found, while the persons with ASD focused on the bottom half of the face—missing about 90% of the socially affective information, which is primarily provided in the top half of the face (Klin et al., 2002a). This pattern of focusing on the less socially informative aspects of the face in watching social interactions holds true in large groups of cases (Klin et al., 2002b) and can be documented in very young children (Chawarska & Shic, 2009). Abnormal patterns of facial viewing can be documented in the brain using fMRI (Schultz et al., 2000) and EEG (McPartland et al., 2011).

The condition known as infantile autism was coined by Leo Kanner, the first child psychiatrist in the United States. In 1943 he described 11 children whom he believed came into the world with a congenital (from birth) lack of interest in others, or autism (Kanner, 1943). He also emphasized that a second feature was their "insistence on sameness," i.e., difficulties in dealing with change in routine or aspects of

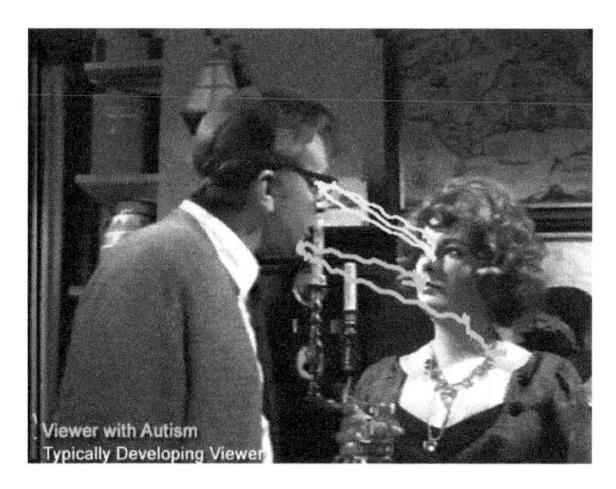

Fig. 1.1 Visual focus of a man with autism (bottom line) as compared to a typically developing viewer observing a short movie clip interested. The typically developing person goes back and forth between the eyes in viewing a social scene; the high-functioning person with autism goes back and forth between the mouths of the speakers missing much of the social–emotional meaning in the scene *Source* Reprinted with permission from Klin et al., (2002a)

the non-social environment. His description notes many of the "classic" features we still see today in children with the condition—stereotyped and repetitive body or hand movements, and **echolalia** (repetition of language) when the child spoke at all (many didn't and never would). Although his description is classic, some aspects were misleading, e.g., he thought that because children with autism seemed to do well on certain (nonverbal) parts of tests of intelligences, they weren't also intellectually disabled/mentally retarded—in point of fact most were, although, with earlier intervention and treatment, that number is decreasing. Kanner's description remains classic and is closely followed in the current DSM-5 definition of autism.

A year after Kanner's report, a Viennese medical student, Hans Asperger, also used the word autism to describe a group of boys who had difficulties forming social relationships. His description of "autistic personality disorder" shared a similarity with Kanner's in his use of the term autism but differed in other respects, e.g., these children were much more verbal, had areas of intense special interest that interfered with other aspects of learning, and their problems were often recognized somewhat later. Asperger's description essentially set the stage for what has been a continuing debate on how narrowly or broadly autism should be defined. The current DSM-5 diagnostic system uses the term autism spectrum disorder (an improvement over the previous term pervasive developmental disorder), but in point of fact it is a narrower definition (see Smith et al., 2015). Interestingly enough, the genetics of autism now support the notion of a broader view of the concept (Yuenn et al., 2019) and this is consistent with a large body of clinical work on the topic (Ingersoll et al., 2014). In popular literature there has also been considerable discussion of this among some advocating for a broader neurodiversity movement that tries to destigmatize differences in learning styles (see Silverman, 2015).

It is undoubtedly the case that children with autism existed well before Kanner or Asperger's work (Donvan & Zucker, 2016). It may, for example, be the case that so-called "feral children" (supposedly left to be reared by animals) were children with autism (Candland, 1995) who had either run away (a common problem even today Volkmar & Wiesner, 2009) or been abandoned by their parents (a practice still used in some developing countries). In their review of the history of autism, Donavan and Zucker (2016) found reports of children who likely had autism in the records of state training schools in the 1800s. But it was the classic descriptions of Kanner and Asperger that focused interest on these individuals and began the field of autism work that has developed so extensively today.

How Does Autism Manifest Itself?

If you think of autism and related conditions as being disorders that involve problems in social learning, a number of consequences follow. Young children have a host of problems that reflect their lack of social engagement, e.g., failures to engage in **joint attention** (the immediate learning from parents about what is important), imitation and **incidental learning** (that comes from just watching others), social routines and the early games of infancy that become the basis of language and conversation, and difficulties in "learning to learn" tasks effectively (a hallmark of usual social interaction where multiple kinds of information are processed selectively in a very efficient and effortless fashion).

These difficulties then have a host of downstream effects on:

- Language and communication (especially social communication)
- Learning effectively
- Engaging in what is referred to as "**executive functions**"—essentially efficient organization and multitasking
- Being overly rule-governed—not making appropriate accommodations to change
- Engaging in repetitive behaviors rather than learning effectively from the environment
- Having difficulties with change
- Having slow processing speed
- Being overly literal and having problems with humor, irony, sarcasm, and idioms

In general, individuals with ASD often learn things in whole chunks ("**gestalt learning**") and as a result have major problems in generalizing knowledge across situations (e.g., a math genius who solves complex equations in his head but can't order a cheeseburger and calculate his change at McDonald's). As we'll discuss, many aspects of this unusual learning style play out in negative ways as individuals with ASD interact with the legal system and contribute to the significantly increased risk for involvement with the law in all kinds of ways. Many individuals with ASD have sensitivities to things like touch, sounds, lights—things that most of us can effectively put out of our minds and largely ignore. The ability to do this is often significantly impaired in autism. Those with autism may have difficulties with changes in routine and their tendency toward overly rigid and rule-governed structures can cause trouble, e.g., the man with a special interest who arrives at a national historic site to discover that it is opening late, despite what the posted times on the website states, and gets arrested after arguing with the security guard!

The manifestations of autism vary tremendously over the age span and across the range of associated intellectual disabilities. The latter is frequently associated with autism and in many states, it is the associated **intellectual disability** ("mental retardation" as it was once termed) that entitles adults to obtain services. (For children, however, the autism label itself is sufficient under federal law.) One of us has taught an undergraduate course on autism for over 30 years and tells the students on the first day that what he expects them to learn from the course is that *when you have met one person with autism you have met one person with autism*. In some ways, this is the most important take-home message from this chapter.

While acknowledging the diversity of syndrome expression, it is also important to note the major commonalities that individuals on the autism spectrum share to some degree—that is, the autism (social information processing difficulties) and rigidity (resistance to change). These can take many forms. You might be asked to consult on a case with a man who is totally nonverbal and whose intellectual ability is unclear, or you might be invited to consult on a case where the client is highly verbal and wants to talk to you constantly about his special interest (the latter may have gotten him into trouble). Getting some quick sense of the client's ability to communicate with you, understand what is going on, and participate actively in his or her case is the first task for the attorney asked to represent a client with autism/Asperger's as well as for others, e.g., prosecutors and court staff working with a person with ASD.

Problems with social interaction and communication remain the hallmarks of autism. In addition, other problems frequently noted, to varying degrees across individuals, can include the following:

- Problems in organization and "**executive functioning**" lead to problems in multitasking efficiently, tendency to be rigid and "lock step"
- Problems in temporal sequencing so that the person can be readily distracted and "lose place" in tasks
- Attentional issues/sensitivities make for problems with what to most would be minimal extraneous distractors—noises, lights, sounds, smells, etc.
- **Gestalt learning style** makes it difficult to generalize knowledge across situations
- **Visual learning style** (particularly in more classic autism) means that auditory information may be less relevant and more difficult to process
- Overreliance on rules can lead to problems when exceptions are needed, and when coping with novelty or adapting to changes in situations and circumstance
- Problems with more complex language, particularly social language (**pragmatic language**) means that figurative language, idioms, understanding sophisticated humor, and implied meaning are difficult to process and the person with ASD

may have overly literal language (e.g., on hearing that "it is raining cats and dogs" the child with autism may look out the window expecting to see cats and dogs!)

- Language can be restricted and repetitive so that the person with ASD may engage in **echolalia** and have trouble with complex language and following instructions
- Problems with **prosody** (musical aspects of language) can lead to a loud monotonic voice with limited inflection and failure to adjust volume to the situation).
- Problems interpreting social cues can cause difficulties in approaching others too closely, not giving a turn for a conversational partner, and droning on about a topic of interest
- Significant delays in social understanding of what can or can't be said frequently lead to difficulties for teenagers with ASD who may say something that is actually true but wildly inappropriate, e.g., commenting on someone's being overweight. "You look like John Kerry but you are too fat!"

As we will discuss there are good treatments to help with these (and the many other) issues that may arise.

How Is Autism Diagnosed?

Although autism is strongly genetic and brain-based disorder, there are not as of yet simple blood or brain tests for the condition, nor is there a biological marker for the condition (although work on this is underway [McPartland et al., 2011; Ruggeri et al., 2014]). Currently, the condition is diagnosed based on other history and current presentation. At the most basic level, this likely reflects a diversity of genetic factors that can predispose to autism (Rutter & Thapar, 2014) and indeed may also be involved in the manifestation of what we now realize are a broader spectrum of related traits and conditions (some of which may well be adaptive in certain contexts—see Ingersoll & Wainer, 2014).

Various diagnostic approaches have been considered over the years (see Volkmar et al., 2021 for a detailed review). Briefly, these include diagnostic guidebooks, which list specific features/symptoms of the condition and rules for diagnosis, e.g., the psychiatric diagnostic books produced by the American Psychiatry Association or DSM—now called DSM-5 (APA, 2013) and the World Health Organization's guide the "International Classification of Diseases 10th Edition" (Organization, 1994). These approaches have their uses as well as their limitations (Volkmar et al., 2021). The DSM-5 system has, in particular, been criticized for adopting an overly stringent approach to diagnosis as a series of studies have shown that more cognitively able people are at risk of "losing" their diagnosis in DSM-5 (Smith et al., 2015). This could have special importance relative to issues of entitlements for services or accommodations in the workplace or at school), and to determinations of when a witness in a legal proceeding is competent to testify, or if a defendant in a criminal proceeding is competent to participate in his or her own defense. A somewhat different approach to diagnosis involves the use of screening or diagnostic assessment instruments that are more dimensional in nature (IbaÑez et al., 2014; Lord et al., 2021). These instruments, now numbering about 30 or so, also have their limitations (see Volkmar & Wiesner, 2018 for a short discussion). All these approaches work best when they are part of an assessment conducted by an experienced clinician or clinical team. Some of these instruments are designed to screen for risk of autism (e.g., based on parent or teacher report or direct observations of the child (IbaÑez et al., 2014), while others focus more on diagnosis as such (Lord et al., 2021). It is important to realize that these instruments are not, of themselves, sufficient and that a competent and experienced examiner and/or clinical team is likely needed. Also, the results of these instruments should be viewed within the broader context of a comprehensive assessment of the individual's psychological and communicative abilities. Volkmar and Wiesner provide a relatively succinct summary of diagnostic procedures and assessment instruments and how results are reported and interpreted (Volkmar et al., 2006).

As a practical matter several things are important. Given how frequently intellectual disabilities and unusual learning styles are seen in autism, intellectual testing is almost always indicated. As noted above, this may also be important in later determination for services as an adult (Volkmar et al., 2014). Psychological testing in this population is best done by an experienced examiner who understands the tests, as well as approaches to the individual with autism that facilitate more valid outcomes. It is not at all uncommon to see a very significant scatter in abilities, e.g., in Asperger disorder, for instance, verbal ability may be significantly higher than visual-spatial abilities. It is also common to see very low processing speed in someone with otherwise intact intellectual ability. Conversely, in more classic autism, verbal abilities may be very low but nonverbal skills may be so high as to inflate the overall IQ score. The latter may be very misleading in this population and results must be interpreted in the context of the full clinical picture. Thus, brief IQ tests and screens are less helpful in a person with autism than tests that assess multiple domains. Also keep in mind that it is possible that a person once (as a child) functioned in the intellectual deficiency range, but as an adult no longer does, at least in terms of IQ. However, adaptive skills, one of the two components of the diagnosis of intellectual deficiency, may remain quite impaired. For example, one young man with Asperger's had an IQ of 140, but his social skills (assessed on the Vineland Adaptive Behavior Scales (a common measure of adaptive skills) were at the four-year old level. This individual had major difficulties with social interactions at college, where he would say things to girls that were literally true but not socially appropriate (commenting on how attractive their breasts were). He ended up being expelled from several colleges before taking online classes to get a degree. In addition to fully assessing intellectual ability, an experienced examiner will be able to do other tests, e.g., of adaptive skills, executive functioning, personality, achieved academic skills, that may complement a full psychological assessment including cognitive and other testing (Tsatsanis & Powell, 2014). The psychologist or psychiatrist involved may also have important insights from interactions with the individual, e.g., what strategies work to help or hurt performance and compliance. Obviously in specific situations (e.g., understanding proceedings, being able to testify as a witness, providing informed consent in legal proceedings, engaging meaningfully with a defense team), this testing may have critical importance. Similarly, a good speech communication examination will move past the obvious simple measures (like receptive and expressive vocabulary) to standard measures assessing pragmatics, figurative language, and so forth. Again, both results and the observations of the examiner may be important. Other disciplines may be involved as well, e.g., neurology in the presence of seizures (see below), occupation and/or physical therapists, special education teachers, vocational counselors, social workers, etc. When there are specific questions that need to be addressed, these should be explicitly asked. If you are unfamiliar with the use and interpretation of psychological tests, several excellent resources for the layperson are available (Hogan, 2002; Volkmar & Wiesner, 2017; Wodrich, 1997).

Diagnostic Complexities

The clinical presentation of the child, adolescent, or adult will vary considerably with age and depending on the response to treatment. Often the youngest children with autism are those with the most "classic" presentation. These children are usually diagnosed in early childhood. In general, by age three years there is reasonable certainty of the diagnosis (Chawarska et al., 2014). Before that time some, but not necessarily all, of the usual diagnostic features required may be present. There is some potential for misdiagnosis at this age (and indeed in all age groups). Sometimes individuals with features of autism will seem to "grow out" of them in early childhood. Some preschool children enrolled in early intervention programs will make remarkable progress (Tager-Flusberg et al., 2014; Vivanti & Duncan, 2017). Children with Asperger disorder and those without conspicuous developmental delays in early childhood typically are diagnosed as they enter preschool or even elementary school and the serious social problems with peers become evident. Diagnosis can be delayed by various factors. There are issues of cultural bias and under-diagnosis in minority groups (see Freeth et al., 2014; Watson & Zhang, 2018) within the United States. In other developed countries children in minority groups and living in poverty may frequently be missed, although this is beginning to improve. Occasionally it becomes clear that an individual has an ASD diagnosis only in adulthood—usually any number of factors have combined to delay or disguise the diagnosis. For example, one young man was sufficiently high functioning as to not need an IEP (Individualized Education Plan) in school, and as a young adult he was volunteering in a day job but lived with his mother who basically took full care of him. Only when she developed Alzheimer's and he had to function on his own did it become clear that he needed tremendous amounts of support and that his significant social problems had been written off to "oddity" with the collaboration of the local educational authority. Similarly, another young man who came into trouble with the legal system had come to this country on vacation (his first) from the Caribbean, where he had a job but lived a very socially isolated existence, pursuing his extensive interest in American history. On coming to Washington DC, he visited a monument specific to his interest, but a construction project delayed the opening (despite the explicitly posted opening time). On his third visit, his anger at the guards for not allowing him to enter led to his arrest. The man was assigned a public defender, but did not inform his attorney that he had Asperger's and should be evaluated until his first appearance in court. While the man may not have met his public defender until that first court appearance, he certainly interacted with a multitude of people in the criminal justice system from the time of his arrest to whom he may have disclosed his condition to no avail. While this man informed his attorney of his diagnosis, one can imagine the man not doing so if he had already told multiple people and nothing was done.In one study by White of students taking an intro Psychology course, between 0.5 and 1% screened positive for possible autism and had never been diagnosed, suggesting that in the more cognitively able college bound population a significant number of cases may be undiagnosed (White et al., 2011)! A diagnosis of autism can also sometimes be missed in a child with attentional difficulties, obsessive concerns, and social anxiety when clinicians fail to appreciate the severity of social difficulties. Conversely, sometimes a misdiagnosis is made in cases, e.g., where the problem is primarily obsessive-compulsive disorder or social anxiety without the profound social learning problems of autism.

Complexities also arise given the importance of autism as a qualification under the IDEA and its successor legislation. Autism was mentioned in the original law (PL-94-142) specifying the mandate for schools to provide services to children with disabilities. Over time, autism has assumed a special status, in some respects, within the education system in that it requires more complex, mutlidisciplinary, and well-coordinated services and is often considered a "Golden Ticket" for educational services. Also, there is more public awareness of and less stigma associated with autism, and the label itself is, in many ways, a more hopeful one than intellectual disability. Accordingly, in some instances, the IEP may use autism as a label rather than an intellectual deficiency (when either could actually be used) or there may be a bias toward over-diagnosis of autism on the part of parents (and professionals) to obtain the most intensive services. Issues of **diagnostic substitution** (see Bishop et al., 2008; Newschaffer, 2006) and **diagnostic overshadowing**, where a diagnosis of autism is missed or "overshadowed" by some other diagnosed condition (Meera et al., 2013), both occur. In general, controversies around diagnosis arise with very young or much older individuals (who have not previously had a diagnosis) and in those with greater degrees of intellectual deficiency or, at the opposite end of that spectrum, among the very high functioning. The latter area is an interest group in its own right, as an increasing number of children have responded to intervention and may, in a technical sense, be thought to "lose" their diagnosis; the so-called "**optimal outcome**" cases may still exhibit social oddity and other conditions like anxiety and depression (Fein et al., 2013; Kelley et al., 2006).

Other issues arise given the awareness of **broader autism phenotype (BAP)** (Ingersoll et al., 2014), i.e., of the many individuals who have some features of autism (e.g., intense special interests, unusual habits or sensitivities, or unusual abilities along with problems in social interaction) but who would not meet current criteria for autism. This problem has been increased by the narrower view of autism adapted in DSM-5 (APA, 2013) and the exclusion of individuals who in the past might have obtained a diagnosis of Asperger's disorder or atypical autism/PDD-NOS. This issue also intersects with the neurodiversity movement—a movement that wants to view differences in conditions like autism, attention deficit disorders, and so forth, as part of the broad range of normalcy (see Silverman, 2015). This is a complex issue in several respects. This view seeks to expand our awareness of the issue of difference rather than disorder, i.e., that autism represents a different style of learning and interaction with the world. Problems can arise with this approach in terms of issues like qualifying for needed services in schools. Another problem arises when more cognitively able and communicatively able people with autism talk about their own experience of autism and then want to generalize this to everyone's experience. Everyone is, of course, entitled to talk about their experience but issues arise when these individuals become advocates and, with the best of intentions, want to speak for the person with ASD who has trouble speaking about his or her own experiences. Parents and siblings may be particularly upset if their experience of their child or sibling's needs is somehow overshadowed by that of someone who doesn't really know their child or sibling. This can be a special issue in decision-making regarding conservatorship, guardianship, trusts, and representing the person who can't easily speak for himself.

The issues of how best to advocate for a more cognitively impaired person do present important challenges. For example, one of us once had the experience of being asked to consult in the case of a minimally verbal man who clearly had both autism and intellectual deficiency and who had been physically abused in his group home. There had not previously been an adequate assessment of the client, and the attorney for the defendant claimed that the person was already so damaged that he could not be further damaged and therefore it was impossible to assess whether he had been damaged at all. However, interviews with the young man by an experienced clinician quickly made it clear that the simple mention of the name of the group home or the abuse would set the young man on a complex tirade of verbal complaints and signs of massive anxiety. In other cases, the client may be making the issue of who best speaks for him or her very complex.

The final set of diagnostic complexities arises with regards to associated or "**comorbid**" conditions noted frequently with autism. As we have noted, the most common one, particularly in the past, is intellectual disability (mental retardation). This continues to be true for some individuals although, over time and with earlier diagnoses and intervention, more and more are able to function within the broad range of normal intellectual ability (Howlin et al., 2014). As noted above, it is possible that some individuals as children functioned in the intellectually deficient range but technically lost this diagnosis as their IQ improved with intervention (often with adaptive skills continuing to be major impairments).

The psychiatric problems associated with autism in adolescents and adults are noteworthy, including increased rates of almost all other psychiatric problems. There are particularly significant increases in rates of anxiety disorders and depression, as well as significant attentional difficulties (Howlin et al., 2014). The issue of co-morbidity is a complex one and presents problems for classification systems (Rutter, 1994; Volkmar et al., 2021; Volkmar & Woolston, 1997). From a practical point of view, the presence of other conditions may have important implications for working with an individual with autism, e.g., relative to very high anxiety levels or the presence of suicidal ideation, and so forth. The presence of additional problems also increases the risk for bullying quite significantly (Maiano et al., 2015; van Schalkwyk et al., 2018; Weiss et al., 2015).

A number of medical co-morbidities with ASD are also observed. The most common of these is seizure disorder. There is an increased risk for developing seizure disorder throughout childhood and adolescence and possibly beyond (Volkmar & Nelson, 1990). Autism is also associated with several strongly genetic conditions, notably Fragile X syndrome and tuberous sclerosis (Rutter et al., 2014; Yuenn et al., 2019). Physical conditions like sleep difficulties and GI problems may also have an impact on the individual's behavior and family life and complicate issues related to educational and vocational programming (Volkmar & Wienser, 2018).

Cognitive Theories of Autism Spectrum Disorder

Since the initial clinical accounts of what is now referred to as autism spectrum disorder by Leo Kanner (1943) and Hans Asperger (1944), many theories have been proposed in attempts to provide a unified understanding of the development and broad symptomatic manifestations of this complex condition. Perhaps the most infamous of these efforts is the once-popular, but now debunked, psychogenic theory known as the *Refrigerator Mother Theory,* which dominated the autism etiology discussion in the 1960s. This theory, which postulated that autism was a mental state of children withdrawing from the external world and into themselves as a result of extreme circumstances created by the emotional abandonment and rejection of their mothers, was championed by Bruno Bettelheim (1959, 1967). The 1970s, however, marked a pivotal turning point for the field of autism, as researchers began to move away from the clinical descriptions and/or theory presentations that previously dominated the landscape of autism literature, and began applying more stringent methodologies to the study of the disorder, thus paving the way for more scientifically grounded theories to be developed and introduced (Irwin et al., 2011).

Reflecting the current zeitgeist of the era, theories of autism based around a core cognitive deficit or variance began to be introduced and gain popularity in the mid-1980s. While these cognitive theories of autism often struggled to account for the broad range of both social and non-social characteristics, as well as the broad spectrum of severity that can be found within this condition, there are a few that have gained popularity and have had an immense impact on the focus of both researchers and practitioners in the field. Perhaps the most notable of the cognitive theories of autism that have been proposed are the Theory of Mind Hypothesis, the Theory of

Executive Dysfunctions, the Weak Central Coherence Theory, and Extreme Male Brain Theory.

Theory of Mind Hypothesis: The term theory of mind describes a set of complex cognitive functions that enable the decoding or inferring of the mental states (including feelings and emotions) of others, as well as the ability to comprehend that the desires, knowledges, beliefs, and intentions of others may differ from one's own (Schlinger, 2009). Colloquially, this can be likened to the concept of "putting yourself into another's shoes." Deficits in theory of mind have been studied as a specific area of impairment in children with autism since the mid-1980s (Baron-Cohen et al., 1985), and the idea that this set of cognitive functions could represent the defining functional impairments of the disorder (the Theory of Mind Hypothesis of autism) began to emerge not long afterward (Baron-Cohen et al., 1997; Happé, 1994). While an extensive body of research has since been produced supporting the fact that theory of mind abilities are a common area of impairment for individuals with autism, there are a few critical issues that challenge its role as a core, defining cognitive deficit for the disorder. First, there is the issue that this hypothesis does not account for the non-social aspects of an autism diagnosis (e.g., sensory sensitivity, repetitive interest, and preoccupations). Second, similar deficits in theory of mind are found in other clinical populations (e.g., individuals with mental retardation or schizophrenia), and therefore are not unique to autism. Finally, there are some individuals with autism who are able to pass the standard theory of mind tasks, and others who will even perform in the normal range on the more recently developed "advanced" theory of mind tasks, thus creating an issue with the universality of this "core deficit" across the entirety of the disorder.

Theory of Executive Dysfunctions: Executive functioning is an umbrella term for a set of higher order cognitive processes that encompass working memory, cognitive flexibility, cognitive inhibition, impulse control, attention shifting, planning and organizing, and initiating behavior. Severe deficits in executive functions are often found in individuals with damage to the frontal lobe area of the brain, resulting in behaviors that include an insistence on sameness/routine, impulse control difficulties, tendencies to perseverate, and problems with attention shifting (Baddeley & Wilson, 1988). The fact that these symptoms are very similar to those that often manifest in individuals with autism led some researchers to propose the Theory of Executive Dysfunctions, which posits that these are the core underlying cognitive deficits of autism (e.g., Ozonoff et al., 1991). As with the Theory of Mind Hypothesis, there is strong empirical support for the relationship between autism and executive dysfunctions in the literature. While this theory has an advantage over the Theory of Mind Hypothesis in that it can account for many of the non-social components of the disorder (including motor behaviors like rocking and hand flapping), it is not without its critiques. Like with the Theory of Mind Hypothesis, this theory is limited by its lack of uniqueness (individuals with schizophrenia, Obsessive-Compulsive Disorder, Attention Deficit Hyperactivity Disorder, and Tourette syndrome all perform similarly to those with autism on executive function tasks) and poor consistency across the disorder, with individuals with autism presenting with different executive dysfunction profiles and some demonstrating no dysfunction in these areas at all (Hill, 2004).

Weak Central Coherence Theory: Central coherence refers to a perceptual-cognitive style relating to how individuals process information and draw meaning from the things in their environment. The Weak Central Coherence Theory suggests that in typical development, individuals will have a tendency toward information processing that will draw together diverse pieces of information and construct them into a coherent whole, allowing them to extract overall meaning (it can be likened to the ability to "see the big picture"). Meanwhile, for individuals with autism, this theory suggests that this processing style is disturbed or absent, resulting in an information processing style that is done in a detail-focused manner, concentrating on the individual parts as opposed to the global whole (Frith, 1989, 2003; Firth & Happé, 1994). More recently, there has been a reframing of this theory suggesting that individuals with autism have superior local processing and poor (but not necessarily absent) global processing (Happé & Booth, 2008). Regardless, an advantage to this theory is that it can account for both social and non-social characteristics associated with autism, including difficulties understanding/interpreting social cues, having circumscribed interests, focusing on parts of objects, insistence on sameness, sensitivity to small changes in the environment, and can even account for the fact that some individuals with autism can demonstrate high levels of skills in detail-oriented fields like mathematics and engineering. This type of information processing was noted even in the first descriptions of autism, with Kanner (1943) writing that individuals with autism have an "...inability to experience wholes without full attention to the constituent parts. ... A situation, a performance, a sentence is not regarded as complete if it is not made up of exactly the same elements that were present at the time the child was first confronted with it" (p. 246). Limitations for this theory include inconsistent findings across studies (e.g., Hoy et al., 2004; Ropar & Mitchell, 2001), suggesting this type of perceptual-cognitive style is not universally found in individuals with autism, and findings of similar central coherence deficits in other clinical groups (e.g., Williams syndrome; Bernardino et al., 2012) suggesting a lack of uniqueness to autism.

Extreme Male Brain Theory: Finally, the most recently proposed cognitive theory of autism is the Extreme Male Brain Theory (Baron-Cohen, 2002). This theory is based around two cognitive styles, "empathizing" and "systemizing," that relate to how individuals attempt to understand and make sense of the world around them. According to Baron-Cohen, "empathizing" is the drive to understand and predict the thoughts and emotions of others, and to produce an emotionally appropriate response. Meanwhile, "systemizing" is the drive to study and analyze the details that make up a system, in order to determine how that system operates. Based on a broad range of studies (including behavioral, brain imaging, and developmental methodologies), Baron-Cohen makes the argument that on average females tend to naturally empathize more than males, and males tend to naturally systemize more than females. The Extreme Male Brain Theory postulates that individuals with autism present with an exaggerated (or "extreme") version of the typical male profile of increased systemizing and reduced empathizing. Similar to the Weak Central Coherence Theory, an "extreme" male brain theory has been suggested since the earliest clinical accounts of autism, with Asperger (1944) writing (translated from German), "The autistic personality is an extreme variant of male intelligence. Even within the normal variation, we find typical sex differences in intelligence… In the autistic individual, the male pattern is exaggerated to the extreme" (p. 129). As empathizing can be likened to components of Theory of Mind, and systemizing can be likened to components of local processing (i.e., weak central coherence), an advantage of this cognitive theory of autism is that it incorporates aspects of two other prominent theories. Critics of this theory suggest that the cornerstone of the theory (sex-based differences in cognitive styles) are based on stereotypes more than proven science, and much of the supportive findings for the theory are based on studies conducted by the theory author (Baron-Cohen) and/or his students and are largely based on instruments developed by the theory author (e.g., the Systemizing Quotient, the Empathizing Quotient).

Limitations of current theoretical approaches: As no single, unified cognitive theory of autism has emerged that has been able to account for the broad and varied autistic profile, it is possible that alternatively a multiple deficit account of autism would be better suited for this population. This aligns with the view that while autism spectrum disorder is currently listed as a unified condition, it may in fact be comprised of a collection of related but unique disorders (or subgroups of autism) that manifest with different cognitive profiles (e.g., Whitehouse & Stanley, 2013). The existence of different subgroups of autism could help to explain the conflicting findings when studying the different proposed cognitive profiles of autism, and, if ever identified, the definition of such subgroups could have important implications for interventions and clinical treatment for individuals with autism.

Treatment Approaches

The earliest attempts to provide treatment for children with autism focused on unstructured psychotherapy. This approach was not particularly effective and in the 1970s, studies (Bartak & Rutter, 1973; Lockyer & Rutter, 1970) began to make it clear that structured teaching and special education was much more effective. A highly influential review for the National Research Council in 2001 (National Research Council, 2001) looked at a number of programs across the U.S. (each of which had at least one peer-reviewed publication demonstrating efficacy) and noted that while these programs had some differences they also had many similarities and were, on balance, effective in treating children with autism. Since that time there has been an explosion of research on treatment.

There are now a number of well-established (with good to very good empirical support) and some emerging (some support in the literature) treatment models. These can be confusing to understand and a few distinctions may be helpful. In the first, place, specific intervention methods may have been well validated in studies. Careful and rigorous scientific evaluation of comprehensive treatment programs is more complex (Odom et al., 2019; Silverman, 2015; Volkmar & Wiesner, 2017). Model treatment approaches often developed in university settings (not surprisingly). Over time the standard for evaluating effectiveness has evolved (and is discussed shortly), but at present there are now several evidence-based models of effective programs and many more studies of specific evidence-based interventions. (see McClure, 2014; Reichow & Barton, 2014; Odom et al., 2018; Volkmar et al., 2014; Wilson et al., 2014). Two organizations, the Cochrane and Campbell Collaborations, are important general resources for looking at the strength of scientific evidence in many kinds of treatment. Schools and school programs increasingly rely on evidence-based treatments in their choice or programs (see Volkmar & Wiesner, 2017 for a summary of effective treatment models).

Many "non-established" treatments are available. A quick search on any of the usual search engines will turn up literally millions of websites, many of which make fantastic (and unfounded) claims based on anecdotes, etc. These can include a host of things. The term complementary treatment is used for non-established treatments that are utilized in addition to evidence-based ones and the term alternative treatment is used when the putative treatment is used instead of an evidence-based one. Given their very nature, of course, the serious scientific literature on these treatments is highly limited with a few noteworthy exceptions where scholars attempt to summarize what is known (see Foxx & Mulick, 2016; Smith et al., 2014; Volkmar & Wiesner, 2017).

In helping families make decisions about treatment or when representing a client with autism who has limited communicative abilities, it is critical that attorneys help the family or individual rely on proven treatments. One of us has seen a family squander a substantial trust fund on a child with autism who, rather than go to a local and appropriate school program, was forced to sit for hours at a time in a wooden box that was supposed to transfer energy to him! It is important to realize that many evidence-based treatments (both medical and psychological) are available for associated conditions of autism, e.g., **CBT (Cognitive Behavior Therapy)** (Reaven et al., 2012) has been modified for children in the autism population and, at least in the general population, works about as well as medications for anxiety.

Outcome

As knowledge of autism and its treatment has increased, so has earlier diagnosis and intervention and, as a result, overall outcomes for those with autism have significantly improved (Magiati & Howlin, 2019). Unfortunately, even with early detection and intervention, some children still don't do well (National Research Council, 2001). But the number of overall individuals requiring 24/7 residential care has decreased dramatically. As a result, more individuals with autism reside in the community at large—increasing chances for legal involvement.

It is hard to predict for very young children what their outcomes will be. However, the two positive signs are the presence of spoken language and nonverbal cognitive ability in the normal range by the time the child is five years of age. The first five years of life is the period when the most absolute progress occurs. Sometimes this is very dramatic (one of us has had a mute child at two and a half years old who, as a teenager, was successfully doing stand-up comedy on national television!).

The term "**optimal outcome**" (Fein et al., 2013) has been used for individuals who "technically" move out of autism (no longer meeting strict criteria for the condition—a possibility made even greater by the recent changes introduced in the DSM-5 guidelines for autism (Smith et al., 2015). Most of the time these individuals still face significant challenges, e.g., in educational, workplace, or social settings. Subtle problems in social interaction or social communication may make life more difficult and there may be a greater risk for depression and anxiety problems sometimes even suicidal ideation (van Schalkwyk et al., 2016).

Transition planning (i.e., from school settings to whatever comes next) should begin early in adolescence and the teenager with ASD should be involved in this process (see Chap. 17). For some individuals, this may involve exploring possible jobs or volunteer opportunities. For others, this may involve thinking about more specialized training programs or moving on to college. A number of programs (a little less than 100 at last count) are designed to help with transitional college supports. All colleges within the United States are required by the ADA and Rehabilitation Act of 1973 act to provide appropriate supports, although this often is a challenge for colleges that are not yet as experienced in dealing with ASD as they are with other problems like ADHD.

While many more students with ASD are moving to college settings, it is important for them and their parents to realize that college presents many challenges—academic (often not the major problem) and nonacademic (often the major problem) (see Gerhardt et al., 2014; Chaps. 22, 16 and 17; White et al., 2017, 2019). For some students, living at home and attending a community college is a good opportunity to have an introductory experience while minimizing the nonacademic demands, although even in these situations the increased expectations for organization and self-monitoring can be a major challenge (see Wenzel & Brown, 2014; Wolff et al., 2009).

There are some critically important issues for students and parents to know:

1. Unlike high school, college is **NOT** a right and students can be expelled (and quickly are these days) for inappropriate behavior. Although, particularly in public institutions, specific rights and aspects of due process and procedure may be mandated.
2. The student (**NOT** the parent) must be the one to identify him or herself as in need of special supports with difficulties related to the manifestations of his or her disability
3. Without permission from the student, college staff do **NOT** talk to parents on a regular basis.
4. College and vocational schools are required to render **appropriate** supports under ADA and other applicable state and federal laws (this is often much less than in high school).

It is important in preparing for college to be sure that the individual works explicitly on adaptive (real life) skills, i.e., can take care of personal hygiene, have a roommate or suitemate, can take medicates independently, etc. A surprising number of parents will tell you that they help their 17- or 18-year-old children get organized in the morning and this must happen independently in college.

Finally, it is important to note that the preparation of first responders of all types (police, firemen, EMT, medical personnel) is an important area of work. The uneducated first responder may have difficulty in understanding the responses and behavior of the person with ASD. For example, the mute person who doesn't respond to verbal instructions, the individual who engages in body rocking, or the person who tries to re-enter a burning building to rescue his rock collection. Given a lack of awareness of social conventions, individuals with autism may exhibit odd behavior that police interpret as threatening, e.g., the child who runs toward the officer or who is overly interested in his gun.

Summary

This chapter provides a concise summary of scientific knowledge regarding autism and related disorders. Other chapters in this Handbook address specific issues. Understandably these are quite varying. They might include issues of legal advocacy for needed education services (Mandlawitz, 2002), of ensuring safety and future planning (Allen et al., 2019), or of forensic evaluation and criminal behavior (Allely et al., 2019). Specific problems can arise in a host of areas/arenas:

- Stalking can be perceived (sometimes quite correctly) when an individual with ASD is preoccupied with making a friend or having a relationship—sometimes without knowing how to approach a person or not being able to understand when the person gives signs that they do not want to make a social connection (Post et al., 2014) (also see Chap. 14).
- Issues of legal rights both in schools (see Chaps. 16), transition planning (Chap. 17), college (Chap. 18), and the workplace (Chap. 19) are very frequent.
- Bullying (see Chap. 9) is particularly common with rates at least double for children with ASD, with risks persisting into adulthood and college or the workplace. Bullying is a complex issue and can take many forms (physical aggression, verbal bullying, relational bully, and cyberbullying). Cyberbullying is particularly pernicious in this population (see Bostic & Brunt, 2011; van Schalkwyk et al., 2018).
- Hostile work environments and bullying can also persist in the workplace (Van Wieren et al., 2008) and see Chap. 18.
- Individuals with autism can, of course, be arrested for a range of actual or potential criminal behaviors (Cashin & Newman, 2009; Freckelton, 2011; Freckelton & List, 2009; Hall et al., 2007; and see Chaps. 9, 10, 11, 12, 13, 14, 15). This can include criminality related to online child pornography and violence, including sexual violence (Bjorkly, 2009; Creaby-Attwood & Allely, 2017; First, 2011; Payne et al., 2019) and see chaps. legal rights both in school 9, 10, and 12.

- Within the judicial system itself other issues arise, e.g., relative to the person with ASD as a victim (Essique, 2018; Mallory, 2014; Sreckovic et al., 2014) and see Chap. 23; as a defendant (Mannynsalo et al., 2009) and see Chap. 6; and as a witness (Maras & Bowler, 2014) and see Chap. 7. Within this context, there is the role of experts in helping courts understand autism in general and in specific cases (Berryessa, 2017); of judges and attorneys to best approach the person with autism as a witness or other participant in the judicial process (Berryessa, 2014, 2016; Brewer & Young, 2018; Freckelton, 2013; Goldfarb & Gonzalez, 2018; Rhodes, 2009); and of courts understanding the implications of an ASD diagnosis is highly relevant to issues of risk assessment, detention (Cashin & Newman, 2009), prevention as well as first responder training are all important (see Chaps. 22, 23 and 25).

Glossary

Broader Autism Phenotype (BAP): The broader range of autism/autism-like traits in the more general population

Cognitive Behavior Therapy (CBT): A form of psychological treatment that is structured and focuses both on behavior and cognitive aspects of conditions like anxiety and depression, has been modified for use in autism.

Comorbid: having more than one condition, e.g., autism with depression

Diagnostic overshadowing: A tendency for major developmental problems like autism or intellectual disability to 'overshadow' other conditions that may be overlooked.

Diagnostic substitution: When more than one diagnostic label can be used a tendency to overlook one of the labels resulting in inflated rates of one disorder, may happen n association with autism being more effective in getting services.

Echolalia: repetition of whole 'chunks' of language rather than a single word, e.g., the sentence "want a cookie want a cookie" is used in place of the word cookie.

Executive functions: Psychological processes involved in forward planning, self-monitoring, organization, and problem solving.

Extreme Male Brain Theory: A theory that suggests a difference between empathizers (often females) and systematizers (often males) with the latter group being more at risk for ASD

Gestalt learning: The tendency to learn things in chunks rather than to break things down to consequent parts, echolalia is one example incidental learning: Learning that happens just from watching others without explicit teaching

Intellectual disability: Previously termed mental retardation and sometimes associated with ASD this term refers to significantly subaverage (IQ70 or below) and similar levels of adaptive (real life) skills.

Joint attention: A process that beginning in infancy as the baby follows the gaze and attention of the parents to learn about what is important or relevant in the world.

Optimal outcome: Individuals who once had a diagnosis of autism according to official diagnostic criteria but who no longer do so (*often still exhibiting some signs o of social oddity).

Pragmatic language: Social language.

Prosody: The musical or 'sing song' aspects of speech.

Theory of Mind: The ability to understand the thoughts, feelings, and intention of others reflecting an ability to put one's self in the other person′s place.

Visual learning style: A tendency to learn best with static visual symbol, pictures, etc. (as opposed to auditory learning).

Weak Central Coherence Theory: A theory of autism that posits that the difficulty in autism in an inability to being various observations (particularly social ones) together in a coherent and unified way.

References

Allen, C., Fehr, K. K., & Nyp, S. S. (2019). Maintaining safety and planning for the future. *Journal of Developmental and Behavioral Pediatrics, 21,* 21.

Allely, C. S., Kennedy, S., & Warren, I. (2019). A legal analysis of Australian criminal cases involving defendants with autism spectrum disorder charged with online sexual offending. *International Journal of Law and Psychiatry, 66,*.

American Psychairc Association. (2013). *Diagnostic and Statistical Manual (DSM-5).* Arlington, VA: American Psychiatric Association.

Asperger, H. (1944). Die "Autistischen Psychopathe" im Kindesalter. *European Archives of Psychiatry and Clinical Neuroscience, 117*(1), 76–136.

Baddeley, A., & Wilson, B. (1988). Frontal amnesia and the dysexecutive syndrome. *Brain and Cognition, 7*(2), 212–230.

Baron-Cohen, S. (2002). The extreme male brain theory of autism. *Trends in Cognitive Sciences, 6*(6), 248–254.

Baron-Cohen, S., Jolliffe, T., Mortimore, C., & Robertson, M. (1997). Another advanced test of theory of mind: Evidence from very high functioning adults with autism or Asperger syndrome. *Journal of Child Psychology and Psychiatry, 38*(7), 813–822.

Baron-Cohen, S., Leslie, A. M., & Frith, U. (1985). Does the autistic child have a "theory of mind"? *Cognition, 21*(1), 37–46.

Bartak, L., & Rutter, M. (1973). Special educational treatment of autistic children: A comparative study. 1. Design of study and characteristics of units. *Journal of Child Psychology and Psychiatry and Allied Disciplines, 14*(3), 161–179.

Bernardino, I., Mouga, S., Almeida, J., van Asselen, M., Oliveira, G., & Castelo-Branco, M. (2012). A direct comparison of local-global integration in autism and other developmental disorders: Implications for the central coherence hypothesis. *PLoS ONE, 7*(6),

Berryessa, C. M. (2014). Judiciary views on criminal behaviour and intention of offenders with high-functioning autism. *Journal of Intellectual Disabilities & Offending Behaviour, 5*(2), 97–106.

Berryessa, C. M. (2016). Brief report: Judicial attitudes regarding the sentencing of offenders with High Functioning Autism. *Journal of Autism and Developmental Disorders, 46*(8), 2770–2773.

Berryessa, C. M. (2017). Educator of the court: The role of the expert witness in cases involving autism spectrum disorder. *Psychology, Crime & Law, 23*(6), 575–600.
Bettelheim, B. (1959). Feral children and autistic children. *American Journal of Sociology*, 455–467.
Bettelheim, B. (1967). *Empty fortress: Infantile autism and the birth of the self*. Simon and Schuster.
Bishop, D. V., Whitehouse, A. J., Watt, H. J., Line, E. A., Bishop, D. V. M., Whitehouse, A. J. O., Watt, H. J., & Line, E. A. (2008). Autism and diagnostic substitution: Evidence from a study of adults with a history of developmental language disorder. [see comment]. *Developmental Medicine and Child Neurology, 50*(5), 341–345.
Bjorkly, S. (2009). Risk and dynamics of violence in Asperger's syndrome: A systematic review of the literature. *Aggression and Violent Behavior, 14*(5), 306–312.
Bostic, J. Q., & Brunt, C. C. (2011). Cornered: An approach to school bullying and cyberbullying, and forensic implications. *Child & Adolescent Psychiatric Clinics of North America, 20*(3), 447–465.
Brewer, N., & Young R. L. (2018). Interactions of individuals with autism spectrum disorder with the criminal justice system: Influences on involvement and outcomes.
Candland, D. C. (1995). *Feral children and clever animals: Reflections on human nature*. Oxford University Press.
Cashin, A., & Newman, C. (2009). Autism in the criminal justice detention system: A review of the literature. *Journal of Forensic Nursing, 5*(2), 70–75.
Chawarska, K., Macari, S., Volkmar, F. R., Kim, S. H., & Shic, F. (2014). ASD in infants and toddlers. In *Handbook of autism and pervasive developmental disorders: Diagnosis, development, and brain mechanisms, Volume 1* (4th ed., pp. 121–147). Wiley.
Chawarska, K., & Shic, F. (2009). Looking but not seeing: Atypical visual scanning and recognition of faces in 2 and 4-year-old children with autism spectrum disorder. *Journal of Autism and Developmental Disorders, 39*(12), 1663–1672.
Creaby-Attwood, A., & Allely, C. S. (2017). A psycho-legal perspective on sexual offending in individuals with autism Spectrum disorder. *International Journal of Law and Psychiatry, 55*, 72–80.
Donvan, J., & Zucker, C. (2016). *In a different key: The story of autism*. Crown Publishers/Random House.
Essique, T. J. (2018). *Gaining a better understanding of bullying behavior and peer victimization: An analysis of personality characteristics of adolescents with an autism spectrum disorder. Dissertation Abstracts International: Section B: The Sciences and Engineering, 78*(9-B(E)): No Pagination Specified.
Fein, D., Barton, M., Eigsti, I.-M., Kelley, E., Naigles, L., Schultz, R. T., Stevens, M., Helt, M., Orinstein, A., Rosenthal, M., Troyb, E., & Tyson, K. (2013). Optimal outcome in individuals with a history of autism. *Journal of Child Psychology and Psychiatry, 54*(2), 195–205.
First, M. B. (2011). The inclusion of child pornography in the DSM-5 diagnostic criteria for pedophilia: Conceptual and practical problems. *Journal of the American Academy of Psychiatry & the Law, 39*(2), 250–254.
Foxx, R. M., & Mullick, J. A. (2016). *Controversial therapies for autism and intellectual disabilities*. Routledge.
Freckelton, I. (2011). Asperger's disorder and the criminal law. *Journal of Law & Medicine, 18*(4), 677–694.
Freckelton, I. (2013). Autism spectrum disorder: Forensic issues and challenges for mental health professionals and courts. *Journal of Applied Research in Intellectual Disabilities, 26*(5), 420–434.
Freckelton, I., & List, D. (2009). Asperger's disorder, criminal responsibility and criminal culpability. *Psychiatry, Psychology and Law, 16*(1), 16–40.
Freeth, M., Milne, E., Sheppard, E., Ramachandran, R., Volkmar, F. R., Paul, R., Rogers, S. J., & Pelphrey, K. A. (2014). Autism across cultures: Perspectives from non-Western cultures and implications for research. In *Handbook of autism and pervasive developmental disorders* (4th ed.). Wiley.
Frith, U., & Happé, F. (1994). Autism: Beyond "theory of mind". *Cognition, 50*(1–3), 115–132.

Frith, U. (1989). Autism and "theory of mind". In *Diagnosis and treatment of autism* (pp. 33–52). Springer.
Frith, U. (2003). *Autism: Explaining the enigma*. Blackwell.
Gerhardt, P. F., Cicero, F., & Mayville, E. (2014). Employment and related services for adults with ASD. In *Handbook of autism and pervasive developmental disorders, Volume 2: Assessment, interventions, and policy* (pp. 907–917). Wiley.
Goldfarb, D., & Gonzalez, A. (2018). Children with autism spectrum disorder in the courtroom: How courts handle testimony today and what we can do in the future.
Hall, A. V., Godwin, M., Wright, H. H., & R. K. Abramson (2007). Criminal justice issues and autistic disorder. In *Growing up with autism: Working with school-age children and adolescents* (pp. 272–292). Guilford Press.
Happé, F. G. (1994). An advanced test of theory of mind: Understanding of story characters' thoughts and feelings by able autistic, mentally handicapped, and normal children and adults. *Journal of Autism and Developmental Disorders, 24*(2), 129–154.
Happé, F. G. E., & Booth, R. D. L. (2008, Jan). The power of the positive: Revisiting weak coherence in autism spectrum disorders [Review]. *Quarterly Journal of Experimental Psychology, 61*(1), 50–63.
Hill, E. L. (2004). Executive dysfunction in autism. *Trends in Cognitive Sciences, 8*(1), 26–32.
Hogan, T. P. (2002). *Psychological testing: A practical introduction*. Wiley.
Howlin, P., Moss, P., Savage, S., Bolton, P., & Rutter, M. (2014). Outcomes in adult life among siblings of individuals with autism. *Journal of Autism and Developmental Disorders*: No Pagination Specified.
Hoy, J. A., Hatton, C., & Hare, D. (2004). Weak central coherence: A cross-domain phenomenon specific to autism? *Autism, 8*(3), 267–281.
IbaÑez, L. V., Stone, W. L., & Coonrod, E. E, Volkmar, F. R., Paul, R., Rogers, S. J., & Pelphrey, K. A. (2014). Screening for autism in young children. In *Handbook of autism and pervasive developmental disorders* (2). John Wiley & Sons, Inc. https://doi.org/10.1002/9781118911389.hautc24.
Ingersoll, B., Wainer, A., Volkmar, F. R., Paul, R., Rogers, S. J., & Pelphrey, K. A. (2014). The broader autism phenotype. In *Handbook of autism and pervasive developmental disorders* (4th ed.). Wiley.
Irwin, J. K., MacSween, J., & Kerns, K. A. (2011). History and evolution of the autism spectrum disorders. In J. L. Matson & P. Sturmey (Eds.), *International handbook of autism and pervasive developmental disorders* (pp. 3–16). Springer.
Kanner, L. (1943). Autistic disturbances of affective contact. *Nervous Child, 2*(3), 217–250.
Kelley, E., Paul, J. J., Fein, D., & Naigles, L. R. (2006). Residual language deficits in optimal outcome children with a history of autism. *Journal of Autism and Developmental Disorders, 36*(6), 807–828.
Klin, A., Jones, W., Schultz, R., Volkmar, F., & Cohen, D. (2002a). Defining and quantifying the social phenotype in autism. *American Journal of Psychiatry, 159*(6), 895–908. https://doi.org/10.1176/appi.ajp.159.6.895.
Klin, A., Jones, W., Schultz, R., Volkmar, F., & Cohen, D. (2002b). Visual fixation patterns during viewing of naturalistic social situations as predictors of social competence in individuals with autism. *Archives of General Psychiatry, 59*(9), 809–816.
Lockyer, L., & Rutter, M. (1970). A five- to fifteen-year follow-up study of infantile psychosis. IV. Patterns of cognitive ability. *British Journal of Social and Clinical Psychology, 9*(2), 152–163.
Lord, C., Rosen, N. E., & Volkmar, F. R. (2021, Feb 24). The Diagnosis of Autism: From Kanner to DSM-III to DSM-5 and Beyond [Review]. *Journal of Autism & Developmental Disorders, 24*, 24. https://doi.org/10.1007/s10803-021-04904-1.
Magiati, I., & Howlin, P. (2019). Adult life for people with autism spectrum disorders. In F. R. Volkmar. *Autism and pervasve developmental disorders* (pp. 220–248). Cambridge University Press.

Maiano, C., Normand, C. L., Salvas, M.-C., Moullec, G., & Aime, A. (2015). Prevalence of school bullying among youth with autism spectrum disorders: A systematic review and meta-analysis. *Autism Research*: No Pagination Specified.

Mallory, S. B. (2014). Factors associated with peer aggression and peer victimization among children with autism spectrum disorders, children with other disabilities, and children without a disability. *Dissertation Abstracts International Section A: Humanities and Social Sciences, 75*(5-A(E)): No Pagination Specified.

Mandlawitz, M. R. (2002). The impact of the legal system on educational programming for young children with autism spectrum disorder. *Journal of Autism and Developmental Disorders, 32*(5), 495–508.

Mannynsalo, L., Putkonen, H., Lindberg, N., & Kotilainen, I. (2009). Forensic psychiatric perspective on criminality associated with intellectual disability: A nationwide register-based study. *Journal of Intellectual Disability Research, 53*(3), 279–288.

Maras, K. L., & Bowler, D. M. (2014). Eyewitness testimony in autism spectrum disorder: A review. *Journal of Autism and Developmental Disorders, 44*(11), 2682–2697.

McClure, I. (2014). Developing and implementing practice guidelines. In N. J. Hoboken (Ed.), *Handbook of autism and pervasive developmental disorders, Volume 2: Assessment, interventions, and policy* (pp. 1014–1035). Wiley.

McPartland, J. C., Webb, S. J., Keehn, B., & Dawson, G. (2011). Patterns of visual attention to faces and objects in autism spectrum disorder. *Journal of Autism and Developmental Disorders, 41*(2), 148–157.

McPartland, J. C., Wu, J., Bailey, C. A., Mayes, L. C., Schultz, R. T., & Klin, A. (2011). Atypical neural specialization for social percepts in autism spectrum disorder. *Social Neuroscience, 6*(5–6), 436–451.

Meera, S., Kaipa, R., Thomas, J., & Shivashankar, N. (2013). Brief report: An unusual manifestation of diagnostic overshadowing of pervasive developmental disorder-Not otherwise specified: A five year longitudinal case study. *Journal of Autism and Developmental Disorders, 43*(6), 1491–1494.

National Research Council. (2001). *Educating young children with autism.* Washington, DC: National Academy Press.

Newschaffer, C. J. (2006). Investigating diagnostic substitution and autism prevalence trends [see comment] [comment]. *Pediatrics, 117*(4), 1436–1437.

Odom, S. L., Morin, K., Savage, M., & Tomaszewski, B. (2018). Behavioral and educational interventions. In F. Volkmar. *Autism and the pervasive developmental disorders* (pp. 176–190). Cambridge University Press.

Odom, S. L., Morin, K., Savage, M., & Tomaszewski, B. (2019). Behavioral and educational interventions. In F. Volkmar. *Autism and the pervasive developmental disorders* (pp. 176–190). Cambridge University Press.

Ozonoff, S., Pennington, B. F., & Rogers, S. J. (1991). Executive function deficits in high-functioning autistic individuals: Relationship to theory of mind. *Journal of Child Psychology and Psychiatry, 32*(7), 1081–1105.

Payne, K.-L., Russell, A., Mills, R., Maras, K., Rai, D., & Brosnan, M. (2019). Is there a relationship between cyber-dependent crime, autistic-like traits and autism? *Journal of Autism and Developmental Disorders, 49*(10), 4159–4169.

Post, M., Storey, K., Haymes, L., Campbell, C., & Loughrey, T. (2014). Stalking behaviors by individuals with autism spectrum disorders in employment settings: Understanding stalking behavior and developing appropriate supports. *Education and Training in Autism and Developmental Disabilities, 49*(1), 102–110.

Reaven, J., Blakeley-Smith, A., Culhane-Shelburne, K., & Hepburn, S. (2012). Group cognitive behavior therapy for children with high-functioning autism spectrum disorders and anxiety: A randomized trial. *Journal of Child Psychology and Psychiatry, 53*(4), 410–419.

Reichow, B., & Barton, E. E. (2014). Evidence-based psychosocial interventions for individuals with autism spectrum disorders. In *Handbook of autism and pervasive developmental disorders, Volume 2: Assessment, interventions, and policy* (pp. 969–992). Wiley.

Rhodes, A. M. (2009). Autism and the courts. *Journal for Specialists in Pediatric Nursing, 14*(3), 215–216.
Ropar, D., & Mitchell, P. (2001). Susceptibility to illusions and performance on visuospatial tasks in individuals with autism. *The Journal of Child Psychology and Psychiatry and Allied Disciplines, 42*(4), 539–549.
Ruggeri, B., Sarkans, U., Schumann, G., & Persico, A. M. (2014). Biomarkers in autism spectrum disorder: The old and the new. *Psychopharmacology (Berl), 231*(6), 1201–1216.
Rutter, M. (1994). Comorbidity: Meanings and mechanisms. *Clinical Psychology: Science and Practice, 1*(1), 100–103.
Rutter, M., & Thapar, A. (2014). Genetics of autism spectrum disorders. In *Handbook of autism and pervasive developmental disorders, Volume 1: Diagnosis, development, and brain mechanisms* (pp. 411–423). Wiley.
Schlinger, H. D. (2009). Theory of mind: An overview and behavioral perspective. *The Psychological Record, 59*(3), 435–448.
Schultz, R. T., Gauthier, I., Klin, A., Fulbright, R. K., Anderson, A. W., Volkmar, F., Skudlarski, P., Lacadie, C., Cohen, D. J., & Gore, J. C. (2000). Abnormal ventral temporal cortical activity during face discrimination among individuals with autism and Asperger syndrome. *Archives of General Psychiatry, 57*(4), 331–340.
Silverman, A. C. (2015). NeuroTribes: The legacy of autism and the future of neurodiversity. Penguin Random House.
Smith, I. C., Reichow, B., & Volkmar, F. R. (2015). The effects of DSM-5 criteria on number of individuals diagnosed with autism spectrum disorder: A systematic review. *Journal of Autism and Developmental Disorders, 45*(8), 2541–2552.
Smith, T., Oakes, L., Selver, K., Volkmar, F. R., Paul, R., Rogers, S. J., & Pelphrey, K. A. (2014). Alternative treatments. In *Handbook of autism and pervasive developmental disorders* (4th ed.). Wiley.
Sreckovic, M. A., Brunsting, N. C., & Able, H. (2014). Victimization of students with autism spectrum disorder: A review of prevalence and risk factors. *Research in Autism Spectrum Disorders, 8*(9), 1155–1172.
Tager-Flusberg, H., Paul, R., & Lord, C. (2014). Language and Communication in autism. In F. R. Volkmar, S. J. Rogers, R. Paul & K. A. Pelphrey *Handbook of autism and pervasive developmental disorders, No 1*, (pp. 335–364). Wiley.
Tsatsanis, K. D., & Powell, K. (2014). Neuropsychological characteristics of autism spectrum disorders. *Handbook of autism and pervasive developmental disorders, Volume 1: Diagnosis, development, and brain mechanisms* (pp. 302–331). Wiley.
van Schalkwyk, G., Smith, I. C., Silverman, W. K., & Volkmar, F. R. (2018). Brief report: Bullying and anxiety in high-functioning adolescents with ASD. *Journal of Autism and Developmental Disorders, 48*(5), 1819–1824.
van Schalkwyk, G. I., Beyer, C., Martin, A., & Volkmar, F. R. (2016). College students with autism spectrum disorders: A growing role for adult psychiatrists. *Journal of American College Health, 64*(7), 575–579.
Van Wieren, T. A., Reid, C. A., & McMahon, B. T. (2008). Workplace discrimination and autism spectrum disorders: The National EEOC Americans with Disabilities Act Research project. *Work, 31*(3), 299–308.
Vivanti, G., & Duncan, E. (2017). *Implementing the group-based early start Denver model for preschoolers with autism*. Springer.
Volkmar, F. R., & Nelson, D. S. (1990). Seizure disorders in autism. *Journal of the American Academy of Child and Adolescent Psychiatry, 29*(1), 127–129.
Volkmar, F., & Wiesner, L. (2009). *A practical guide to autism*. Wiley.
Volkmar, F. R., & Wiesner, L. (2017). *Essential guide to understanding and treating autism*. Wiley.
Volkmar, F., & Wiesner, E. (2018). *Essential clinical guide to understanding and treating autism*. Wiley.

Volkmar, F. R., Booth, L. L., McPartland, J. C., & Wiesner, L. A. (2014). Clinical evaluation in multidisciplinary settings. *Handbook of autism and pervasive developmental disorders: Assessment, interventions, and policy, Volume 2* (4th ed., pp. 661–672). Wiley.
Volkmar, F., Siegel, M., Woodbury-Smith, M., King, B., McCracken, J., & State, M. (2014). Practice parameter for the assessment and treatment of children and adolescents with autism spectrum disorder [Literature Review]. *Journal of the American Academy of Child & Adolescent Psychiatry, 53*(2), 237–257. https://doi.org/10.1016/j.jaac.2013.10.013.
Volkmar, F. R., Wiesner, L. A., & Westphal, A. (2006). Healthcare issues for children on the autism spectrum. *Current Opinion in Psychiatry, 19*(4), 361–366.
Volkmar, F. R., & Woolston, J. L. (1997). Comorbidity of psychiatric disorders in children and adolescents. In S. Wetzler & W. C. Sanderson. In *Treatment strategies for patients with psychiatric comorbidity An Einstein psychiatry publication, No 14* (pp. 307–322). Wiley.
Volkmar, F. R., Woodbury-Smith, M., Macari, S. L., & Oien, R. A. (2021, Mar 15). Seeing the forest and the trees: Disentangling autism phenotypes in the age of DSM-5. *Development & Psychopathology*, 1–9. https://doi.org/10.1017/S0954579420002047.
Watson, L. R., & Zhang, W. (2018). In search of culturally appropriate autism interventions: Perspectives of Latino caregivers. *Journal of Autism and Developmental Disorders, 48*(5), 1623–1639.
Weiss, J. A., Cappadocia, M., Tint, A., & Pepler, D. (2015). Bullying victimization, parenting stress, and anxiety among adolescents and young adults with autism spectrum disorder. *Autism Research*: No Pagination Specified.
Wenzel, C., & Brown, J. T. (2014). Beyond academic intelligence: Increasing college success for students on the autism spectrum. In *Handbook of autism and pervasive developmental disorders, Volume 2: Assessment, interventions, and policy* (pp. 918–931). Wiley.
White, S. W., Elias, R., Capriola-Hall, N. N., Smith, I. C., Conner, C. M., Asselin, S. B., Howlin, P., Getzel, E. E.., & Mazefsky, C. A. (2017). Development of a college transition and support program for students with autism spectrum disorder. *Journal of Autism and Developmental Disorders, 47*(10), 3072–3078.
White, S. W., Ollendick, T. H., & Bray, B. C. (2011). College students on the autism spectrum: Prevalence and associated problems. *Autism, 15*(6), 683–701.
White, S. W., Smith, I. C., Miyazaki, Y., Conner, C. M., Elias, R., & Capriola-Hall, N. N. (2019). Improving transition to adulthood for students with autism: A randomized controlled trial of steps. *Journal of Clinical Child and Adolescent Psychology*: No Pagination Specified.
Whitehouse, A. J., & Stanley, F. J. (2013). Is autism one or multiple disorders. *Medical Journal of Australia, 198*(6), 302–303.
Wilson, C., Roberts, G., Gillan, N., Ohlsen, C., Robertson, D., & Zinkstok, J. (2014). The NICE guideline on recognition, referral, diagnosis and management of adults on the autism spectrum. *Advances in Mental Health and Intellectual Disabilities, 8*(1), 3–14.
Wodrich, D. L. (1997). *Children's psychological testing: A guide for nonpsychologists*. Brookes.
Wolff, L. E., Brown, J. T., & Bork, G. R. (2009). *Students with Asperger syndrome: A guide for college personnel*. Shawnee Mission, KS, APC Publishing.
World Health Organization. (1994). *Diagnostic criteria for research*. Geneva: World Health Organization.
Yuenn, R. K. C., Szatmari, P., & Vorstman, J. A. S. (2019). The genetics of autism spectrum disorders. In F. R. Volkmar. *Autism and the pervasive developmental disorders* (pp. 112–128). Cambridge University Press.

Fred R. Volkmar M.D. is the Irving B. Harris Professor of Child Psychiatry, Pediatrics, and Psychology at the Yale Child Study Center, Yale University School of Medicine and the Dorothy Goodwin Family Chair in Special Education at Southern Connecticut State University. An international authority on Asperger's disorder and autism, Dr. Volkmar was the primary author of the DSM-IV autism and pervasive developmental disorders section. He has authored several hundred scientific papers and has co-edited numerous books, including Asperger Syndrome, Healthcare for Children on the Autism Spectrum: A Guide to Medical, Nutritional, and Behavioral Issues, and the recently released third edition of The Handbook of Autism and Pervasive Developmental Disorders. He serves as an Associate Editor of the Journal of Autism, the Journal of Child Psychology and Psychiatry, and the American Journal of Psychiatry. He also served as a Co-Chairperson of the autism/MR committee of the American Academy of Child and Adolescent Psychiatry. Since 2007 he has served as the Editor of the Journal of Autism and more recently of the Encyclopedia of Autism.

Scott Jackson Ph.D., M.Res., is the Director in the Office of Assessment and Planning at Southern Connecticut State University and an Assistant Clinical Professor at the Yale Child Study Center.

Brian Pete J.D. is a graduate of New York University School of Law. He is a Labor & Employment partner in the New York office of Lewis Brisbois Bisgaard & Smith LLP and was formerly outside counsel to New Jersey public school districts.

Chapter 2
The Autism Diagnosis

Rachel Loftin

Autism Spectrum Disorder (ASD) is a neurodevelopmental disorder that is typically evident in infancy or childhood and is characterized by persistent difficulties with social-communication, as well as restricted interests, repetitive behaviors, and atypical responses to sensory stimulation. Measuring those domains, as well as non-diagnostic areas that may be impacted, is a challenging but critical process in determining eligibility for services, designing interventions, evaluating civil matters, and evaluating factors that may be relevant in criminal cases. Chapter 21 focuses specifically on how psychological testing may be used in legal cases, while this chapter focuses on the diagnosis of ASD, the developmental course as it relates to diagnosis, difficulties with diagnosis that can arise in legal cases, and the best practice procedures for obtaining a diagnosis.

How ASD Is Diagnosed

There are no diagnostic medical tests for autism, and the diagnosis is not made using any single behavioral instrument or observation in isolation. Rather, ASD is diagnosed based on data collected about an individual's early developmental history and current presentation and, when possible, this information is collected from multiple sources. There are a number of clinicians who may be qualified to make a diagnosis; typically, though, diagnosis is made by a pediatrician, neurologist, psychiatrist, or

R. Loftin (✉)
Department of Psychiatry and Behavioral Sciences, Northwestern University Feinberg School of Medicine, Chicago, IL, USA
e-mail: Rachel.loftin@northwestern.edu

F. R. Volkmar et al. (eds.), *Handbook of Autism Spectrum Disorder and the Law*,
https://doi.org/10.1007/978-3-030-70913-6_2

psychologist. At many centers, a multidisciplinary team is able to coordinate evaluations in order to provide medical, psychological, speech and language, and occupational therapy evaluations that contribute information about functioning. Diagnostic criteria from the Diagnostic and Statistical Manual 5th edition (DSM-5, APA) and ICD-10 (WHO, 2004) are used most often, although eligibility for educational programs is somewhat different (see Chap. 15). The current DSM-5 system has been somewhat controversial as some researchers fear it excludes more cognitively able individuals, who previously would have received diagnoses of Autistic Disorder, Aspergers Disorder, or PDD-NOS in the DSM-IV. In one study, about half of the more cognitively able individuals with autism did not meet the new DSM-5 criteria and for the other two categories and 80–90% lost their diagnosis (McPartland et al., 2012). As a result, a provision was made so that persons who had earlier established diagnoses could retain them, essentially muddling the present diagnostic situation (Volkmar & McPartland, 2014).

In most countries, there are limited national guidelines for diagnosis. Penner and colleagues (2018) found among the national autism guidelines they could find among English-speaking countries with single-payer healthcare systems, only New Zealand and the United Kingdom covered the whole lifespan, instead of focusing on early childhood and childhood. The United States does not have national guidelines (or, indeed, a single-payer healthcare system) and, like many countries, relies on guidelines set out by particular professional groups, which can differ greatly in their quality. Diagnostic guidelines from the United Kingdom's National Institute on Healthcare and Guidance (Pilling et al., 2012) specify that all staff working with adults with autism should have an understanding of "the nature, development, and course of autism; the impact on personal, social, educational, and occupational functioning; the impact of the social and physical environment; assessment for autism." However, while most clinicians are familiar with ASD, many clinicians do not have training and experience consistent with the breadth of those guidelines.

Finally, guidelines developed for Australia (Whitehouse & Evans, 2018) clearly advocate a person-centered approach, which prioritizes a comprehensive assessment to understand an individual's unique presentation, rather than relying on a categorical diagnosis alone. This is an important aspect of evaluation, but one that can be time-consuming and difficult to apply in widespread use without significant policy changes in countries like the United States that rely on private health insurance. Some limitations of this approach have, however, been noted (see Vivanti & Volkmar, 2019).

Developmental Course and Age of Diagnosis

Although ASD is more conspicuous in some individuals than others, a comprehensive diagnostic evaluation is essential for accurate diagnosis because the differential diagnosis can be quite challenging. ASD is a neurodevelopmental disorder in the way it presents over an individual's lifetime. Thus, the way a toddler presents with

ASD is significantly different from how the same individual presents as a school-age child, adolescent, and adult. Likewise, the differential diagnoses and commonly co-occurring conditions can vary over the lifespan. Clinicians who are experienced at one point of the development may not be adept with ASD presentation at other points.

While cases of ASD in infancy have been documented (i.e., Volkmar et al., 2005), reliable behavioral markers have not been identified in children under 12 months (Zwaigenbaum et al., 2015). Promising attempts are being made to find early possible markers of the conditions (Chawarska & Volkmar, 2020). The age of initial diagnosis is typically much earlier for children with marked developmental disabilities, such as children who do not develop oral language. Children with intact intellectual ability and verbal skills, on the other hand, may not be diagnosed until well into elementary school or even middle school, when the impact of social deficits becomes more apparent.

For the most part, once someone is diagnosed with ASD, they do not lose the diagnosis. However, the course of development is not always predictable with accuracy, and diagnoses sometimes change over time (see, for instance, Davidovitch et al., 2015; Fein et al., 2013). This means that students who did not qualify for special education services under an Autism eligibility at one point in time, such as in kindergarten, may meet criteria later in life, such as in fourth grade when the increased social and academic pressures make the symptoms more apparent in school. Alternately, a very young autistic child who receives intervention may progress to a point that the signs of autism are subtle and, thus, no longer qualify for services. The developmental course of the disorder can be confusing for educational and clinical staff who are not ASD specialists, and more subtle signs of ASD are often missed. Finally, some subgroups can be particularly difficult to diagnose and may, in turn, receive an initial diagnosis later in life. One clear example is verbal autistic girls without intellectual disability who have learned to mask their symptoms and tend to present somewhat differently from the boys, whose symptoms largely defined the original signs of the diagnosis (Dean et al., 2017).

Less commonly, an ASD diagnosis may be missed entirely in childhood and made for the first time in adolescence or even adulthood. Such later in life diagnoses can be controversial. Understandably, some autism specialists, courts, and prosecutors have expressed concern about the potential over-application of the diagnosis in instances where there is clear benefit to the individual to have the diagnosis applied, such as when an individual is seeking eligibility for disability benefits or when a person is first diagnosed after criminal charges are brought against them. At the same time, there are many reasons why an initial diagnosis of ASD may not be made until adulthood. For many older adults with intact language and intellectual ability, the diagnosis of autism would not have been considered during childhood. Rather, it was only in the last 30 years or so that these cases (often referred to as "higher functioning") were diagnosed. In some cases, a diagnosis was missed in childhood because the autistic person did not have a caregiver advocating for evaluation and supports. In a student without externalizing behavior, the school district would be unlikely to pursue evaluation, and an autistic person without developmental delays may not come to the attention of a pediatrician. People from racial and ethnic groups that differ from the dominant culture may be missed or symptoms may be misinterpreted. An autistic adult may only realize that they should be evaluated after experiencing challenges at work or in an intimate relationship that causes them to recognize the extent of social challenge. Finally, an initial diagnosis is sometimes made in a parent who pursues an evaluation after completing an evaluation for their autistic child and realizing that they possess many of the same traits.

Ableism and related experiences of bias against neurodiverse people may also affect whether an adult pursues the diagnostic process. Autistic adults who were first diagnosed later in life reported fear of not being believed about their symptoms (Lewis, 2017), and it is reasonable to assume that others elected not to seek diagnosis based on such fears. Thus, even once an individual is old enough to seek diagnosis for himself, there may be a reluctance to do so.

Finally, although a post-arrest diagnosis of ASD may be appropriate, there is likely to be bias against criminal defendants who receive a post-arrest diagnosis. There are no known studies of post-arrest diagnosis in ASD, defendants with post-traumatic stress disorder (PTSD) who received their PTSD diagnosis after their arrest, were found guilty more often and had fewer opportunities for diversion than defendants who had a PTSD diagnosis prior to their arrest (Smith, 2018).

Diagnostic Process

Clinicians are generally reliable when determining whether someone is "on the spectrum" or not, but rating individual ASD traits or assigning a designation within the ASD spectrum is not very reliable (see Klin et al., 2000; Taylor et al., 2017; Lord, Petkova, et al., 2012). (This is why, at least in part, the DSM-5 moved to an autism spectrum disorder designation, rather than separate disorders under the umbrella of autism.)

The diagnostic process includes establishing that the signs of ASD are present and with sufficient intensity to meet diagnostic criteria. However, there are rare medical conditions which may cause ASD-like symptoms that can resolve with appropriate treatment, and these conditions would preclude an ASD diagnosis. (These are discussed under Medical Evaluation, below.)

Differential Diagnosis

A primary task of diagnosing ASD is separating it from other, similar-appearing disorders or combinations of symptoms.

In young children, differential diagnoses typically include language delays without ASD, global developmental delays, sensory impairments (such as deafness), attention deficit-hyperactivity disorder (ADHD), and learned behaviors. In school-age children, language disorders, anxiety disorders, intellectual disability, ADHD, and behavior disorders may be difficult to distinguish from ASD. The risk of mood and anxiety disorders increases in adolescence. Adults can have many of the same differential diagnoses as school-age children and adolescents. Additionally, particular caution should be made when diagnosing psychotic disorders in ASD. Certainly, ASD and psychosis can co-occur. However, particularly for those who are less familiar with ASD, the core features of autism can be misinterpreted as psychosis (Van Schalkwyk et al., 2015).

Throughout the lifespan, diagnostic overshadowing can occur. Diagnostic overshadowing refers to when the disorder with the more dominant features masks the other condition(s) in the same individual (Volkmar et al., 2012). When this occurs, the subtler problem is often missed, which can be a significant problem because it is not addressed. Take for example, post-traumatic stress disorder (PTSD). Emerging research suggests that people with ASD may be particularly vulnerable to traumatic events (Haruvi-Lamdan et al., 2018), yet the trauma-related signs may be attributed to the ASD diagnosis and may not be adequately treated.

When psychiatric comorbidities are diagnosed in an autistic adult, it is important for clinicians to know that autistic adults may disagree with the added diagnoses. This often stems from concern that the clinician does not appreciate the characteristics of ASD which may present in similar ways to mental health diagnoses (Au-Yeung et al., 2019). Rather, the mental health challenges were viewed as resultant from ASD. Lack of autism awareness and inadequate communication can present barriers in diagnostic evaluation.

Components of Evaluation

Through the evaluation process, information is collected about functioning in specific domains. These data, taken together, can confirm the diagnosis and also be used to set goals and identify needed accommodations and modifications.

When eligibility for services or confirmation of diagnosis is a question, there are key components that should be part of the evaluations, regardless of additional referral questions that may be posed. The key components include (see Saulnier & Ventola, 2012; Volkmar, Booth, et al., 2014 for more information):

- Search for associated medical conditions;
- Assessment of co-occurring psychiatric concerns;
- Gathering information about the early developmental history;
- an estimate of intellectual ability (or developmental level in a very young child);
- a measure of adaptive skills;
- direct assessment of the individual's social-communication presentation.

The key areas for assessment are outlined in more detail below:

Medical evaluation: A thorough physical examination is required. This may include a pediatrician or general physician performing an examination, in concert with other professionals who complete measures of psychological testing. In university medical centers, multidisciplinary teams typically include physicians, psychologists, speech and language specialists, occupational therapists, and others who are each responsible for portions of the evaluation.

Vision and hearing screens are essential, particularly in young children. Common signs of autism, such as not responding to one's name or nonverbal cues, could result from a child with a visual or hearing disorder.

Genetic testing, specifically a chromosomal microarray, is typically recommended as part of the diagnostic process for ASD and other developmental disorders (Miller et al., 2010). In an increasing number of cases, a known genetic cause of ASD can be identified, and some of these syndromes are associated with particular health risks or known medication responses. Neurologist consults are often warranted as well. There is a high co-occurrence of seizure disorders in ASD (one systematic review found a mean prevalence of epilepsy in ASD of 16.2%; Lukmanji et al., 2019). Rarer neurological conditions (e.g., tuberous sclerosis) can also co-occur at higher rates than in the general population, and physicians who specialize in ASD will typically perform a Wood's lamp test for that disorder.

In very rare cases, an untreated medical problem can look like autism. For instance, metabolic disorders can mimic the social deficits of ASD (e.g., Wolfenden, Wittkowski, Hare, 2017), as can acquire epileptic syndromes, such as Landau Kleffner (Zafari et al., 2018). One case study also mentioned a seizure disorder which led to catatonia symptoms similar to the unresponsiveness in autism (Creten et al., 2011). A thorough history of the development of the symptoms, as described in the Developmental History section below, is critical for tracking the course of the disorder and determining whether the ASD diagnosis is appropriate.

Psychiatric Evaluation. Further, given the high rate of psychiatric comorbidity in ASD throughout the lifespan (see Brookman-Frazee et al., 2018; Buck et al., 2014; Joshi et al., 2013), it is appropriate to screen for the most commonly co-occurring psychiatric conditions, including attention deficit-hyperactivity disorder (ADHD), mood disorders, and anxiety disorders.

Developmental History. One of the key features which separates ASD from other conditions with similar features is its developmental course. ASD is present at birth or soon after and, although it may not be apparent until later childhood, most autistic people show signs in early childhood. For many, clear developmental differences are evident, including speech delays and atypical behaviors (e.g., lining up toys, flapping hands). Many do not show such clear-cut signs and a detailed developmental interview is needed to draw out details about early social-communication skills, play, and the presence of restricted and repetitive behaviors and interests and unusual sensory responses.

The developmental history can be collected in interviews with caregivers or other people intimately familiar with the individual during childhood. Rating scales, such as the *Social Communication Questionnaire*, may also be helpful. Because it is extremely thorough, research studies often employ the *Autism Diagnostic Interview, Revised* (ADI-R, Rutter and LeCouteur et al., 2003) to collect the developmental history. The ADI-R is a standardized interview measure of early developmental history and current behavior across the domains of reciprocal social interactions, language and communication, and restricted and stereotyped behaviors and interests. However, the ADI-R requires a caregiver with intimate knowledge of the individual's early years and can take a long time to administer.

Intellectual Ability. In making a diagnosis of ASD, it is essential to understand the individual's intellectual level. Someone with a marked intellectual disability may demonstrate social deficits similar to those of a person with ASD but still possess social-communication skills that commiserate with ability-based expectations, in which case diagnosis of ASD would not be appropriate. There are many test options when assessing intellectual ability. The psychologist administering the IQ test will select the most appropriate measure based on background information (communication skills, in particular) of the person being evaluated.

Brief measures of intellectual ability may be sufficient in situations with a time constraint, but more comprehensive measures are generally needed. Unusual and uneven cognitive profiles are well documented in autism, and brief measures of intellectual ability typically do not capture the significant range of abilities that is often present.

Comprehensive measures of intelligence include the Wechsler Scales, which include preschool, school-age and adult measures (WPPSI, Wechsler, 2012; WISC V, Wechsler, 2014; WAIS IV, Wechsler, 2008), the *Stanford Binet Intelligence Scales, Fifth Edition* (SBIS 5, Roid, 2003), and the *Differential Ability Scales, Second Edition* (DAS-2; Elliott, 2007) for children and adolescents. For some individuals with ASD, particularly those with an intellectual disability or substantial language delays, nonverbal IQ tests are more appropriate. There are fully nonverbal IQ tests, such as the *Test of Nonverbal Intelligence, Fourth Edition* (TONI-4; Fopiano, 2013) and the *Raven's Progressive Matrices, Second Edition* (Raven's; Raven et al., 2018). Alternately, some measures, such as the DAS-2 can yield nonverbal composites.

For very young children or those with marked intellectual disability who cannot complete items on standard IQ tests, developmental measures, which do not yield IQ scores, may be more appropriate. Developmental measures include the *Mullen Scales of Early Learning* (Mullen, 1995) and *Bayley Scales of Infant Development, Third Edition* (Bayley, 2006).

Adaptive Function. Assessment of daily adaptive functioning across such areas as communication, daily living skills, and socialization is also important. Typically, the adaptive function of a person with ASD is much lower than their intellectual potential, and the adaptive behavior scores provided a better snapshot of how the person actually functions in everyday environments than scores obtained in structured testing. An adaptive behavior assessment also helps identify skill deficits that interfere with independent functioning, as well as reliance on caregiver support.

There are many adaptive measures available. A widely used adaptive behavior scale, with a long history of use by clinicians who specialize in ASD, is the *Vineland Adaptive Behavior Scales, Third Edition* (Vineland-3, Sparrow et al., 2016). Alternatives include the *Adaptive Behavioral Assessment System, Third Edition* (ABAS 3, Harrison & Oakland, 2015), and the *Scales of Independent Behavior, Revised* (SIB-R, 1995). Further, some government agencies and school districts have their own checklists, comprised of lists of specific adaptive skills, which can be incorporated in a test battery.

Direct Assessment of ASD features. Clinicians who regularly diagnose ASD report the helpfulness of standardized measures, along with concern about their validity with certain populations, particularly females (Rogers et al., 2016).

Clinicians can feel overwhelmed by the range of measures available, as well as by the varying recommendations from professional organizations and agencies (Hayes et al., 2018; Penner et al., 2018). Both semi-structured and unstructured methods, as well as rating scales, are used. Regardless of the specific tests, it is important to collect direct observation of social-communication challenges, not just reports. There are various methods for obtaining the direct assessment, but the combination of a standardized measure and expert clinical judgment is most helpful for obtaining valid and reliable estimates of ASD symptoms.

The *Autism Diagnostic Observation Schedule, Second Edition* (ADOS-2, Lord et al., Lord, Rutter, et al., 2012) is the most widely used structured direct observation method. Although the procedures are standardized, the ADOS-2 sets up a social context that is meant to feel natural and includes many tasks and activities, with separate modules based on language and developmental level. Thus, a good sample of social-communication before can be obtained.

A comprehensive battery can also include rating scales or checklists to assess the presence and severity of other symptoms of an ASD, although an ASD diagnosis should never be made on the basis of rating scales alone (or, indeed, any single components of the assessment battery). A commonly used rating scale is the *Social Responsiveness Scale, Second Edition* (SRS-2, Constantino & Gruber, 2012) which measures social behavior via parent or teacher report for children or by caregiver or self-report for adults. *The Autism Spectrum Quotient* (AQ; Baron-Cohen et al., 2001) and its related child and adolescent versions and the *Childhood Autism Rating Scale–Second Edition* (CARS-2; Schopler et al., 2010) are also frequently used. There are numerous other rating scales with varying psychometric properties. For a chart of options, see Volkmar et al. (2014).

Summary

Accurate and reliable diagnosis is important for obtaining services and entitlements, as well as for understanding an individual in a court case. The process of ASD diagnosis is complicated by debate about the current DSM-5 criteria, difficulty securing accurate diagnosis, delays in diagnosis, and challenges in differential diagnosis. In many cases, particularly in atypical or otherwise challenging cases, evaluations by clinicians who specialize in ASD are needed.

References

Au-Yeung, S. K., Bradley, L., Robertson, A. E., Shaw, R., Baron-Cohen, S., & Cassidy, S. (2019). Experience of mental health diagnosis and perceived misdiagnosis in autistic, possibly autistic and non-autistic adults. *Autism, 23*(6), 1508–1518. https://doi-org.turing.library.northwestern.edu/10.1177/1362361318818167.

Baron-Cohen, S., Wheelwright, R., Skinner, J. M., & Clubley, E. (2001). The Autism Spectrum Quotient (AQ): Evidence from Asperger syndrome/high functioning autism, males and females, scientists and mathematicians. *Journal of Autism and Developmental Disorders, 31*, 5–17.

Bayley, N. (2006). *Bayley Scales of Infant and Toddler Development*. PsychCorp, Pearson.

Brookman-Frazee, L., Stadnick, N., Chlebowski, C., Baker-Ericzén, M., & Ganger, W. (2018). Characterizing psychiatric comorbidity in children with autism spectrum disorder receiving publicly funded mental health services. *Autism, 22*(8), 938–952.

Buck, T. R., Viskochil, J., Farley, M., Coon, H., McMahon, W. M., Morgan, J., & Bilder, D. A. (2014). Psychiatric comorbidity and medication use in adults with autism spectrum disorder. *Journal of Autism and Developmental Disorders, 44*(12), 3063–3071.

Chawarska, K., & Volkmar, F. R. (2020). *Autism spectrum disorder in the first years of life*. Guilford Press.

Constantino, J. N., & Gruber, C. P. (2012). *Social Responsiveness Scale: SRS-2*. Torrance, CA: Western Psychological Services.

Creten, C., Van der Zwaan, S., Blankespoor, R., Maatkamp, A., Nicolai, J., Van Os, J., & Schieveld, J. (2011). Late onset autism and anti-NMDA-receptor encephalitis. *The Lancet, 378*(9785), 98.

Davidovitch, M., Levit-Binnun, N., Golan, D., & Manning-Courtney, P. (2015). Late diagnosis of autism spectrum disorder after initial negative assessment by a multidisciplinary team. *Journal of Developmental and Behavioral Pediatrics, 36*(4), 227–234.

Dean, M., Harwood, R., & Kasari, C. (2017). The art of camouflage: Gender differences in the social behaviors of girls and boys with autism spectrum disorder. *Autism, 21*(6), 678–689.

Elliott, C. D. (2007). *Differential ability scales—Second edition (DAS-II)*. San Antonio, TX: The Psychological Corporation.

Fein, D., Barton, M., Eigsti, I.-M., Kelley, E., Naigles, L., Schultz, R. T., Stevens, M., Helt, M., Orinstein, A., Rosenthal, M., Troyb, E., & Tyson, K. (2013). Optimal outcome in individuals with a history of autism. *Journal of Child Psychology and Psychiatry, 54*(2), 195–205.

Fopiano, J. (2013). Test of nonverbal intelligence (TONI-4). *Encyclopedia of Autism Spectrum Disorders*. New York: Springer, 3089–3092.

Groth-Marnat, G. (2009). *Handbook of psychological assessment*. John Wiley & Sons.

Harrison, P. L., & Oakland, T. (2015). *ABAS-3*. Torrance: Western Psychological Services.

Haruvi-Lamdan, N., Horesh, D., & Golan, O. (2018). PTSD and autism spectrum disorder: Co-morbidity, gaps in research, and potential shared mechanisms. *Psychological Trauma: Theory, Research, Practice, and Policy, 10*(3), 290.

Hayes, J., Ford, T., Rafeeque, H., & Russell, G. (2018). Clinical practice guidelines for diagnosis of autism spectrum disorder in adults and children in the UK: A narrative review. *BMC Psychiatry, 18*(1). Retrieved from https://link-gale-com.turing.library.northwestern.edu/apps/doc/A547059445/AONE?u=northwestern&sid=AONE&xid=960dc79c.

Joshi, G., Wozniak, J., Petty, C., Martelon, M. K., Fried, R., Bolfek, A., ... & Caruso, J. (2013). Psychiatric comorbidity and functioning in a clinically referred population of adults with autism spectrum disorders: a comparative study. *Journal of autism and developmental disorders, 43*(6), 1314–1325.

Klin, A., Lang, J., Cicchetti, D. V., & Volkmar, F. R. (2000). Brief report: Interrater reliability for clinical diagnosis and DSM-IV criteria for autistic disorder: Results of the DSM-IV autism field trial. *Journal of Autism and Developmental Disabilities, 30*, 163–178. https://doi.org/10.1023/A:1005415823867 .

Lewis, L. (2017). A mixed methods study of barriers to formal diagnosis of autism spectrum disorder in adults. *Journal of Autism and Developmental Disorders, 47*(8), 2410–2424.

Lord, C., Petkova, E., Hus, V., Gan, W., Lu, F., Martin, D. M., ... & Algermissen, M. (2012). A multisite study of the clinical diagnosis of different autism spectrum disorders. *Archives of general psychiatry*, *69*(3), 306–313.
Lord, C., Rutter, M., DiLavore, P.C. et al. (2012). *Autism Diagnostic Observation Scale, Second Edition* (ADOS-2). Western Psychological Services.
Lukmanji, S., Manji, S. A., Kadhim, S., Sauro, K. M., Wirrell, E. C., Kwon, C. S., & Jetté, N. (2019). The co-occurrence of epilepsy and autism: A systematic review. *Epilepsy & Behavior, 98*, 238–248.
Maenner M. J., Shaw, K. A., Baio J., et al. (2020). Prevalence of autism spectrum disorder among children aged 8 years—Autism and developmental disabilities monitoring network, 11 Sites, United States, 2016. MMWR Surveill Summ, *69*(No. SS-4),1–12. https://doi.org/10.15585/mmwr.ss6904a1.
McClure, I., Volkmar, F. R., Paul, R., Rogers, S. J., & Pelphrey, K. A. (2014). Developing and implementing practice guidelines. In *Handbook of autism and pervasive developmental disorders* (4th ed.). John Wiley & Sons, Inc.
McPartland, J. C., Reichow, B., & Volkmar, F. R. (2012). Sensitivity and specificity of proposed DSM-5 diagnostic criteria for autism spectrum disorder. *Journal of the American Academy of Child & Adolescent Psychiatry, 51*(4), 368–383.
Miller, D. T., Adam, M. P., Aradhya, S., Biesecker, L. G., Brothman, A. R., Carter, N. P., ... & Faucett, W. A. (2010). Consensus statement: chromosomal microarray is a first-tier clinical diagnostic test for individuals with developmental disabilities or congenital anomalies. *The American Journal of Human Genetics*, *86*(5), 749-764.
Mullen, E. M. (1995). *Mullen Scales of Early Learning* (AGS ed.). Circle Pines, MN: American Guidance Service Inc.
Penner, M., Anagnostou, E., Andoni, L. Y., & Ungar, W. J. (2018). Systematic review of clinical guidance documents for autism spectrum disorder diagnostic assessment in select regions. *Autism, 22*(5), 517–527. https://doi.org/10.1177/1362361316685879.
Pilling, S., Baron-Cohen, S., Megnin-Viggars, O., Lee, R., Taylor, C., & Guideline Development Group. (2012). Guidelines: Recognition, referral, diagnosis, and management of adults with autism: Summary of NICE guidance. *BMJ: British Medical Journal, 345*(7865), 43–45. Retrieved April 18, 2020, from www.jstor.org/stable/23279273.
Raven, J., Rust, J., Chan, F., & Zhou, X. (2018). *Raven's 2 progressive matrices, clinical edition (Raven's 2).* Pearson.
Rogers, C., Goddard, L., Hill, E., Henry, L., & Crane, L. (2016). Experiences of diagnosing autism spectrum disorder: A survey of professionals in the United Kingdom. *Autism, 20*(7), 820–831.
Roid, G.H. (2003). Stanford-Binet Intelligence Scale-5 (SB-5). CA: Western Psychological Services.
Saulnier, C. A., & Ventola, P. E. (2012). *Essentials of autism spectrum di orders evaluation and assessment* (Vol. 83). Wiley.
Schopler, E, Van Bourgondien, M. E., Wellman, et al. (2010). *Children Autism Rating Scale 2* (CARS 2). Western Psychological Services.
Simms, M. D. (2017). When autistic behavior suggests a disease other than classic autism. *Pediatric Clinics, 64*(1), 127–138.
Simonoff, E., Pickles, A., Chandler, S., et al. (2008). Psychiatric disorders in children with autism spectrum disorders: prevalence, comorbidity, and associated factors in a population-derived sample. *Journal of the American Academy of Child and Adolescent Psychiatry, 47*, 921–929.
Smith, B. A. (2018). Impact of veteran status and timing of PTSD diagnosis on criminal justice outcomes. *Healthcare (Basel), 6*(3):80. Published 2018 Jul 12. https://doi.org/10.3390/healthcare6030080.
Sparrow, S. S., Cicchetti, D. V., & Saulnier, C. A. (2016). *Vineland Adaptive Behavior Scales.* (3rd ed.). Pearson Education Inc.

Taylor, L., Eapen, V., Maybery, M., Midford, S., Paynter, J., Quarmby, L., . . . Whitehouse, A. (2017). Brief report: An exploratory study of the diagnostic reliability for autism spectrum disorder. *Journal of Autism and Developmental Disorders, 47*(5), 1551–1558.
Van Schalkwyk, G. I., Peluso, F., Qayyum, Z. et al. (2015). Varieties of misdiagnosis in ASD: An illustrative case series. *Journal of Autism and Developmental Disorders, 45*, 911–918. https://doi.org/10.1007/s10803-014-2239-y.
Vivanti, G., & Volkmar, F. R. (2019). Review: National guideline for the assessment and diagnosis of autism spectrum disorders in Australia (Whitehouse, Evans et al. 2018). *Journal of Autism & Developmental Disorders,20,* 20.
Volkmar, F. R., Reichow, B., & McPartland, J. (2012). Classification of autism and related conditions: progress, challenges, and opportunities. *Dialogues in Clinical Neuroscience, 14*(3), 229.
Volkmar, F. R., Booth, L., McPartland, J., & Wiesner, L. (2014). Clinical evaluation in multidisciplinary settings. In *Handbook of autism and pervasive developmental disorders: Assessment, interventions, and policy , Volume 2* (pp. 661–672) (4th ed.). Wiley.
Volkmar, F., Chawarska, K., & Klin, A. (2005). Autism in infancy and early childhood. *Annual Review of Psychology, 56*, 315–336.
Volkmar, F. R., & McPartland, J. C. (2014). From Kanner to DSM-5: autism as an evolving diagnostic concept. *Annual Review of Clinical Psychology, 10*, 193–212.
Volkmar, F., Siegel, M., Woodbury-Smith, M., King, B., McCracken, J., & State, M. (2014). Practice parameter for the assessment and treatment of children and adolescents with autism spectrum disorder. *Journal of the American Academy of Child & Adolescent Psychiatry, 53*(2), 237–257.
Wechsler, D. (2008). *Wechsler Adult Intelligence Scale- Fourth Edition (WAIS-IV)*. Pearson Educational Resources.
Wechsler, D. (2014). *Wechsler Intelligence Scale for Children, Fifth Edition (WISC-V)*. Pearson Educational Resources.
Wechsler, D. (2012). *Wechsler Preschool and Primary Scale of Intelligence—Fourth Edition*. The Psychological Corporation San Antonio.
Wiggins, L., Baio, J., Schieve, L., Lee, L.-C., Nicholas, J., & Rice, C. (2012). Retention of autism spectrum diagnoses by community professionals: Findings from the autism and developmental disabilities monitoring network, 2000 and 2006. *Journal of Developmental & Behavioral Pediatrics, 33*, 387–395. https://doi.org/10.1097/DBP.0b013e3182560b2f.
Wolfenden, C., Wittkowski, A., & Hare, D. J. (2017). Symptoms of autism spectrum disorder (ASD) in individuals with Mucopolysaccharide Disease Type III (Sanfilippo Syndrome): A systematic review. *Journal of Autism and Developmental Disorders, 47*, 3620–3633.https://doi.org/10.1007/s10803-017-3262-6.
World Health Organization. (2004). *ICD-10: international statistical classification of diseases and related health problems*. Tenth revision.
Zafari, A., Karimi, N., Taherian, M., & Taherian, R. (2018). Landau Kleffner syndrome and misdiagnosis of autism spectrum disorder: A mini-review. *International Clinical Neuroscience Journal, 5*(1), 3–6.
Zwaigenbaum, L., Bauman, M., Stone, W., Yirmiya, N., Estes, A., Hansen, R., . . . Wetherby, A. (2015). Early Identification of autism spectrum disorder: recommendations for practice and research. *Pediatrics, 136 Suppl 1*(S1), S10–S40.

Rachel Loftin is an autism specialist trained in school and clinical psychology. She maintains a private practice that offers diagnosis and assessment, therapy, and consultation on educational and legal cases. She is an adjunct faculty in the psychiatry departments in the psychiatry departments of Northwestern and Yale University. She was previously an Associate Professor in the Department of Psychiatry at Rush University Medical Center, where she was the Clinical Director of the autism program. Dr. Loftin completed fellowship training in developmental disorders at Yale.

Chapter 3
Expert Evidence about Autism Spectrum Disorder

Ian Freckelton

Introduction

All expert evidence has as its object the provision of assistance to a court and the enhancement of the understanding of the trier of fact—whether that be a judge, a magistrate or a jury (Freckelton, 2019b). As it was put by Lord President Cooper in *Davie v Magistrates of Edinburgh* (1953), the duty of the expert witness.

> is to *furnish the judge or jury with the necessary scientific criteria for testing the accuracy of their conclusions*, so as to enable the Judge or jury to form their own independent judgment by the application of these criteria to the facts proved in evidence.

In *Kennedy v Cordia (Services) LLP* (2016), the United Kingdom Supreme Court similarly identified four factors that govern the admissibility of expert evidence in civil proceedings:

1. Whether the proposed evidence will assist the court in its task;
2. Whether the witness has the necessary knowledge and experience;
3. Whether the witness is impartial in his or her presentation and assessment of evidence; and
4. Whether there is a reliable body of knowledge or experience to underpin the expert's evidence.

Thus, there should be an imparting of knowledge by expert witnesses on matters not otherwise within the ken of the court and there can be the provision of an informed

---

Some material in this chapter has previously been published in more extensive form in Freckelton (2011, 2020a, 2020c). It is reproduced with permission.

I. Freckelton (✉)
Queen's Counsel, Melbourne, VIC, Australia
e-mail: I.Freckelton@vicbar.com.au

University of Melbourne, Melbourne, VIC, Australia

F. R. Volkmar et al. (eds.), *Handbook of Autism Spectrum Disorder and the Law*,
https://doi.org/10.1007/978-3-030-70913-6_3

perspective on how evidence as to facts should be interpreted by the trier of fact. Another role of the expert, which is especially important in cases dealing with autism spectrum disorder ("ASD") is educative—the giving of counter-intuitive evidence to reduce the potential that erroneous reasoning processes will be employed by the trier of fact; for instance, to address the risk that it will be inferred from their manner that a person with ASD is indifferent to the harm that they have caused or to the seriousness of court proceedings.

ASD, and Asperger's Syndrome/Disorder are specialist areas of clinical and forensic practice. On occasion, they are diagnoses which are not identified by practitioners in the forensic context, or in the clinical context, in part because they can overlap with other conditions such as ADHD, intellectual disability, obsessive–compulsive disorder (Freckelton, 2020b) and personality disorders (see Freckelton, 2019; Freckelton & List, 2009). This means that there can be a conflict between experts in the area, who are consulted for a forensic analysis or even who are treaters, and mental health professionals who are generalists and who have not been sensitised to the diagnostic criteria for ASD.

This chapter reviews a range of cases in England, Scotland, Ireland, Australia, New Zealand and Canada where expert evidence has been prominent in relation to ASD. It endeavours to identify where the evidence has been effective in facilitating a better informed decision by courts and what has led in others to courts not adopting or appreciating the nuances of the evidence that has been given in forensic reports or in viva voce evidence. In this regard, the aspiration is to provide assistance to mental health professionals in relation to where they should direct their investigations and their analyses, and also to legal practitioners in relation to how they should commission expert reports and where they should focus their questioning of expert witnesses.

Expert Evidence

There are three forms of expert evidence: expert evidence of fact, expert evidence in the form of opinions, and expert evidence of conjecture (*HG v The Queen*, 1999), the last of which is generally not permissible. While there is not a complete dichotomy between evidence in the form of facts and evidence in the form of opinions, in essence expert evidence in the form of opinions consists of inferences drawn from facts otherwise proved (see Freckelton, 2019b).

There are occasions when a psychologist or psychiatrist makes observations of a person whom they are assessing or even treating. It may be close to the time of the commission of a criminal offence, whether or not the person with ASD is a suspect or a victim, or it may be later, at the time of a forensic assessment. It may be at the time of trial or later for the purposes of an appeal. Such evidence, even though inevitably it incorporates some amount of subjective evaluation, is regarded as in the form of facts. More commonly, though, mental health professionals utilise their clinical skills of observation, analysis and interpretation to arrive at a diagnosis. This tends to be only part of the forensic challenge in ASD cases, however, as the major issue in respect of which courts need assistance is the extent to which the symptomatology of the person assessed impacted upon their conduct or upon how they behaved in relevant circumstances. Both aspects of such evidence are evidence in the form of opinions and they deal with areas of specialised knowledge, well beyond the awareness of laypersons unless provided with expert assistance.

Little controversy attaches to the expertise of psychologists or psychiatrists in diagnosing ASD. However, there are two further issues. First, expertise in ASD is generally a specialised subset of general expertise as a mental health professional—by corollary, many mental health practitioners could not properly be regarded as having expertise in ASD (Berryessa, 2017). Secondly, it is important for the credibility of a diagnosis that the expert witness make clear and transparent the bases upon which they have arrived at a diagnosis—under the DSM or the ICD. A failure to do so has the potential to render opinions inadmissible or at least of reduced probative value. This means that the employment of any tests, scales or measures should be identified specifically and explained within a forensic report. Adoption of such a procedure also enables a trier of fact to understand the particular symptoms that are prominent in a person's diagnosis, how pronounced they are, and therefore what impact they may have had upon the person's offending behaviour.

For the sentencing phase of a criminal trial, the key issues for mental health professionals giving evidence about ASD are whether the convicted person is a suitable medium for deterrence, general or specific, or for punishment, as well as whether the person is plausibly amenable to rehabilitative measures. Overall, the protection of the community (including by reducing the potential for recidivism) is the aim of sentencing but factors such as whether the convicted person will struggle to cope in a custodial environment, including whether their symptomatology will be exacerbated by confinement can also be relevant issues upon which mental health practitioners can provide helpful opinions to courts.

The most significant challenge facing mental health professionals expressing opinions about the ramifications of ASD, though, is to go beyond the mere provision of a labelling diagnosis and to take the decision-makers in a court—a judge, a jury or a magistrate—inside the internal world of the person with ASD so that the trier of fact can acquire a better appreciation of how differently the person is likely to have experienced stimuli and to have made decisions on the basis of such experiences. Inevitably, this encompasses the assumption of an educative role by the witness (see Berryessa, 2017), and the provision of a level of explication that is more extensive and more subtle than is often necessary for expert evidence in other contexts. It can extend to disabusing the court of erroneous inferences they might draw by what is, in effect, counter-intuitive evidence (see *Merritt v The Queen*, 2018: at [46]–[49]).

Expert Evidence as to Impairment of the Capacity for Reasoning

The symptoms of ASD can inhibit the capacity of a person from reasoning through the consequences of their behaviour. In principle, this can mean that they may not be criminally responsible for their behaviour or, at least, their moral culpability may be significantly diminished.

Davies v The Queen. These difficulties were identifiable in *Davies v The Queen* (2019) where the Victorian Court of Appeal in Australia heard a multifaceted appeal brought against a sentence of 14 years imprisonment with a non-parole period of 12 years and 3 months on five counts of arson. Two psychologists gave evidence. The first, Ms. Matthews, expressed the view that Davies had Asperger's disorder which impacted on his "thought stream, focus of interest and interpersonal relatedness". She thought that it would be difficult but not impossible to ameliorate his condition through pharmacological or counselling treatments but that he did not appear to be coping within the challenging environment within the prison (at [630]).

Another forensic psychologist, Mr. Watson-Munro, concurred that Davies had Asperger's disorder but also considered that he had post-traumatic stress disorder and high levels of depression and anxiety. He expressed the view that Davies' ASD "had led to an impairment of his judgment, which in turn impacts upon his culpability. In saying this I am not for a moment suggesting that he is unaware of his criminality" (at [633]). He was more optimistic that treatment in the form of cognitive behaviour therapy might ameliorate the risk of Davies' reoffending.

When cross-examined, Mr. Watson-Munro emphasised the limitation in Davies' self-control by reason of ASD and asserted that: "… he's not functioning as a normal person. His level of functioning is reduced by virtue of his condition" (at [637]).

In spite of the expert evidence, though, the trial judge concluded that the only factor relevant to sentencing Davies as a person with impaired mental functioning was that he would find a term of imprisonment harder than others would: "your moral culpability remains very high and is not, in my view, to be seen as diminished by reason of any aspect of your impaired mental functioning of anxiety, post-traumatic stress disorder or autism taken separately or in combination. You knew precisely what you were doing by committing each of the arsons and that it amounted to what you intended which is a deliberate attack on our community. It was a considered, deliberate campaign all planned and executed by you. There was, and is, no causal connection or link between your post-traumatic stress disorder, anxiety or your autism and these five fires" (at [666]).

However, in this regard the trial judge was found on appeal to have erred as the evidence established a link between Davies' ASD and the views he held, and espoused in various YouTube videos that he generated, and thus the motivation that led him to engage in the arson offences: "To that extent, his disorder affected his reasoning processes" (at [688]). The Court of Appeal noted that the view of Mr. Watson-Munro was that Davies' ASD affected his exercise of judgement. This meant that Davies' congenital psychological disorder played a material role in his offending: "it was erroneous for the prosecutor to suggest, and the judge to accept, that the applicant's moral culpability was not diminished by reason of his impaired mental functioning, and in particular, by reason of his autism spectrum disorder" (at [698]). The result was that the Court of Appeal reduced Davies' sentence to 12 years and three months imprisonment with ten years and three months set as a non-parole period. It was the impairment in the capacity to exercise judgement that resulted in the reduced moral culpability on the part of Davies and thus the appropriateness of a reduced sentence of imprisonment.

R v Peake. In a 2017 manslaughter by criminal negligence case involving the death of the accused woman's mother, Vanstone J of the South Australian Supreme Court was persuaded to accept expert evidence that Peake was precluded by her symptomatology of autism from appreciating the need of her mother for medical intervention, when such a need would have been apparent to others (*R v Peake*, 2017). Key to the acceptance by Vanstone J was the evidence from a clinical evidence with a particular interest in autism that Peake's autism had impacted adversely on her ability to appreciate the nature of the risks posed to her mother and to feel a need to respond with urgency. Thus she lacked the necessary mental element to have committed the offence charged.

R v Walker. In a 2008 case before the New Zealand High Court at first instance (*R v Walker*, 2008) the accused's Asperger's disorder was found central to the sentence to be imposed upon him (see further Freckelton, 2011). Walker pleaded guilty to a series of computer fraud offences committed when he was aged between 16 and 18 years. He developed and used software that enabled him to control infected computers remotely via a robot network, known as a "bot net". He installed a code on tens of thousands of computers, automatically disabling antivirus software. The court was informed that Walker's code was considered by international cyber-crime investigators to be among the most advanced bot programming to that time generated, although it had not been deployed to effect fraud.

Walker had no previous convictions and had a good background and reputation. He had been tentatively diagnosed as having a mild form of Asperger's Syndrome as a child, although latterly his symptoms had decreased in conjunction with his being encouraged to socialise more. He described his offending as having been motivated principally by curiosity—"to see what he could do". He showed signs of remorse and was prepared to pay reparation. A psychologist, Mr. Laven, classified him as being of low to medium risk of reoffending.

Justice Potter accepted that Walker had a "diminished understanding in relation to the nature of his offending" (*R v Walker*, 2008: [17]), partly because of having Asperger's disorder. He concluded that Walker's conduct was carried out simply to demonstrate to himself that he could inflict the kind of harm that resulted—"he was unaware of the nature of the harm that his activities could cause and was immature to the extent that he was unable, or failed, to set proper boundaries for himself in relation to his undoubted ability and expertise in the use of computers" (*R v Walker*, 2008, at [25]). He also took into account that Walker had received offers of employment from large corporations active outside New Zealand and also that the New Zealand Police were interested in employing him. Justice Potter formed the view that Walker had a "potentially outstanding future" (*R v Walker*, 2008: [37]) and discharged him without conviction.

Expert Evidence about Impaired Capacity for Empathy

If a person by reason of their symptomatology of ASD is unable to empathise with the distress or harm that they are causing to another, this has the potential to reduce their level of culpability for their conduct.

Gray (a Pseudonym) v The Queen. An argument in this regard was heard by the Victorian Court of Appeal in *Gray (a Pseudonym) v The Queen* (2018) (see further Freckelton, 2020c). Tom Gray had pleaded guilty in the Victorian County Court to a series of charges relating to sexual assaults. He was a man of superior intelligence and held a doctoral degree in quantum physics. He was sentenced to 19 years imprisonment with a non-parole period of 15 years.

On the plea, evidence was called on behalf of Gray from Associate Professor Andrew Carroll, a consultant forensic psychiatrist, who expressed the view that Gray met the criteria for a diagnosis of ASD. He said that Gray had profound impairments in vocational and interpersonal functioning, commenting that "a significant core problem in Asperger's disorder is impaired capacity to empathise with the thoughts and feelings of other people", so that it was "possible" that Gray "was unable to appreciate the full extent of the impact of his behaviours upon the victim" (at [29]). The tentative wording that Associate Professor Carroll utilised in this respect was ultimately viewed as important.

A consultant clinical neuropsychologist, Professor Warwick Brewer, agreed with Associate Professor Carroll, observing that a key feature of Asperger's disorder is the compromised ability of those with the condition to relate to another person emotionally. His view on balance was that Gray's Asperger's disorder did not cause his criminal conduct but was a "significant contribution to the offending and the nature of the offending". As the offending continued on the second day of Gray's infliction of sexual assaults upon his victim, Gray's anxiety and distress "had continued to compound", and "his ability to formulate rational and reasoned behaviour, or to even respond to what the victim was expressing in terms of distress … was becoming further [and] more significantly reduced as his distress exacerbated". With respect to Gray's level of executive functioning throughout the offending, Associate Professor Brewer thought that Gray did have "analytical skills" to plan and organise, but his "socioemotional executive function" was subject to a "significant developmental delay, if not arrest, of those features of socioemotional self". As a consequence, Gray's socio-emotional executive functioning was "significantly compromised"; put another way, he had "lost the capacity for that normal ability in his cognitive executive function to regulate his socioemotional executive function" (at [33]).

The trial judge accepted that at times during the period when Gray offended his symptoms facilitated his regression into a fantasy world and that his mental state was further compromised by insomnia and depression to some degree in the aftermath of a relationship break-up. She concluded that his deficits facilitated his remaining wilfully egocentric as regards his desires, and in that sense inhibited his ability to think clearly and exercise appropriate judgement: "The nature of your illness, and to a lesser extent your depression, facilitated you viewing what you were engaged in only within the confines of your desires" (at [44]). However, she rejected the proposition that Gray's deficits were causally related to his offending.

The Court of Appeal found this analysis "beyond any legitimate criticism". It observed, without demur, that the trial judge concluded that Gray was not incapable of appreciating the victim's emotional perspective, but "rather sought to exploit it so as to prevent his crimes coming to light (for example, by use of the video recording), whilst obtaining twisted gratification from her suffering. Importantly, the judge found that Gray was conscious of the effect of his depredations on the hapless victim 'in terms of physical pain and the disgusting nature of the acts'" (at [46]). In short, therefore, while there was some measure of acceptance by the sentencing judge, and on appeal, that the socio-emotional functioning of Gray was compromised by ASD, he was found to have sufficient awareness of the harm that he was inflicting that his condition did not mitigate his culpability.

Expert Evidence about the Consequences of a Conviction

In some scenarios the rigidity of thinking of a person with ASD may not only lead to obsessionality of thinking and conduct, but preclude the capacity to understand why they should be convicted of criminal offending. This affects the relevance of deterrent purposes in sentencing. In turn the imposition of a conviction in such circumstances may have deleterious consequences for the mental state and social integration of such a person, rendering the imposition of a conviction counter-productive and, in particular, counter-therapeutic. For such potential consequences to be arguable, expert evidence is essential.

Glover v Police. An illustrative New Zealand decision on the potential relevance of Asperger's disorder for the criminal law is that of the High Court in *Glover v Police* (2009) (see further Freckelton, 2011). Glover had damaged the victim's property on two separate occasions. He described himself as a "road safety activist". Glover was of the view that a footpath needed to run past the front of his property. However, to his considerable consternation the Council had licensed the victim to use a garden area at the front of the victim's property as part of his front garden.

In purported assertion of his and others' rights to the use of the area in front of the victim's house, Glover interfered with and caused damage to the victim's garden area. At his trial Glover argued that he had acted with lawful justification, excuse or a "claim of right" to do what he had done. However, his defence was not accepted, he was convicted and he was ordered to pay reparation and to undertake 40 hours of community work. He appealed against the sentence.

The issue before the courts at first instance and then on appeal was the relevance of the fact that Glover suffered from Asperger's disorder. It was argued that both the gravity of his offending and the direct and indirect consequences of a conviction need to be considered in light of the nature of the syndrome and its effects on his behaviour. A psychologist, with expertise on ASD, Professor Tony Attwood (see Attwood, 2008) contended that a conviction would lead to an increase in Glover's alienation, frustration and despair.

The sentencing judge had viewed Glover's offending as lying at the more serious end of the scale, having regard to the fact that his conduct was repeated, the victim was 86 years of age, the distress caused to the victim and the degree of premeditation on the part of Glover. He declined to place much weight on Glover's Asperger's disorder. He took into account Glover's three earlier convictions and a previous discharge without conviction, as well as the fact that Glover had exhibited no remorse, indicating that he would continue his conduct, regardless of the orders of the court.

On appeal Clifford J was provided with a report from a forensic psychiatrist, Dr. Justin Barry-Walsh. He accepted that the syndrome was relevant for the assessment both of the gravity of his offending and of the consequences for him of conviction. Justice Clifford concluded that Glover's rigidity of thought and inflexibility contributed to his offending behaviour and that Glover's offending "must be regarded as significantly less than that of a healthy and rationally thinking person" (*Glover v Police*, 2009: [21]; see too possibly *R v Burkett*, 2006). He found Glover's strong interest in road safety to be a manifestation of his "syndrome" and concluded that Glover was not motivated by criminal intent or malice (see also *R v Walker*, 2008) but by his position on road safety matters.

Justice Clifford also found that Glover's Asperger's went "a considerable way to explain his failure to express remorse or to offer to make amends, which appear to be a result of his rigidity of mind and egocentric perspective" (*Glover v Police*, 2009: [23]). He classified the property damage as "in effect minor and easily remedied" and that his offending was of relatively minor gravity. Dr. Barry-Walsh expressed the view that:

> He is vulnerable to depression and more sensitive to apparently minor grievances and setbacks than other people. His response to such setbacks may be disproportionate and severe. It is likely Mr Glover would have difficulty in accepting a conviction was reasonable and further in accepting the reasonableness of any sentence. Further, he lacks the capacity to adopt a pragmatic, flexible approach to the circumstance and therefore I think it unlikely he would put aside his strong sense of entitlement and injustice. Consequently I believe it likely that the impact of a sentence upon Mr Glover would be greater than it would be towards other people. It is possible he would experience an increase in frustration and despair …; it is also plausible that he would not be able to accept the conviction or sentence and would continue to consider he had been wronged and to ruminate upon such findings. It is possible that he would become depressed. (*Glover v Police*, 2009: [27])

Justice Clifford noted that Dr. Barry-Walsh's views about depression were conditional, in the sense that he was expressing no more than the potential for depressive consequences to flow from a conviction for Glover. He stated that he had been informed that the incidents had also provided the opportunity for Glover to consider his behaviour carefully and to ensure that his road safety initiatives in the future would be carried out within a lawful framework—"notwithstanding his subjective views as to the appropriateness of that framework" (*Glover v Police*, 2009: [30]). Accordingly, he determined that given the centrality to Glover's life of those interests, it was appropriate to place considerable reliance on the significance of his having Asperger's disorder in assessing the consequences to him from the imposition of a conviction. He held that convictions would have an effect "out of all proportion to the gravity of his offending" and discharged him without conviction, thereby quashing the order for community work.

Expert Evidence about Alertness to Risks, Social and Sexual Cues

An aspect of ASD can be that those with the disorder are insensitive or inadequately sensitive to the risks of their conduct. In addition, persons may not respond appropriately to cues and other forms of communication that persons in whom they develop a romantic and/or sexual interest do not reciprocate or which they misinterpret. This can have an outcome in a variety of proceedings in which expert evidence plays a vital role in attuning the court to the propensity of the person with ASD to draw erroneous inferences. However, for a court to reach such a conclusion, expert evidence assisting the impact of the characteristics of ASD in relevant respects is essential.

DPP v Borg. In *DPP v Borg* (2016), the Victorian Court of Appeal heard an appeal brought by the Director of Public Prosecutions against a decision by an intermediate court to impose a community corrections order, rather than imprisonment, for two charges of dangerous driving causing death and two charges of dangerous driving causing serious injury. The deaths and injuries had been caused by driving that resulted from the accused man falling asleep. He was 20 years of age at the relevant time. Borg had not been driving at an excessive speed or been affected by alcohol or drugs. His IQ was assessed at 83 and he had significant symptoms of autism. A psychologist testified that Borg's level of fatigue and autistic functioning would have combined to reduce his self-awareness of physical and psychological functioning. In addition, the sentencing judge accepted that Borg was vulnerable in the sense that he would experience real difficulty in the prison environment and was at risk of committing suicide. The Court of Appeal declined to interfere with the "merciful" sentence imposed below.

Parish v DPP. In *Parish v DPP* (2007) a person with Asperger's disorder appealed against a decision of a magistrate in Victoria, Australia, who had found him guilty of two common assaults upon a woman whom he met on a train (see further Freckelton, 2011).

Proceedings before the Magistrate. At first instance, a Magistrate accepted the complainant's evidence that at about 5.00 p.m. she took a train from the city to a suburban station. Prior to entering the train, she noticed Parish looking at her. On entering a relatively empty carriage, Parish sat diagonally opposite her and soon after the train started its journey pushed his calf against hers. She tried to move her leg away from his. He also changed positions and sat directly in front of her, with his hands over his knees. He then placed his hands on top of her knees. At this stage she was looking out the window, trying to ignore him. He then rubbed his hands on top of her knees. She did not speak to him or attempt to change seats.

When she got to her destination, she waited back and allowed Parish to alight first. She stood beside the train to make sure that Parish was not close. She then took the escalator but felt a hand on top of her leg. She turned around and noticed that it was Parish. He was standing on he step below her and, as the escalator was going up, he rubbed her lower back and her upper buttocks. She gave evidence that she was scared and was unable to move through the people surrounding her on the escalators. She made a complaint to the police and Parish was identified from CCTV photographs.

At interview, Parish denied any recollection of the events and said he had no memory of the alleged incident with the complainant. However, he did admit that he had rubbed his leg against girls on trains before. He said:

> I put my leg close to her and see if she doesn't mind. And if she kind of does then I won't do it anymore. She didn't seem - - - I suppose at the time she didn't seem - - - she probably didn't seem to mind. (*Parish*, at [10])

He was asked whether it had occurred to him that perhaps the complainant might have been frightened and not known what to do? He answered: "Err no at the time it didn't" (*Parish*: at [11]). He was further asked: "Why did you rub her leg with yours?" His answer was: "It was kind of ... I'm not as you say a very confident person, I'm more of a touchy feely sort of person and that was kind of my way of trying to get to know her a little bit" (*Parish*: at [11]). He was then asked if such behaviour excited him and he responded: "It wasn't, it wasn't sexual. It wasn't for excitement or sexual. It was more a way of me trying to get to know her, to see if something would come out of it; a relationship or something" (*Parish*: at [11]).

Parish was charged with indecent assault and unlawful assault in relation to events on the train and indecent assault and unlawful assault in relation to his conduct on the escalator.

Parish's defence arose out of his having been recently diagnosed with Asperger's disorder. Evidence was given by Dr. Nicole Reinhardt, who had been treating Parish, about the nature of the disorder, including that "a person born with Asberger's (sic) is born without the brain capacity to understand, interpret and act in the social world – they have to be taught in a concrete way the rules of social behaviour". Further, she said, people affected by the disorder are unable to pick up non-verbal cues—a subtle cue probably would not even register. Dr. Reinhardt expressed the view that Mr. Parish would have been unlikely to have been aware that the complainant was not consenting to his actions:

> ... Phillip had no understanding of how ... he has no understanding of how to make same sex friends, just in a friendship way. For example, he doesn't know how long it is you have to speak to somebody before they might be your friend. Or is that they have to offer their phone number to establish that they might be your friend. In terms of meeting a potential partner of the opposite sex, Phillip has no idea how that would happen or how he would come to have a sexual encounter with a person of the opposite sex. He had this idea that perhaps ...

> he's not good, he knows he's not good at expressing himself verbally. Pragmatics, part of the disorder, he was aware he's not good with words, so had an idea that perhaps the way that you do it is you might use your hands ... and that might be a way of ... and if somebody doesn't object, that might mean that they want to be your girlfriend. He didn't know, when he had discussions about this, that you would interact with that person verbally, and that all the sophisticated steps that are involved in meeting a potential partner. He had no idea, so again, an early primary school aged concept. (at [16])

Under cross-examination, Dr. Reinhardt said:

> The interpretation of that behaviour for a person with Asberger's disorder ... might be: M'hm, she might be interested, she might have enjoyed sitting next to me, em, I'll follow her and see if I can get any more data to enter into my information about that social interaction ... em ... again unless there was this pronounced verbal and non-verbal communication that this isn't OK in concert ... would he have understood that this wasn't OK for that person. Remembering at the same time that a person with Asberger's disorder cannot interpret and understand other subtle cues that we would have. So, for example, tense body posture that the person, the victim, would have been no doubt showing ... where her eyes were looking ... all of that would have just been ... it wouldn't have even gone into Phillip's thinking, ... (indistinct) (long pause). I might just add, I'm giving you clinical anecdotes and observations, but em there are hard empirical data to show that people with Asberger's disorder cannot pick up cues. (at [17])

The magistrate found Mr. Parish not guilty of the first charge of indecent assault as the prosecution had not established a sexual connotation to the assault or that Mr. Parish's intent was sexual. He also found in relation to the further charge of indecent assault that the prosecution had not proved beyond reasonable doubt that Mr. Parish did not believe that the victim was consenting or might have been consenting to his overtures. However, he found the common assault to be in a different category and that the charges were made out.

The Appeal. Justice Robson found that the magistrate had made an error of law in finding the common assault charges proven. He allowed the appeal and quashed the finding of guilt in relation to the escalator assault but proceeded to hear further submissions about the train assault in respect of which the magistrate made no finding related to Parish's awareness. He stressed that his decision was confined to the circumstances of Mr. Parish's disability—"his being a sufferer of Asberger's (sic) Syndrome and the unfortunate impact that it has on Mr Parish's ability to deal with other people. I would expect that in the case of a person who was not suffering from Asberger's Syndrome or having a similar disability, that the prosecution would be able to easily establish the necessary awareness on the part of any person who did what Mr Parish did" (*Parish*: at [126]).

The decisions both at first instance and on appeal, therefore, constitute examples of how the symptomatology of ASD, as interpreted by an appropriate clinician, can exercise an impact upon assessment by a court of the capacity of a defendant to form the necessary intent for criminal offences to be established.

PLP v McGarvie. A 46-year-old solicitor, PLP, ran his own suburban practice. The complainant, who was a conveyancer, undertook practical legal training after obtaining her law degree, including a placement at PLP's practice. PLP was found guilty by the Victorian Civil and Administrative Tribunal (VCAT) of both sexual harassment (*GLS v PLP*, 2013) and of engaging in professional misconduct (*Legal Services Commissioner v PLP*, 2014) by making multiple sexual advances towards the complainant and of having set up cameras at his office in the hope of covertly videoing have sexual relations with the complainant.

A clinical and forensic psychologist, Dr. David List, who treated PLP noted that PLP reported numerous symptoms consistent with high-functioning autism, including:

(a) I can't take jokes—I'm not sure what's funny;
(b) I can't read cues, like [the complainant's], it's confusing, she seemed in control;
(c) I feel lost when things are not in order;
(d) All through my life I've said things and didn't understand how they would be perceived; and
(e) I need structure in my day, my life, like the whole day has to be planned or things get lost. (*Legal Services Commissioner v PLP*, 2014: at [25])

He referred PLP for assessment by a psychologist, Ms. Langford, who was an expert in the area of Asperger's and ASD. She administered the Adult Asperger Assessment of Baron-Cohen, Wheelwright, Robinson and Woodbury Smith, and the Gilliam Asperger's Disorder Scale (GADS). The results showed that PLP had the propensity to experience heightened anxiety in some situations, and a low need for interpersonal closeness, as well as difficulties with interpreting others' opinions of himself. She classified these characteristics as typical of an individual with Asperger's Disorder:

> He also seeks acceptance and appeasement of others but without the interpersonal knowledge that would aid his protection. He has often appeared vulnerable and naive to others. [PLP's] background of lack of social and interpersonal experiences has significantly contributed to his current charges and he has been unable to protect himself or his firm and determine a reasonable course of action.
>
> The behavioural assessment indicated the presence of many features consistent with Asperger's Disorder. The primary difficulties were found in the areas of social interaction (understanding conventions and reading the thoughts and feelings of others), preoccupation with restricted patterns of interest, difficulty with being receptive to multiple perspectives of a situation or problem and impairments in verbal and non-verbal communication. (at [30])

Ms. Langford found that PLP had been able to minimise the level of impairment his condition had imposed on his life through his vocational success and dedication; his "primary impairment appears to manifest in the form of social interaction and communication difficulties, factors likely to impact on his close interpersonal relationships and his extreme difficulties with ascribing motives and intentions to others" (at [30]). She noted that for persons with Asperger's difficulties in appreciating the subtle nuances of social communication can lead to anxiety, misunderstandings and sometimes conflict. She observed that a common coping mechanism is a retreat into isolative special interests. In addition, she said: "greater preoccupation with specific interests often leads to negative social experiences, further enhancement of social anxiety and increased withdrawal, placing the individual at a greater risk of developing a reactive depression. Therefore, stress management plays an important part in coping with daily life and preventing further difficulties" (at [30]).

However, Judge Jenkins found many unsatisfactory aspects to the psychologists' opinions and was not satisfied that the diagnosis had been established. The primary reason for this was that the diagnosis was substantially dependent on the veracity of the account given by PLP about his own history and his recounting of his emotions, perceptions, interpretations and reactions towards the complainant's conduct. Judge Jenkins also found that the reliability of Dr. List's diagnosis was seriously brought into question both by the fact he had a treating relationship with PLP and that he had relied on the diagnosis by Ms. Langford. Judge Jenkins was also uncomfortable with accepting the diagnosis of Ms. Langford because, once again, it was reliant upon the accounts given by PLP which Judge Jenkins regarded as self-serving. In particular, Judge Jenkins had major reservations about the view of Ms. Langford that PLP was unable to dissemble, and was eccentric, vulnerable, preoccupied with subjects of personal interest and naïve to others:

> Asperger's Disorder is a condition that exists on the Autism spectrum. It may be difficult or impossible for a person with no genuine Asperger's symptoms to create a history and persona consistent with the condition. However, even if the Respondent exhibits certain personality traits that are consistent with Asperger's, equally such symptoms are not exclusively apparent only in a person with a discernable autism spectrum disorder. (at [54])

Judge Jenkins was not satisfied that PLP presented a low risk of reoffending and concluded that the evidence before the Tribunal gave a conflicted picture of PLP's level of insight and genuine remorse in relation to the nature and gravity of his conduct. She cancelled his registration and precluded him from reapplying for a period of eight months.

The Court of Appeal found no appealable error in the reasoning of Judge Jenkins in respect of the psychologists' evidence about Asperger's, although it reduced the PLP's sanctions on other grounds.

The decision is an example of judicial officers' reservations in accepting clinicians' evidence about a condition with which they are not familiar, such as ASD, when they are concerned that a diagnosis may be affected by advocacy by a clinician or when it may be affected by an account or presentation by the person most likely to benefit from the diagnosis, the offender. Significantly, the fact that the expert on ASD had administered the Baron-Cohen et al. assessment and the Gilliam Asperger's Disorder Scale was not enough to reassure Judge Jenkins, possibly because of contaminating factors including that the patient was intelligent and was found to have engaged in highly discreditable sexual harassment of a staff member. The judgement highlights the need for clinicians to identify rigorously the bases upon which they arrive at a diagnosis, as well as the aspects of the diagnosis that have forensic relevance from their perspective.

Expert Evidence about Awareness of Consequences of Conduct

In computer hacking charges, arson cases and violence allegations, issues have arisen with some regularity about the capacity of accused persons with ASD to appreciate the consequences of their conduct. Expert evidence directed towards the particular symptoms of the accused person which might be regarded as mitigating their capacity for the relevant foresight and appreciation is vital.

R v Marinovich. In *R v Marinovich* (2020) Justice Walker of the New Zealand High Court was called upon to sentence a male who had been convicted by a jury of the murder of his mother. Marinovich had argued at trial that he had not intended to kill his mother when he put his hands around her neck and that he had believed she was dead when he struck her with a hammer. He had a very close and supportive relationship with his mother but in the period leading up to her death she had become ill with a lower respiratory tract infection, influenza and lithium toxicity. At hospital when visiting, Marinovich had been observed to be acting strangely and very agitated. He told a close friend of his mother that he could not cope any more. He had been depressed for some months, had been prescribed antidepressant medication and had experienced difficulty sleeping. After assaulting (and killing) his mother in the course of an argument, he telephoned the police and informed them that he thought he had killed his mother.

In a pre-sentence report an experienced forensic psychiatrist, Dr. Duff, diagnosed Marinovich as suffering from moderate severity ASD, explaining that it is:

> a multifactorial disorder with many potential causes including a genetic predisposition and exposure to medication prior to [your] birth are likely to be the causative factors in this case. Autistic spectrum disorder arises from before birth and is not a consequence of lifestyle choices but rather a pervasive and intrinsic difference in the way an individual brain is 'hardwired' to interpret and interact with the World. (at [25])

Dr. Duff explained that Marinovich's ASD had not previously been identified because he was at the high-functioning end of the spectrum. She said that although he had "good intellectual functioning", his thinking was linear and rigid—without cognitive flexibility. Dr. Duff considered that he had significant deficits in his social communication skills, a "narrowed repertoire of interests, and a limited range of coping strategies" (at [26]). He led a routine-driven life, repeating patterns of activities such as chores, shopping and making meals with a self-imposed timetable. His life was also insular with no social life or friends outside his home, although he did not regard himself as lonely.

Dr. Duff observed that Marinovich's life had been "blighted" by his "moderately severe impairment that has rendered him unable to adapt when a culmination of stressors occurred in February 2019,,, creat[ing] a perfect storm that exceeded his capacity to cope" (at [27]).

Justice Walker approached the sentencing task in the context of being obliged to impose a life sentence with a minimum period of imprisonment of 17 years unless such a sentence would be manifestly unjust for a brutal murder. He took into account that the deceased was particularly vulnerable. However, he was satisfied that Marinovich was remorseful for his actions although "the expression of remorse may be communicated less emotionally than ordinarily expected because of the characteristics of your autism" (at [41]). He also noted that it was Marinovich's first criminal offence and that it was not characterised by premeditation or planning.

Justice Walker concluded that the particular characteristics of ASD played a significant role in his conduct:

> Clearly, you have grave difficulty managing emotions and handling situations. Your lack of capacity to respond appropriately to the stress of your living situation became acute in the days or even weeks leading up your offending. Even before then, you were in an intolerable situation for a young man, with a heavy responsibility. You had socially isolated yourself; this explains why no one else was able to pick up the signs of your disorder. You were unable to reach out for assistance as a consequence. (at [44])

He accepted Dr. Duff's evidence that people with ASD may often have problems with both verbal and non-verbal social communication, difficulties in interpreting others' emotions, and are more likely to live in a rigid, repetitive and very structured way. He observed that: "Courts recognise that ASD may reduce the moral culpability, as distinct from an offender's legal responsibility, provided there is some causative link between the illness or condition and the offending. It will not fully exculpate a defendant. But I accept that it provides important context and sheds light on the appropriate sentence" (at [46]). He concluded that Marinovich's lack of life experience and maturity, as well as his ASD, meant that his minimum sentence should be confined to 14 years.

R v Sokaluk. In *R v Sokal*uk (2012) Justice Coghlan of the Victorian Supreme Court presided over a trial of a man diagnosed with ASD and a mild intellectual disability who was convicted of ten counts of arson causing death in a rural location, each offence carrying a maximum term of imprisonment of 25 years (see also Hooper, 2019; Freckelton, 2020c). Sokaluk had been found guilty by a jury of intentionally lighting a fire, not with the intention of killing, but recklessly and with the knowledge that his actions would cause damage to property. A senior forensic psychologist, Professor James Ogloff, observed that Sokaluk was distant from others, including his parents. At the time of his offending he was aged 42 and had no forensic history. Professor Ogloff concluded that Sokaluk met the criteria for a diagnosis of ASD:

> his disorder has affected his social and adaptive functioning all of his life. He does not meet the criteria for a diagnosis of a major mental illness or personality disorder at present, although he has been treated with medication in the community for depression and in prison for lowered mood and anxiety.
>
> Whilst his overall level of intellectual functioning is in the borderline range, his verbal capacity is more limited and, in fact, falls in the intellectually disabled range. Conversely, his perceptual capabilities are much better, falling in the low average range. This suggests that while Mr Sokaluk has been able to hold a job, operate a motor vehicle, and live on his own, his level of intellectual reasoning and verbal comprehension is very impoverished. He has been dependent on his parents for maintaining his finances, cleaning his house, and providing him with meals. It takes him much longer to acquire information or to learn a task than would be the case for most others and his abstract reasoning capacity is very limited. His presentation, reasoning, receptive and expressive language are affected by the confluence of

his Autism Spectrum Disorder and decreased level of intellectual functioning. For example, he is a very concrete and literal thinker. (at [55])

Notably, Professor Ogloff, a very experienced forensic psychologist, offered no specific evidence on the extent to which Sokaluk's ASD or intellectual disability would have mitigated his capacity to understand the consequences of his behaviour nor how amenable he might be to behaviour modification of a kind that might thenceforth protect the community. It is highly unlikely that this was an oversight on the part of the expert witness. Nonetheless the absence of such evidence meant that the diagnosis of the two conditions is likely to have had relatively little impact upon the sentencing process, save to have removed as a factor the proposition that Sokaluk should be used as a vehicle to deter others from similar conduct.

Professor Ogloff's evidence led Justice Coghlan to conclude that Sokaluk had a mental impairment and for that reason regarded him as having "reduced moral culpability and therefore moderated general deterrence as a sentencing factor, rather focussing upon the need for deterring Sokaluk from similar conduct". He sentenced him to 17 years and 9 months imprisonment, with a direction that he serve 14 years of the sentence before becoming eligible for parole.

The Director of Public Prosecutions appealed the sentence, contending that it was manifestly inadequate (*DPP v Sokaluk*, 2013). However, the Court of Appeal did not interfere with the sentence imposed by Justice Coghlan.

Expert Evidence about the Consequences of Imprisonment

In *R v Marinovich* (2020), Justice Walker received submissions that the ASD of Marinovich would render a sentence of imprisonment particularly burdensome for him. Ultimately, he did not accept this argument, finding instead that while Marinovich's ASD may make it more difficult for him to manage social situations in prison, reports suggested that Marinovich had settled well into the routines of prison. Accordingly, this did not constitute a factor which significantly mitigated the appropriateness of the length of the incarceration imposed at sentencing (at [51]; see too *R v Scarrott*, 2020 at [23]).

However, there are cases where offenders with ASD experience their sentence of imprisonment as particularly harsh. An example in this regard is the decision of the Court of Appeal of England and Wales in *Cleland v The Queen* (2020), which came before the Court through a referral by the Criminal Cases Review Committee. Leave was sought (and granted) to rely upon a post-trial diagnosis of ASD. Cleland was 16 years of age when he committed the offence of attempted murder. His victim with whom he was infatuated was aged 12. In the lead-up to his offending Cleland became depressed at losing contact with the victim and used an online chat forum, Childline, to ventilate his feelings, including that he wanted to rape her because her life was too good and he wanted to balance things out. Ultimately he ambushed her. He was wearing latex gloves, threatened to rape and attempted to stab and strangle her, ultimately though only causing minor physical injuries. He was sentenced to life imprisonment with a minimum term of seven years.

However, Cleland experienced great difficulty with life in prison and a consultant forensic psychiatrist concluded that there was very strong evidence that Cleland had ASD and that the ASD was a "highly significant contributory factor" in his offending. He recommended that Cleland receive treatment in hospital and be dealt with by the mental health pathway release scheme. Another psychiatrist concurred with the diagnosis and opined that ASD was a "highly significant contributory factor" in Cleland's conduct. The Court of Appeal accepted that the new expert evidence established that Cleland suffered at all material times from a mental illness, namely ASD. It concluded that Cleland would need lifelong treatment for his ASD and accepted that his offending was "in significant part, though certainly not wholly, attributable to his ASD" (at [52]). While it was satisfied that there were serious features of his crime for which Cleland was culpable, the Court of Appeal found that his "ASD no doubt provided the explanation for his thinking that murder was a logical solution to his own problems, but it did not in our view reduce the seriousness of the careful planning and preparation which he put into the offence, or of his conduct in abandoning the knife which did not serve his purpose and resorting instead to attempting to kill by manual strangulation" (at [52]). It focused on the ongoing risk posed by Cleland, observing that Cleland's ASD was not treatable in the sense of there being a cure which could bring it to an end. However, it found that he could "by specialist treatment and supervision be assisted to manage his disorder and to control his aggressive behaviour. It is clear from the fresh evidence which we have accepted that the pervasive and persistent nature of the disorder means that there will be a risk in the future of aggressive behaviour, in particular towards women. That risk will be increased should the appellant for any reason feel under stress or pressure. This is not, therefore, a case in which it could be said that once treated, the appellant will not in any way be dangerous" (at [58]). It concluded that Cleland would remain in hospital for a considerable period, regardless of the order which it made. Its focus in resentencing was upon the need to guard against the risk of Cleland engaging in further violent behaviour linked to a lesser or greater degree with his ASD. Taking into account that it was not expected that Cleland's future treatment would be based on medication, and thus did not depend upon his adherence to prescribed pharmacotherapy, it found that the interests of the public would best be served by expert treatment and monitoring which would reduce the risks arising from his ASD. Thus, it quashed the sentence of life imprisonment and substituted a mental health order requiring him to be detained in hospital and restricting the circumstances in which he could be discharged.

In a series of high profile English (*McKinnon v United States of America*, 2007; *McKinnon, R (on the application of) v Secretary of State for Home Affairs*, 2009; *Love v The Government of the United States of America*, 2018; see Freckelton, 2011, 2020b, 2020c) and Irish (*Attorney-General v Davis*, 2016; *Attorney-General v Davis*, 2017; *Attorney-General v Davis*, 2018) judgements, the appropriateness of extradition of a citizen with ASD to the United States for trial on computer offences was the subject of assertive contest. The well-known expert on autism spectrum disorder,

Simon Baron-Cohen (see Baron-Cohen, 2006, 2008), Professor of Developmental Psychopathology at the University of Cambridge and Fellow at Trinity College, Cambridge, and Director of the Autism Research Centre (ARC) gave evidence in each of the cases.

The most significant of the early judgements in terms of expert evidence was that in 2014 involving Gary Davis who was arrested in Ireland on an extradition warrant issued by a New York magistrate alleging he had engaged in a conspiracy to distribute narcotics, commit computer hacking and launder money utilising the Silk Road website. The application went before Justice McDermott of the Irish Supreme Court. It was opposed on a number of grounds, including that his extradition, as a person suffering from Asperger's Syndrome, would place his health and life at grave risk by resulting in his being detained in a maximum security prison which would be highly damaging to his mental health. A forensic psychiatrist, Professor Michael Fitzgerald, in a report for a different matter involving Davis, possession of cannabis for the purposes of sale, had found that he met the criteria for Asperger's Syndrome (under ICD-10), depressive disorder and generalised anxiety disorder:

> He is described as a loner, problems with social know how, naive and immature. He has narrow interests, obsessed with computers, so much that growing up he would soil himself rather than go to the toilet because he was so fixated on the computer.
>
> Problems sharing, controlling and dominating, speaks with a monotonous tone of voice, preservation of sameness, sensory issues. This gives you Asperger's Syndrome ICD10 which could be helped by pragmatic language therapy, social skills therapy, mind reading skills therapy, help in social know how, help in seeing things from other people's perspective. (*Attorney-General v Davis*, 2016: at [87])

Further reports were submitted by Professor Baron-Cohen. He agreed with the diagnosis made by Professor Fitzgerald and observed that Davis' self-reported symptoms of obsessive behaviour, avoidance of noisy social situations, limited interaction with others and focus on computers were classic signs of Asperger's Syndrome. He observed that while depression is not a sign of Asperger's Syndrome, it is a common consequence of it. He expressed concern that if extradited, Davis would experience high levels of stress in a United States prison by reason of sensory overload, unfamiliarity and his vulnerability as a potential victim of bullying by reason of his odd social behaviour: "He would also likely be less able to defend himself against such victimisation because people with AS, … lack the 'street smarts' or social skills to evade or resist aggression" (*Attorney-General v Davis*, 2016, at [96]). In a follow-up report, Professor Baron-Cohen emphasised Davis' "extremely high score" on the Autism Spectrum Quotient and low score on the Empathy Quotient, as well as his "extremely low score" on the Childhood Autism Spectrum test completed by his mother. He expressed concern about the risk of Davis attempting to commit suicide.

Significantly, Davis was also examined by Professor Harry Kennedy, Consultant Forensic Psychiatrist and Executive Clinical Director of the Central Mental Hospital and Professor of Forensic Psychiatry at Trinity College Dublin, who also wrote a forensic report for the court. Professor Kennedy accepted that a diagnosis of Autism Spectrum Disorder/Asperger's Syndrome had the potential to be correct in relation to Mr. Davis, but expressed the view that with Davis it was so mild as to be of no practical significance. He criticised the absence of sources of contemporary, independent and validated observations concerning childhood and adolescent development which, if available, might lend considerable support to the diagnosis made. School records had not been supplied. No childhood tests or public health nurse records of developmental checks had been made available. He noted that while the diagnostic criteria relevant to Asperger's Syndrome include abnormal or impaired development evident at or after the age of three in language used in social communication, the development of selective social attachments and functional or symbolic play, there was no evidence of any of these traits in Davis. He found there to be no evidence of any qualitative abnormality in reciprocal social interaction or communication or restricted repetitive or stereotypical patterns of behaviour, interests and activities.

Professor Kennedy did not regard Davis' preoccupation with technology and computers as extreme enough to merit the diagnosis; no specific examples had been given of clearly abnormal behaviour concerning failure to use eye to eye gaze adequately, failure to develop peer relationships, lack of socio-emotional reciprocity or lack of spontaneity in seeking to share enjoyment, interests or achievement with other people. He noted, on the contrary, that Davis described normal social development of relationships with girlfriends and appeared on his own account to have been able to support an extensive use of cannabis over a period of time by dealing with friends. There were no specific examples of abnormally delayed spoken language. Nor were there examples of relevant failure on the past of Davis to initiate or sustain conversational interchange and the professor considered that he conversed normally during a long interview.

Professor Kennedy identified that the suicide rate in United States prisons was reported to be as low or lower than in the community. Professor Kennedy's affidavit prompted a response from Professor Baron-Cohen who argued that Professor Kennedy had used as a reference point "classic autism" rather than Asperger's Syndrome which was his diagnosis:

> One does not expect to see the symptoms Dr Kennedy lists (such as total lack of development of spoken language) in Asperger's Syndrome, and simply by listing such symptoms … and the subsequent sections, Dr Kennedy is revealing his lack of expertise in this field. Saying that no examples of abnormally intense preoccupations have been shown to be present in Gary's behaviour … makes no sense given that earlier Dr Kennedy noted that as a child, Gary would become so preoccupied on the computer that he would soil himself, because he did not want to stop playing on the computer to go to the bathroom. Surely such examples are abnormal in their intensity. (*Attorney-General v Davis*, 2016, at [107])

In a further affidavit, Professor Kennedy added that:

> Prof. Baron-Cohen may wish to consider the necessity in normal clinical practice as well as forensic practice of obtaining independent objective evidence. It is normal clinical practice not to rely on subjective self report evidence. It is also normal clinical practice to make assessments based on information specific to the individual in hand (including observation, signs and symptoms) and not a generalisation. (*Attorney-General v Davis*, 2016, at [110])

In yet another affidavit Professor Baron-Cohen stated that he found Professor Kennedy's suggestion that Davis might be malingering "surprising" and questioned whether Professor Kennedy could be regarded art as an expert on Asperger's Syndrome.

No effort was made to cross-examine Professor Fitzgerald, Professor Baron-Cohen or Professor Kennedy in respect of any of their diagnostic and other differences of opinion, a consideration about upon which the Court commented pointedly during the course of the hearing. Very surprisingly, the Court was provided with no affidavit evidence from Davis, any person who knew him or had been in contact with him during his childhood, adolescence or short working life, or from his family concerning his behaviour and disposition over those years. No evidence was adduced of any ongoing active treatment or counselling offered to, or availed of, by Davis in respect of his depression or anxiety which was said to involve suicidal ideation. Basic records concerning Davis's education, school attendance and attendance with his doctor had to be requested by the Court and were only procured and furnished after a considerable lapse of time.

Ultimately, Justice McDermott accepted that Davis had Asperger's Syndrome although "most of the material is self-reported and a number of unexplained inconsistencies have been identified by Prof Kennedy" (*Attorney-General v Davis*, 2016, at [114]). He was not satisfied, though, that the medical evidence established as a matter of probability that Davis suffered from depression accompanied by suicidal ideation of such a level and intensity that his trial should be stayed on the basis of unfitness to be tried. He noted that in respect of the concern that if Davis were extradited, he might be so unable to cope by reason of Asperger's Syndrome and so depressed that he may attempt to commit suicide, no attempt had been made to assist him; nor had Davis sought any help from Professor Fitzgerald or anyone else in relation to this anticipated deterioration in his health.

Ultimately, Justice McDermott stated that he was satisfied that "though pre-trial detention in the United States involves a number of challenges for the respondent and for the prison administration, reasonable and adequate provision has been made within MCC [Metropolitan Correction Centre in Lower Manhattan, New York] to receive and accommodate those who have Asperger's Syndrome and/or suffer from depression" (*Attorney-General v Davis*, 2016, at [138]). He stated that he was "satisfied to accept the evidence given by officials of the United States Federal Bureau of Prisons and Mr Turner as an Assistant United States Attorney on these matters. The court also regards this evidence as a solemn assurance to the court by the Government of the United States that all reasonable and necessary care and treatment will be given to the respondent during all periods of imprisonment while in the United States" (*Attorney-General v Davis*, 2016, at [138]). He was not persuaded that if extradited to the United States Davis would be at risk of being exposed to treatment of an inhuman or degrading nature by reason of the conditions under which he would be imprisoned or the fact that he had Asperger's Syndrome and suffered from depression and generalised anxiety with thoughts of suicide prompted and exacerbated by a fear of isolation and separation if imprisoned in the United States (*Attorney-General v Davis*, 2016, at [145]).

Davis appealed the decision of Justice McDermott to the Irish Court of Appeal (*Attorney-General v Davis*, 2017; see too *Attorney-General v Marques*, 2015). However, the Court of Appeal found no error of law in the decision below, commenting only that: "It is to be hoped that the extent to which the issue relating to the appellant's diagnosis of Asperger's Syndrome has been debated and considered in these proceedings, and the assurances provided by the US authorities will reduce those concerns to an appreciable degree" (*Attorney-General v Davis*, 2017: at [42]).

Davis then appealed to the Irish Supreme Court (*Attorney-General v Davis*, 2018). The Supreme Court emphasised that "imprisonment is inherently distressing for any person and unlikely in the vast majority of cases to improve one's health or wellbeing, irrespective of their medical condition. Accordingly, the suggestion that any deterioration in a person's health as a result of imprisonment will amount to a violation of their rights cannot be sustained. Secondly, it is a matter of high probability that a person with Asperger's Syndrome will find imprisonment, particularly in a foreign jurisdiction, more difficult than would someone without such condition: though relevant, this is not an end in itself" (*Attorney-General v Davis*, 2018: at [89]).

The Supreme Court made no criticism of the analysis of the expert evidence by Justice McDermott and commented that "it is difficult to understand why no attempt at cross-examination of the relevant witnesses was undertaken, particularly those based in this country" (*Attorney-General v Davis*, 2018: at [100]). It found that Professor Baron-Cohen and Professor Kennedy each appeared to have made "*prima facie* valid criticisms of the other's methodology and conclusions":

> Though the interviews with the appellant and his sister were clearly highly influential in the diagnosis made by Professor Baron-Cohen, the same also seemed to rely at least in some measure on self-reporting and on test scores which were liable to manipulation. It must also be acknowledged that on any reading of the relevant reports, there are a number of unexplained inconsistencies in the appellant's background history. The conclusion reached by Professors Baron-Cohen and Fitzgerald also seems at odds with the manner in which the appellant presented in interview with Professor Kennedy. On the other hand, one could not but agree with Professor Baron-Cohen that Professor Kennedy appears to have used a number of one-off instances of conduct or behaviour to drawing rather sweeping conclusions that do not necessarily logically follow from the premise. For example, the suggestions that developing a relationship with a girlfriend soon after the suicide of his brother-in-law means that he was not clinically depressed, or that his failure to name his cannabis dealer to the Garda for fear of reprisals for being a "rat" shows that he has normal social awareness, seem to distort the overall picture. Professor Kennedy's view that there are no examples of encompassing preoccupation of abnormal intensity is directly at odds with his earlier acknowledgement that the appellant used to be so preoccupied with playing computer games as a child that he would soil himself rather than go to the bathroom. The Court will not express a view on whether Professor Kennedy was purposefully discrediting the appellant, as Professor Baron-Cohen suggests, but would agree that some of his more pointed comments regarding malingering seem unwarranted. Given the marked divergences in professional opinion, these matters, at the very least, could usefully have been explored on cross-examination. (*Attorney-General v Davis*, 2018: at [101])

The series of decisions in relation to Davis, and before him in relation to Gary McKinnon in England (see Freckelton, 2011; Mann et al., 2017), highlight the fact that even expert evaluations that a person satisfies the diagnostic criteria for ASD can be subject to robust professional disagreement. More than taking at face value the assertions or accounts of the person the subject of diagnosis is necessary. The more that objective tests which command the confidence of the relevant expert community, are utilised, the more likely it is that expert clinicians' opinions will be accepted by courts. Put another way, if such opinions are not the product of psychometric assessments, and are "merely" the outcome of clinical impressions, substantially based on histories provided by the patient, they are at risk of being rejected or discounted.

In addition, where what is contended on behalf of a person with ASD is that the consequences of their being diagnosed with ASD are not just that they are prone to engage in inappropriate computer behaviours such as hacking (see Hollin, 2017; Hayhurst, 2017), an assertion that needs to be justified in general and in the individual case, but that their condition will render them prone to risk in a custodial environment (see Ledingham & Mills, 2015), including overseas, strong bases for such contentions will need to be established.

These various lessons were effectively learned and a sophisticated forensic strategy deployed in *Love v The Government of the United States*, 2018; see further Freckelton, 2020b) to oppose extradition of a man charged with computer offences who had Asperger syndrome. Lauri Love was charged with making a series of cyber-attacks on computer networks and United States government agencies. The Home Secretary of England and Wales ordered his extradition from England to face the charges. Ultimately the matter went on appeal before Lord Chief Justice Burnett and Justice Ouseley of the Court of Appeal.

Professor Baron-Cohen diagnosed Love as having "extremely severe" Asperger's, as well as stress-related eczema, asthma and depression. He expressed the view that Love would attempt suicide if it were finally determined he was to be extradited to the United States and that his mental health was dependent upon his being in England with his parents. Professor Kopelman, an Emeritus Professor of Neuropsychiatry, agreed, expressing the view that there was a very high risk that, if extradited, Love would not be fit to stand trial in the United States:

> There would be a severe deterioration in both his physical and his mental state. His eczema, his asthma, gastrointestinal symptoms, and palpitations, would certainly become far worse, and he might lose his hair again (alopecia), thereby causing further deterioration in his mental state. Mr Love would not be able to cope with separation from his family and friends, nor would he cope with the likely isolation in a United States facility. His depression would become far worse, and he would be very likely to develop psychotic symptoms (as he has during past severe depressions). His suicide risk would become very high as a result of the exacerbation of his clinical depression and a deterioration in his physical health. In such circumstances, Mr Love's ability to concentrate and sustain attention would, in consequence, be severely affected. His ability to cope with the proceedings in the trial, to make rational decisions, and to give evidence in a satisfactory manner, would be severely compromised in such circumstances. In brief, it this were to occur, he would no longer be fit to plead or to stand trial in the United States. (*Love v The Government of the United States*, 2018: at [32])

The Court of Appeal found that this evidence could not be rejected as conjectural and, while not definite, created a significant risk factor that told against extradition being in the interests of Mr. Love's victims to the extent that there was at least a significant risk that there would not be able to be a trial at all by reason of his being unfit to stand trial in the United States.

The Court also heard from Professor Kopelman on the issue of whether the extradition of Love would be oppressive that the proposed suicide prevention programme for Love in the United States would involve his wearing a suicide smock and being monitored 24 h a day, without an unapproved personal items. The Court concluded that:

> That would leave Mr Love feeling extremely isolated in the absence of an internet connection and undoubtedly would have a severe adverse effect on his mental state. Social isolation was known to precipitate psychotic experiences, including psychotic depression, and increase suicidal ideas. A severe deterioration in clinical depression, a likely recurrence of psychotic ideas, a severe deterioration in his physical health with an exacerbation of eczema and asthma, should be anticipated in such circumstances. Suicidal risk would increase to 'very high' in consequence, exacerbating rather than reducing the risk of suicide. His mental condition would remove his mental capacity to resist the impulse to commit suicide. His ability to cope with the trial would be severely compromised. (*Love v The Government of the United States*, 2018: at [87])

Other evidence from Dr. Kucharski, an experienced forensic psychologist who had worked at the relevant United States facilities, suggested that Love would experience high levels of stress in isolation in a United States prison and that this would exacerbate his depression and substantially increase his risk of committing suicide.

The Court of Appeal ultimately concluded that the fact of extradition would bring on severe depression in Love and that he would probably become determined to commit suicide before extradition or upon extradition. If he were extradited to the United States he would be very vulnerable and a target for bullying and intimidation by other prisoners. In all the circumstances, Lord Chief Justice Burnett and Justice Ouseley found that it would be oppressive to extradite Love and quashed the decision that he be removed to the United States. The decision constitutes an exemplar for how a court can be enabled by high-quality expert evidence to be informed about the diverse adverse consequences of autism spectrum disorder for a person if removed from their accustomed environment and placed in a custodial setting which for them would be highly psychologically oppressive.

Counter-Intuitive Expert Evidence

An important issue that can arise in cases that involve persons with autism spectrum disorder is the risk that those unfamiliar with the condition may misconstrue the conduct or impressions given by the person with ASD. Expert evidence has the potential to disabuse such impressions and to educate laypersons about the internal world of the person with ASD and the risks of too readily drawing adverse inferences from how they present. However, the courts have been resistant to receiving such counter-intuitive evidence. Four decisions are particularly illustrative.

Sultan v The Queen. In *Sultan v The Queen* (2008) the Court of Appeal of England and Wales heard an appeal from a Crown Court jury's conviction of a man of one count of rape and one of indecent assault on his former wife, Ms. Haque. At the trial Sultan maintained that the sexual contact with his former wife was consensual but behaved strangely, including reading a book while the complainant gave her evidence.

Between the time of the trial and the appeal Dr. Nigel Blackwood, a forensic psychiatrist and senior lecturer in forensic mental health science at the Institute of Psychiatry, formed the view that Sultan met the criteria for Asperger's Syndrome. Dr. Blackwood had the care of Sultan since 2006. He found Sultan to have a significant discrepancy between his verbal IQ (117) and his performance IQ (87), which he informed the Court of Appeal was a neuropsychological profile often seen in persons with Asperger's Syndrome. He reported that Sultan's speech had an "odd prosody with an almost telegraphic quality" (*Sultan v The Queen*, 2008: at [20]).

Dr. Blackwood's diagnosis went to whether Sultan misinterpreted the cues from his ex-wife and also to his conduct in court. A psychiatrist who had treated Sultan for some years was of the view that he suffered from delusional jealousy but conceded that he had no expertise in Asperger's Syndrome. The Court of Appeal stated that it was unable to affirm that Dr. Blackwood's diagnosis was established but found it to have sufficient cogency to require a retrial:

> the new evidence could have affected the trial in one or more of three ways. First, it would have enabled a defence for the first time to be based on the requirements of *mens rea*. Secondly, it would have enabled the jury to view the defendant before them not solely on the basis of whether what he said happened was at all credible, but more importantly on the basis of whether he was honest about what he believed to have been the situation, even if the facts were otherwise as Ms Haque said them to be. Thirdly, it might have gone some way to explain to the jury why the appellant was behaving so oddly at trial, such as reading a book during Ms Haque's evidence. (*Sultan v The Queen*, 2008: at [34])

McGraddie v McGraddie. A similar issue in terms of anomalous conduct in court arose in *McGraddie v McGraddie* (2009). Lord Brodie of the Scottish Court of Sessions heard a familial property dispute. A key issue in the resolution of the case was the assessment of the credibility of the first defender who was diagnosed by Professor Mackay as having Asperger's Syndrome. Professor Mackay (in a Minute of Amendment) emphasised that the condition can generate difficulties in communication and comprehension of context.

He stated that McGraddie had problems with communication including a "relative failure to sustain a conversational interchange in which there is a reciprocal responsiveness to the communications of the other person" (at [19]).

A question that arose was whether Professor Mackay's Minute of Amendment should be received. Lord Brodie declined to do so although he noted that McGraddie's presentation was "casual", even when speaking about his mother's terminal illness and:

> He did not appear to engage with his counsel's questioning. He was abrupt. He gave the impression of being wearily exasperated at the questions he was being asked. Perhaps to his credit, he did not seem overly concerned to present himself in a favourable light. (at [19])

Lord Brodie accepted that it was appropriate to have regard to the possibility McGraddie may have an autistic spectrum disorder but ultimately did not find this perspective of particular utility:

> Asperger's syndrome may be the explanation for the way in which the first defender gave his evidence. It may not. However, whatever the reason for the first defender responding to questions in the way that he did, taking his responses as a whole I have felt bound to conclude that he was not a witness upon whom I could rely. This is particularly so when it came to his accounts of interactions with other people and the inferences to be drawn from these interactions. To an extent this case is about the reasonable interpretation of what was said and done in a particular social context. (at [19])

McGraddie appealed the decision of Lord Brodie to the Extra Division, Inner House, Court of Session (*McGraddie v McGraddie*, 2012), among other things, on the basis that the expert evidence had not been admitted. The ground of appeal was not permitted on a number of grounds. The attempt to lead the evidence had been to bolster the credibility of the first defender, which was problematic and had the potential to proliferate expert evidence on the issue. In addition, the attempt was at a late juncture in the proceedings, and after the first defender had been cross-examined on the basis that he did not have Asperger's Syndrome.

Approaches to the admissibility of expert evidence whose purpose is counter-intuitive or myth-dispelling differ from one country to another (see Freckelton, 2019b), with jurisdictions such as Canada and New Zealand being more amenable to such evidence than others such as Australia and the United Kingdom. However, where an expert attempts to provide educative assistance to a court so as to avoid misinterpretations being made of the conduct or demeanour of a person with ASD, it is necessary for the witness/report writer to explain that many persons with ASD are not very aware of the impressions that they give, that they can be quite self-absorbed and anxious, and that they may lack empathy and insight into non-verbal behaviours. Then it is necessary to go to the next step and explain that the person before the court fits into that category and to give concrete examples of matters, such as their absence of self-awareness.

The State of Western Australia v Mack. In *The State of Western Australia v Mack* (2012) the issues needing to be determined by Justice McKechnie. were whether the accused man with autism was fit to plead and whether he should have a judge-alone trial. He was facing a charge of murder. His counsel attested Mack to have a robotic manner and not to engage in eye contact. Justice McKechnie made similar observations of him in court. Two psychiatrists testified—one each for the defence and the prosecution. Justice McKechnie commented of Mack: "My observation of the accused certainly confirms that his behaviour is unusual. I am satisfied that the accused has a mental impairment due to autism. The question is whether his detachment from his trial process manifested by apparent nonresponsiveness is primarily due to his autism" (*The State of Western Australia v Mack* (2012) at [41]). He noted that "The accused also raises the possibility that the accused's unusual personal characteristics may cause him some prejudice in that the jury are distracted by his behaviour or draw adverse inferences against him as a result of such behaviour" (*The State of Western Australia v Mack* (2012) at [44]). Justice McKechnie did not accept this submission as he concluded that a jury, properly instructed, would be able to put aside such matters and focus on the evidence in the case. However, he did accept that because of the accused man's autism and its impact on the trial process, the interests of justice required a judge-alone trial. At a level, therefore, this constituted an acceptance of concerns raised by expert evidence on behalf of the accused.

Thompson v The Queen. In *Thompson v The Queen* (2014) the Court of Appeal of England and Wales quashed convictions for sexual assaults upon young boys in part on the basis that had expert evidence about Thompson's ASD been available at the trial it could have been of value to the jury in determining whether, on the one hand, Thompson was evading questions or, on the other, as a result of his ASD traits he was reluctant to be deflected from his preoccupation with matters of detail (at [33]).

A Court Warning about Post-conviction Autism Diagnoses

In 2020 the Court of Appeal of England Wales delivered a pointed set of warnings in *Roddis v The Queen* (2020) about the provision of expert evidence about ASD as a basis for reconsidering a conviction. The Criminal Cases Review Commission referred to the convictions of Roddis for placing a hoax bomb and engaging in the preparation of an act of terrorism for which he had been sentenced to seven years imprisonment.

The appeal by Roddis was on the basis that he had latterly been diagnosed as having ASD. The facts of his conduct were uncontested. In 2007, Roddis, dressed in an obviously false beard and thick glasses left a hoax bomb in a bus. It was composed of bags of sugar, along with wires and an alarm clock. It was packed with nails and a message was attached that was written in Arabic: "There is no god but Allah, Mohammed is the messenger of Allah. God is great, God is great, God is great, Britain must be punished". It purported to be signed by "The Al Qaeda organisation of Iraq". Two months later Roddis met with work colleagues and produced a number of railway fog signals (small explosive devices used to alert railway workers of an advancing train) which he said were landmines, along with some imitation bullets. They alerted police who raided his accommodation and found bottles of hydrogen peroxide and acetone, which, if combined with sulphuric acid, could be used to make the explosive TATP. The police discovered that Roddis had made inquiries on the internet about buying sulphuric acid and making explosives. They also recovered extensive material from his telephone and computer relating to the war in Iraq, insurgency and terrorism. In particular, he had 19 graphic video clips of beheadings, including the execution of a hostage, stored on his telephone. He had filmed footage from a television or computer screen of the bombing of the Iraq Parliament, the murder of an Iraqi parliamentarian and the detonation of an explosive device. There was a folder containing material downloaded and printed from the internet on how to make explosives. The police found a word document created by Roddis which included observations on bombs "to hit" Rotherham, a bomb in Rotherham market and a "second bomb", with related comments on "electric alarm clock, electric motor, wire, explosive ingredients".

At trial Roddis maintained he had no intention to engage in terrorism, although he had an interest in terrorism and had engaged in attention-seeking behaviour with his work colleagues. At trial mental health expert evidence was adduced. A clinical forensic psychologist was called on behalf of Roddis. He noted Roddis' account that what he had done was a practical joke and expressed the view that Roddis was not diagnosable with a mental disorder or a learning disability; instead he was very immature and was psychologically vulnerable. He may have been acting out a fantasy of being an Islamic militant while not intending to do anything harmful, although that was not his defence. A forensic psychiatrist called at trial diagnosed Roddis as having a personality disorder characterised by a variety of abnormal traits—schizoid, histrionic and dependent.

For another trial in another matter in 2014 Roddis was the subject of a detailed autism assessment. A multitude of autism traits was identified and a psychologist in a separate assessment found Roddis to have a high-functioning ASD (Asperger's Syndrome) due to difficulties with social interaction, social communication, flexibility of thought and sensory experience. A senior clinical psychologist, Dr. Rachael Collins, on 25 October 2015 confirmed the diagnosis of autism and suggested that it appeared to have impacted adversely on all areas of Roddis' life including at school, at home, with his peers and as regards his own mental health and well-being: "He has found it difficult to fit in and has tried to impress others. He has struggled with social communication and he has what are described as 'excessive interests'" (at [29]).

On appeal evidence from a psychiatrist, Dr. Blackwood, was adduced. He stated that: "The absence of an understanding of his impaired appreciation of the social world and his fixed interests, abnormal in intensity and focus, clearly impacted upon the conduct of his defence. This potentially calls the safety of the original convictions into question" (at [23]). The Court of Appeal noted Dr. Blackwood's view that Roddis "struggles fully to understand other peoples' position and he fails to appreciate the effect on others of his clownish and prankish behaviour. This is because he is dominated by his own mental state with the result that he does not take into account his effect on others. In the context of a hoax, therefore, he would not necessarily understand or think about how frightening this behaviour would be. [Roddis] may have thought that his activities on the bus were a joke from the outset" (at [32]). It also took into account the view expressed by Dr. Blackwood that Roddis's inability to "understand the effect he has on others may explain why he is indiscreet in his actions, such as adopting his unusual costume on the bus and making seemingly unguarded statements to colleagues at work" (at [33]).

However, it observed that while the diagnosis of ASD "has seemingly given a broader understanding" of Roddis' clinical position, in many respects the main elements of Dr. Blackwood's conclusions were known before the 2008 trial. Importantly, it identified common features of ASD and the mixed personality disorder diagnosed at Roddis' trial. It also observed that when an expert is called, their evidence cannot be limited artificially by the party calling the witness: "Once in the witness box, the psychologist or psychiatrist would have been available [at trial] to be questioned about all relevant matters, and in this case that included the likely conclusion that the defendant was acting out a terrorist fantasy, as he had previously acted out the fantasy of being a soldier" (at [40]). It noted that Roddis could not sensibly have called evidence that would have directly contradicted his own case—he rejected the suggestion that he was acting out any fantasy. Although it was impossible 12 years after the event to know exactly what evidence would have been called if the ASD diagnosis had been available at the time of his trial, there was no suggestion that the experts who gave evidence at trial were incorrect in their conclusions in relation to Roddis acting out an Islamic fantasy. The Court of Appeal was influenced by the fact that "Dr Blackwood has proceeded on the erroneous basis that the defence case included the assertion that he was a lone fantasist, influenced by Islamic or Al Qaeda literature" (at [40]). Rather, the Court of Appeal found that the relevant material was available at trial and, whatever was the diagnosis for Roddis, he understood the potential impact of his hoax.

The Court expressed frustration that Dr. Blackwood had insufficiently taken into account the importance of the detail of Roddis' defence. Dr. Blackwood classified Roddis' interests in Islam as fixated—abnormal in their intensity and focus, as typically is to be observed with autism. He regarded Roddis as a "simple, isolated fantasist" wanting to shock but without any deeply held beliefs. However, that was inconsistent with what Roddis had communicated to the jury—he said he simply had an academic concern or idle curiosity in such matters.

The Court also noted that Dr. Blackwood had given significant emphasis to Mr. Roddis' interest in terrorist material as being research that was within his rights and that he would not have been alert to the potential concerns of others about his conduct. However, such insights were irrelevant to the intentions of Roddis—the perceptions of others were not relevant to the charges he was facing. In dismissing Roddis' appeal, the Court commented that:

> when, following a trial, there is a diagnosis of autism and consideration is given to mounting an appeal on this basis, it is important to focus on the issues in the case and the extent to which the new diagnosis relates to those issues. Additionally, there needs to be careful examination as to whether the relevant "behaviour" or "behaviours" may have been revealed in expert reports in advance of the trial, possibly in the context of a different diagnosis (which may, in turn, overlap with the new diagnosis). (at [53])

Conclusions

Through the use of examples from decided cases (mostly at appellate level) in England and Wales, Scotland, Ireland, Australia, New Zealand and Canada, this chapter has identified where expert evidence by both psychiatrists and psychologists has succeeded and failed in communicating to courts aspects of persons with ASD that have been potentially relevant to both their criminal responsibility and their culpability. It is apparent that many judicial officers are not receptive to such evidence (especially in relation to sexual matters) unless it is rigorously presented in such a way as to establish not just that the diagnosis is well-founded and that the witness has the expertise to make it, but that the diagnosis has real relevance for the charges that the accused person is facing. It does not follow merely from the making of a diagnosis that criminal responsibility is impaired or that culpability is reduced (see *R v Grant-Murray*, 2017), at [62]). The question, ultimately, in any given case is whether the person's particular experience of symptomatology of ASD and any comorbidities, either on its own or in combination with them, has had a significant effect upon their mental state at the time of committing the criminal act (which may go as far as their *mens rea*) (see *Elster and Parsi*, 2020) or that their symptoms render them an inappropriate vehicle for punishment, specific deterrence or general deterrence. In that context the ongoing risk that they might be regarded as posing to the community, in the absence of effective clinical intervention, is also important for sentencing purposes, as is the fact that penal confinement may be experienced by them as frightening and oppressive in a way that it is not for those without the disorder.

At the heart of the giving of effective expert evidence (see Freckelton, 2013) about ASD is the capacity of the clinician to communicate the distinctive experience of the world for the person the subject of their opinions. It may incorporate an element of the reconstructive in relation to the accused person's state of mind or ability to respond suitably in a particular situational matrix. It also needs to be the product of an overall evaluation of the person's presenting features which may well incorporate indicia of other conditions.

The expert evidence needs to be grounded in more than the accused person's own narrative and should be replete with examples of their limitations and eccentricities which are illustrative of the extent to which their symptoms/characteristics render them different from others who appear before the criminal courts. Thus, at the heart of expert opinion evidence should be the pedagogical provision of counter-intuitive or myth-dispelling information (see Berryessa, 2017) which enables a better rounded and more personalised appreciation of why a person with ASD has behaved in a way which would otherwise be regarded as anti-social, criminal and culpable. Often this will relate to matters such as their obsessionality in engaging in cyber activities, whether that be hacking into sites, collecting pornographic images that are illegal, or their focus upon fire-lighting or upon a particular person upon whom they become fixated. On other occasions, it will arise from their failure to read and understand the significance of presenting scenarios or communications to them, whether those be verbal or more subtle physical cues. On occasions too it will be necessary to explicate the fear and anxiety which has generated an otherwise inexplicable response to stimuli which are experienced as oppressive or disorienting by a person with ASD. Finally, on some occasions, it will be necessary to educate a court that what it might otherwise interpret as offensive or indifferent behaviour by a person with ASD, from which it might draw adverse inferences, in fact has another plausible explanation grounded in their condition. Each of these expert opinions by clinicians must be embedded in demonstrable and long-standing patterns of dealing with the complexities of the world by the particular individual with ASD.

References

Attorney-General v Davis [2016] IEHC 497.
Attorney-General v Davis [2017] IECA 50.
Attorney-General v Davis [2018] IESC 27.
Attorney-General v Marques [2015] IEHC 798.
Attwood, T. (2008). *The complete guide to Asperger's syndrome.* Jessica-Kingsley.
Baron-Cohen, S. (2006). *Asperger syndrome: A different mind.* Jessica Kingsley.
Baron-Cohen, S. (2008). *Autism and Asperger syndrome.* Oxford University Press.
Berryessa, C. M. (2017). Educator of the court: The role of the expert witness in cases involving autism spectrum disorder. *Psychology, Crime and Law., 23*(6), 575–600.
Cleland v The Queen [2020] EWCA Crim 906.
Davie v Magistrates of Edinburgh [1953] SC 34.
Davies v The Queen [2019] VSCA 66.
DPP v Borg [2016] VSCA 53.
DPP v HPW [2011] VSCA 88.
DPP v Sokaluk [2013] VSCA 48.
Elster, N., & Parsi, K. (2020). Like autism, representation falls on a spectrum. *American Journal of Bioethics, 20*(4), 405.
Freckelton, I. (2019a). Attention deficit hyperactivity disordser (DHD) and the criminal law. *Psychiatry, Psychology and Law, 26*(6), 817–840. https://doi.org/10.1080/13218719.2019.1695266.
Freckelton, I. (2019b). *Expert evidence: Law, practice, procedure and advocacy* (6th ed). Thomson Reuters.
Freckelton, I. (2011). Autism spectrum disorders and the criminal law. In M.-R. Mohammadi (Ed.), *A comprehensive book on autism spectrum disorders* (InTech) (pp.249–272).
Freckelton, I. (2013). Autism spectrum disorder: Forensic issues and challenges for mental health professionals and the courts. *Journal of Applied Research in Intellectual Disabilities, 25*(5), 420–434.
Freckelton, I. (2020a). Obsessive compulsive disorder and obsessive compulsive personality disorder and the criminal law. *Psychiatry, Psychology and Law, 27*, 831–842. https://doi.org/10.1080/13218719.2020.1745497.
Freckelton, I. (2020b). Autism spectrum disorder and suitability for extradition. *Psychiatry, Psychology and Law, 27*(2), 181–219. https://doi.org/10.1080/13218719.2020.1727645.
Freckelton, I. (2020c). Dilemmas for the criminal justice system in dealing with diagnoses for neuropsychiatrically impaired offenders. *Forensic Research and Criminology International Journal, 8*(2), 64–75.
Freckelton, I., & List, D. (2009). Asperger's disorder, criminal responsibility and criminal culpability. *Psychiatry, Psychology and Law, 12,* 16–40.
GLS v PLP [2013] VCAT 221.
Gray (a Pseudonym) v The Queen [2018] VSCA 163.
Hayhurst, C. (2017, April 3). Scientists to study a potential link between autism-like personality traits and cyber crime. *The Independent.* https://www.independent.co.uk/news/science/autism-link-cyber-crime-personality-trait-scientist-research-university-bath-dark-web-a7663086.html.
HG v The Queen [1999] 197 CLR 414.
Hollin, G. (2017). Failing, hacking, passing: Autism, entanglement, and the ethics of transformation. *Biosocieties, 12*(4), 611–633.
Hooper, C. (2019). *The Arsonist: A mind on fire.* Penguin.
Ledingham, R., & Mills, R. (2015). A preliminary study of autism and cybercime in the context of international law enforcement. *Advances in Autism, 1,* 1–10.
Legal Services Commissioner v PLP [2014] VCAT 793.
Love v The Government of the United States of America [2018] EWHC 172 (Admin); [2018] 1 WLR 2889.

Mann, M., Warren, I., & Kennedy, S. (2017). The legal geographies of transnational cyber-prosecutions: Extradition, human rights and forum shifting. *Global Crime, 19*(2), 107–124.
McGraddie v McGraddie [2009] ScotCS CSOH 142.
McGraddie v McGraddie [2012] ScotCS CSIH 23.
McKinnon v United States of America [2007] EWHC 762 (Admin).
McKinnon, R (on the application of) v Secretary of State for Home Affairs [2009] EWHC 20121 (Admin).
Merritt v The Queen [2018] NZCA 610.
PLP v McGarvie and VCAT [2014] VSCA 253.
R v Burkett [2006] NZHC 800.
R v Grant-Murray [2017] EWCA Crim 1228.
R v Kagan [2007] NSSC 215.
R v Kagan [2009] NSCA 43.
R v Marinovich [2020] NZHC 1160.
R v Peake [2017] SASC 10.
R v Scarrott [2020] EWCA Crim 1435.
R v Sokaluk [2012] VSC 167.
R v Walker [2008] NZHC 1114.
Roddis v The Queen [2020] EWCA 396.
Sultan v The Queen [2008] EWCA Crim 6.
The State of Western Australia v Mack [2012] WASC 127.
Thompson v The Queen [2014] EWCA Crim 836.

Ian Freckelton is an experienced Queen's Counsel with a national practice in Australia. He works as a barrister from Crockett Chambers in Melbourne, undertaking trial and appellate litigation, as well as advisory work, including internationally.

Chapter 4
Neuroscience of Autism in the Legal Context

Stephanie Yarnell-Mac Grory, Mark Mahoney, and Alexander Westphal

Neuroscience of Autism

Since the earliest clinical descriptions of ASD in the 1940s, theories have been posited to explain the etiology of the differences that define ASD. Many of these, including a number of psychodynamic theories, such as Bruno Bettelheim's claim that autism results from a lack of maternal affective warmth, the so-called "refrigerator mother" theory, have been discounted with the movement toward conceptualizing ASD as a neurodevelopmental condition.

Currently, the consensus is that an array of genetic and environmental risk factors, either together or separately, create atypical brain development, which alters the trajectory of social development (among other things), and is manifest in the condition. This is supported by a burgeoning literature on environmental and genetic risk factors, coupled with neuroimaging studies from a variety of modalities that demonstrate fundamental differences in the way in which people with ASD process information, in particular information relevant to social interactions.

In addition, clear neurological differences, for example, higher rates of seizure disorder, as well as a number of so-called neurological "soft signs," such as toe-walking, suggest atypical brain development. Cognitive theories have suggested possible abnormalities in frontal lobe functioning including: executive dysfunctions, theory of mind, and weak central coherence. Biological theories have suggested

S. Yarnell-Mac Grory (✉) · A. Westphal
Division of Law and Psychiatry, Yale University, New Haven, CT, USA
e-mail: stephanie.yarnell@yale.edu

A. Westphal
e-mail: alexander.westphal@yale.edu

M. Mahoney
Harrington & Mahoney Buffalo, NY, USA
e-mail: mjm@harringtonmahoney.com

F. R. Volkmar et al. (eds.), *Handbook of Autism Spectrum Disorder and the Law*,
https://doi.org/10.1007/978-3-030-70913-6_4

abnormalities in areas such as the frontal lobe, temporal lobe, corpus callosum, cerebellum, and amygdala, as well as gross differences such as increased total brain volume (TBV) and abnormal connectivity of white matter tracts (Koyama, 2009).

Our Inherited Tools for Social Understanding and Social Survival

A constant theme in theories has been that some failure in theory of mind, so-called *mindblindness*, underlies ASD. In their introduction to Simon Baron-Cohen's seminal "Mindblindness – An essay on Autism and Theory of Mind," (1995), John Tooby and Leda Cosmides show us where the path begins: in our own minds. We look at an apple. The apple is red. Or, our brain tells us that the apple is red. But, for those with some form of "colorblindness," the apple may be green, or shades of gray. And even thus, under different conditions the apple might seem to change colors. We live our lives with the feeling that color is an inherent property of things, but we accept it when forced to, that objects actually have no color, and what we perceive as color is the operation of our brain responding to the ability of cells in our retina to differentiate light frequencies allowing us to attribute the color to things. And we understand that not all living things have color vision, that some living things have better coloration than we do. Seeing color is a function of natural selection, giving those who have it, among other things, the ability to tell which are the poison berries and which are the ones that are safe to eat.

Just as intuitive as the idea that color is an independent property of objects, or, say, that the sun goes around the earth, is the feeling that our comprehension of the social world is the product of that world having come to us, "pre-packaged" and it "acted though the senses and through general-purpose learning mechanisms to build our concepts, interpretative frameworks, and mental organization." In other words, in this "folk psychology" we feel we know the world and how it works because it presented itself to us as infants and our senses and intelligence taught us what it all meant.

But in the latter decades of the twentieth-century scientists discovered "face cells" in the brains of monkeys that were dedicated exclusively to detecting a face—a monkey face, a human face, even a "face" carved on a pumpkin! (Bruce et al., 1981). And while we assume that we have simply learned the ability to detect that someone has made eye contact with us, or detect the direction of another's gaze, or that we and they are giving "shared attention" to some other thing, in fact there are cells in our human brain dedicated to these and other social tasks. Indeed, our survival as a species depended on living in groups, or conquering groups, and for that our brains had to develop tools to "understand and participate in complex social interactions" and did so over millions of years as the frontal lobe of the brain tripled in size to perform these advanced social tasks (Baron-Cohen, 1995). And this, Tooby and Cosmides tell us, gives us at birth a wide array of neurological tools

> designed to solve adaptive problems endemic to our hunter-gatherer ancestors. Each of these devices has its own agenda and imposes its own exotic organization on different fragments of the world. There are specialized systems for grammar induction, for face recognition, for dead reckoning, for construing objects, and for recognizing emotions from the face. There are mechanisms to detect animacy, eye direction, and cheating. There is a "theory of mind" module, and a multitude of other elegant machines.

Just as our brain paints the world with color to give us a richer life, the mental and social world that is so rich for us is enabled by "battalions of evolved, specialized neural automata" each of which "makes its own distinctive contribution to the cognitive model of the world that we individually experience as reality." Thus we have "Theory of Mind," a "mind-reading" skill, "a universal, evolved language of the eyes, which is mutually intelligible to all members of our species, can bring two separate minds into an aligned interpretation of their interaction." But these neural tools operate so automatically that we are not aware of them, and

> we mistake the representations they construct (the color of a leaf, the irony in a tone of voice, the approval of our friends, and so on) for the world itself—a world that reveals itself, unproblematically, through our senses.

"Yet," Tooby and Cosmides write, "even well-designed machinery can break down." And those who are impaired in neural areas of the brain which enable us to speak this "language of the eyes," become

> blind to the existence of other minds, while still living in the same physical, spatial, visual, and many-hued world as unimpaired people do. For beings who evolved to live woven into the minds of mothers, fathers, friends, and companions, being blind to the existence of others' minds is a catastrophic loss.

This is the neurodevelopmental problem of ASD; an impairment in evolved neurocognitive tools designed to allow us to perceive, understand, and survive in the social world. The practical problem is that those not familiar with this feeling that the world "reveals itself, unproblematically, through our senses" and that those who are both percipient and intelligent could figure the world out on their own.

Failure to "See" the Social World

The most salient consequence of the disruption of these inherited social tools is that the person with ASD simply does not see those countless signals in expressions, intonation, and "body language" that give meaning to social interactions and social scenes. This was demonstrated using eye tracking technology, comparing the gaze patterns of persons with autism to the gaze patterns of typically developed individuals while looking at a movie scene from "Who's Afraid of Virginia Woolf" (Klin et al., 2005).

The typically developed viewers looked at the faces of the actor speaking, George Segal, and the person spoken to, Elizabeth Taylor, and Richard Burton, playing her husband, in the background. This was to be expected because the impact of the scene derives from the inviting, flirtatious nature of Elizabeth Taylor's interaction with George Segal, and we expect the viewer to have natural curiosity as to how Richard Burton will react. In contrast, the viewers with autism focused on the mouth of the person speaking, with only a glance toward the body of the person spoken to. Thus, the individuals with autism were not seeking out the nonverbal information which would be the key to the scene's meaning and the understanding of the dynamic plot of the movie. Instead, they were trying to capture the words of the speaker to understand what was going on.

Similarly, in another scene, where two of the actors display visibly shocked expression, with their mouths open and their eyes wide, but not speaking, persons with autism still looked at the mouths, with no words coming out to interpret, disregarding the balance of their wide-eyed facial expressions.

Something was happening in the brain of the individuals with autism that was preventing their eyes from seeking out the social meaning of what they were watching. Numerous studies replicate this tracking of mouths over eyes.

As a result, those with ASD are significantly worse than the controls in recognizing emotions in others, which is a predictor of impairment in perceiving and learning from the social world (Ashwin et al., 2006; Corden et al., 2008) This is corroborated by research that shows marked difficulty in identifying emotions and mental states in pictures or from context (Ashwin et al., 2006; Baez et al., 2012).

Consequently, those with ASD may have trouble recognizing and distinguishing faces, holding the memory of faces, and even find themselves unable to tell gender from faces (Behrmann et al., 2006; Njiokiktjien et al., 2001). Research has even shown that for those with ASD, faces tend to be seen as objects, made up of parts; they do not show a normative decrement in performance when matching upside-down faces compared to their performance when matching right-side-up faces (Schultz et al., 2000).

What we are seeing in this research is the effect that the brain's difficulty in processing the critical nonverbal information (which typically developed brains process effortlessly and unconsciously) has on the person with ASD. The effect is as if, in order to avoid utter confusion, the brain is simply avoiding this information. Thus we see the lack of "social visual engagement" that is "pathognomonic" for children with autism (Constantino et al., 2017).

What is the effect of this lack of "social visual engagement" on the individual with ASD? To understand this we have to consider what the benefit is to typically developed person of the reciprocal social interactions they experience. From social interactions our mind learns how to instantly "read" other people from all the countless nonverbal cues in their facial expression, intonation, and "body language." We develop the intuitive ability to conceptualize how the other person feels, and what her intentions are. We can predict what others will do, and we can imagine, and do imagine, what their experience feels like. In a reciprocal way we also learn about our own feelings and how to express them (Goffman, 1959). Collectively these experiences give us a sense of how others feel about us, about others, and about what behaviors are appropriate. We develop intuition as to how the social rules we learn will be applied in novel situations. It is from thousands of reciprocal social interactions, from birth to adulthood, that we learn social mores, taboos, and develop "common sense" as to what is appropriate and inappropriate behavior. We become who we are today!

So then the task is to consider what would we be like if, instead of that life experience of processing myriad social cues over thousands of social interactions that gave us our "social common sense," we had none of that input, none of that reciprocity, and no developed intuition about the feelings and intentions of others or the social rules that society sets, or how to apply them to every new social situation. It is very hard to imagine. But it is from that perspective that one has to consider the problem at hand, judging the person with ASD who appears to have engaged in proscribed social misbehavior. The "mindblindness" in autism is the result of the brain interfering with the perception and processing of the social cues essential to social competence which typically developed individuals take for granted and mistakenly assume to be innate.

To really explain the scope of the problem for persons with autism, it is very useful to examine the mental operations on which typically developed individuals rely in their daily lives. As part of his Nobel Prize-winning work, Daniel Kahneman, makes exactly the same connection as autism researchers between the ability to perceive social information and the development of intuitive thinking abilities about the social world. In his best-selling book recapping his work, "Thinking, Fast and Slow," Kahneman describes the natural human inclination to see the social, the mental, and the psychological everywhere in the world around us. He refers to the work of psychologists Heider and Simmel in the 1940s.

> They made a film, which lasts all of one minute and forty seconds, in which you see a large triangle, a small triangle, and a circle moving around a shape that looks like a schematic view of a house with an open door. Viewers see an aggressive large triangle bullying a smaller triangle, a terrified circle, the circle and the small triangle joining forces to defeat the bully; they also observe much interaction around a door and then an explosive finale. . . . All this is entirely in your mind, of course. Your mind is ready and even eager to identify agents, assign them personality traits and specific intentions, and view their actions as expressing individual propensities. Here again, the evidence is that we are born prepared to make intentional attributions: infants under one-year old identify bullies and victims, and expect a pursuer to follow the most direct path in attempting to catch whatever it is chasing.

In the midst of this observation, where the ellipses appear above, Kahneman observes as matter of fact that, "The perception of intention and emotion is irresistible; *only people afflicted by autism do not experience it.*"

The centrality of the importance of perception of the social world for Kahneman is evidenced at the beginning of his book. The first chapter opens with a picture of the face of an obviously angry woman.

> Your experience as you look at the woman's face seamlessly combines what we normally call seeing and intuitive thinking. As surely and quickly as you saw that the young woman's hair is dark, you knew she is angry. Furthermore, what you saw extended into the future. You sensed that this woman is about to say some very unkind words, probably in a loud and strident voice. A premonition of what she was going to do next came to mind automatically

> and effortlessly. You did not intend to assess her mood or to anticipate what she might do, and your reaction to the picture did not have the feel of something you did. It just happened to you. It was an instance of fast thinking.

This "fast thinking" is what Kahneman "System 1" or "Type1" thinking. This is automatic, intuitive, effortless, and often unconscious, thought, reflections impossible to control, and thinking though practiced tasks like driving or speaking. Contrasting with this is what Kahneman calls "System 2" or "Type 2" thinking which involves orderly computation, doing things in stages, remembering and applying rules; it is controlled, effortful, logical. He describes how infants of less than one-year old have intuitive thinking. He describes how this intuition derives from the perception of the social world.

But in describing "Type 1" thinking, Dr. Kahneman is describing capabilities that a typical infant would have but that those with ASD do not have—but that are essential to social survival. And without those perceptions of "the other," and the intuitive thinking that can only grow out of that, the autistic person has to figure some other way to mediate to the world. One of the ways is by grasping at rules they are taught or can try to discern:

> In this context, individuals with AS were said to mediate their social and emotional exchange through explicit verbal and logical means, cognitively, rigidly, and in a rule-governed fashion. (Klin et al., 2005)

The enormity of the problem for the autistic individual suddenly becomes apparent when Dr. Kahneman tells us that "most of the work," 90% of what our mind does during the day is easy, unconscious thinking, intuitions, and predictive abilities that come from social perception. Clearly he is talking about "Theory of Mind" here, something that is generally impaired in ASD. Because we have that intuition to get us by most tasks, only a relatively small amount of effort and time is expended implementing the more difficult, deliberate step-by-step logical thinking directed by whatever rules and evidence we have at hand.

For the individual with ASD this mental workload is stood on its head. Without those perception-based intuitions which typically developed people can get by with most of the day, this person has to rely on laborious Type 2 thinking most of the time in the social world: everything social is an exhausting mental struggle. This is merely a part of what Cosmides and Tooby called the "catastrophic loss."

Autism: A "Social Learning Disorder"

When psychologists were first pushed to define the parameters of autism, in 1978, by the parents of children with autism—the National Society for Autistic Children ("NSAC")—one of the suggested criteria for the condition was "Disturbed Quality to relate appropriately to people, events and objects." The inability to develop social competence is the leading factor in the failure of most adults with autism to attain even a minimal level of quality in their lives (Howlin & Goode, 2000). It was widely understood and problematic that individuals with ASD see the concrete and do not grasp or "appreciate these unwritten rules of social engagement." "Everything that is not explicit, everything that is unstructured, everything that is not defined and expressly supported is a difficulty for individuals with Asperger Syndrome." Rather, their behavior may appear "inappropriate or embarrassing when, in addition to failing to use these social niceties, they violate clear social conventions," which oftentimes results from an unawareness of other people's feelings or point of view. They often engage in behavior that is completely alien to, and therefore usually misunderstood by, mainstream society, which expects adolescents or young adults exhibiting normal intelligence and language abilities to "act their age" (Mesibov et al., 2001).

Without Social Perception and Intuitive Social Thinking, Social Norms and Taboos Are Often Not Evident to the Person with ASD

Lack of awareness of social norms and taboos, which figures into both domains of the diagnostic criteria for ASD, arises directly and inevitably from the absence of social intuition and its antecedent, "social visual engagement," with its neurodevelopmental underpinnings (Gutstein & Whitney, 2002; Loveland, 1991; Venter et al., 1992).

Even if the young man with ASD is not "completely naïve about the fact that their behaviour is inappropriate, they have not internalized the extent to which it is against the conventions of society" (Lindsay, 2009). Although they may also "understand something of the illegality or inappropriate sexual behavior, they may not have a full comprehension of the extent of which such practices are condemned by society" (Craig & Lindsay, 2010).

Those with ASD see the concrete and may not grasp or "appreciate [the] unwritten rules of social engagement," and their behavior may "violate clear social conventions," often resulting from an unawareness of other people's feelings or point of view (Mesibov et al., 2001). As a result, "the social and emotional deficits within ASDs may be salient during incidents of *unintended criminal . . . behavior*" (Lerner et al., 2012).

The problem is not that these individuals do not "know right from wrong," but rather that what is regarded as right and wrong is often unwritten, untaught, and implicit, and therefore not apparent to many young men with autism whose social learning is most severely affected:

> Takeda et al. found intact external (subject to predetermined rules) moral reasoning, but impaired internal (autonomous) moral reasoning, particularly higher-level autonomous-altruistic moral reasoning, among children and adolescents with HFASDs relative to typical peers.
>
> * * *

> Individuals with HFASDs appear to learn specific behaviors most effectively via explicit, rules-based instruction; this type of learning appears to apply to the domain of moral reasoning and behavior as well. (Lerner et al., 2012)

Lacking in Social Intuition, Young Men with ASD Are Vulnerable to Unwitting Sexually Offensive Behaviors

Sociosexual norms and taboos are often the least taught, and most difficult to apply across different situations. This implicates issues of "age of consent," and age differential in adolescence, and the very concept of consent. Researchers have noted for some time that, although young men with ASD are not more prone to criminality of any sort, including sex offenses, than their neurotypical peers, they seem susceptible to a range of offensive behaviors because they are unaware of these implicit rules (Mogavero, 2016). Researchers have noted that the effects of ASD itself "has a critical role among the minority who commit sexually-related offenses," because of its effects on understanding social norms (Mogavero, 2016; see also Lindsay et al., 2014).

Without Social Intuition, the Individual with ASD May Not See the Implication of Social Scenes, in Life and in Photographs

Social competence for adolescents and adults involves not only knowing the untaught social rules, but also how to interpret social situations in order to apply the rules. The problem is that the same neurological deficits which filter out the nonverbal social information in personal encounters also impair the ability to interpret whole social scenes. These individuals are not just missing what we see in others' eyes, or facial expressions. They are missing the entire social scene, in multiple social cognition domains. This includes social scenes in photographs (Baez et al., 2012).

As discussed above, Daniel Kahneman, in "Thinking, Fast and Slow" described how the typically developed mind looks for the social and mental implications of social scenes—including scenes without explicit social cues, as in the animation by Heider and Simmel in the 1940s. Kahneman said there that, "The perception of intention and emotion is irresistible; *only people afflicted by autism do not experience it.*"

Using the same video from the 1944 research on which Kahneman comments, Klin (2000) demonstrated that those with ASD are significantly less able than their typically developed peers at recognizing the social cues in the video, even when prompted, and even with age. Often they see none of these cues.

The above research adds breadth to the fundamental eye tracking research by demonstrating that those with ASD do not just have a *brain* that filters out nonverbal social cues, and the meaning of social scenes. They also have a *mind* that is not even looking for them, and, even when prompted, are markedly poor in recognizing them in scenes where others cannot avoid seeing them.

This has enormous significance in addressing the problem of online sex offending. We confront two assumptions, or "heuristics," when it comes to persons who are viewing sexual images of underage persons. First, that they are aware of the social rules related to viewing such images, and how that behavior is viewed by others. Second, that in viewing such images, persons are cognizant of the social implications of the scene, and the perspectives of the persons therein, and that this would deter a person who is not deviant or antisocial from viewing the material even if he was not aware of the social opprobrium against viewing it. The first heuristic is addressed by the problem of often not being aware of the taboo against viewing such material to begin with. The second is addressed by the difficulty of interpreting the social scenes within the images or videos. These assumptions simply do not hold true for those with autism.

While Autism Makes Young Men Vulnerable to Unwittingly Transgressing Social Norms, Their Autism Renders Them Generally "Rule Bound" and Assiduous at Following the Social Rules They Are Told About

The inability to develop socially intuitive thinking leaves most of those with ASD desperate to figure out the important social rules that they are unable to intuit and which no one has expressly told them. DSM-5 observes that being rule bound is a trait under both domains of diagnostic criteria. This is a trait which all clinicians and all teachers and others who work with those with ASD are very familiar.

Being rule bound can be a serious problem for children, and frustrate their efforts to play with others. They will insist on adherence to rules, regardless of more or less accurate understanding of the rules, and complain about others violating the rules. But when it comes to assessing risk for future offending, being rule bound is an asset which prosecutors and judges can and do rely on. Research supports this.

> Youth with ASDs were also less likely to be charged with probation violations. This may be due to several factors, including increased rule adherence in youth with ASD, the fact that youth with ASD are less likely to be prosecuted, and therefore less likely to serve probation, or because youth with ASD may be more closely supervised by adults than youth without a developmental disability. (Cheely et al., 2012)

This same paper notes the frequency with which cases involving those with ASD are diverted out of appreciation of this phenomenon:

> We also found significant differences in outcomes between youth with ASD and comparison youth, such that youth with ASD were less likely to be prosecuted and were more likely to have their charges diverted than comparison youth. (Cheely et al., 2012)

Thus, despite its role in obscuring social boundaries, and exposing these young persons to the criminal justice system, ASD can also provide assurance against the risk of reoffending, once they have learned the rules, especially where being rule bound is well developed in the developmental history.[1]

Neuroimaging

Neuroimaging has found differences in brain functioning in areas classically associated with ToM in individuals with ASD. Positron emission tomography (PET) studies have found differences between healthy controls and individuals with ASD in areas classically associated with ToM paradigm, such as: the medial prefrontal cortex (Gallagher et al., 2000) and the ventral frontal region (Happe et al., 1996). Similar emotional inference tasks in Functional Magnetic Resonance Imaging (fMRI) studies have also shown distinct differences in the amygdala (Baron-Cohen et al., 1999), superior temporal gyrus (Baron-Cohen et al., 1999), and the orbital frontal cortex (OFC) (Carper & Courchesne, 2005; Chung et al., 2005; Girgis et al., 2007; Jiao et al., 2010). The OFC, in particular, has been associated with social cognition and ToM (Girgis et al., 2007).

Executive Function and the Frontal Lobes

"Executive functions," classically associated with the frontal lobes, is an umbrella term generally used when referring to so-called higher level functions such as: planning, initiation, inhibition, cognitive flexibility, and working memory (Koyama, 2009). Research has indicated that individuals with ASD often suffer from difficulties in one or more of these tasks, though it is important to note, not all individuals with ASD show such deficits (Koyama, 2009). Numerous researchers have examined the connection between ASD and executive functioning difficulties from a number of perspectives (Ozonoff et al., 1991; Perner & Lang, 2000; Sabbagh et al., 2006).

In criminal cases executive functioning is critical in two major respects (1) understanding behaviors of those with autism and (2) evaluating competency. It can be bewildering to observers how a young man with ASD can persist in the pursuit of an objective, or in the use of certain means, without noticing otherwise obvious signals that the objective or the means, or both, are unwelcome, inappropriate, or illegal. This is partly a problem of executive functioning and is most evident in cases of stalking, sexting with minors, or trolling behavior which becomes obsessive and perseverative.

[1] While there can be a significant occurrence of Oppositional Defiant Disorder or Conduct Disorder, or their symptoms in conjunction with ASD, is not clear the extent to which these conditions actually militate against rigid adherence to social rules considered to be morally important, once learned.

Impairments in executive function also point directly to concerns about legal competence. Competence implicates the ability to utilize whatever knowledge the accused with ASD has about the legal process, or the facts of the case, and bring it to bear in properly assisting in the defense. It bears critically on the ability to understand tactics and strategy and autonomously make important choices, or even participate in making important choices, in the conduct of his defense, or any of the essential decisions that are his alone to make.

Neuroimaging studies indicate potential frontal cortical anomalies in individuals with ASD (Hardan et al., 2004; Levitt et al., 2003). Specifically, studies have shown enlargement of the amygdala, temporal cortex, and frontal lobes as a whole (Courchesne et al., 2011; Wolff et al., 2018); within the frontal lobe, increase surface area has been noted in the dorsolateral and medial frontal regions (Carper & Courchesne, 2005) and prefrontal cortex (PFC) white matter (Herbert et al., 2004), while the decreased surface area has been reported in the OFC (Ecker et al., 2013).

Central Coherence and Sensory Perception

It has been suggested that individuals with ASD spend significantly more time processing sensory level stimuli and less time with executive functions, particularly those mediated by the PFC which is needed for holistic integration of sensory stimuli (Ring et al., 1999). This disconnect in individuals with ASD is referred to as Central Coherence. In support of this theory, functional studies have shown individuals with ASD showed greater activation in ventral occipito-temporal areas and decreased activation in prefrontal cortical areas (an area associated with Executive Functioning as above) (Ring et al., 1999). Indeed, studies have shown that, as early as ages 6–12 months, children who will go on to have ASD undergo expansion of cortical surface area starting with the areas associated with sensory domains such as audio and visual processing (Hazlett et al., 2017; Shen et al., 2013).

Brain Regions and Findings Potentially Involved in Autism

The temporal lobe, as a whole, is involved in processing sensory information and includes the areas responsible for: language, face recognition, audition, and memory. It is perhaps not surprising then that temporal lobe abnormalities have frequently been reported in ASD (Baron-Cohen et al., 1999; Boddaert et al., 2002, 2003; Boddaert, Chabane, Belin, et al., 2004; Courchesne et al., 2011; Dougherty et al., 2016; Hadjikhani et al., 2006; Ogai et al., 2003; Pierce et al., 2001; Ring et al., 1999; Scheel et al., 2011; Wolff et al., 2018; Zilbovicius et al., 2000). Specific temporal lobe deficits noted include issues with speech-related issues, social gaze, mirror neurons, and social cognition. PET studies have shown bilateral temporal lobe dysfunction and hypo-perfusion (under-performance) (Boddaert et al., 2002; Zilbovicius et al.,

2000), with particular deficits in speech-related areas in the left temporal cortex in both adults and children with ASD (Boddaert et al., 2003; Boddaert, Chabane, Belin, et al., 2004). Individuals with ASD are also frequently reported to be inattentive to social stimuli such as gaze (Kylliainen & Hietanen, 2004); functional neuroimaging studies of face processing demonstrated qualitative differences between ASD individuals and controls (Ogai et al., 2003; Pierce et al., 2001) suggesting individuals with ASD spend less time processing faces. Finally, adults with ASD have been found to have cortical thinning in areas associated with the mirror neuron system and other areas responsible for social cognition, such as the: middle and inferior temporal gyrus (Hadjikhani et al., 2006) and posterior superior temporal sulcus in high-functioning individuals (Scheel et al., 2011).

Total Brain Volume

Increased total brain volume (TBV) is a consistent structural finding in ASD with many individuals suffering from macrocephaly as a result of TBV (Koyama, 2009); these results have been heavily published and are reviewed by Koyama (Koyama, 2009). In ASD, it is believed that shortly after birth brain size is below average to average (Courchesne et al., 2003; Hazlett et al., 2005; Nordahl et al., 2011). However, a period of increased brain growth occurs thereafter (Langen et al., 2014), though the exact age of onset for this brain growth remains debated (Langen et al., 2014; Nordahl et al., 2011). As mentioned above, starting between the ages of 6 and 12 months, children who will go on to develop ASD show an expansion of cortical surface area, starting in sensory domains underlying auditory and visual processing, followed by more global overgrowth from the ages of 12–24 months (Hazlett et al., 2017; Shen et al., 2013). From the ages of 2–4 years, TBV in children with ASD remains enlarged compared with those of their peers (Courchesne et al., 2011; Redcay & Courchesne, 2005). By school age, brain growth has slowed, with TBV of typically developing children approaching that of children with ASD (Courchesne et al., 2011; Redcay & Courchesne, 2005).

Cerebellum

The cerebellum, perhaps best known for its role in sequencing and integration of motor functions, is also involved in cognitive functions (Koyama, 2009). Individuals with cerebellar cortical atrophy have been found to display executive function, visuospatial, language, and affective deficits (Koyama, 2009). The cerebellum has been implicated in ASD, because at the macroscopic level, ASD is associated with decreased size of the cerebellar cortical volume (Ciesielski et al., 1997; Courchesne et al., 1994, 1988, 2001; Murakami et al., 1989; Sparks et al., 2002). Neuroimaging studies suggest cerebellar size may be increased up to ages 2–4 years (Courchesne et al., 2001; Sparks et al., 2002), but volume decreases thereafter through adulthood (Courchesne et al., 2001). The first MRI studies looking at the cerebellum in ASD found hypoplasia in lobules VI-VII (Courchesne et al., 1988; Murakami et al., 1989) and reduced cerebellar hemisphere size (Murakami et al., 1989). Subsequent studies confirmed these findings (Ciesielski et al., 1997; Courchesne et al., 1994, 2001).

Though most studies of the cerebellum in ASD have mostly noted reductions in the cerebellum as a whole or cerebellar sub-regions, these results are not universal. Indeed, one study found persistently increased cerebellar volume into adulthood (Piven, Saliba, et al., 1997). The lack of consistency has led some to hypothesize that these findings may be related to IQ and therefore reflecting a level of cognitive impairment not specific to autism (Koyama, 2009). Another complicating finding, adults with high-functioning ASD were reported to have reduced grey matter volume in cerebellar regions (McAlonan et al., 2002), while children were found to have reduced white matter volume (Boddaert, Chabane, Gervais, et al., 2004; Brun et al., 2009; Carper & Courchesne, 2000; McAlonan et al., 2005; Scott et al., 2009; Stanfield et al., 2008).

Amygdala

Another brain area that has inconsistent findings is the amygdala. Most ASD studies have shown amygdala overgrowth (Abell et al., 1999; Baron-Cohen et al., 1999; Courchesne et al., 2011; Howard et al., 2000; Munson et al., 2006; Schumann et al., 2004; Sparks et al., 2002; Wolff et al., 2018), and after adjusting for methodological differences (Koyama, 2009) there is a strong trend for amygdala size to be increased, rather than decreased in autism (Koyama, 2009). Enlargement of the amygdala can be found as early as age 2–4 in individuals who will develop ASD (Nordahl et al., 2012); indeed, the extent of the bilateral amygdalar overgrowth has been found to correlate with severity of social impairment in toddlers (Schumann et al., 2009). There is some evidence suggesting that amygdalar volume may normalize in adolescence (Barnea-Goraly et al., 2014).

Corpus Callosum

The corpus callosum (CC) has a role in processes that require integrating sensory and motor stimuli, including: visual attention shifting, procedural learning, and bimanual motor coordination—all issues that have been reported in ASD. MRI studies have found a consistent pattern of overall decrease in CC size in individuals with ASD (Alexander et al., 2007; Boger-Megiddo et al., 2006; Egaas et al., 1995; Frazier & Hardan, 2009; Freitag et al., 2009; Haar et al., 2016; Hardan et al., 2000; Just et al., 2007; Manes et al., 1999; Piven, Bailey, et al., 1997; Saitoh et al., 1995; Vidal et al.,

2006; Waiter et al., 2005), including overall decreases in the midsagittal area (Boger-Megiddo et al., 2006; Manes et al., 1999; Vidal et al., 2006) and subregional areas such as the anterior (Hardan et al., 2000; Just et al., 2007; Vidal et al., 2006), middle (Egaas et al., 1995; Piven, Bailey, et al., 1997), and posterior (Just et al., 2007; Piven, Bailey, et al., 1997; Saitoh et al., 1995; Waiter et al., 2005) portions of the CC. These findings are consistent with white matter-based theories, leading some to postulate if autism may be a disorder of connectivity.

Connectivity

Brain connectivity refers to the pattern of linkages between distinct units within the nervous system and brain. An oversimplified analogy would be roads; the brain must have a "road" or route of roads connecting 2 regions in order for them to properly communicate with one another. ASD is associated with abnormalities of white matter tracts, the so-called roads (Koyama, 2009). Recent neuroimaging studies have found that high-risk infants, 6-months of age, who will later develop ASD, already exhibited abnormal connectivity patterns (Emerson et al., 2017; Lewis et al., 2017; Wolff et al., 2012, 2018). The abnormal connectivity patterns particularly affect low-level sensory processing at this early stage (Lewis et al., 2017) and the degree of atypical connectivity at 6-months was found to correlate with future symptom severity (Lewis et al., 2017; Wolff et al., 2018).

Resting state analysis data obtained from fMRI studies found individuals with ASD had a predominance of hypoconnectivity of long-range cortical-cortical and interhemispheric projections compared with age-matched controls (Di Martino et al., 2014). Meanwhile these same individuals demonstrated subcortical hyperconnectivity of local connections (Di Martino et al., 2014; Muhle et al., 2018). Together, these data suggest that ASD depresses high-order brain functions involving communication between and across brain regions in preference of local circuits which could become overactive and difficult to inhibit (Muhle et al., 2018).

The Possible Usefulness of Neuroimaging in the Legal Context

Given the importance of neuroscience in the development of our understanding of autism, beginning with Charles Gross' discovery of "face cells," and later "modules" in the brain dedicated to social survival, it only seems logical that neuroscience and neuroimaging have someplace in explaining ASD and its effects on individuals in legal contexts where their behavior is at issue. In the larger picture, neuroscience is already in the courtroom, and there is an ongoing debate about how much it will be able to contribute. Maybe it has "many things to say, but not nearly as much as people would hope" (Morse, 2011). Maybe it presents "a fundamental paradigm shift in which neuroimaging is becoming a highly significant part of the criminal justice process," in addition to being an ethically mandated tool for criminal defense lawyers to use, at least in the most serious cases (Gaudet & Marchant, 2016; ABA, 2003). Maybe it "will shape the future of legal theory and create a more biologically informed jurisprudence" (Ebert, 2012).

In the case of ASD, neuroscience and neuroimaging can be powerful tools to illustrate that there are real neurological differences that correlate to the traits and deficits we see behaviorally in those with ASD, even tied to areas of the brain dedicated to social learning. That is, that ASD is "real," to be taken seriously, and not simply a hypothesis. So, group neuroimaging investigations, and the images they produce, may be helpful, albeit depended on the deduction that these same neurological differences are present in that individual.

The problem comes with the usefulness of neuroimaging of the individual. In the trial of John Hinckley, *United States v. Hinckley*, 525 F. Supp. 1342 (D.D.C. 1981), a psychiatrist testified for the defense that Hinckley was not criminally responsible for shooting the President of the United States because he was "suffering from a major depressive disorder and from process schizophrenia" (Caplan, 1984). To tip the scales in their direction Hinckley's defense team introduced neuroimaging showing atrophy of Hinckley's brain that was consistent with schizophrenia—among other conditions. The uproar over Hinckley's acquittal which precipitated drastic changes in federal and state laws concerning the insanity defense, had little to do with the use of neuroimaging. The evidence was admissible and relevant to the opinion offered, and thoroughly and capably challenged (Kulynych, 1996). The victim of the furor over the verdict was the legal burden of the government to prove that Hinckley was sane, meaning that his insanity acquittal could be compelled merely by his raising a reasonable doubt about his sanity. But the legal lore of the time was that the neuroimaging evidence swayed the jury (DeBenedictis, 1990). While successful in the hands of elite defense counsel in that case, one can only be cautiously optimistic that such evidence can responsibly and effectively be used in others.

It is not possible to conceptualize substantial reliance on neuroimaging in proving a diagnosis of ASD, no matter how many apparent neurological correlates, from group studies, appear to be present in an individual. But perhaps imaging has a useful role in supporting a diagnosis, or ruling out a differential diagnosis, or challenging an incorrect diagnosis, or perhaps most importantly, as an additional pedagogic aid in persuading prosecutors and judges that ASD is *real in this individual* defendant.

Functional Limitations

In summary, this chapter discussed a number of brain differences between individuals with ASD and typical people. But there are limitations to what can be concluded from this information. First, many of these findings are shared with other conditions. There is a significant degree of overlap between neuroimaging findings in ASD and ADHD

(Johnson et al., 2015), as well as significant overlap in brain regions for ASD and OCD (Carlisi et al., 2017). While there are multiple possible explanations for why different diagnostic syndromes may share common early life predictors (Johnson et al., 2015), the problem remains—in order for any particular brain finding to be meaningful on its own, it needs to be unique or characteristic in the constellation in which it appears. To date, this has not been established for ASD. Thus, an image of cerebellar dysfunction does not in itself indicate that the individual has ASD, and must be interpreted with caution. Further complicating this issue, the results of these brain studies may differ significantly by age and gender (Lai et al., 2017), again limiting any universal statements regarding the findings.

Second, the methodological limitations of these studies make interpretation of these findings difficult. For example, a number of studies compared children with ASD to healthy adults (Zürcher et al., 2015). Others enrolled siblings of individuals with ASD as controls despite knowledge that siblings of individuals with ASD have a higher number of autistic traits than other healthy controls (Zürcher et al., 2015). Further, low-functioning children were frequently scanned while sedated or asleep while high-functioning adults and children were awake (Zurcher et al., 2015). The risk/benefit of sedating young participants to avoid motion artifacts is a known barrier to recruiting children. In numerous institutions, it is also considered unethical to sedate healthy controls. This leads to a situation where all children with ASD were sedated, but only a fraction of the control children were sedated leading to potential confounders (Zurcher et al., 2015). In the past, people have also discussed the relatively low number of people scanned in these studies as highly problematic, but recent studies have included larger cohorts decreasing concern for this bias.

Taken together, while the studies themselves are improving, there is still no 'smoking gun' on brain imaging and current methodology remains complicated for a variety of reasons. Although neuroimaging research is advancing our understanding of the biology of ASD, there is no evidence to support routine neuroimaging in autistic individuals (Filipek et al., 2000; Johnson & Myers, 2007).

Interpreting Neuroimaging in Court—The Group to Individual Conundrum

In the court room, few things can be as powerful as a picture; after all, they do say, "a picture is worth a thousand words" The ability to show a brain scan with gorgeous, multi-hued sulci and gyri is both impressive and impactful. Indeed, previous studies have shown just how influential a pretty picture or charismatic speaker can be to a jury—even when the evidence being presented is wrong (Oullier, 2012; Stern, 2014).

In ASD, it would be relatively easy to do a brain scan and produce a brain image for the court showing differences in the frontal lobes, temporal lobes, corpus callosum, cerebellum, and/or amygdala for a defendant. An expert witness could point to the red blob in the frontal lobe and talk about how the defendant did not have proper impulse control or was not processing information in the usual manner. In this fashion, the brain image could be quite helpful in convincing the jury that this defendant needs to be given special considerations. While this scenario sounds good and does indeed happen in court, there is a problem. The trouble is that armed only with a brain scan and no other information (e.g., clinical data), the results of a brain scan are almost meaningless to any one individual, including the defendant. The problem is not with the accuracy of the prior autism studies; those brain regions were discovered after comparing hundreds of brains. Instead, there is a fundamental problem with applying information gleaned from aggregated data to any particular individual.

Much of science works by evaluating averages. If asked, for example, to establish the weight of the average American, with enough patience and the right methodology, one would be able to come up with an accurate number. The weights of all individuals sampled would be pooled to create an average. The same is true of brain imaging studies such as fMRI. However, just as any particular individual's weight may differ from that of the average person, so too do brains differ. No two brains look exactly the same, but which difference means something clinically and which is just a product of age, gender, race, head size, etc.? The fewer subjects the greater the chance that individual variability, rather than a class difference, may account for any given difference discovered. To control for these normal variations, the data must be pooled to create an average. As more and more data points are added, a result becomes increasingly valid. Often it takes a large number of data points to begin to resolve findings from the noise of individual variability.

Group level analysis is precisely what was done in the brain imaging studies reviewed in this chapter. The scanned brains of individuals with ASD were pooled and compared to the pooled brain scans of the controls. These "averaged" brains have allowed scientists to find substantial differences between the average autistic brain and that of the "typical" control. Findings such as these have allowed scientists to make progress on understanding what happens in neurodevelopment that leads to ASD. However, while it is certainly true that group level brain differences exist between individuals with ASD and those without, science is not yet able to discern if these findings hold true in any one particular individual. If the findings discussed above are to conclusively show an individual has ASD, the neuroimaging marker needs to be unique to ASD, but, as discussed above, many of the brain features discovered for ASD are shared by other conditions such as ADHD (Johnson et al., 2015) and OCD (Carlisi et al., 2017). More troubling, even within the ASD group, the brain findings may differ based upon an individual's age or gender (Lai et al., 2017). Thus, although neuroimaging research is advancing our understanding of the biology of ASD, there is no evidence to support routine neuroimaging in autistic individuals (Filipek et al., 2000; Johnson & Myers, 2007) and no evidence that ASD-specific findings are close at hand.

Individual variability is at the core of why neuroimaging results should have a very narrow application in the legal setting. Neuroimaging's lack of specificity does not integrate well into the legal system; this science is not best suited to saying anything definitive about individuals, while courts desire categorical, dichotomous information—either (s)he has it or (s)he does not; (s)he is a risk or (s)he is not; (s)he can be rehabilitated or (s)he cannot. The problem lies in applying what is known about groups of people to individuals. This class of problems has been termed the Group to Individual (G2i) problem. An article by Faigman, Monahan, and Slobogin (Faigman et al., 2014) describes it in the legal context:

> A fundamental divide exists between what scientists do as scientists and what courts often ask them to do as expert witnesses. Whereas scientists almost invariably inquire into phenomena at the group level, trial courts typically need to resolve cases at the individual level. In short, scientists generalize while courts particularize. A basic challenge for trial courts that rely on scientific experts, therefore, concerns determining whether and how scientific knowledge derived from studying groups can be helpful in the individual cases before them.

The process can backfire. Returning to the hypothetical scenario of a defendant with ASD and using the same brain scan image indicating frontal lobe dysfunction, a prosecutor could argue a different interpretation: that the defendant is sociopathic and incapable of controlling his or her behavior, and, thus, is a permanent risk to society necessitating that he or she be locked away for societal protection. Such arguments are reminiscent of the testimonial style of Dr. James Grigson, known a "Dr. Death," memorialized in the Supreme Court case of *Barefoot v. Estelle*, 463 U.S. 880 (1983). Grigson, a forensic psychiatrist, gave testimony regarding risk of future danger to the community—successfully leading to the death penalty in Mr. Barefoot's case and over 100 others. Dr. Grigson successfully convinced juries that there were fundamental differences in the defendant's brain, and, in turn, behavior, from normal people, making him dangerous.

Thus, care must be used when considering using individual neuroimaging in court because it may not be definitive and can be misinterpreted as a result. While legal decision-making wants categorical answers (yes or no), scientific and medical experts frequently provide statistical answers. Responsible experts frequently do bring data-based statistics into the courtroom to try to answer questions about an individual. This is frequently done through measurement tools, such as a risk assessment. However, even still, the kind of statistical statements made by experts does not integrate well with the need the court has for categorical, dichotomous information, because, once again, they are not designed to be used to say anything so definitive about individuals. As with the average American weight, what is known about groups, no matter how precise, does not mean one can confidently or accurately predict the outcome of individual cases.

The G2i problem has been described as a key issue at the intersection of science and the law. However, it has received very little attention from either the legal or scientific communities, something attributed to the "intractability of the problem" A consortium of scholars, supported by the MacCarthur Foundation, and led by David Faigman, was formed to study the problem further, and guidelines have been set out in Faigman's paper (Faigman et al., 2014). The overarching point, however, is that neuroimaging findings of the type discussed in this chapter should not lightly be used in a trial setting as the basis on which to render an opinion to a reasonable degree of medical or psychological certainty as to a diagnosis or the etiology or severity of the relevant deficits of the accused.

Nevertheless, neuroimaging results, if properly qualified, and not improperly relied on for rendering an expert opinion, may satisfy requirements for legal relevance in the courtroom, in a corroborative role, to support diagnoses and other opinions about the condition of the accused that have been independently arrived at by accepted and empirical means, especially when imaged neurological correlates of a diagnosis or condition, albeit just in this individual, are more reliable than the contrary evidence which often is no more than that apparently deviant or intentional acts demonstrate a deviant or purposeful mind.

Neuroimaging Out of Court

As pointed out in relation to online offenses, Chap. 16, and true in many other criminal cases as well, the best results for those with ASD, under current jurisprudence, may come about not as a result of criminal trials, but as a result of the exercise of prosecutorial discretion, in light of what we know about autism and its presentation in the accused. In this setting, the demonstration, through imaging, of expected neurological correlates of ASD can help to fairly persuade prosecutors, skeptical of mental "excuses" to criminality, to understand that indeed the demonstrated group characteristics of those with autism inhabit the accused, as independently attested to in whatever diagnostic reports and developmental history and standardized testing.

And the biggest point may be what is *not* revealed in neuroimaging. For example, what might really decide the fate of a young man with autism is the best guess by an assistant district attorney, with no experience or prior understanding of developmental disabilities, as to whether the conduct of the accused was that of antisocial predator, or someone who simply had not learned pertinent sociosexual taboos, and whose ASD impaired his cognitive empathic abilities. Imaging evidence reasonably supporting the clinical conclusion the accused is not antisocial could be determinative in the mind of a prosecutor or judge.

So, neuroimaging investigations of autism and antisociality demonstrate diagnostically specific aberrant cortical brain structure: thinner temporal and parietal cortices during adolescence and adulthood in high-functioning individuals with ASD (Hadjikhani et al., 2006; Scheel et al., 2011; Wallace et al., 2010), while antisocial disorders during adulthood (Yang & Raine, 2009) and disruptive behavior disorders during childhood (Fahim et al., 2011) correlate with thinner prefrontal and cingulate cortices. This has shown to be the case also in a non-clinical large sample population of TD youth, and to remain stable into early adulthood (Wallace et al., 2012). These aberrant structures only slightly overlap in the affected areas of the brain. Thus, there are dissociable neural signatures for these diametrically opposite social traits. That neuroimaging of the accused might demonstrate cortical correlates of autism but not of antisocial traits may provide powerful support for the effort to persuade the prosecutor to take a more empirical rather than intuitive approach to making her decision. If there is a way to make this comparison just within the individual's own brain (cortical thinning here, but not there) or in comparison to groups tested in population samples, such as in the above imaging investigations, this could be an important tool in avoiding injustice.

Bibliography

ABA. (2003). *Guidelines for the appointment and performance of defense counsel in death penalty cases 31*. American Bar Association.

Abell, F., Krams, M., Ashburner, J., Passingham, R., Friston, K., Frackowiak, R., … Frith, U. (1999). The neuroanatomy of autism: A voxel-based whole brain analysis of structural scans. *Neuroreport, 10*(8), 1647–1651.

Alexander, A. L., Lee, J. E., Lazar, M., Boudos, R., DuBray, M. B., Oakes, T. R., … Bigler, E. D. (2007). Diffusion tensor imaging of the corpus callosum in Autism. *Neuroimage, 34*(1), 61–73.

Ashwin, C., Chapman, E., Colle, L., & Baron-Cohen, S. (2006). Impaired recognition of negative basic emotions in autism: A test of the amygdala theory. *Social Neuroscience, 1*(3–4), 349–363. https://doi.org/10.1080/17470910601040772.

Baez, S., Rattazzi, A., Gonzalez-Gadea, M. L., Torralva, T., Vigliecca, N., Decety, J., … Ibanez, A. (2012). Integrating intention and context: Assessing social cognition in adults with Asperger syndrome. *Frontiers in Human Neuroscience, 6*, 302.

Barnea-Goraly, N., Frazier, T. W., Piacenza, L., Minshew, N. J., Keshavan, M. S., Reiss, A. L., & Hardan, A. Y. (2014). A preliminary longitudinal volumetric MRI study of amygdala and hippocampal volumes in autism. *Progress in Neuro-Psychopharmacology and Biological Psychiatry, 48*, 124–128.

Baron-Cohen, S. (1995). *Mindblindness: An essay on autism and theory of mind*. MIT Press.

Baron-Cohen, S. (2006). Impaired recognition of negative basic emotions in autism: A test of the amygdala theory. *Social Neuroscience, 1*(34), 349–363.

Baron-Cohen, S., Ring, H. A., Wheelwright, S., Bullmore, E. T., Brammer, M. J., Simmons, A., & Williams, S. C. (1999). Social intelligence in the normal and autistic brain: An fMRI study. *European Journal of Neuroscience, 11*(6), 1891–1898.

Behrmann, M., Thomas, C., & Humphreys, K. (2006). Seeing it differently: Visual processing in autism. *Trends in Cognitive Sciences, 10*(6), 258–264.

Boddaert, N., Belin, P., Chabane, N., Poline, J. B., Barthélémy, C., Mouren-Simeoni, M. C., … Zilbovicius, M. (2003). Perception of complex sounds: Abnormal pattern of cortical activation in autism. *American Journal of Psychiatry, 160*(11), 2057–2060.

Boddaert, N., Chabane, N., Barthelemy, C., Bourgeois, M., Poline, J. B., Brunelle, F., … Zilbovicius, M. (2002). Bitemporal lobe dysfunction in infantile autism: Positron emission tomography study. *Journal de radiologie, 83*(12 Pt 1), 1829.

Boddaert, N., Chabane, N., Belin, P., Bourgeois, M., Royer, V., Barthelemy, C., … Zilbovicius, M. (2004). Perception of complex sounds in autism: Abnormal auditory cortical processing in children. *American Journal of Psychiatry, 161*(11), 2117–2120.

Boddaert, N., Chabane, N., Gervais, H., Good, C. D., Bourgeois, M., Plumet, M. H., … Brunelle, F. (2004). Superior temporal sulcus anatomical abnormalities in childhood autism: A voxel-based morphometry MRI study. *Neuroimage, 23*(1), 364–369.

Boger-Megiddo, I., Shaw, D. W., Friedman, S. D., Sparks, B. F., Artru, A. A., Giedd, J. N., … Dager, S. R. (2006). Corpus callosum morphometrics in young children with autism spectrum disorder. *Journal of Autism and Developmental Disorders, 36*(6), 733–739.

Bruce, C., Desimone, R., & Gross, C. G. (1981). Visual properties of neurons in a polysensory area in superior temporal sulcus of the macaque. *Journal of Neurophysiology, 46*(2), 369–384. https://doi.org/10.1152/jn.1981.46.2.369.

Brun, C. C., Nicolson, R., Leporé, N., et al. (2009). Mapping brain abnormalities in boys with autism. *Human Brain Mapping, 30*(12), 3887–3900.

Caplan, L. (1984). *The insanity defense and the trial of John W. Hinckley, Jr.* David R. Godine
Carlisi, C. O., Norman, L. J., Lukito, S. S., Radua, J., Mataix-Cols, D., & Rubia, K. (2017). Comparative multimodal meta-analysis of structural and functional brain abnormalities in autism spectrum disorder and obsessive-compulsive disorder. *Biological Psychiatry, 82*(2), 83–102.
Carper, R. A., & Courchesne, E. (2000). Inverse correlation between frontal lobe and cerebellum sizes in children with autism. *Brain, 123*(4), 836–844.
Carper, R. A., & Courchesne, E. (2005). Localized enlargement of the frontal cortex in early autism. *Biological Psychiatry, 57*(2), 126–133.
Cheely, C. A., Carpenter, L. A., Letourneau, E. J., Nicholas, J. S., Charles, J., & King, L. B. (2012). The prevalence of youth with autism spectrum disorders in the criminal justice system. *Journal of Autism and Developmental Disorders, 42*(9), 1856–1862. https://doi.org/10.1007/s10803-011-1427-2.
Chung, M. K., Robbins, S. M., Dalton, K. M., Davidson, R. J., Alexander, A. L., & Evans, A. C. (2005). Cortical thickness analysis in autism with heat kernel smoothing. *NeuroImage, 25*(4), 1256–1265.
Ciesielski, K. T., Harris, R. J., Hart, B. L., & Pabst, H. F. (1997). Cerebellar hypoplasia and frontal lobe cognitive deficits in disorders of early childhood. *Neuropsychologia, 35*(5), 643–655.
Cohen, D. J., & Volkmar, F. R. (1997). *Handbook of autism and pervasive developmental disorders.* John Wiley & Sons Inc. (Fred R. Volkmar, Rhea Paul, Ami Klin, Donald J. Cohen, "Asperger Syndrome," Chapter 4).
Constantino, Kennon-McGill, Weichselbaum, Marrus, Haider, Glowinski, Gillespie, Klaiman, Klin & Jones (2017). Infant viewing of social scenes is under genetic control and is atypical in autism. *Nature, 547*(7663), 340–344. https://doi.org/10.1038/nature22999. Epub 2017 July 12.
Corden, B., Chilvers, R., & Skuse, D. (2008). Avoidance of emotionally arousing stimuli predicts social-perceptual impairment in Asperger's syndrome. *Neuropsychologia, 46*(1), 137–147.
Courchesne, E., Campbell, K., & Solso, S. (2011). Brain growth across the life span in autism: Age-specific changes in anatomical pathology. *Brain Research, 1380,* 138–145.
Courchesne, E., Carper, R., & Akshoomoff, N. (2003). Evidence of brain overgrowth in the first year of life in autism. *JAMA, 290*(3), 337–344.
Courchesne, E., Karns, C. M., Davis, H. R., Ziccardi, R., Carper, R. A., Tigue, Z. D., … Lincoln, A. J. (2001). Unusual brain growth patterns in early life in patients with autistic disorder: An MRI study. *Neurology, 57*(2), 245–254.
Courchesne, E., Saitoh, O., Yeung-Courchesne, R., Press, G. A., Lincoln, A. J., Haas, R. H., & Schreibman, L. (1994). Abnormality of cerebellar vermian lobules VI and VII in patients with infantile autism: Identification of hypoplastic and hyperplastic subgroups with MR imaging. *AJR. American Journal of Roentgenology, 162*(1), 123–130.
Courchesne, E., Yeung-Courchesne, R., Hesselink, J. R., & Jernigan, T. L. (1988). Hypoplasia of cerebellar vermal lobules VI and VII in autism. *New England Journal of Medicine, 318*(21), 1349–1354.
Craig, L., Lindsay, W. R. (2010). Sexual offenders with intellectual disabilities: Characteristics and prevalence. In L. Craig, W. R. Lindsay, W. R., & K. D. Browne (Eds.), *Assessment and treatment of sexual offenders with intellectual disabilities* (pp. 13–36). Wiley-Blackwell.
DeBenedictis, D. J. (1990). Criminal minds. *ABA Journal, 76,* 30.
Di Martino, A., Yan, C. G., Li, Q., Denio, E., Castellanos, F. X., Alaerts, K., … Deen, B. (2014). The autism brain imaging data exchange: Towards a large-scale evaluation of the intrinsic brain architecture in autism. *Molecular Psychiatry, 19*(6), 659–667.
Dougherty, C. C., Evans, D. W., Myers, S. M., Moore, G. J., & Michael, A. M. (2016). A comparison of structural brain imaging findings in autism spectrum disorder and attention-deficit hyperactivity disorder. *Neuropsychology Review, 26*(1), 25–43.
Ecker, C., Ginestet, C., Feng, Y., Johnston, P., Lombardo, M. V., Lai, M. C., … Williams, S. C. (2013). Brain surface anatomy in adults with autism: The relationship between surface area, cortical thickness, and autistic symptoms. *JAMA Psychiatry, 70*(1), 59–70.

Elbert, J. M. (2012). A mindful military: Linking brain and behavior through neuroscience at court-martial. *Army Law, 2012,* 4.
Egaas, B., Courchesne, E., & Saitoh, O. (1995). Reduced size of corpus callosum in autism. *Archives of Neurology, 52*(8), 794–801.
Emerson, R. W., Adams, C., Nishino, T, et al. (2017). Functional neuroimaging of high-risk 6-month-old infants predicts a diagnosis of autism at 24 months of age. *Science Translational Medicine, 9*(393): eaag2882.
Faigman, D. L., Monahan, J., & Slobogin, C. (2014). Group to individual (G2i) inference in scientific expert testimony. *The University of Chicago Law Review*, 417–480.
Filipek, P. A., Accardo, P. J., Ashwal, S., Baranek, G. T., Cook, E. H., Dawson, G., ... & Levy, S. E. (2000). Practice parameter: Screening and diagnosis of autism: report of the Quality Standards Subcommittee of the American Academy of Neurology and the Child Neurology Society. *Neurology, 55*(4), 468–479.
Frazier, T. W., & Hardan, A. Y. (2009). A meta-analysis of the corpus callosum in autism. *Biological Psychiatry, 66*(10), 935–941.
Freitag, C. M., Luders, E., Hulst, H. E., Narr, K. L., Thompson, P. M., Toga, A. W., ... Konrad, C. (2009). Total brain volume and corpus callosum size in medication-naive adolescents and young adults with autism spectrum disorder. *Biological Psychiatry, 66*(4), 316–319.
Gallagher, H. L., Happé, F., Brunswick, N., Fletcher, P. C., Frith, U., & Frith, C. D. (2000). Reading the mind in cartoons and stories: An fMRI study of 'theory of mind' in verbal and nonverbal tasks. *Neuropsychologia, 38*(1), 11–21.
Gaudet, L. M., & Marchant, G. E. (2016). Under the radar: Neuroimaging evidence in the criminal courtroom. *Drake Law Review, 64,* 577.
Girgis, R. R., Minshew, N. J., Melhem, N. M., Nutche, J. J., Keshavan, M. S., & Hardan, A. Y. (2007). Volumetric alterations of the orbitofrontal cortex in autism. *Progress in Neuro-Psychopharmacology and Biological Psychiatry, 31*(1), 41–45.
Goffman, E. (1959). The presentation of self in everyday life, doubleday.
Gutstein, S. E., & Whitney, T. (2002) Asperger Syndrome and the development of social competence. *Focus on Autism and Other Developmental Disabilities, 17*(3, Fall), 161–171.
Haar, S., Berman, S., Behrmann, M., & Dinstein, I. (2016). Anatomical abnormalities in autism? *Cerebral Cortex, 26*(4), 1440–1452.
Hadjikhani, N., Joseph, R. M., Snyder, J., & Tager-Flusberg, H. (2006). Anatomical differences in the mirror neuron system and social cognition network in autism. *Cerebral Cortex, 16*(9), 1276–1282.
Happe, F., Ehlers, S., Fletcher, P., Frith, U., Johansson, M., Gillberg, C., ... Frith, C. (1996). 'Theory of mind' in the brain. Evidence from a PET scan study of Asperger syndrome. *Neuroreport, 8*(1), 197–201.
Hardan, A. Y., Jou, R. J., Keshavan, M. S., Varma, R., & Minshew, N. J. (2004). Increased frontal cortical folding in autism: A preliminary MRI study. *Psychiatry Research: Neuroimaging, 131*(3), 263–268.
Hardan, A. Y., Minshew, N. J., & Keshavan, M. S. (2000). Corpus callosum size in autism. *Neurology, 55*(7), 1033–1036.
Hazlett, H. C., Gu, H., Munsell, B. C., Kim, S. H., Styner, M., Wolff, J. J., ... Collins, D. L. (2017). Early brain development in infants at high risk for autism spectrum disorder. *Nature, 542*(7641), 348–351.
Hazlett, H. C., Poe, M., Gerig, G., Smith, R. G., Provenzale, J., Ross, A., ... Piven, J. (2005). Magnetic resonance imaging and head circumference study of brain size in autism: Birth through age 2 years. *Archives of General Psychiatry, 62*(12), 1366–1376.
Herbert, M. R., Ziegler, D. A., Makris, N., Filipek, P. A., Kemper, T. L., Normandin, J. J., ... Caviness Jr., V. S. (2004). Localization of white matter volume increase in autism and developmental language disorder. *Annals of Neurology, 55*(4), 530–540.

Howard, M. A., Cowell, P. E., Boucher, J., Broks, P., Mayes, A., Farrant, A., & Roberts, N. (2000). Convergent neuroanatomical and behavioural evidence of an amygdala hypothesis of autism. *Neuroreport, 11*(13), 2931–2935.
Howlin, P., & Goode, S. (2000). Outcome in adult life for people with autism and Asperger's syndrome. *Autism, 4*(1), 63–83.
Jiao, Y., Chen, R., Ke, X., Chu, K., Lu, Z., & Herskovits, E. H. (2010). Predictive models of autism spectrum disorder based on brain regional cortical thickness. *Neuroimage, 50*(2), 589–599.
Johnson, M. H., Gliga, T., Jones, E., & Charman, T. (2015). Annual Research Review: Infant development, autism, and ADHD–early pathways to emerging disorders. *Journal of Child Psychology and Psychiatry, 56*(3), 228–247.
Johnson, C. P., & Myers, S. M. (2007). Identification and evaluation of children with autism spectrum disorders. *Pediatrics, 120*(5), 1183–1215.
Just, M. A., Cherkassky, V. L., Keller, T. A., Kana, R. K., & Minshew, N. J. (2007). Functional and anatomical cortical underconnectivity in autism: Evidence from an FMRI study of an executive function task and corpus callosum morphometry. *Cerebral Cortex, 17*(4), 951–961.
Klin, A. (2000). Attributing social meaning to ambiguous visual stimuli in higher-functioning autism and Asperger syndrome: The social attribution task. *Journal of Child Psychology and Psychiatry, 41*(7), 831–846.
Klin, A., McPartland, J., & Volkmar, F. R. (2005). Asperger syndrome In Fred R. Volkmar, R. Paul, A. Klin, & Donald J. (Eds.), *Cohen Handbook of autism and pervasive developmental disorders*, (Vol. 1, Diagnosis, Development, Neurobiology, and Behavior, 3rd Ed., pp. 105). Wiley.
Koyama, A. (2009). A review on the cognitive neuroscience of autism. *Activitas Nervosa Superior, 51*(4), 125–139.
Kulynych, J. (1996). Brain, mind, and criminal behavior: Neuroimages as scientific evidence. *Jurimetrics, 36*(3), 235–244.
Kylliäinen, A., & Hietanen, J. K. (2004). Attention orienting by another's gaze direction in children with autism. *Journal of Child Psychology and Psychiatry, 45*(3), 435–444.
Lai, M. C., Lerch, J. P., Floris, D. L., Ruigrok, A. N., Pohl, A., Lombardo, M. V., & Baron-Cohen, S. (2017). Imaging sex/gender and autism in the brain: Etiological implications. *Journal of Neuroscience Research, 95*(1–2), 380–397.
Langen, M., Bos, D., Noordermeer, S. D., Nederveen, H., van Engeland, H., & Durston, S. (2014). Changes in the development of striatum are involved in repetitive behavior in autism. *Biological Psychiatry, 76*(5), 405–411.
Lerner, M. D., Haque, O. S., Northrup, E. C., Lawer, L., & Bursztajn, H. J. (2012). Emerging perspectives on adolescents and young adults with high-functioning autism spectrum disorders, violence, and criminal law. *Journal of the American Academy of Psychiatry and the Law Online, 40*(2), 177–190.
Levitt, J. G., Blanton, R. E., Smalley, S., Thompson, P. M., Guthrie, D., McCracken, J. T., … Toga, A. (2003). Cortical sulcal maps in autism. *Cerebral Cortex, 13*(7), 728–735.
Lewis, J. D., Evans, A. C., Pruett Jr, J. R., Botteron, K. N., McKinstry, R. C., Zwaigenbaum, L., … Dager, S. R. (2017). The emergence of network inefficiencies in infants with autism spectrum disorder. *Biological Psychiatry, 82*(3), 176–185.
Lindsay, W. R. (2009). *The treatment of sex offenders with developmental disabilities.* Wiley-Blackwell.
Lindsay, W. R., Carson, D., O'Brien, G., Holland, A. J., Taylor, J. L., Wheeler, J. R., & Steptoe, L. (2014). A comparison of referrals with and without Autism Spectrum Disorder to forensic intellectual disability services. *Psychiatry, Psychology and Law, 21*(6), 947–954.
Loveland, K. (1991). Social affordances and interaction II: Autism and the affordances of the human environment. *Ecological Psychology, 3,* 99–120.
Manes, F., Piven, J., Vrancic, D., Nanclares, V., Plebst, C., & Starkstein, S. E. (1999). An MRI study of the corpus callosum and cerebellum in mentally retarded autistic individuals. *The Journal of Neuropsychiatry and Clinical Neurosciences, 11*(4), 470–474.

McAlonan, G. M., Cheung, V., Cheung, C., Suckling, J., Lam, G. Y., Tai, K. S., … Chua, S. E. (2005). Mapping the brain in autism. A voxel-based MRI study of volumetric differences and intercorrelations in autism. *Brain, 128*(2), 268–276.

McAlonan, G. M., Daly, E., Kumari, V., Critchley, H. D., Amelsvoort, T. V., Suckling, J., … Schmitz, N. (2002). Brain anatomy and sensorimotor gating in Asperger's syndrome. *Brain, 125*(7), 1594–1606.

Mesibov, G. B., Shea V, & Adams L. W. (2001). *Understanding Asperger syndrome and high-functioning autism.* The Autism Spectrum Disorders Library 1. Kluwer Academic/Plenum Publishers.

Mesibov, G., Shea, V., & Adams, L. (2001). Understanding Asperger syndrome and high-functioning autism. In G. Mesibov (Ed.), *The autism spectrum disorders library* (Vol. 1, p. 10). Heidelberg: Springer.

Mogavero, M. C. (2016). Autism, sexual offending, and the criminal justice system. *Journal of Intellectual Disabilities and Offending Behaviour.*

Morse, S. J. (2011). The status of NueroLaw: A plea for current modesty and future cautious optimism. *The Journal of Psychiatry & Law, 39,* 595.

Muhle, R. A., Reed, H. E., Stratigos, K. A., & Veenstra-VanderWeele, J. (2018). The emerging clinical neuroscience of autism spectrum disorder: A review. *JAMA Psychiatry, 75*(5), 514–523.

Munson, J., Dawson, G., Abbott, R., Faja, S., Webb, S. J., Friedman, S. D., … Dager, S. R. (2006). Amygdalar volume and behavioral development in autism. *Archives of General Psychiatry, 63*(6), 686–693.

Murakami, J. W., Courchesne, E., Press, G. A., Yeung-Courchesne, R., & Hesselink, J. R. (1989). Reduced cerebellar hemisphere size and its relationship to vermal hypoplasia in autism. *Archives of Neurology, 46*(6), 689–694.

Njiokiktjien, C., Verschoor, A., de Sonneville, L., Huyser, C., Op het Veld, V., & Toorenaar, N. (2001). Disordered recognition of facial identity and emotions in three Asperger type autists. *European Child & Adolescent Psychiatry, 10*(1), 79–90. https://doi.org/10.1007/s007870170050.

Nordahl, C. W., Lange, N., Li, D. D., Barnett, L. A., Lee, A., Buonocore, M. H., … Amaral, D. G. (2011). Brain enlargement is associated with regression in preschool-age boys with autism spectrum disorders. *Proceedings of the National Academy of Sciences, 108*(50), 20195–20200.

Nordahl, C. W., Scholz, R., Yang, X., Buonocore, M. H., Simon, T., Rogers, S., & Amaral, D. G. (2012). Increased rate of amygdala growth in children aged 2 to 4 years with autism spectrum disorders: A longitudinal study. *Archives of General Psychiatry, 69*(1), 53–61.

Ogai, M., Matsumoto, H., Suzuki, K., Ozawa, F., Fukuda, R., Uchiyama, I., … Takei, N. (2003). (2003). fMRI study of recognition of facial expressions in high-functioning autistic patients. *Neuroreport, 14*(4), 559–563.

Oullier, O. (2012). Clear up this fuzzy thinking on brain scans. *Nature, 483*(7387), 7–7. https://www.nature.com/news/clear-up-this-fuzzy-thinking-on-brain-scans-1.10127.

Ozonoff, S., Pennington, B. F., & Rogers, S. J. (1991). Executive function deficits in high-functioning autistic individuals: Relation to theory of mind. *Journal of Child Psychology and Psychiatry, 32*(7), 1081–1105.

Perner, J., Lang, B. (2000). Theory of mind and executive function: Is there a developmental relationship? In S. Baron-Cohen, H. Tager-Flusberg, & D. Cohen (Eds). *Understanding other minds: Perspectives from autism and developmental cognitive neuroscience* (2nd ed., pp. 150–181). England: Oxford University Press; Oxford.

Pierce, K., Müller, R. A., Ambrose, J., Allen, G., & Courchesne, E. (2001). Face processing occurs outside the fusiform face area'in autism: Evidence from functional MRI. *Brain, 124*(10), 2059–2073.

Piven, J., Bailey, J., Ranson, B. J., & Arndt, S. (1997). An MRI study of the corpus callosum in autism. *American Journal of Psychiatry, 154*(8), 1051–1056.

Piven, J., Saliba, K., Bailey, J., & Arndt, S. (1997). An MRI study of autism: The cerebellum revisited. *Neurology, 49*(2), 546–551.

Redcay, E., & Courchesne, E. (2005). When is the brain enlarged in autism? A meta-analysis of all brain size reports. *Biological Psychiatry, 58*(1), 1–9.
Ring, H. A., Baron-Cohen, S., Wheelwright, S., Williams, S. C., Brammer, M., Andrew, C., & Bullmore, E. T. (1999). Cerebral correlates of preserved cognitive skills in autism: A functional MRI study of embedded figures task performance. *Brain, 122*(7), 1305–1315.
Sabbagh, M. A., Xu, F., Carlson, S. M., Moses, L. J., & Lee, K. (2006). The development of executive functioning and theory of mind. A comparison of Chinese and U.S. preschoolers. *Psychological Science, 17*(1), 74–81. https://doi.org/10.1111/j.1467-9280.2005.01667.x.
Saitoh, O., Courchesne, E., Egaas, B., Lincoln, A. J., & Schreibman, L. (1995). Cross-sectional area of the posterior hippocampus in autistic patients with cerebellar and corpus callosum abnormalitiGs. *Neurology, 45*(2), 317–324.
Scheel, C., Rotarska-Jagiela, A., Schilbach, L., Lehnhardt, F. G., Krug, B., Vogeley, K., & Tepest, R. (2011). Imaging derived cortical thickness reduction in high-functioning autism: Key regions and temporal slope. *Neuroimage, 58*(2), 391–400.
Schultz, R. T., Gauthier, I., Klin, A., Fulbright, R. K., Anderson, A. W., Volkmar, F., Skudlarski, P., Lacadie, C., Cohen, D. J., & Gore, J. C. (2000). Abnormal ventral temporal cortical activity during face discrimination among individuals with autism and Asperger syndrome. *Archives of General Psychiatry, 57*(4), 331–340. https://doi.org/10.1001/archpsyc.57.4.331.
Scott, J. A., Schumann, C. M., Goodlin-Jones, B. L., & Amaral, D. G. (2009). A comprehensive volumetric analysis of the cerebellum in children and adolescents with autism spectrum disorder. *Autism Research, 2*(5), 246–257.
Schumann, C. M., Barnes, C. C., Lord, C., & Courchesne, E. (2009). Amygdala enlargement in toddlers with autism related to severity of social and communication impairments. *Biological Psychiatry, 66*(10), 942–949.
Schumann, C. M., Hamstra, J., Goodlin-Jones, B. L., Lotspeich, L. J., Kwon, H., Buonocore, M. H., … Amaral, D. G. (2004). The amygdala is enlarged in children but not adolescents with autism; the hippocampus is enlarged at all ages. *Journal of neuroscience, 24*(28), 6392–6401.
Shen, M. D., Nordahl, C. W., Young, G. S., Wootton-Gorges, S. L., Lee, A., Liston, S. E., … Amaral, D. G. (2013). Early brain enlargement and elevated extra-axial fluid in infants who develop autism spectrum disorder. *Brain, 136*(9), 2825–2835.
Sparks, B. F., Friedman, S. D., Shaw, D. W., et al. (2002). Brain structural abnormalities in young children with autism spectrum disorder. *Neurology, 59*(2), 184–192.
Stanfield, A. C., McIntosh, A. M., Spencer, M. D., Philip, R., Gaur, S., & Lawrie, S. M. (2008). Towards a neuroanatomy of autism: A systematic review and meta-analysis of structural magnetic resonance imaging studies. *European Psychiatry, 23*(4), 289–299.
Stern, M. J. (2014, June). Serving on the jury? The scientific forensic evidence you'll hear isn't scientific. *Slate Magazine.*
Venter, A., Lord, C., & Schopler, E. (1992). A follow-up study of high-functioning autistic children. *Journal of Child Psychology & Psychiatry & Allied Disciplines, 33*(3), 489–507
Vidal, C. N., Nicolson, R., DeVito, T. J., Hayashi, K. M., Geaga, J. A., Drost, D. J., … Toga, A. W. (2006). Mapping corpus callosum deficits in autism: An index of aberrant cortical connectivity. *Biological Psychiatry, 60*(3), 218–225.
Waiter, G. D., Williams, J. H., Murray, A. D., Gilchrist, A., Perrett, D. I., & Whiten, A. (2005). Structural white matter deficits in high-functioning individuals with autistic spectrum disorder: A voxel-based investigation. *Neuroimage, 24*(2), 455–461.
Wallace, G. L., Dankner, N., Kenworthy, L., Giedd, J. N., & Martin, A. (2010). Age related temporal and parietal cortical thinning in autism spectrum disorders. *Brain, 133,* 3745–3754.
Wallace, G.L., Shaw, P., Lee, N.R., Clasen, L.S., Raznahan, A., Lenroot, R.K., Martin, A., & Giedd, J.N. (2012). Distinct cortical correlates of autistic versus antisocial traits in a longitudinal sample of typically developing youth. *The Journal of Neuroscience, 32*(14), 4856–4860.
Wolff, J. J., Gu, H., Gerig, G., Elison, J. T., Styner, M., Gouttard, S., … Evans, A. C. (2012). Differences in white matter fiber tract development present from 6 to 24 months in infants with autism. *American Journal of Psychiatry, 169*(6), 589–600.

Wolff, J. J., Jacob, S., & Elison, J. T. (2018). The journey to autism: Insights from neuroimaging studies of infants and toddlers. *Development and Psychopathology, 30*(2), 479.
Yang, Y., & Raine, A. (2009). Prefrontal structural and functional brain imaging findings in antisocial, violent, and psychopathic individuals: A meta-analysis. *Psychiatry Research, 174,* 81–88. https://doi.org/10.1016/j.pscychresns.2009.03.012.
Zilbovicius, M., Boddaert, N., Belin, P., Poline, J. B., Remy, P., Mangin, J. F., ... Samson, Y. (2000). Temporal lobe dysfunction in childhood autism: A PET study. *American Journal of Psychiatry, 157*(12), 1988–1993.
Zürcher, N. R., Bhanot, A., McDougle, C. J., & Hooker, J. M. (2015). A systematic review of molecular imaging (PET and SPECT) in autism spectrum disorder: Current state and future research opportunities. *Neuroscience and Biobehavioral Reviews, 52,* 56–73.

Stephanie Yarnell-Mac Grory is on faculty at the Yale School of Medicine within the Department of Psychiatry. Yarnell-Mac Grory is dual fellowship trained in Addiction Psychiatry and Forensic Psychiatry.

Mark Mahoney is exclusively defending person with social learning differences on criminal accusations in the United States. He is currently a Partner at Harrington & Mahoney, Buffalo, NY. Previously: Lecturer, University of Buffalo Law School; Founder, President, New York State Association of Criminal Defense Lawyers; Board of Directors, National Association of Criminal Defense Lawyers (USA).

Alexander Westphal is on faculty at the Yale School of Medicine within the Department of Psychiatry. Westphal is dual fellowship trained in Child and Adolescent Psychiatry and Forensic Psychiatry.

Chapter 5
Trauma in Individuals with Autism Spectrum Disorder: An Empirically Informed Model of Assessment and Intervention to Address the Effects of Traumatic Events

Alexia Stack and Joseph Lucyshyn

The study of traumatic events and their effects on individuals has received increased attention in the literature. For the purposes of this chapter, trauma is defined as a psychological injury that causes damage or harm to the person, and which varies in terms of its permanency, severity, and longevity (Kerns et al., 2015). A trauma may occur as a single event or can occur repeatedly, both of which can harm an individual psychologically if the experience was perceived to be threatening. Traumas can be placed on a spectrum of severity of experience. On one end of the spectrum, a trauma can be minor and easily overcome. On the other end of the spectrum, trauma can be severe. The repercussions of severe trauma are alterations in one's life-functioning (Kerns et al., 2015), and disease and morbidity in adulthood (Felitti et al., 1998). When psychological trauma occurs, feelings of helplessness, intense fear and horror (Sherin & Nemeroff, 2011) can lead to the development of post-traumatic stress disorder (PTSD) (Copeland et al., 2007), and Complex-Post Traumatic Stress Disorder (CPTSD) (Courtois, 2008). A range of sequelae such as depression, anxiety, addiction, medical problems, difficulties with relationships and dissociation may develop (Copeland et al., 2007; Courtois, 2008). As such, exposure to a single traumatic event or repeated traumatic events is a public health risk given the potential long-term consequences on the development and long-term functioning of the individual (Hibbard & Desch, 2007; Kerns et al., 2015).

Children in general are more vulnerable to maltreatment as they are dependent on the care of adults. Individuals with developmental disabilities may be at a greater

A. Stack (✉)
A Block Above Behavioral Consulting, North Vancouver, BC, Canada
e-mail: alexia@ablockabove.com

J. Lucyshyn
University of British Columbia, Vancouver, BC, Canada
e-mail: joe.lucyshyn@ubc.ca

F. R. Volkmar et al. (eds.), *Handbook of Autism Spectrum Disorder and the Law*,
https://doi.org/10.1007/978-3-030-70913-6_5

risk for being maltreated as compared to their typical peers (Hibbard & Desch, 2007; Kerns et al., 2015). Children with developmental disabilities struggle with their communication skills, are more likely to be socially isolated, and are prone to experiencing high levels of familial stress. These factors are common in individuals with Autism Spectrum Disorder (ASD), and make them more susceptible to maltreatment (Sullivan & Knutson, 2000). ASD is a developmental disorder characterized by social and communication deficits, restricted interests and behaviors, and intellectual disability in 33% of cases (Maenner et al., 2020). Other common characteristics of children, youth, and adults with ASD are that they are socially naive and inappropriate, which may make them more prone to victimization (Berg et al., 2016; Hoover, 2015; Kerns et al., 2015, 2017). All of these characteristics taken together potentiate the risk of maltreatment and exposure to traumatic life events in children with ASD. Despite the many factors that make children with ASD more prone to the experience of trauma, there is a paucity of research in the field. Accurate attribution of the symptoms of trauma to individuals with ASD is difficult to make due to the associated behavioral problems common in individuals on the spectrum. The observable behavior problems associated with some children with ASD, such as self-injury, also are common to individuals who have suffered from trauma, thereby making a diagnostic discrimination between ASD and the side effects of trauma clinically challenging (Brenner et al., 2017). Additionally, evidence-based treatment of trauma in children with ASD has not been established (Brenner et al., 2017).

For society to protect this highly vulnerable population, the assessment and treatment of trauma caused by some form of abuse by another person have implications for the individual's civil rights. If trauma due to abuse cannot be proven because the child lacks the ability to provide oral evidence of the abusive event that led to child's traumatic responses, then justice is not served and the individual who engaged in abuse is free to do so again. Rather than expecting a child to be able to speak in order to report abuse, accommodating the child's disability in court ought to be the solution so that the child can communicate to a jury. Although the court system has improved in its openness to accommodations, there is much work to be done in this area (Goldfarb & Gonzalez, 2018). Prosecutors need to have an understanding of the social and communication challenges of children with ASD, why children on the spectrum are more prone to abuse, and how to help children with Autism communicate their experiences of abuse (American Bar Association, 2013). The prosecutor's role also becomes to familiarize themselves with how an individual client communicates, and to file for special accommodations in court (Rainville, 2013). As well, if the effects of such abuse require treatment and a perpetrator is found guilty, then the court can mandate treatment. The purpose of this chapter is multifold. We will briefly review the literature regarding the effects of trauma on child development; examine why children with ASD may have an increased vulnerability to trauma and the present understanding of how symptoms of trauma and PTSD are expressed; provide an overview of the assessment and treatment of trauma in typically developing children; and suggest a modified treatment model for working with trauma in children with ASD followed by a case study of the application of the treatment model to a child on the autism spectrum.

Trauma and Its Effects on Development

The age at which children are first traumatized, the frequency of the trauma, and the role of the caregiver in the event itself have an impact on the severity of the psychological damage (van der Kolk, 2003). Trauma responses in children are most likely to occur within the context of intimate relationships, such as in cases of neglect and abuse (Koerner, 2012; van der Kolk & Najavits, 2013). The American Psychiatric Association (2013) holds that children suffering from PTSD experience intense feelings of fear, helplessness, or horror as a result of being exposed to a traumatic event, resulting in behavior that is disorganized and agitated. Behavior problems are a common feature of children who have suffered a trauma (American Psychiatric Association, 2013). Generally speaking, exposure to traumatic events in childhood may have nocuous effects on the child's neurobiological, emotional, and cognitive development (Perry et al., 1995).

Neurobiological Effects

Exposure to repeated traumatic events or chronic trauma can cause changes in a person's neural structures and sensory systems. Environmental threats are detected by the prefrontal cortex, amygdala, and hippocampus (McEwan, 2007). When a psychosocial stress is perceived, the hippocampus and prefrontal cortex activate the firing of the amygdala. The amygdala then triggers the locus coeruleus, which in turn activates the sympathetic nervous system (i.e., the fight vs. flight response; Danese & McEwen, 2012). These are the brain structures that are in turn affected in individuals with PTSD (Sherin & Nemeroff, 2011). Systems most affected by traumatic stress are those that are critical for mediating arousal states, executive functioning, behavioral regulation, and memory.

The amygdala plays a role in emotional processing and in acquiring fear responses (Sherin & Nemeroff, 2011). The amygdala evaluates whether stimuli are potentially threatening. For example, when one sees a potential aggressor and perceives what may be dangerous intention on his/her part, the amygdala initiates a series of behavioral, emotional, and hormonal responses (Yehuda, 2006). Thus, it initiates responses within the sympathetic and parasympathetic nervous systems (van der Kolk, 2003; Yehuda, 2006). Signals that are sent by the amygdala to the brain stem begin startle responses and initiate defensive behaviors. Therefore, when trauma occurs early in a child's development, or, as Courtois (2008) suggests, in unfavorable conditions throughout one's life, the repeated activation of the amygdala results in the conditioning of fear responses.

When trauma occurs during development, the limbic system is affected. The limbic system is comprised of the hypothalamus, amygdala, and hippocampus (see Fig. 5.1). It ensures that the regulatory functions of the hypothalamus and brain stem are fine-tuned, and acts as a filter that helps to determine what sensory information requires

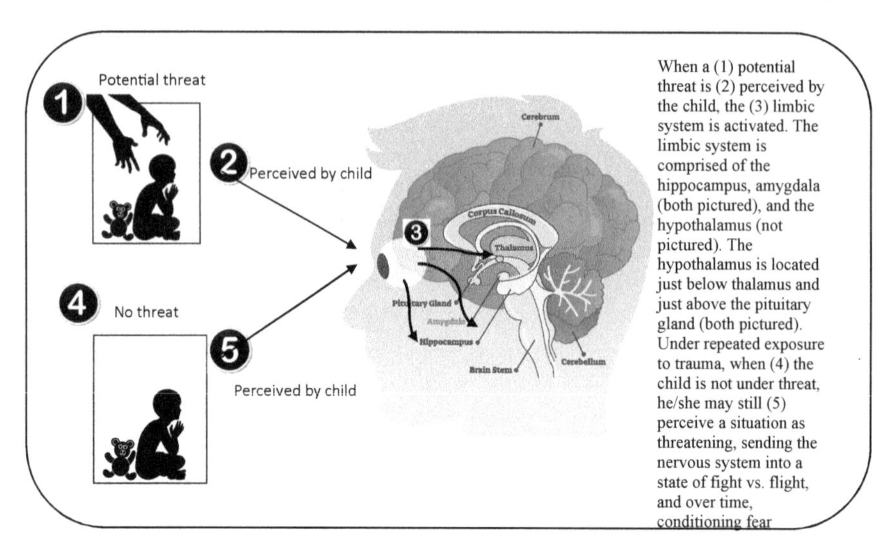

Fig. 5.1 The limbic system when exposed to trauma or under threat as perceived by the child (Reproduced from Stack & Lucyshyn, 2018)

further processing (Sherin & Nemeroff, 2011; van der Kolk, 2003). In infants, the hippocampus develops gradually in the first 5 years, resulting in the central nervous system (CNS) not being fully developed in early childhood (van der Kolk, 2003). Consequently, when a child experiences a threat, the limbic system is activated much faster than the prefrontal cortex is able to evaluate the nature of the stimulus (see Fig. 1.1 in Chap. 1). Although controversial, van der Kolk (2003) argues that the role of primary caregivers is to mediate threat within the infant's environment. If the amygdala is sending signals to the organism to activate the fight or flight response, the caregiver can act as mediator in the infant's response to a threat by helping to calm the nervous system (van der Kolk, 2003). Further adding to the debate, van der Kolk (2003) maintains that most functions are mediated by caregivers until the CNS is fully developed. For example, when children are not soothed when under extreme duress, they develop problems with impulse control, aggression, emotion regulation, and cognition. Additionally, research has demonstrated that reduced hippocampal volume is a feature of PTSD. The hippocampus plays a role in responses to stress, explicit memory, and fear conditioning (Sherin & Nemeroff, 2011). Decreased hippocampal volume may both promote the onset and the failure to terminate stress responses. Additionally, reduced volume in the hippocampus may contribute to conditioned fear responses, and difficulties with discriminating unsafe versus safe situations (Sherin & Nemeroff, 2011).

Emotion regulation. Emotion regulation (ER) can be best understood within the framework of a biopsychosocial model. ER refers to a group of processes that work together so that the individual can appropriately react and modify one's emotional response to meet a variety of situational demands (Gross & Thompson, 2007). Samson et al. (2015) describe two primary paths that individuals employ to regulate their emotions: (a) cognitive reappraisal, and (b) expressive suppression. Cognitive reappraisal is a strategy that involves cognitive changes and is adaptive. Expressive suppression occurs when the person modulates the expression of the emotional response. When used as a primary method of emotion regulation, it is believed to be maladaptive (Samson et al., 2015). In those who have experienced trauma, van der Kolk and Najavits (2013) describe a range of possible emotional responses on a spectrum from states of hypoarousal to hyperarousal. Living in a state of hypoarousal involves dissociation. Dissociation occurs when an individual is experiencing a traumatic event (e.g., victimization, abuse, crime), and leads to a disconnection between the person and his or her environment in circumstances where the trauma is more than one can bear (APA, 2013). An individual can dissociate the memory of the place in which the trauma occurred, the memory of the trauma, and the emotions about the event. The prolonged use of maladaptive emotion regulation strategies such as emotional arousal, emotional numbing, and rumination are believed to contribute to other negative life outcomes such as difficulties with social functioning, anxiety, and depression (Mazefsky et al., 2014).

Cognitive Development

Cognitive development can be delayed in children who have incurred or who are experiencing trauma. Past or ongoing trauma may interfere with one's ability to learn. van der Kolk (2003) argues that a calm physiological state is required for optimal learning conditions. Given that neurobiological systems are activated for survival even when children are safe, the heightened states can lead to learning challenges (van der Kolk, 2003). Children who are traumatized may overly attend to sources of threat in their environment, leaving them in states of hyperarousal for extended periods of time, in turn leading to generalized learning problems and struggle with overall academic achievement. At times, novel information can lead to physiological arousal, leaving the child overstimulated, feeling threatened, and dissociated, incapable of learning (Streek-Fischer & van der Kolk, 2000). From the perspective of the traumatized child, the world is a terrifying place, and as such, there is little desire to explore it, resulting in inflexibility and an insistence on sameness (Streek-Fischer & van der Kolk, 2000).

Enlow et al. (2012) conducted the first longitudinal study measuring the long-term effects of interpersonal trauma (IPT) on cognitive functioning experienced by children from birth to 5 years of age. They defined IPT as being witness to maternal partner violence or experiencing physical, emotional, sexual abuse, or neglect. The study included 206 participants from the Minnesota Longitudinal Study of Parents and Children. Measures of exposure to IPT occurred via home observations, maternal interviews, laboratory visits, reviews of child protection records, and medical records. At 24, 64, and 96 months of age, child intelligent quotient (IQ) scores were measured. IPT, particularly during the first 2 years of life, was found to have had significant and long-lasting detrimental effects on cognitive development.

Autism and Trauma

What we know of typical development in children who have experienced trauma tells us that there are detrimental effects on their neurobiological, emotional, and cognitive development. Children diagnosed with ASD may be at increased risk for exposure to traumatic life events (Berg et al., 2016; Hoover, 2015; Kerns et al., 2015, 2017; Rigles, 2016). Yet, whether children with ASD have an increased predisposition to trauma, are more vulnerable to trauma, or may develop symptoms of PTSD is not well understood. The literature is in its infancy, leaving more questions than answers (Brenner et al., 2017; Kerns et al., 2015). For example, is the sudden emergence of self-injury in a child with ASD a symptom of his/her ASD or a result of exposure to trauma? Kerns et al. (2015) point out that the symptoms of traumatic stress and ASD are behaviorally defined, resulting in potential diagnostic overlap with one another. This may lead to difficulties in discriminating the effects of trauma on individuals with ASD. They ask, are hyperarousal, flattened affect, difficulties with attention, self-injury, and inflexibility the resulting effects of ASD or trauma? Are the core symptoms of ASD made worse in children who have incurred trauma or who have a comorbid diagnosis of PTSD (Brenner et al., 2017)? Are the preexisting symptoms of ASD exacerbated in cases where the individual has suffered trauma(s)? What are the vulnerabilities or effects on neurobiology, cognitive development and processes, emotion regulation, and behavioral symptoms? Below we discuss some of what is presently known in the literature regarding vulnerability to trauma and how the symptoms associated with trauma or PTSD may be expressed in persons with ASD.

Neurobiology

The limbic-hypothalamic–pituitary–adrenal (LHPA) axis, whose role it is to regulate stress and other bodily functions such as emotion, mood, immune responses, and digestion, has been shown to be dysregulated in individuals with ASD and those who have experienced trauma (Danese & McEwen, 2012). Children with ASD have higher levels of salivary cortisol in response to novel and threatening stimuli (Corbett et al., 2008). Examples of stimuli that may cause elevated cortisol levels are psychosocial stress or sensory stimuli (Corbett et al., 2008). Additionally, children with ASD exhibit elevations in salivary cortisol levels when anticipating reexposure to perceived stressors (Corbett et al., 2008). These pre-existing, inherently weak stress responses may increase vulnerability to the future experience of trauma, or increase traumatic responses to environmental stimuli in individuals with ASD. Such responses may in turn initiate a cycle of biological and behavioral dysregulation (Kerns et al., 2015).

As has been demonstrated in the literature with typically developing children exposed to trauma, the stress imposed on the amygdala leads to the emergence of conditioned fear responses, and increased perceptions of threat (Courtois, 2008; van der Kolk, 2003; Yehuda, 2006). In individuals with ASD, the prefrontal cortex and amygdala, areas associated with emotion regulation, have been shown to have alterations in functional connectivity (Mazefsky et al., 2013). Kerns et al. (2015) suggest that these correlates may offer understanding into the particular vulnerabilities of children with ASD and the development of trauma-related pathology.

Cognitive Development and Processes

Another potential predisposition to the development of traumatic stress is differences in cognitive processes in individuals with ASD (Kerns et al., 2015). These differences may lead to a limited ability to use effective coping strategies such as cognitive reappraisal or problem-solving in response to trauma. The cognitive deficits of individuals with ASD such as impairments in the processing of information, emotional insight, and difficulties with goal-directed behavior may reduce the use of strategies that are adaptive in terms of ER. This can in turn lead to a heightened trauma response (Mazefsky et al., 2013; Wood & Gadow, 2010). Kerns et al. suggest that individuals with ASD may struggle to shift their thoughts in relation to their traumatic experiences, ruminating on the memories of the trauma, or they may be unable to think flexibly about their experience.

Research pertaining to the long-term effects on cognitive functioning has yet to be extended to individuals with ASD. The emergent literature in typically developing children has demonstrated that IQ is significantly affected as a result of being exposed to IPT in the first 5 years of life (Enlow et al., 2012). Given that children with ASD have a range of learning challenges, and in some cases, lower than average IQ's (Centers for Disease Control and Prevention, 2016), it may too be the case that IPT, as well as other traumatic experiences could lead to significant changes in IQ in this population. Future research in this area is needed, as it may inform education and treatment of trauma in children with ASD.

Emotion Regulation

Given that the experience of trauma leads to difficulty with emotion regulation (Koerner, 2012), it is surprising that so little is known in regard to emotion regulation in individuals with ASD who have been exposed to traumatic life events. Increasingly it is recognized that ASD involves problems with ER in terms of the frequency, duration, and intensity with which emotion is experienced (Samson et al., 2015). Gross (2013) suggests that some individuals with ASD fail to regulate their emotions altogether, whereas others use strategies that are not adaptive. Samson et al. (2015) found that participants with ASD, aged 8–20, were less likely to use cognitive reappraisal as an ER strategy, which in turn led to increases in negative emotion and higher levels of maladaptive behavior. Some research also suggests that individuals with ASD may have biological vulnerabilities that increase the likelihood of impaired

ER, such as atypical neural reactivity (Pitskel et al., 2014) and heart rate variability that is atypical (Guy et al., 2014).

Behavioral Symptoms

Brenner et al. (2017) conducted the first exploratory study, examining the behavioral symptoms of PTSD with a sample of children with ASD, with parent/caregiver reported histories of abuse. Results from their study found that children with ASD with a reported history of abuse and a comorbid diagnosis of PTSD, reported more fear, tantrums, intrusive thoughts, and upsetting memories than their peers with a caregiver reported history of abuse, but without a diagnosis of PTSD (Brenner et al., 2017). The data suggest that children with ASD experience similar symptoms to those that meet the diagnostic criteria for PTSD, but that there is an overlap in symptoms in children with ASD who do and do not have reported histories of abuse, making the discrimination of symptoms challenging (Brenner et al., 2017). Additionally, it was found that some symptoms commonly associated with PTSD (i.e., sleep difficulties, fear, anger, problems with attention, and irritability) did not differ significantly between children with and without abuse histories, possibly because these symptoms also are common in children with ASD (Brenner et al., 2017). Brenner et al. (2017) argue that diagnostic overshadowing may have been at play in this population when diagnosing PTSD in this sample of children, as children with ASD in general present with complex emotional and behavioral symptoms. This in turn may have led clinicians to inadvertently impose a higher threshold for diagnosing PTSD (Brenner et al., 2017). Further research is needed to further develop a deeper understanding of vulnerabilities to trauma, the symptoms of traumatic stress, and PTSD in children with ASD. This can in turn lead to the development of ASD-specific assessment and treatment.

Assessment of Trauma in Children

To effectively plan for treatment, it is imperative to implement assessments that are developmentally appropriate and psychometrically sound (King et al., 2017). To date, a number of assessments have been developed to assess for history and symptoms of trauma in children. Assessment of trauma can be completed by the child as informant or by the parent or caregiver as informant (Lanktree et al., 2008). Examples of the child as informant assessment instruments include: (a) Trauma Symptom Checklist (TSCC; Briere, 1996); (b) UCLA PTSD-Reaction Index (Steinberg et al., 2004); and (c) Angie/Andy Cartoon Trauma Scales (ACTS; Praver et al., 2000). Examples of parent/caregiver as informant assessment instruments include: (a) Abuse Dimensions Inventory (ADI; Chaffin et al., 1997); and (b) Trauma Symptoms Checklist for Young Children (TSCYC; Briere, 1996).

Lanktree et al. (2008) evaluated the psychometric properties of the TSCC and TSCYC. Participants were 335 children and their primary caretakers. Children completed the TSCC and primary caretakers, the TSYC. Convergent validity was found across the TSCC and TSCYC scales in their measurement of sexual concerns, anxiety, depression, and dissociation. In addition, discriminant validity was found between the TSCYC PTSD and TSCC PTS (Posttraumatic Stress) scales.

King et al. (2017) noted that child as informant assessments ought to take into consideration shorter attention spans, varied verbal abilities, and difficulties with abstract thinking. King et al. (2017) addressed problems with the developmental appropriateness of assessments by developing and evaluating a novel pictorial assessment, The Cameron Complex Trauma Interview (CCTI). They argued that the use of pictorial assessments may improve children's engagement with the assessment process. The CCTI was developed for children between the ages of 5 and 11, and assesses for history of complex trauma and associated symptoms. In selecting items for the CCTI, language was modified to ensure developmental appropriateness for children as young as the age of 5. The CCTI is comprised of two parts. The first part measures a history of trauma across a range of events such as physical abuse, domestic violence, sexual abuse, medical trauma, violence in the community, neglect, traumatic loss, and natural disaster. The second part includes 21 questions that measure impairment related to attachment, biology, affect regulation, dissociation, behavioral regulation, cognition, self-concept, and post-traumatic symptoms. A preliminary evaluation of the CCTI found it to be internally consistent ($a = 0.931$), and to have convergent validity, as shown by strong correlations between the CCTI and UCLA PTSD-RI symptomatology and trauma history scales ($r = 0.819$, and 0.677, respectively; King et al., 2017).

Assessment of Trauma in Children with ASD

As with the dearth of literature on autism and trauma, there are no psychometrically validated assessment instruments used to evaluate for history of trauma or symptoms of trauma in children with autism. Kerns et al. (2015), however, have offered general recommendations. They note that the quality of traumatic events and responses to trauma may vary in children with ASD. Therefore, measures designed to assess a broader array of trauma-related symptoms may be more relevant than those that are more specific. For example, the TSCC and the TSCYC may be more appropriate assessment tools compared to tools designed to measure specific PTSD criteria. Additionally, guidelines for the assessment of PTSD in young children suggest that assessment criteria should be behaviorally based and developmentally sensitive to detect trauma in young children with ASD who may have delayed abstract cognitive and verbal expression abilities. Symptoms such as flattened affect and social detachment may be difficult to discriminate as symptoms of trauma in children with ASD, as many individuals on the autism spectrum do not express emotions and are socially isolated. In addition to recommendations made by Kerns et al., some of the other adaptations that should be considered in the assessment of trauma in children with ASD include the use of simplified language to address language deficits and the use of pictures to facilitate comprehension of trauma-related concepts.

Treatment of Trauma in Children

Historically, when treating trauma in children, therapies have relied on the use of language to make meaning of trauma or on the use of medication to regulate the neurobiological effects of trauma (van der Kolk, 2003). van der Kolk and Najavits (2013) argue that such treatments are insufficient for treating traumatic symptoms in children. As well, they note that there is a lack of treatments that address affective arousal, the ability to concentrate, and social engagement difficulties that develop. Memory research has shown that memories are like a quickly drawn sketch; imprecise stories that people tell themselves so that they can make meaning and create a narrative of their life experiences (van der Kolk, 2014). Memories are not precise recollections of images, sensations in the body, odors, or muscular actions. However, when individuals experience trauma resulting in the development of PTSD or CPTSD, the body and the brain form a "blueprint" of particular pictures, scents, body sensations, and muscular actions. Re-experiencing traumatic memories in the form of flashbacks can occur for years following the event itself (van der Kolk, 2014). van der Kolk states that treatment approaches should ideally help individuals process the past without fully re-experiencing it. When treating trauma, the approach cannot exclude knowledge of neurobiology because of the effect trauma has on the brain and the body. van der Kolk and Najavits (2013) further assert that effective treatment must teach individuals to regulate their autonomic arousal system. Physiological arousal must be calmed before one can access one's executive functioning system to engage in adaptive emotional regulation and problem-solving strategies. van der Kolk (2003) argues that children must develop the capacity to withstand trauma-related body sensations and their associated emotional states. It is not until the child has developed an internal state of control over his/her various arousal states that he/she can start to learn from novel experiences and to respond flexibly to new situations. Below we review two common evidence-based treatments for a range of mental illnesses such as anxiety, depression, and trauma in typically developing children: (a) Cognitive Behavior Therapy (CBT); and (b) Trauma-Focused Cognitive Behavior Therapy (TF-CBT).

Cognitive Behavior Therapy

CBT is well established in the literature as an evidence-based practice for the treatment of a variety of mental health disorders including depression, anxiety, and obsessive–compulsive disorder in children and adults (Barrett et al., 2001; Kendall et al.,

2004; Oar et al., 2017; Rapee et al., 2009). The aim of CBT is to teach individuals to change their thoughts and behaviors, so that they become more realistic and adaptive, resulting in improvements in quality of life (Coffey et al., 2015). CBT treatment packages typically include the following strategies: identification of problematic thoughts; challenge of thoughts and beliefs by the therapist; teaching of alternative adaptive thoughts; relaxation; problem-solving; scheduling of fun events in order to increase positive reinforcement in the person's environment; and exposure to negative thoughts, physiological sensations, and situations to decrease the person's avoidance of and arousal associated with environmental stimuli (Coffey et al., 2015; Fréchette-Simard et al., 2018).

Trauma-Focused CBT

CBT has been extended to the treatment of trauma in children in what is known as Trauma-Focused CBT (TF-CBT) with modifications (Coffey et al., 2015). The results of a recent meta-analysis, including 39 psychological treatments for symptoms of PTSD in children, indicated that TF-CBT interventions can effectively decrease PTSD symptomatology when compared to wait list and active control conditions (Morina et al., 2016). TF-CBT is a multicomponent treatment model that includes a manualized treatment protocol (Cohen et al., 2010). The components of the model are ascribed in the acronym "P.P.R.A.C.T.I.C.E": (a) psycho-education, to teach about trauma and trauma responses; (b) positive parenting skills and behavior management skills; (c) relaxation skills, to teach management of physiological response to trauma; (d) affective modulation skills; (e) cognitive coping skills, to make clear the connection between one's thoughts, feelings, and behaviors; (f) trauma narrative and processing to correct cognitive distortions that are the result of trauma; (g) in vivo mastery of trauma triggers to reduce generalized fear; (h) conjoint sessions with child and parent; and (i) enhanced safety and plans for safety in the future. Ideally, TF-CBT is provided in parallel child and parent/primary caregiver sessions, with conjoint child–parent sessions that are added on later in treatment. Additionally, Cohen et al. (2010) suggest that flexible implementation of the model, with early focus on the positive parenting component, can accommodate cases that are complex and include externalizing behavior problems. They note that externalizing behaviors often are the reasons why parents initially seek treatment for their children; not for PTSD/C-PTSD symptomatology. Therefore, one of the benefits of the TF-CBT model is that it treats both behavior problems and trauma symptoms. As part of the treatment package, explicit behavior management plans and ongoing monitoring of behaviors are required. Behavioral rehearsal and practice between sessions are expected of clients. Research evaluating TF-CBT indicates that it can ameliorate the symptoms of children who have incurred trauma (e.g., Cohen et al., 2005; Morina et al., 2016). Although significant modifications may be needed to adapt TF-CBT for children with ASD, the approach has a number of components that are likely to be appropriate and efficacious for children with ASD. We will review these components in our model below.

Treatment Modifications for Children with ASD

There is a scarcity of literature as it pertains to the treatment of trauma in individuals with ASD. Presently, there is only one case study that reports treatment modifications made for an adolescent with ASD who suffered a trauma (King & Desaulnier, 2011). Although there is a well-established literature supporting the use of TF-CBT as an evidence-based practice for treatment of trauma in children (Cohen et al., 2010; Morina et al., 2016), to date there has been no extension of the research to children with ASD. However, there is an emergent body of literature that has looked at the application of CBT with individuals with ASD to teach ER (Scarpa & Reyes, 2011; Shaffer et al., 2018; Thomson et al., 2015; Weiss et al., 2018) and to treat symptoms of anxiety (Chalfant et al., 2007; Ung et al., 2015; Wood et al., 2015). We believe that examining modifications to CBT with children on the autism spectrum to teach ER and to treat anxiety may be helpful in the development of a model to treat symptoms of trauma in children with ASD, given the commonalities of shared symptoms with typically developing children who have incurred trauma. Therefore, we will next look at potential treatment modifications found in the CBT literature aimed at teaching ER and treating anxiety in individuals with ASD.

Modified CBT to Teach Emotion Regulation

Research applying CBT to teach ER skills to children with ASD is emergent (Scarpa & Reyes, 2011; Shaffer et al., 2018; Thomson et al., 2015; Weiss et al., 2018). In these studies, treatment protocols with modifications were used to teach children with ASD to recognize and regulate their own emotions in group settings. Modifications included: (a) decreasing session length; (b) use of songs, stories, and play activities; (c) inclusion of parent training sessions; (d) skill building via psycho-education regarding affect, stress management, and understanding emotion expression; (e) highly structured sessions on specific topics; (f) parent group meetings to provide psycho-education concurrent with the children's sessions; (g) progress checks; (h) use of multimedia to teach skills; (i) modeling and role-playing to practice skills being taught; (j) mindfulness and relaxation exercises; (k) promotion of generalization to home and school environments; and/or (l) token economies to reinforce skill development (Scarpa & Reyes, 2011; Thomson et al., 2015). In order to extend the literature and address the urgent need to treat maladaptive ER, Shaffer et al. (2018) developed and conducted an initial evaluation of the Intensive Outpatient Program for Emotion Regulation Treatment (IO-PERT). IO-PERT is comprised of components from CBT, mindfulness practices, and Applied Behavior Analysis

(ABA). IO-PERT also involves caregiver training that is founded in CBT, mindfulness, and ABA. Initial results suggest a high level of parent satisfaction, and IO-PERT appears to have a positive impact in teaching coping skills (Shaffer et al., 2018). Weiss et al. (2018) conducted a randomized wait list-controlled trial of a manualized CBT program, Secret Agent Society: Operation Regulation (SAS: OR) to teach ER to a group of children with ASD. Components of the treatment package included teaching emotion naming in self and others, using relaxation techniques in challenging situations, and systematic exposure to increasingly distressing situations. Results indicated moderate to strong effects based on caregiver ratings of the intervention; however, child reports showed no change (Weiss et al., 2018). Weiss et al. argued that the lack of reported change was expected, given similar findings in a recent meta-analysis by Weston et al. (2016).

Modified CBT to Treat Anxiety

The second body of literature that may prove useful in the development of a treatment model for trauma is the treatment of anxiety in children and youth with ASD. Anxiety, a common result of exposure to trauma in typically developing children (Copeland et al., 2007; Courtois, 2008; Mazefsky et al., 2014; Streek-Fischer & van der Kolk, 2000), frequently emerges as a comorbid disorder in individuals on the spectrum. Modified CBT, implemented in groups or with individuals, has emerged as a commonly used treatment of anxiety with children with ASD (Chalfant, et al., 2007; Wood, 2009; Wood et al., 2015). A systematic review and meta-analysis reported by Ung et al. (2015) reported moderate effects of group implemented CBT in this population.

As with the implementation of CBT to teach ER to children with ASD, the application to treating anxiety in this population requires modifications. Chalfant et al. (2007) modified the "Cool Kids" curriculum to treat anxiety in a group of forty-seven children with high-functioning ASD. Modifications included: (a) increased number of sessions; (b) adapted material to teach identification of anxious feelings; (c) adapted material to teach somatic responses to anxiety; (d) simplified cognitive restructuring exercises; (e) adapted gradual exposure exercises to fearful stimuli; (f) planned relapse prevention; (g) increased use of visual supports; (h) structured worksheets; (i) modified exercises to teach relaxation skills; and (j) planned weekly exposure tasks to be completed as homework. Chalfant et al. examined the effectiveness of the modified CBT treatment using an experimental comparison group design. The forty-seven children were assigned to either an experimental group or wait list control group. Group sessions for the experimental group were conducted over a period of 12 weeks. Results showed that the CBT treatment group experienced statistically significant reductions in symptoms of anxiety compared to the wait list control group.

More recent modifications to CBT for the treatment of anxiety in children and youth with ASD have involved implementing modular CBT (Wood et al., 2015).

Modular CBT involves administering the treatment protocol individually instead of in groups. Individual implementation allows for individualizing treatment, matching the intervention to the unique learning characteristics of the child. For example, Wood et al. (2015) implemented Behavioral Interventions for Anxiety in Children with Autism (BIACA; Wood et al., 2009), in individual sessions, allowing clinicians to select modules on a session-by-session basis, in order to better tailor intervention to the needs of the child. Components such as: behavioral activation, cognitive restructuring, in vivo exposure, and parent training remained part of the treatment. Taken together, modular CBT, which allows for individualization of a treatment protocol, along with modifications to teach ER to children with ASD (Scarpa & Reyes, 2011; Shaffer et al., 2018; Thomson et al., 2015; Weiss et al., 2018), and modifications to treat anxiety in children with ASD (Chalfant et al., 2007; Wood et al., 2009) begin to provide a model from which to build a protocol for the treatment of trauma in children with ASD.

Trauma Treatment Model for Individuals with ASD

Currently, there is no evidence-based practice for the treatment of trauma in individuals with ASD. In the following section, we propose a multicomponent treatment package that draws on evidence-based practices in the treatment of trauma in other populations, while considering modifications and individualization of treatment for children with ASD (see Fig. 5.2). The model is comprised of components from TF-CBT for typically developing children and modified CBT to teach ER and treat anxiety symptoms in individuals with ASD. Individualization of the treatment package should be considered on a case by case basis given the variability in learning styles of children and adults with ASD. Components of the modified TF-CBT package are presented Fig. 5.1. We first explicate components of the package as applied to children, and second expand on the treatment components for parents. Variables affecting individualization of the treatment are addressed, and examples of how to individualize treatment are suggested, followed by a case study example of the model applied to a victimized child.

Assessment

Although at present there are no valid diagnostic assessments of trauma in children with ASD, as Kerns et al. (2015) recommend, measures such as the TSCC and TSYC that assess a broad array of trauma-related symptoms can be implemented with modifications to determine if trauma has occurred and the nature of the trauma. The ACTS or CCTI, which are both pictorially based assessments of trauma, may prove to be useful in the assessment of trauma in children with ASD as well. For chronologically young children and children with significant language deficits or severe cognitive impairments, simplifying the language used as part of the assessment is recommended. Adding visual supports for these children also may be beneficial. For example, pairing questions that assess for the occurrence of different traumas with a picture representing the specific type of trauma may lead to accurate disclosures of trauma by children with ASD.

Functional Behavior Assessment (FBA)

Many children who have incurred trauma and are referred for treatment engage in problem behavior (Cohen et al., 2010). Furthermore, it is well documented that many children with ASD engage in problem behavior as a result of their language impairment. Therefore, Cohen et al. (2010) recommend the completion of an FBA to determine the function of problem behavior. FBA results then inform the development of a behavior support plan. Cohen et al. argue that it is important to determine the relationship, if any, between behavior problems and the child's trauma. The FBA can identify specific antecedent triggers for trauma-related problem behavior and also the function of trauma-related behavior. For example, self-harm, substance abuse, or risky sexual behavior triggered by memories of trauma may have the immediate function of reducing the trauma-related memories. Cohen et al. recommend assessing whether or not problem behavior occurred prior to the trauma or if problem behavior emerged following the traumatic experience. Additionally, if the behavior problems predated the trauma, assessing for changes in regard to rate, intensity, or topography is recommended. For instance, completion of an FBA may inform the practitioner that self-harm in the form of hitting oneself in the head occurred prior to the trauma, however, a novel self-injurious behavior, in the form of scratching one's arm emerged following the trauma. Further, the FBA may determine that scratching may serve the function of escaping from traumatic memories.

Teach Emotion Regulation

To address emotion dysregulation, a core symptom of trauma, teaching ER skills through training in mindfulness practices (e.g., body scans, breath awareness; Scarpa & Reyes, 2011; Thomson et al., 2015) and Progressive Muscle Relaxation (PMR) should be components of intervention. The use of multimedia (Scarpa & Reyes, 2011; Thomson et al., 2015), such as videos to guide mindfulness practices should be incorporated. A mindfulness practice that may be used to teach emotion regulation is *Meditation on the Soles of the Feet*. This meditation practice directs individuals to focus on the soles of one's feet, and to maintain attention on this neutral body part (Singh et al., 2003). *Meditation on the Soles of the Feet* teaches the individual to stop, bring attention to the body, calm down, and then decide how to respond to the situation that triggered the emotional arousal (Singh et al., 2003). A variable to consider for individualization when teaching this practice may be that of the ability to maintain one's attention. Therefore, it will be important to ensure that the initial duration of mindfulness exercises is brief, gradually increasing the time spent on this practice. When working with children with severe cognitive impairments, the use of visual supports when teaching PMR skills is recommended. When teaching flexing and relaxing of muscles, one can use photos of high preference characters (e.g., the Incredible Hulk) flexing and relaxing their muscles to model these actions. Finally, to extend the application of reinforcement procedures in the IO-PERT model for managing problem behavior (Shaffer et al., 2018), it will be necessary to create individualized plans to reinforce newly learned emotion regulation skills. Individualized token economies should be developed and implemented. For example, one child may be expected to earn three tokens before acquiring a backup reinforcer while another child may be expected to earn two tokens before acquiring a backup reinforcer for the completion of mindfulness or PMR exercises within sessions.

Teach Emotion Recognition

Another component of a modified TF-CBT treatment package should include teaching children to name their emotions. When emotional suppression or dysregulation results from exposure to trauma, teaching children to name their emotional states may serve as a cue to engage in adaptive ER skills. For example, "I am angry—I should try to flex and relax my muscles" or "I feel scared—I should practice my breathing exercises." A variable to consider for individualization is child preference. To help increase motivation to learn, one may include the learner's highest preference characters as part of the materials being used (e.g., if the learner prefers Mickey Mouse, one could include exemplars of him feeling happy, calm, sad, or angry). An additional variable to consider is generalization difficulties of some learners on the autism spectrum. To promote generalization across stimuli, general case analysis is a systematic method for selecting and sequencing teaching exemplars (Cooper et al., 2007). General case analysis requires selecting and teaching examples that adequately sample the full range of stimulus situations that may occur in the natural environment (Cooper et al., 2007). For example, if teaching a child to label the emotion of anger, one ought to plan to teach the emotion across multiple exemplars by arranging the instructional materials so that they represent the full range of stimuli. A selection of materials, all representing the feeling of anger may include: Mickey Mouse feeling angry (or any cartoon character), a photo of the child her/himself feeling angry, a photo of a parent feeling angry, a line drawing of a person feeling angry, and a photo of a teacher feeling angry.

Graduated Exposure

Graduated exposure is a common component of a TF-CBT treatment package (Cohen et al., 2005, 2010) and in the treatment of anxiety in children with ASD (Wood et al., 2009, 2015). Extending its application to the treatment of trauma in children with ASD is recommended. Exposure can systematically teach the child to tolerate stimuli that remind them of their trauma and gradually decrease the physiological distress associated with their experience. A trauma hierarchy should be created, in which environmental triggers are identified from least to most distressing. Children work their way up the hierarchy as part of graduated exposure exercises (Wood et al., 2009). Children's successful use of effective ER strategies in the face of environmental triggers is positively reinforced. Planning graduated exposure exercises between sessions can help with the promotion of generalization across environments (Chalfant et al., 2007). Although a common component of TF-CBT, individualization of this component of the package is important to emphasize. For example, providing opportunities to practice the same exposure exercise multiple times, across multiple environments, paired with child-specific reinforcers for successful use of ER strategies in the face of distressing events should be considered. Further, in children with impaired language and cognitive abilities, it may be helpful to add a within-activity schedule to provide increased structure and predictability around exposure exercises. Following the within-activity schedule step-by-step, may increase the child's understanding of the process, and help the child to predict when it will end. Caution when implementing graduated exposure must be taken with individuals who have not developed sufficient emotion regulation skills, as exposure therapy can cause re-traumatization, leading to severe symptoms such as suicidal ideation or attempts, and depression (Courtois, 2004, 2008). In cases where exposure therapy is contraindicated, the goal of therapy becomes teaching children to discriminate between dangerous and non-dangerous situations, and to use skills to problem-solving about how to cope with both types of situations (Cohen et al., 2010).

Cognitive Restructuring

Trauma narrative and processing aim to correct cognitive distortions that are the result of trauma. Additionally, cognitive coping skills aim to make clear the connection between one's thoughts, feelings, and behavior (Cohen et al., 2010). In cases where individuals with ASD have severe cognitive impairments, cognitive restructuring exercises may require individualization or removal from the treatment package altogether. Similar to modifications found in the treatment of anxiety for children with ASD (Chalfant, et al., 2007; Wood et al., 2009, 2015), increased use of visual supports is recommended for children who require them. The use of simplified language along with visual supports to teach concepts may help children understand the concepts being taught in cognitive restructuring exercises. In cases where a child cannot generate his or her own responses verbally, worksheets upon which he/she answers written questions or completes fill in the blank exercises can be created and implemented. As well, re-scripting the traumatic narrative, simplifying language, adding pictures to help make meaning of the story, and adding visuals of happier endings for the child may be a way to individualize cognitive restructuring for learners with language delays or severe cognitive impairments. When working with young children, focusing on teaching ER and implementing exposure therapy may be most relevant to treatment, while forgoing components of treatment such as cognitive restructuring.

Psycho-Education About Trauma and Trauma Responses

Another component of TF-CBT for individuals with ASD should be psycho-education regarding what trauma is and people's responses to trauma. The literature regarding teaching emotion regulation to children with ASD recommends parent education as a component of the treatment package (Scarpa & Reyes, 2011; Shaffer et al., 2018; Thomson et al., 2015; Weiss et al., 2018). We further recommend that psycho-education be implemented for both children and their parents. Cohen et al. (2010) found it beneficial to provide psycho-education about the connection between behavior problems and trauma. In addition, it is important to teach parents that changing their own behavior and changing the environment are crucial components for their child's behavior change. For children with ASD, psycho-education about trauma and responses to trauma also should be included. However, factors for individualization should again be considered. As the literature on the treatment of anxiety in this population recommends, simplified language and visual supports should be added to instruction (Chalfant et al., 2007; Wood et al., 2015). Additionally, individualization of treatment may require consideration of child preferences when creating lesson materials. For example, when teaching children about how their bodies respond to trauma, one can create simple cartoons of the fight or flight response to threat, with developmentally appropriate language to teach this concept. An additional consideration for individualization may be a child's endurance to learn. Scheduling breaks away from task demands during psycho-education sessions is recommended for children who cannot attend to task demands for extended periods of time. Finally, as the literature on teaching emotion regulation and treating anxiety recommends, the use of reinforcement strategies (Shaffer et al., 2018; Wood et al., 2015) also should be extended to the psycho-education about trauma and trauma responses. Consideration of child preferences when planning the use of reinforcers should be considered as well. If a token economy is used to reinforce active responding in sessions about the effects of trauma, then tokens can be customized to include child preferences. For example, if a child has a strong preference for vehicles, then tokens could be customized with images of vehicles.

Dosage Level and Between-Session Support

When considering dosage level of treatment, interventionists should plan for an increase in the number of sessions and a decrease in session length to accommodate the learning difficulties of individuals on the autism spectrum. This has commonly been a component of both treatment packages to teach ER and treat anxiety in children with ASD (Chalfant et al., 2007; Scarpa & Reyes, 2011; Shaffer et al., 2018; Thomson et al., 2015; Weiss et al., 2018). In addition, providing support between sessions may prevent attrition rates when treating trauma. A brief between-session phone call, lasting 5–15 min, can be implemented to answer questions or concerns that clients may have or to ensure homework exercises are being completed (Koerner, 2012).

Safety Plan

A safety plan should be developed to enhance the safety of the child when he/she perceives their safety is threatened or to prevent future occurrences of the traumatic event. Developing a trusting working relationship with the therapist, identification of safe adults who can support the child, along the development of emotion regulation skills must be prioritized (Cohen et al., 2012). Developing a trusting relationship with a child with ASD may be challenging as a result of idiosyncratic preferences, challenges with language skills, and impaired social and play skills. Therefore, ensuring child preferences are incorporated into therapy sessions is recommended.

An additional safety strategy is to help the child identify adults who are safe and who can support the child outside of therapy (Cohen et al., 2011, 2012). Adults who can support the child outside of therapy can provide support both in times of perceived threat, or when the child may have experienced a novel trauma (Cohen et al., 2011, 2012). The child with ASD may require more than the identification of safe adults in a therapy session. He/she may benefit from the creation of a visual support, that can be taken home, which includes: (a) a photo of each person identified as safe; (b) the name of the individual written on the visual; (c) contact information for the individual; and (d) explicit rules written on the visual that state when he/she should seek support from the person. Additional modifications can be made to the visual support depending on the particular level of need of the child. The use of the visual support should then be role-played in therapy, and paired with reinforcers contingent on correctly participating in the role-play activity. As well, the use of reinforcers should be applied to the natural environment to increase the likelihood that the child will use the safety visual when needed. Specifically, when the child uses the visual support to get adult support when feeling threatened, or if experiencing a new threat, he/she should earn a reinforcer for seeking support from a safe person in the natural environment. Finally, as Courtois (2004, 2008) has argued, exposure therapy can lead to severe side effects such as re-traumatization, and the emergence of symptoms such as suicidal thoughts and attempts. In these cases, graduated exposure should be immediately terminated, and a shift in treatment should be made to further develop emotion regulation skills.

Data Monitoring and Ongoing Evaluation of Outcomes

Assessments of trauma symptomatology should be implemented prior to the onset of intervention, post-intervention, and at 3–12 months follow-up to evaluate outcomes. Additionally, within sessions, a data-collection system should be designed and used to monitor the effectiveness of the approach, and data-based decisions should be made on an ongoing basis to evaluate progress. Daily session data should be collected and evaluated for changes in: (a) the number of times the child uses an appropriate ER strategy; (b) the number of times the child engages in problem behavior in response to trauma associated stimuli; (c) the number of trauma-related triggers the child forbears using ER strategies (as per the trauma hierarchy); and (d) parent and child self-report of the emergence, continuation, or intensification of severe symptoms of trauma such as depression, self-injury or suicidal ideation.

Program for Generalization and Maintenance

In children with ASD, generalization and maintenance of treatment effects cannot be assumed, therefore these effects need to be systematically promoted. Generalization can be promoted by: (a) selecting and teaching across a wide range of exemplars and skills (e.g., different triggers at the same level in a trauma hierarchy; a variety of ER or mindfulness strategies to neutralize the effects of triggers for trauma-related problem behavior); (b) mediating generalization by teaching the child to use a self-monitoring and self-management checklist to prompt ER skills or mindfulness practices in the face of stimuli associated with past trauma; (c) providing opportunities for the child to use ER skills and mindfulness practices across a range of situations in which trauma-related problem behavior has occurred in the home, school, or community; and (d) arranging the environment so that the child receives positive reinforcement contingent on using ER skills and mindfulness practices to successfully self-regulate their behavior in the face of trauma-related stimuli. Maintenance can be systematically promoted by: (a) providing ongoing opportunities for exposure and practice of ER skills and mindfulness practices; and (b) delivering robust positive reinforcement (i.e., praise paired with tangible reward) for demonstration of appropriate ER skills and mindfulness practices in the face of triggers for trauma-related problem behavior.

Behavior Support Plans and Behavioral Skills Training for Parents

For typically developing children who engage in problem behavior, after the completion of an FBA, development of a function-based multicomponent behavior support plan that is both technically sound and contextually appropriate is recommended (Cohen et al., 2010). This behavior support plan development process also should be applied to children with ASD, as they may present with worsening of preexisting problem behavior or the emergence of new problem behavior resulting from traumatic experiences. Goals of intervention should include reducing child problem behavior and increasing child use of alternative communication responses and emotion regulation skills. As with typically developing children (Cohen et al., 2010), the development of behavior support plans should be a collaborative process, informed by parents and their child. Once a technically sound and contextually appropriate plan has been developed, parents should be taught to implement plan components with fidelity. To do so, the interventionist should employ behavioral skills training (BST) procedures such as role-play, coaching, and feedback. In addition to BST, training sessions should: (a) educate parents about trauma and the effects of trauma; (b) identify the nature of the trauma and create a trauma hierarchy; (c) plan for exposure homework exercises between sessions; and (d) review homework completion logs (Cohen et al., 2010).

Case Study

The following case study illustrates the application of the treatment model described above to a child with ASD. Emphasis throughout is on how the treatment is individualized to the child.

Anna is a 10-year-old girl with a diagnosis of ASD. Anna is a charming and well-liked girl who has been in an ABA-based home intervention program since the age of four. Anna's developmental age is equivalent to that of an 8-year old. She is able to communicate her needs, thoughts, likes, and dislikes orally. She has a range of preferences that include playing with her friends at school, watching cartoons on T.V, listening to pop music, and playing sports. She attends her local elementary school in Vancouver, British Columbia, and is included in the regular education program. Since early childhood Anna has struggled to regulate her emotions. When upset, she typically cries, yells, and walks away from adults.

In the past week, when Anna arrives home from school, she is greeted by her mother and her home-based behavior interventionist who ask her about her school day. She unexpectedly starts to cry. Concerned about what may have happened at school that day, her mother and the behavior interventionist follow-up with another question. Anna then screams, jumps from her chair, and hides under her desk, curled up with her face pressed against her knees. Anna spends the next 20 min under her desk, dissociated and inconsolable. She also has been observed scratching her arm with her fingernails. Although Anna has a history of struggling to regulate her emotions, similar to many individuals with ASD, she has never been observed to hide under furniture or curl up her body in apparent fear. Nor has she previously engaged in self-injurious behavior. The behavior analyst assigned to her case hears of this day from Anna's mother and behavior interventionist. Anna's mother further discloses with the behavior analyst that when left alone in her room, she experiences flashbacks, emotional dysregulation, dissociation and engages in self-injurious behaviors. She wonders if Anna may have experienced a traumatic event of which her family and team are unaware. Anna's behavior analyst raises this concern with the family, and recommends she see a specialist to assess for trauma and to develop an individualized treatment plan if needed.

Anna is taken to see a psychologist (Carolyn) who specializes in the treatment of trauma in children and who works with children with ASD. The initial session is spent interviewing her father and building rapport with Anna. Carolyn and Anna watch short video clips on YouTube of Anna's favorite T.V show, Scooby-Doo, and play with Scooby-Doo figurines simultaneously. While they are playing together, Carolyn observes Anna's body shaking at times and sees her subtly scratching her arm. Following the initial appointment Carolyn confirms the behavior analyst's concern about the possibility that Anna has recently experienced a traumatic event. She recommends a follow-up appointment in which she intends to continue building rapport with Anna and to conduct an assessment to determine whether Anna has experienced trauma.

Anna's next appointment continues as planned; Carolyn pairs herself with Anna's preferred activities to further build rapport. Prior to initiating an assessment of trauma, Carolyn determines what may be the most effective approach given Anna's disability and developmental level. Although Anna is 10 years old, her language skills are delayed. Similar to other children with ASD, Anna presents as a younger child of about 8 years of age. Given that there is currently no ASD-specific tool for the assessment of trauma in this population, Carolyn decides to implement a pictorial assessment for complex trauma, the CCTI (King et al., 2017). Once completed, it becomes clear that Anna has experienced an abusive event, and has developed trauma-related symptoms as a result. It is unclear as to who the perpetrator is, but Anna's response to the question, "Has a grown up hurt you really bad? Choked you, pushed you, shook you, or beat you up?" indicates that one of these events likely occurred. In response to the question, Anna became emotionally dysregulated (i.e., screamed, hid under a table in the office, and curled up into a ball), dissociated, and engaged in self-harm (i.e., scratched her arm).

A treatment plan is developed collaboratively with Anna's parents and her counsellor. It is decided that Anna will attend sessions until she no longer experiences the associated symptoms from her trauma, but session length will remain 60 min in length. The team decides that there is no need to implement an FBA at the onset of therapy, however, if needed, one will be implemented to determine the functions maintaining Anna's problem behavior. The following components are included in her treatment plan: (a) mindfulness practices, such as body scans and breath awareness, enhanced with video models to teach emotion regulation; (b) teaching emotion labels in pictures, with high preference characters represented in the picture sets; (c) development of a trauma hierarchy; (d) graduated exposure to a hierarchy of trauma memories to teach Anna to gradually tolerate stimuli that trigger flashbacks (e) cognitive restructuring to teach Anna the connection between her thoughts, feelings, and behaviors, supplemented with visual supports and simplified language to match Anna's language abilities; (f) re-scripting of the trauma narrative, including images of her favorite cartoon characters as part of the story; (g) psycho-education about trauma, supplemented with visuals that teach Anna about the fight-flight-freeze response and the relationship between her trauma and self-injurious behaviors; and (h) support between therapy sessions in the form of one 15-min phone call between Anna and Carolyn, or Anna's parents and Carolyn.

In regard to evaluation, data is collected weekly and evaluated monthly to make data-based decisions on the effectiveness of the multicomponent treatment package. Specifically, data is collected on the number of trauma-related symptoms observed in and out of treatment sessions. During home-based sessions with the behavior interventionist, data collection includes tracking the number of correct and incorrect emotions labeled during lessons on emotion recognition. In addition, Anna's parents are being taught to take data in the family's natural environment when they observe dissociation or self-injurious behavior.

In regard to the promotion generalization and maintenance, Anna is being taught a range of mindfulness practices with the support of multiple video exemplars, or individualized visual supports (i.e., Meditation on the Soles of the Feet, Breath Awareness, and Body Scans). As well, Anna is being taught to apply these practices across a broad range of situations to regulate her emotions. Anna is also being taught to accurately label emotions across a wide range of exemplars. To promote generalization of ER skills outside of therapy sessions, Anna is being taught to self-manage and self-monitor her use of mindfulness practices at home, in school, and in the community. Maintenance is being promoted by ensuring that Anna comes into contact with potent positive reinforcers when she either is observed using ER skills at home or in the community with family members or accurately reports using ER skills at school or in the community.

Weekly parent training sessions are being conducted simultaneously with Anna's weekly treatment sessions with the psychologist Carolyn. Parent sessions include: (a) behavioral skills training to teach Anna's parents how to collect data on her trauma symptoms and how to help Anna engage in mindfulness practices when she is emotionally dysregulated; (b) psycho-education about trauma and Anna's trauma responses; and (c) weekly 15-min phone calls, as needed, to offer consultative support in between weekly therapy sessions with the psychologist.

Implications

Since individuals with ASD are more prone to victimization than their typical peers (Hibbard & Desch, 2007; Kerns, 2015), both judges and lawyers should be keenly aware of the struggles this population has with communication, as this is a variable that makes them more prone to maltreatment (Sullivan & Knutson, 2000). An individual with delayed communication skills may not be able to make sense of their experience of trauma, as they may have insufficient symbolic language to understand their experience (Stack et al., 2020). Alternatively, they may have challenges with communication, which may make it difficult for the individual with ASD to report on their traumatic experience. Keeping these impairments in mind, it is recommended that professionals assessing for trauma in this population attend to the worsening of preexisting behavior problems or the emergence of novel behaviors that can be the result of a trauma, and not symptomatic of ASD. For example, if the individual of concern previously engaged in self-injury in the form of hitting oneself in the head, has this behavior worsened after a suspected traumatic event? This may take the form of the individual hitting their head more frequently on a daily basis compared to how often they did so prior to the suspected trauma. Worsening may take the form of an increase in intensity of the behavior; that is an increase in the force of the head hitting. In addition to assessing for the worsening of preexisting behaviors, one also will assess for the emergence of novel behaviors. For example, is the individual suddenly engaging in aggressive behavior toward other people? Do they engage in new self-injurious behavior? Is the individual destroying property? Is the individual engaging in novel sexual behaviors such as masturbation in front of others? Finally, one will want to assess for changes in emotion regulation. Have there been changes in the individual's ability to cope with stressful circumstances, such that they now engage in more intense emotional dysregulation (Stack et al., 2020)?

In addition to assessing for behavioral changes within the individual, when evaluating formal assessment measures of trauma, lawyers and judges will want to consider what assessment tool was used. As we mentioned previously, there are no psychometrically validated assessments for trauma in individuals with ASD, making assessment at this point in time challenging. Nevertheless, it is highly recommended that modifications be made to assessment tools that are used with the neurotypical population. Modifications should include: (a) simplifying the language in the assessment, and matching language to the developmental level of the individual; (b) adding pictures to augment the questions being asked in the assessment (e.g., if asking a child if they have been hit by a parent or adult, pairing the verbal question with an image of what that looks like); and c) using behaviorally based assessments for trauma.

Finally, when considering the treatment of trauma in individuals with ASD, we must note with caution that there are no empirically validated treatments for this population. In this chapter, we recommend drawing from evidence-based practices in the treatment of anxiety and trauma in typically developing children, and the treatment of anxiety in children with ASD. Based on these literatures, we offer a modified multicomponent treatment package, along with variables to consider for individualization of treatment (see Fig. 5.2). It is important to note that all individuals with ASD are precisely that, individuals. As such, the variables on the right-hand side of Fig. 5.2 should be considered on a case by case basis. For example, one might ask, given that a child has been sexually abused by a caregiver, is graduated exposure needed as a component of the treatment package? If the child does not have sufficient emotion regulation ability, then exposing them to their trauma memories may lead to re-traumatization, thus doing more harm than good. In such a case, it may be advantageous to simply teach the child to regulate their emotions more effectively. Another consideration, not mentioned in the variables for individualization in Fig. 5.2, is comorbid disorders. For example, consider a case in which a youth has received a diagnosis of ASD and has incurred trauma persistently throughout their life, resulting in a second diagnosis of Dissociative Amnesia? When one is diagnosed with Dissociative Amnesia, one has no recollection of one's past, making visual memories of past traumas inaccessible. Yet, there trauma-induced problem behavior occurs throughout the individual's life, causing havoc with emotion regulation, ability to learn, and development of social skills and executive functioning skills. In such a case, treatment must be carefully titrated to ensure that the youth can tolerate the treatment protocol. In such a case, learning to regulate one's emotions in order to tolerate increasingly distressing situations will be critical, as will the creation of a robust behavior support plan for the individual's family and team, as the severity of problem behaviors may be quite intense. Again, in such a case, graduated exposure to the trauma memories would be contraindicated in such a case. Lawyers and judges should be keenly aware that variables for individualization in any treatment package must be carefully considered in the development of a treatment plan for an individual with ASD who has experienced trauma in their life.

Conclusion

A collaborative research approach is needed to advance scientific knowledge of how to assess and treat trauma in children with ASD to ameliorate the immediate symptoms of trauma and to prevent long-term side effects such as learning challenges, emotion dysregulation, dissociation, anxiety, depression, and self-harm. To date, TF-CBT has been demonstrated in the literature to be an evidence-based treatment of trauma in typically developing children (Cohen et al., 2010; Morina et al., 2016). However, there has been no extension in research on the treatment of trauma to children and youth with ASD. This chapter proposes a modified TF-CBT model for the treatment of trauma in children and youth with ASD. However, research is required to evaluate the efficacy and acceptability of the proposed multicomponent treatment package when implemented with children with ASD. Given the positive results of empirically investigated treatments for typically developing children who have experienced trauma, and for adapted versions of CBT and ER training for children with ASD and anxiety, research on an adapted multicomponent model of treatment for trauma in children with ASD holds much promise.

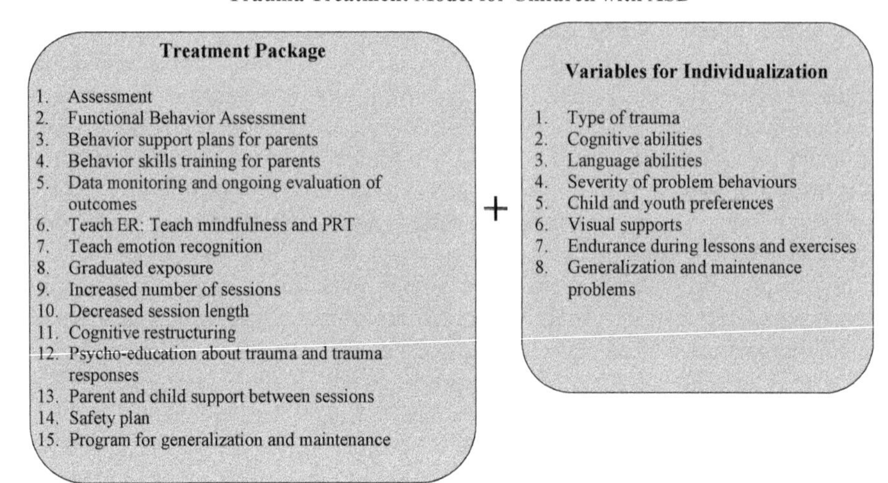

Fig. 5.2 Treatment model for children with ASD who have suffered trauma(s) rooted in CBT and TF-CBT (Reproduced from Stack & Lucyshyn, 2018)

References

American Bar Association. (2013). *Prosecuting cases for children on the autism spectrum*. https://www.americanbar.org/groups/public_interest/child_law/resources/child_law_practiceonline/child_law_practice/vol_32/april-2013/prosecuting-cases-for-children-on-the-autism-spectrum/.

American Psychiatric Association. (2013). *Diagnostic and statistical manual of mental disorders*. (5th ed.). American Psychiatric Publishing.

Barrett, P. M., Duffy, A. L., Dadds, M. R., & Rapee, R. M. (2001). Cognitive-behavioral treatment of anxiety disorders in children: Long-term (6-Year) follow-up. *Journal of consulting and clinical psychology, 69*(1), 135–141.

Berg, K. L., Shiu, C., Acharya, K., Stolbach, B., & Msall, M. (2016). Disparities in adversity among children with autism spectrum disorder: A population-based study. *Developmental Medicine & Child Neurology, 58,* 1124–1131.

Brenner, J., Pan, Z., Mazefsky, C., Smith, K. A., & Gabriels, R. (2017). Behavioral symptoms of reported abuse in children and adolescents with autism spectrum disorder in inpatient settings. *Journal of Autism and Developmental Disorders*. https://doi.org/10.1007/s10803-017-3183-4.

Briere, J. (1996). *Trauma symptom checklist for children: Professional manual*. Psychological Assessment Resources Inc.

Chaffin, M., Wherry, J. N., Newlin, C., Crutchfield, A., & Dykman, R. (1997). The abuse dimensions inventory: Initial data on a research measure of abuse severity. *Journal of Interpersonal Violence, 12*(4), 569–589.

Chalfant, A. M., Rapee, R., & Carroll, L. (2007). Treating anxiety disorders in children with high functioning autism spectrum disorders: A controlled trial. *Journal of Autism and Developmental Disorders, 37,* 1842–1857.

Coffey, S., Banducci, A., & Vinci, C. (2015). Common questions about cognitive behavior therapy for psychiatric disorders. *American Family Physician, 92*(9), 807–812.

Cohen, J. A., Mannarino, A., Kliethermes, M., & Murray, L. K. (2012). Trauma-focused CBT for youth with complex trauma. *Child Abuse and Neglect, 36,* 528–541.

Cohen, J. A., Mannarino, A., & Murray, L. K. (2011). Trauma-focused CBT for youth who experience ongoing traumas. *Child Abuse and Neglect, 35,* 637–646.
Cohen, J. A., Berliner, L., & Mannarino, A. (2010). Trauma focused CBT for children with co-occurring trauma and behavior problems. *Child Abuse and Neglect, 34,* 215–224.
Cohen, J. A., Mannarino, A. P., & Knudsen, K. (2005). Treating sexually abused children: 1 year follow-up of a randomized controlled trial. *Child Abuse and Neglect, 29,* 135–145.
Cooper, J. O., Heron, T. E., & Heward, W. L. (2007). *Applied behavior analysis.* Pearson Education.
Copeland, W. E., Keelar, G., Angold, A., & Costello, J. (2007). Traumatic events and posttraumatic stress in childhood. *Archives of General Psychiatry, 64,* 577–584.
Corbett, B. A., Mendoza, S., Wegelin, J. A., Carmean, V., & Levine, S. (2008). Variable cortisol circadian rhythms in children with autism and anticipatory stress. *Journal of Psychiatry and Neuroscience, 33*(3), 227–234.
Courtois, C. A. (2004). Complex trauma, complex reactions: Assessment and treatment. Psychotherapy: Theory, Research, Practice, Training, *41*(4), 412–425.
Courtois, C. A. (2008). Complex trauma, complex reactions: assessment and treatment. *Psychological Trauma: Theory, Research, Practice and Policy, 41*(4), 86–100.
Danese A., & McEwen, B. S. (2012). Adverse childhood experiences, allostasis, allostatic load, and age-related disease. *Physiology and Behavior, 106,* 29–39.
Enlow, M. B., Egeland, B., Blood, E. A., Wright, R. O., & Wright, R. J. (2012). Interpersonal trauma exposure and cognitive development in children to age 8 years: A longitudinal study. *Journal of Epidemiological Health, 66,* 1005–1010.
Felitti, V. J., Anda, R. F., Nordenberg, D., Williamson, D. F., Spitz, A. M., Edwards, V., Koss, M. P., & Marks, J. S. (1998). Relationship of childhood abuse and household dysfunction to many of the leading causes of death in adults: The adverse childhood experiences (ACE) study. *American Journal of Preventive Medicine, 14*(4), 245–256.
Fréchette-Simard, C., Plante, I., & Bluteau, J. (2018). Strategies included in cognitive behavioral therapy programs to treat internalized disorders: A systematic review. *Cognitive Behaviour Therapy, 47*(4), 263–285.
Goldfarb, D., & Gonzalez, A. (2018). Children with autism spectrum disorder in the courtroom: How courts handle testimony today and what we can do in the future. In J. G. Johnson & P. C. Mundy (Eds.), *The Wiley handbook of memory, Autism spectrum disorder, and the law* (pp. 340–357). Wiley.
Gross, J. J. (2013). Emotion regulation: Taking stock and moving forward. *Emotion, 13*(3), 359–365.
Gross, J. J., & Thompson, R. A. (2007). Emotion regulation: Conceptual foundations. In J. J. Gross (Ed.), *Handbook of emotion regulation* (pp. 3–24). Guilford Press.
Guy, L., Souders, M., Bradstreet, L., DeLussey, C., & Herrington, J. D. (2014). Brief report: Emotion regulation and respiratory sinus arrhythmia in autism spectrum disorder. *Journal of Autism and Developmental Disorders, 44,* 2614–2620.
Hoover, D. W. (2015). The effects of psychological trauma on children with autism spectrum disorders: A research review. *Review Journal of Autism and Developmental Disorders, 2,* 287–299.
Hibbard, R., & Desch, L. (2007). Maltreatment of children with disabilities. *Pediatrics, 119*(5), 1018–1025.
Kendall, P. C., Safford, S., Flannery-Schroeder, E., & Webb, A. (2004). Child anxiety treatment: Outcomes in adolescence and impact on substance use and depression at 7.4-year follow-up. *Journal of Consulting and Clinical Psychology, 72*(2), 276–287.
Kerns, C., Newschaffer, C., Berkowitz, S., & Lee, B. K. (2017). Brief report: Examining the association of autism and adverse childhood experiences in the national survey of children's health: The important role of income and co-occuring mental health conditions. *Journal of Autism and Developmental Disorders, 47,* 2275–2281.
Kerns, C., Newschaffer, C., & Berkowitz, S. (2015). Traumatic childhood events and autism spectrum disorder. *Journal of Autism and Developmental Disorders, 45*(11), 3475–3486.

King, R., & Desaulnier, C. (2011). Commentary: Complex post-traumatic stress disorder. Implications for individuals with autism spectrum disorders- part 3. *Journal on Developmental Disabilities, 17*(1), 47–59.

King, J. A., Solomon, P., & Ford, J. D. (2017). The cameron complex trauma interview (CCTI): Development, psychometric properties, and clinical utility. *Psychological Trauma: Theory, Research, Practice, and Policy, 9*(1), 18–22.

Koerner, K. (2012). *Doing dialectical therapy: A practical guide.* New York: Guilford Press.

Lanktreea, C. B., Gilbert, A. M., Briere, J., Taylor, N., Chen, K., Maida, C. A., & Saltzmane, W. R. (2008). Multi-informant assessment of maltreated children: Convergent and discriminant validity of the TSCC and TSCYC. *Child Abuse and Neglect, 32,* 621–625.

Maenner, M. J., Shaw, K. A., & Baio, J (2020). Prevalence of Autism spectrum disorder among children aged 8 years—Autism and developmental disabilities monitoring network, 11 Sites, United States, 2016. *MMWR Surveillance Summaries, 69*(4).

Mazefsky, C. A., Borue, X., Day, T. N., & Minshew, N. J. (2014). Emotion regulation patterns in adolescents with high-functioning autism spectrum disorder: Comparison to typically developing adolescents and association with psychiatric symptoms. *Autism Research, 7,* 344–354.

Mazefsky, C. A., Herrington, J., Siegel, M., Scarpa, A., Maddox, B. B., Scahill, L., & White, S. W. (2013). The role of emotion regulation in autism spectrum disorder. *Journal of the American Academy of Child and Adolescent Psychiatry, 52*(7), 679–688.

McEwan, B. C. (2007). Physiology and neurobiology of stress and adaptation: Central role of the brain. *Physiological Review, 87,* 873–904.

Morina, N., Koerssen, R., & Pollet, T. V. (2016). Interventions for children and adolescents with post-traumatic stress disorder: A meta-analysis of comparative outcome studies. *Clinical Psychology Review, 47,* 41–54.

Oar, E. L., Johnco, C., & Ollendick, T. H. (2017). Cognitive behavioral therapy for anxiety and depression in children and adolescents. *Psychiatric Clinics of North America, 40,* 661–674.

Perry, B. D., Pollard, A. R., Blakley, T. L., Baker, W. L., & Vigilante, D. (1995). Childhood trauma, the neurobiology of adaptation, and "use-dependent" development of the brain: How "states" become "traits." *Infant Mental Health Journal, 16*(4), 271–291.

Pitskel, N. B., Bolling, D. Z., Kaiser, M. D., Pelphrey, K. P., & Crowley, M. J. (2014). Neural systems for cognitive reappraisal in children and adolescents with autism spectrum disorder. *Developmental Cognitive Neuroscience, 10,* 117–128.

Praver, F., DiGiuseppe, R., Pelcovitz, D., Mandel, F. S., & Gaines, R. (2000). A preliminary study of a cartoon measure for children's reactions to chronic trauma. *Child Maltreatment, 5*(3), 273–285.

Rainville, C. (2013). Prosecuting cases for children on the autism spectrum. *ABA Child Law Practice, 32*(4), 49–64.

Rapee, R. M., Schniering, C. A., & Hudson, J. L. (2009). Anxiety disorder during childhood and adolescence: Origins and treatment. *Annual Review of Clinical Psychology, 5,* 311–341.

Rigles, B. (2016). The relationsuhip between adverse childhood events, resiliency and health among children with autism. *Journal of Autism and Developmental Disorders, 47,* 187–202.

Samson, A., Hardan, A., Lee, I., Phillips, J., & Gross, J. (2015). Maladaptive behavior in autism spectrum disorder: The role of emotion experience and emotion regulation. *Journal of Autism and Developmental Disorders, 45*(11), 3423–3432.

Scarpa, A., & Reyes, N. (2011). Improving emotion regulation with CBT in young children with high functioning autism spectrum disorders: A pilot study. *Psychotherapy, 39,* 495–500.

Shaffer, R. C., Wink, L. K., Ruberg, J., Pittenger, A., Adams, R., Sorter, M. Erickson, C. A. (2018). Emotion regulation intensive outpatient programming: Development, feasilbility, and acceptability. *Journal of Autism and Developmental Disorders.* https://link-springer-com.ezproxy.library.ubc.ca/journal/10803.

Sherin, J. E., & Nemeroff, C. B. (2011). Post-traumatic stress disorder: The neurobiological impact of psychological trauma. *Dialogues in Clinical Neuroscience, 13*(3), 263–278.

Singh, N. N., Wahler, R. G., Adkins, A. D., & Myers, R. E. (2003). Soles of the feet: A mindfulness-based self-control intervention for aggression by an individual with mild mental retardation and mental illness. *Research in Developmental Disabilities, 24,* 158–169.

Stack, A., Hoadley, B., & Schneider, A. (2020, March). *Identifying and supporting trauma in complex cases of ASD.* Paper presented at 12th annual British Columbia-ABA Conference, University of British Columbia, Vancouver.

Stack, A., & Lucyshyn, J. (2018). Autism spectrum disorder and the experience of traumatic events: Review of the current literature to inform modifications to a treatment model for children with autism. *Journal of Autism and Developmental Disorders, 49*(4), 1613–1625.

Steinberg, A. M., Brymer, M. J., Decker, K., & B., & Pynoos, R. S. . (2004). The university of California at Los Angeles post-traumatic stress disorder reaction index. *Current Psychiatry Reports, 6,* 96–100.

Streek-Fischer, A., & van der Kolk, B. A. (2000). Down will come baby, cradle and all: Diagnostic and therapeutic implications of chronic trauma on child development. *Australian and New Zealand Journal of Psychiatry, 34,* 903–918.

Sullivan, P., & Knutson, J. (2000). Maltreatment and disabilities: A population-based epidemiological study. *Child Abuse & Neglect, 24*(10), 1257–1273.

Thomson, K., Riosa, P. B., & Weiss, J. (2015). Brief report of preliminary outcomes of an emotion regulation intervention for children with autism spectrum disorder. *Journal of Autism and Developmental Disorders, 45*(11), 3487–3495.

Ung, D., Selles, R., & Small., B. J. & Storch. E. A.. (2015). A systematic review and meta-analysis of cognitive-behavioral therapy for anxiety in youth with high-functioning autism spectrum disorder. *Child Psychiatry and Human Development, 46*, 533–547.

van der Kolk, B. (2014). *The body keeps the score: Brain, body, and mind in the healing of Trauma.* Penguin Group.

van der Kolk, B. (2003). The neurobiology of childhood trauma and abuse. *Child and Adolescent Psychiatric Clinics of North America, 12*, 293–317.

van der Kolk, B., & Najavits, L. (2013). Interview: What is PTSD really? Surprises, twists of history, and the politics of diagnosis and treatment. *Journal of Clinical Psychology in Session, 69*(5), 516–522.

Weiss, J. A., Thomson, K. Riosa, P. B., Albaum, C., Chan. C., Maughan, A., Tablon, P., & Black, K. (2018). A randomized waitlist-controlled trial of cognitive behavior therapy to improve emotion regulation in children with autism. *Journal of Child Psychology and Psychiatry, 59*(10), 1–12.

Weston, L., Hodgekins, J., & Langdon, P. E. (2016). Effectiveness of cognitive behavioral therapy with people who have autistic spectrum disorders: A systematic review and metaanalysis. *Clinical Psychology Review, 49,* 41–54.

Wood, J., & J., Drahota, A., Sze, K., Har, K., Chiu, A., & Langer, D. A. (2009). Cognitive behavioral therapy for anxiety in children with autism spectrum disorders: A randomized, controlled trial. *The Journal of Child Psychology and Psychiatry, 50*(3), 224–234.

Wood, J.J., Ehrenreich-May, J., Alessandri, M., Fujii, C., Renno, P., Laugeson, E., Piacentini, J. C., S De Nadai, A. S., Arnold, E., Lewin, A. B., Murphy, T. K., & Storch, E. A. (2015). Cognitive behavioral therapy for early adolescents with autism spectrum disorders and clinical anxiety: A randomized, controlled trial. *Behavior Therapy, 46*(1), 7–19.

Wood, J. J., & Gadow, K. D. (2010). Exploring the nature and function of anxiety in youth with autism spectrum disorders. *Clinical Psychology: Science and Practice, 17*(4), 281–292.

Yehuda, R. (2006). Biology of posttraumatic stress disorder. *Journal of Clinical Psychiatry, 61,* 14–21.

Alexia Stack is the Clinical Director and Board Certified Behavior Analyst (BCBA) at A Block Above Behavioral Consulting in Vancouver, British Columbia. Alexia is a BCBA with 20 years of experience working with toddlers, children, teens, and adults with Autism Spectrum Disorder (ASD), developmental and behavioral disorders, and histories of trauma. She has published a review of how trauma impacts individuals with ASD, and has developed a model for the assessment and treatment of trauma in the Journal of Autism and Developmental Disabilities. She will be completing a second Master's degree in Counselling Psychology starting September 2021, where she plans to further develop her clinical skills in the treatment of trauma in both the neuro-diverse and neuro-typical populations.

Joseph Lucyshyn is an Associate Professor and Board Certified Behavior Analyst (BCBA-D) in the Faculty of Education at University of British Columbia. He teaches courses in positive behaviour support, single case research, and ethics for behaviour analysts. He has published research on positive behaviour support with families in peer-reviewed journals including the Journal of Child and Family Studies, Journal of Consulting and Clinical Psychology, and Journal of Positive Behavior Interventions. His current research focuses on group parent training models of positive behaviour support with families, mindfulness training with children with ASD and their parents, and culturally responsive positive behaviour support with families of diverse cultural backgrounds.

Chapter 6
Legal Defense in Criminal Cases

Eileen T. Crehan and Frederic S. Ury

Introduction

The criminal courts are ill-equipped to deal with autistic defendants. Inadequate funding, understaffed State Attorneys' offices in the United States, and perhaps most significantly a lack of appreciation for the nuances of autism spectrum disorder (ASD) all contribute to the difficulties counsel face in leading an autistic individual through the criminal justice system. Regardless, early intervention with the police, close collaboration with a trusted mental health professional, and avoiding a trial if at all possible can result in an outcome that, if not successful in the traditional sense, at least minimizes potential negative results. This chapter will focus on five distinct phases of the criminal justice process: criminal investigation, arrest, pretrial, trial, and post-conviction processes. Before delving into each phase, overarching considerations that impact autistic defendants, families, supports, and legal counsel are discussed. The more knowledge of the symptoms and characteristics of ASD that one has in combination with knowledge of the specific defendant, the easier navigating this process will be. This chapter provides a broad overview for attorneys, clinicians, and caregivers. Additional information about legal defense of people with ASD is found in Chap. 13. While that chapter covers a particular type of criminal charge (i.e., sexual images of children), it includes information that applies to other areas of autism and criminal defense.

E. T. Crehan (✉)
Eliot-Pearson Department of Child Study & Human Development, Tuft University, 105 College Avenue, Medford 02155, MA, USA
e-mail: eileen.crehan@tufts.edu

F. S. Ury
Ury & Moskow, Fairfield, Connecticut, CT, USA
e-mail: Fred@urymoskow.com

F. R. Volkmar et al. (eds.), *Handbook of Autism Spectrum Disorder and the Law*,
https://doi.org/10.1007/978-3-030-70913-6_6

General Recommendations

Understanding a Defendant's Autism

It is essential, particularly in cases involving defendants with autism, that counsel in criminal cases meet with the family to try to understand how the defendant's autism affects their everyday living. Carefully examine how traits associated with autism could be a contributing factor to the alleged criminal activity. This ideally would include information about social relationships, restricted interests, repetitive behaviors, language comprehension and expression, and cognitive profile. While the presence of unlawful behavior is not particularly high among those with ASD, those with ASD who do commit crimes can exhibit inappropriate attempts at forming relationships and illegal behaviors that occur in fulfillment of a special interest (Woodbury-Smith & Dein, 2014).

To provide more context for behaviors such as these, counsel should meet with medical providers, teachers, and caregivers to learn more about potential contributing factors, such as communication needs, sensory profile, behavior, restricted interests, social development, and developmental and clinical history. When possible, getting releases signed to gather detailed information from relevant professionals can help expedite the process of data collection. Assuming permission, share the facts of the alleged crime with these individuals to investigate possible connections between the criminal behavior and the defendant's autism. Although a medical professional may not be able to definitively determine how ASD may or may not be related to the criminal activity, they can recognize and interpret behaviors in the context of the defendant's profile and history. Spending time with the medical professionals who know the client well and have an established clinical relationship is invaluable. Reports from relevant medical professionals and supporting information from caregivers, teachers, and any additional established relationships in the individual's life can be used at the pretrial level to determine if there is a way to resolve the case short of trial. It is very important to make sure that the client and their family understand it is necessary to share the basic facts of the case with the medical professionals that treat the defendant in order to understand if there is any relationship between the alleged crime and the client's autism.

Anticipating and Managing Anxiety

The criminal justice process is full of unknowns and, potentially, fear for defendants. Magnifying this is the high rate of anxiety in ASD (White et al., 2009). Responding negatively to change is a common characteristic of autism (Weiss et al., 2014). The legal system can be confusing, filled with change and uncertainty, and perhaps leading to negative outcomes for autistic defendants. For anxious individuals, anxiety can reduce communication abilities (Lewin et al., 1996) which could be problematic for anxious autistic defendants who are reliant on language in the criminal justice process. Further, anxiety in autistic individuals increases repetitive behaviors (which may be calming for the defendant but may impact how they are perceived by a jury and judge) and, in children, resulted in increased insistence on sameness (Rodgers et al., 2012). These behavioral manifestations of anxiety can appear, at best, as odd to those not familiar with ASD and, at worst, as a lack of cooperation or suggestion of guilty behavior. With this in mind, predicting anxiety-provoking situations and implementing plans or coping strategies proactively is strongly recommended.

To help alleviate anxiety, it is recommended to use visuals and timelines/flowcharts as much as possible. In both school and medical settings, providing schedules has been found to reduce anxiety for autistic children (Chebuhar et al., 2013; Lytle & Todd, 2009). Even if the exact time frame of what happens next is not known, mapping out the likely order of what comes next and what factors impact the timing will help to assuage some anxiety. Writing out an expected order of events and reviewing it with the client may reduce anxiety and increase cooperation in the process.

Sensory Sensitivities

Sensory sensitivities are another common aspect of ASD. Sensitivity to sound, touch, and light in particular may be activated during many points of legal proceedings. An awareness of the defendant's sensory sensitivities and preferences may be helpful to avoid environmental triggers, which may increase the risk of aggression (King & Murphy, 2014). Work with defendants and the system to try to make reasonable accommodations for this either through the actions of the defendant or by altering the environment, e.g., wearing hats or sunglasses in rooms with fluorescent lighting, using headphones to attenuate sound, or working to minimize physical contact as possible between justice system employees and the autistic person.

On the other hand, capitalizing on sensory-seeking behaviors may offer easy ways to help an autistic person remain calm (or at least, calmer) during proceedings. Having a small piece of fabric to stroke, or a fidget toy, or experiences of physical pressure may be useful; communicate with the defendant about tools used successfully in the past and, if helpful or possible, family members or significant others who may be able to identify additional calming strategies.

These are broad strategies to implement across any stage of the criminal justice process. The following provides a more in-depth examination of the stages of the legal process. At each step, the previous recommendations will lend additional support and help to make the process more navigable.

Criminal Investigation

A criminal investigation is filled with potential landmines for autistic clients. It is important to note at this point that oftentimes a lack of diagnosis or misdiagnosis can make this process even more challenging to navigate. Combined with the fact that some individuals with developmental disabilities are practiced at appearing more "competent" than they perhaps are (Bonnie, 1990), this can create confusion for law officers and lawyers alike, resulting in gaps in accommodations that otherwise may be afforded to an individual. When possible, information about an ASD diagnosis should be provided to investigators.

For this reason, a criminal defense attorney well serves their client by intervening with the police as early in the process as possible. This is an important consideration because it runs contrary to the training given to and instincts developed by defense counsel which is to avoid as much interaction with the police as possible. If engaged early enough so that charges have not yet been brought, defense attorneys should accompany their client to interrogations to ensure that law enforcement has a clear understanding of the challenges faced by the client as a result of their autism. By indicating a willingness to cooperate while simultaneously attempting to limit external stressors that could worsen the individual's responses to questioning, the attorney can potentially head off at the pass the worst of charges and minimize extra upset experienced by the defendant.

When those on the spectrum exhibit clear signs of significant aberrant social behavior, it is, unfortunately, easier in some ways to get recognition of the fact that the defendant may be impaired. When verbal or social abilities are not noticeably impaired, however, more significant hurdles may present themselves. For instance, it can be helpful to know that verbal and reading expression oftentimes develop faster than comprehension for autistic individuals, and thus some may be using words they heard in similar contexts (e.g., criminal television shows) without a true meaning of what those words mean (Randi et al., 2010). Thus, the initial perception of their comprehension of a situation may be overestimated.

Some autistic individuals may give answers that they hope will end an interaction most quickly. This clearly could create issues for autistic individuals either by saying things they may not mean and need to later explain (thus seeming untrustworthy) or by unintentionally implicating themselves. Defendants should be given time to process and respond to questions; providing written support may help.

Problems experienced by autistic individuals are easily misperceived by law enforcement in the context of a criminal investigation and prosecution. For instance, "freezing" or high levels of anxiety in novel situations, both common in autism, can look like lackluster participation. Literal interpretation, minimal eye contact, or correcting the vague language of others oftentimes comes across as being rude or oppositional. Even in the presence of intact cognitive abilities, autistic individuals have been shown to display slower processing speed (although there is a question on whether or not this difference is driven by motor demands; (Kenworthy et al., 2013) and slower response times or taking an extra moment to understand a question can feel like resistance to the untrained eye.

Due to challenges with theory of mind and gleaning communicative intent, answering and asking questions may be challenging for an autistic defendant, as will pragmatic language (Baron-Cohen et al., 1999; Eales, 1993; Simon Baron-Cohen, 1988). These facts make close interaction with the mental health professional essential; both to have a medical diagnosis, and understanding of the treatment and medications the individual is taking. At a minimum and as available, these reports should include developmental history, current adaptive functioning, history of social communication, restricted interests, repetitive behaviors, and sensory sensitivities, cognitive abilities, and past school supports. In addition, the attorney needs to talk with the medical professional to discuss the necessity of reports and potentially their participation as a witness at preliminary hearings or a trial.

Criminal Investigation Highlighted Recommendations

- Engage law enforcement early and proactively provide education on autism and developmental disorders, as well as about specific individuals
- Incorporate past educational, developmental, and behavioral information
- Clearly explain expectations and nonverbal communication strategies to the defendant.

Arrest

This stage has a particularly high rate of potential sensory and communication pitfalls for autistic clients. The uncertainty of the process generally, the possibility of physical contact, and exposure to various members of law enforcement who may not have experience with autism. Not knowing or understanding what will come next can be challenging for anyone who is arrested. However, changes in routine and coping with unpredictability are extremely challenging for autistic individuals (Gillott & Standen, 2007). In fact, autistic individuals demonstrate increased sensitivity to threat and uncertainty even at baseline compared to non-autistic individuals (Chamberlain et al., 2013). Further, autistic individuals report greater distress and show greater brain activation when they perceive rule violations when compared to typically developing individuals (Bolling et al., 2011). In combination with the black-and-white and limited insight that is common for autistic individuals and low insight, perception that they are being treated unfairly may cause a larger-than-usual response from autistic individuals. This tendency toward higher sensitivity and greater distress despite potentially appearing emotionally flat should be taken into consideration by those working with autistic defendants.

An arrest can happen in two different ways. First, someone can be arrested at the scene of an alleged crime or the arrest can take place after an investigation and a warrant is signed by a judge. The arrest at the scene will involve the defendant being taken to the police station and charged.

Some autistic individuals may react in physical ways when stressed, such as during an arrest. Whether caused by fear, sensory reaction, or not realizing the negative consequences of this type of reaction, without proper preparation of what is to come, aggressive behavior may emerge (Howlin, 2004). Especially for autistic defendants with comorbid intellectual disability, self-injurious behavior can be a significant problem (Smith & Matson, 2010).

For defendants who respond physically when stressed, it is important to avoid incurring another charge by assaulting the police or acting out in a way that is interpreted as interfering with a police officer which just results in another serious charge. To best combat this, depending on the individual, it may be helpful to develop some guidelines about what to do when approached by a police officer, similar to developing a plan if an emergency or fire occurs in the household. Roleplay and video modeling may be useful. Individual plans may vary but include items such as identification cards and medical bracelets which list autism as a current medical condition. Identification cards, unfortunately, carry with them the need to reach into one's pocket to share with a police officer so this tool may not be beneficial especially for autistic individuals of color. From the law enforcement side, there are programs that can proactively help officers prepare for interactions with autistic citizens. Training and awareness programs for police officers can also help them to approach interactions with autistic individuals with appropriate care and caution.

Some states have optional registries for people with disabilities or communication challenges and individuals should check with their local police and fire departments, as well as a registry of motor vehicles, to learn more about possibilities in their area. These registries can take the form of sharing critical information (such as someone's aversion to being touched) that will pop up on a screen when 911 is called.

In the United States, bail will be determined by the police. If the defendant is released on a promise to appear, they will be required to come to court on a specific date. A promise to appear does not require any cash or surety bond. If a bond is set, then the defendant will be held in jail until they are able to pay the bond. Generally, the defendant is taken to court the next day if a bond is set and the defendant cannot pay it. Once in court, the defendant will appear before a judge. If they cannot afford an attorney a public defender will be appointed. Sometimes this appointment is just for a bail hearing but in some instances for the entire case. If private counsel is hired by the defendant or their family then counsel will appear with the defendant and have the opportunity to argue the amount of the bond at this time.

The second way in which a defendant can be arrested is on a warrant. If counsel knows about an investigation and a potential arrest, then they can proactively call the police. If the police have a warrant for the arrest of their client, the lawyer can offer to produce the client at the police station so that the defendant can be processed. It is good practice for counsel to give the police their cell phone number and ask that they call as soon as they get a warrant. Ask the police to avoid sending a police car to the defendant's house to arrest them; instead, make an appointment and bring the client in. In most instances, the police will have an idea of whether there will be a bond and, if so, how much it will be. If there is going to be a bond, then one should make sure that a bond person will be at the police station to bond the defendant out immediately after the arrest process is completed. The goal here is to minimize discomfort for the defendant and maximize pre-existing knowledge of what is to come.

Remember that literal or rigid interpretations of offhanded comments can cause upset, such as saying something will happen in a few minutes or days, and individuals interacting with autistic individuals should work to be as precise in their language as possible (Vicker, n.d.). Additionally, sensory sensitivities can often lead to strong emotional reactions or feelings of discomfort for autistic individuals. Settings should be assessed for sound and light demand (e.g., is there a flickering light? Are there loud, unexpected banging noises?). Simple supports such as having the person wear headphones or sunglasses may make a big difference in a person's ability to engage in the process.

It is particularly important for the autistic client to review in detail what is going to happen at the police station. Although the examination of autism supports in legal settings is not available in the literature, effective social communication supports and anxiety-reducing techniques from other settings would likely be useful. For instance, supports that benefit students in school can be a stepping stone for developing legal system supports. Visual schedules and social stories can help prepare individuals for novel situations, especially if these individuals have been exposed to these learning tools beforehand (Myles et al., 2007). Giving examples of what is going to happen next, such as getting their picture and fingerprints taken and that they are asked questions will help to contain anxiety (Dettmer et al., 2000). Providing scripts to ask for breaks or for clarification is also recommended. Additionally, providing explanations for why each step is happening and clear behavioral expectations can help an autistic individual navigate a new situation with as much independence and as little fear as possible (Müller et al., 2008).

Police stations rarely allow counsel to accompany clients while they are being booked because this process is primarily administrative and not an opportunity to ask questions or interrogate the defendant which would be a time when counsel would be allowed to be present. Because counsel during this part of the process is not present, make it a point to inform the arresting officers of your client's particular dislikes; for example, that the client does not like certain things such as touching them. Other factors to consider sharing are repetitive movements or motions, such as rocking, and communication style. To inform what information is shared, details from the defendant themselves, their family, or a knowledgeable psychologist/psychiatrist who knows the defendant should be consulted. Defendants who are receiving or who were recently receiving school supports via an Individualized Education Program (IEP) may have a copy of that document that should include recommendations about teaching and learning profiles that are most effective for the individual.

Arrest Highlighted Recommendations

- Proactively have conversations or role play about interactions with law enforcement.
- Integrate use of identifications cards or medical bracelets to help provide information about autism for unexpected interactions with law enforcement. Meeting local law enforcement in calm settings is another way to mitigate future situations from escalating.
- Increase training opportunities for law enforcement especially on sensory sensitivities to avoid escalating situations.

Pretrial

After the arrest, the prosecution must determine if they will file charges on the accused. If the prosecution decides not to file charges, the accused is released. If the prosecution has sufficient evidence and decides to file charges, the accused will appear before a judge to be told their rights and what they are being charged with. The judge then determines if the accused will be held in jail or released on bail before the arraignment. A preliminary hearing will occur, during which evidence will be presented to the judge to determine if the accused should be indicted or released. If the accused is being charged of a felony, the evidence may be presented among a jury of their peers, a grand jury. An arraignment will occur if the judge or grand jury decides to indict the accused. During the arraignment, the accused is formally informed of the charges and may plead guilty, not guilty, or no contest. These options and outcomes should be carefully explained to the defendants, with an emphasis on the "why" of certain decisions and actions and context is oftentimes limited to intuit for autistic individuals (Vermeulen, 2015). If the accused pleads guilty or no contest, the case will not go to trial and the individual will be sentenced later. If the individual pleads not guilty, the trial process begins.

When deciding whether to charge a person with a crime, prosecutors will examine several factors, including the seriousness of the offense and strength of evidence. It may be in the best interest of the defendant to avoid a trial by jury, given the sensory, communication, and stress-related demands. Due to communication and behavioral differences, individuals with ASD may be perceived negatively by jury members if they are not properly educated on what ASD is (Allely & Cooper, 2017). Pretrial is an opportunity for the defense counsel to meet alone with the prosecutor or with the prosecutor and a judge. It is at this stage that discussions with the prosecutor and judge allow the attorney to begin to prepare the case for trial. At this time, counsel will obtain copies of police report, surveillance videos and any other documents the state is going to use to try to prove their case. All of these materials should be reviewed with the defendant and their family if requested.

Criminal liability rests on two pieces; the first, that an act was committed (actus reus) and the second that there was intent to commit that crime (mens rea). The insanity plea can be used to counteract mens rea. The use of the insanity plea in ASD is complicated. On the one hand, some characteristics of ASD mean that behavior that is deemed criminal may not have been intended or planned that way. For instance, repetitive behaviors or highly motivating restricted interests may appear to others as aggressive behaviors. A lack of insight into one's own behavior, a common characteristic of autism, can make "criminal intent" difficult to prove. On the other hand, many autistic individuals have extremely high IQs, hold jobs, maintain personal relationships, and function completely independently, making it difficult to establish a lack of competency to commit a crime.

Once releases are acquired, the council should meet with medical providers, teachers, and caregivers to learn more about potential contributing factors to the case regarding the individual. Those with ASD who are accused of a crime should specifically be prepared for the indictment that will occur if the prosecution decides to file charges. The individual with ASD will appear before a judge to be told their rights and what they are being charged with. This will most likely be a very fast-paced process; preparation for this process can help mitigate an overwhelming courtroom environment. It is particularly important to prepare the accused, and their family, to hear the indictment out loud. Both at this stage and at the trial stage, preparation using established teaching tools for ASD is recommended. Although legal process-system supports have not been studied, a meta-analysis of tools used to support intervention implementation demonstrates that instructional videos (includes video modeling), written instructions, verbal instructions, practice, modeling, role-playing, and direct feedback (Rispoli et al., 2011).

The individual with ASD will need to plead guilty or not guilty at this point. Plans must be made in order for the accused to communicate their desired plea. Spontaneously connecting today's actions with long-term outcomes may not be a strength for many autistic defendants (Fullerton & Coyne, 1999) and legal counsel should clearly write out and describe what pleading guilty or not guilty means in terms of specific charges and past actions, as well as how their plea and behavioral presentation during this stage may be related to next steps (e.g., a literal defendant may take issue with pleading guilty if it is not clear that they are being charged for one very specific incident). The accused, their family, and their attorney must understand the charges presented and have a plan to proceed to optimize outcomes following the indictment.

It is very important that justice system staff interacting directly with the individual understands that individuals exhibiting the ASD symptomology such as a lack of emotional reciprocity, egocentricity, and social impairments may be confused for such anti-social traits, and may influence how the CJS handles them. One displaying such behaviors may lead authorities, judges, and prosecutors to assume that one is guilty and remorseless (Allely & Cooper, 2017). On the other hand, Mayes (2003) cautioned that a diagnosis of ASD does not exempt someone from prosecution and punishment, but suggested that professionals compare the nature and severity of one's impairment to the legal standards for competency or capacity. Overall, training mandates should be broadened to include employees in the CJS, including prosecutors, judges, and correctional staff to better ensure that they handle individuals with ASD properly and justly throughout all sectors of the CJS, particularly while they are preparing for trial.

Pretrial Highlighted Recommendations

- Carefully and fully explain options to defendants and their families. Write out the "why" or "consequences" of different decisions the defendant has, even if their verbal abilities are strong.

Trial

Trials are incredibly complex matters for prosecutors, judges, defense lawyers, and especially autistic defendants. It is important to take the time to explain every facet of what is going to happen. Prior knowledge of an autistic defendant's sensory and behavioral needs can help prepare a legal team for a trial. For instance, if an autistic defendant has a particular area they prefer to sit or type of chair that upsets them, suggesting possible accommodations to a judge can help an autistic defendant most fully participate in the legal process. The use of flow charts or visuals aids to prepare a client for a trial with or without a jury can be useful. Depending on the social knowledge of the individual, it may be worthwhile to discuss the behavioral expectations (e.g., not speaking out until told to do so), especially if a defendant trends toward black-and-white thinking or impulsivity and may be likely to call out if, for example, a witness says something that the defendant believes to be untrue. In the courtroom, limited perspective-taking, a common characteristic of autistic individuals, can take the form of thinking that judges, witnesses, and lawyers are "lying" when in fact they may have a different interpretation of past events. The intent of the communication of others participating in a trial may not be easily discernible for someone with autism (Hobson, 2012). Reasoning through this with an autistic defendant is not a reasonable expectation but rather in preparation for trial, clear expectations about when to speak and why different perspectives may be presented should be laid out for autistic defendants.

If the accused pleads not guilty and the case will be moved to trial, various measures should be taken to prepare. Upon developing an understanding of functional communication methods through information gathered from meetings with caregivers, medical professionals, and teachers, the lawyer should meet with the individual with ASD to practice communicating until both feel comfortable with the process. This will provide insight into how the communication method may function within a courtroom, and determine any necessary accommodations for the individual accommodations for the individual to testify. Communication with the individual with ASD can be mediated through a variety of methods, including sign language, writing, or letter boards. Questions should be phrased in a clear, literal manner with yes or no answers. It is also important to consider the sensory stimulation of the courtroom and any adaptations that could be made for the individual with ASD, including the lights, noises, and any smells they may experience and any way to regulate the overstimulation. There are several additional accommodations that may be beneficial to an individual with ASD while going through the trial process (Rainville, 2013). The individual could testify outside of the courtroom, via video conferencing. An interpreter (sign language, autism specialist, etc.) could serve as a valuable communication asset for the individual. If the case moves to trial, it is a good idea to file a motion in advance of the trial to raise the issue with the judge to ensure the trial process is as clear as possible.

Characteristics of ASD have important implications for providing as well as listening to testimony. Some autistic individuals have strong memory skills while others do not (Johnson et al., 2018). Cued recall is stronger than open-ended recall for autistic adults reporting on recent experiences, which could inform how lawyers approach questioning for defendants (Hare et al., 2007). Neuropsychological testing which assesses memory may provide useful context about an individual but memory in more emotional or socially salient situations may not be directly comparable. In particular, the understanding and use of language in relaying testimony is an area that can be challenging for autistic individuals, who may use or respond to words in unconventional ways (Maras & Bowler, 2014). Reviewing terms and proactively recognizing how literal interpretation of language could cause difficulties for an autistic individual should be incorporated into preparation for providing testimony.

During the trial, there may be testimony that is upsetting to the client. The question is whether the client should be allowed to sit in the room. They may not want to hear some of the things that are said by certain witnesses or, based on past history, the client's team may recognize that listening to testimony could cause a large emotional response. Whether the defendant is present is always a very complex question. The defendant has the constitutional right to hear all of the evidence presented against them. A decision to allow a defendant to remain out of the courtroom during certain testimony should only be allowed if there is some medical reason why hearing certain testimony is going to cause the defendant some harm.

There is a common fear that juries will negatively perceive autistic defendants, although the data is not clear on this point. It is important to note that education about autism and implications for social-emotional learning and presentation (e.g., low levels of expressed emotion, avoiding emotionally laden questions) provides juries with important context about a client. First impressions of autistic adults were found to be more positive when others were provided information about their autism diagnosis (Sasson & Morrison, 2019). Especially in situations where recall of events may not be clear and possibly perceived as a "guilty conscience," providing information about autism is recommended. In a study of children with autism and a mock jury, for autistic children who struggled with recall of events, providing information about autism to the jury resulted in a more favorable response to the child. For an autistic child with more sound recall, the impact of autism information or not did not have a significant effect (Crane et al., 2018). The most efficient way forward in this area is for legal professionals, such as special educationlawyers, to collaborate with autism specialists to meet the needs of families and individuals navigating the system.

Trial Highlighted Recommendations

- Listening to and providing testimony are socially laden experiences. Prepare defendants for what they may say or hear and give a way to express frustration or upset in ways that will not be viewed poorly by a judge and jury
- Provide education about autism broadly and for the particular defendant as possible to juries and judges.

Post-Conviction

Post-conviction is where much of the hard work is done by lawyers and professionals but this is especially true with autistic offenders. Prisons are especially challenging for autistic individuals due to the intense sensory experiences and social dynamics which make up prison life. There is no specialized prison for autistic offenders in the United States, although these do exist in other countries. Few if any prisons have segregated areas for those with the disorder, and few guards have adequate training or understanding of the individuals affected. Prison can be especially challenging for autistic individuals due to social naivety and increased likelihood of bullying. Perceptions of being anti-social and coping with comorbid mental health issues only exacerbate an already challenging setting (Paterson, 2008). Similarly, psychiatric hospitals are not specifically equipped to deal with the needs of this population. Parole officers are not necessarily trained. There is a great need for increased training. Currently, some brief online articles and PowerPoint presentations are searchable online but in-person trainings by psychologists and mental health professionals who can answer questions may be the best resource.

Autistic individuals found guilty of sex crimes are usually placed in probation programs with individuals who are not on the spectrum. These programs are usually a one size fits all type of program which can present challenges for autistic individuals. First, the program content itself may not be useful to the autistic individual. The qualitative differences in criminal behavior between autistic and neurotypical populations should be considered when post-conviction programs are a possibility. For instance, there is consistent evidence that crimes committed by autistic individuals are less likely to be related to drugs or alcohol, and that oftentimes there is very little personal gain from the illegal act (O'Brien, 2002). Browning and Caulfield (2011) summarize a number of studies that identify social skills and explicit description of expected and unexpected behaviors as critical pieces of successful criminal justice programs.

Second, learning in a group setting more generally may not be the ideal setting for an autistic individual. Psychiatric comorbidities such as anxiety or ADHD, both common with ASD, impact engagement in groups. Social communication deficits associated with ASD such as literal interpretation of language, lack of understanding of nonverbal cues, and a need for direct and close-ended questions can make group curricula challenging; it is unlikely that a group probation program would be tailored to meet the learning needs of enrolled autistic adults.

The data available on probation and autism shows that autistic individuals are significantly less likely to violate probation than their neurotypical peers (King & Murphy, 2014). Given all of the above, it is important for families, counsel, and the medical professionals to become creative in crafting sentencing proposals as well as probation programs. Prior to sentencing, the court usually orders a pre-sentence investigation (PSI). A PSI is done by a probation officer who will interview the defendant with counsel, past employers, family, victims and other individuals who the probation officer feels would be helpful in providing him or her with information about the defendant so that the probation officer can make a sentence recommendation to the court. This is the counsel's opportunity to provide as much information as necessary to give the probation officer a full picture of the challenges this client faces every day with their autism.

Sentencing is such an important part of the process because, as said above, there are no special programs or facilities for autistic individuals. As a result, it is incumbent upon counsel and the defendant's family and medical professionals to provide as much information about the defendant so that the court has a good understanding of the defendant that being sentenced. For researchers, this is a critical yet overlooked area of study.

Post-conviction Highlighted Recommendations

- Carefully consider intervention and incarceration options for defendants.
- Proactively engage programs in training and awareness around ASD issues and presentations.

Conclusions

Research demonstrates that individuals with ASD are more likely to be victims rather than perpetrators (Mayes, 2003). Consequently, it is vital that prosecutors understand why individuals with ASD may be victimized. Mansell et al. (1998) note that rates of sexual abuse for children with developmental disabilities are nearly two times greater than for typical children. It is speculated that sexual abuse cases are not prosecuted as frequently as they should be due to misperceptions that children with ASD are not reliable reporters (Rainville, 2013) because communication impairments may restrict one's ability to report victimization (National Research Council, 2001; Phipps & Ells, 1995). There is great speculation that these individuals may be victimized because disabilities inhibit them in recognizing tasks, understanding social boundaries, and knowing what to do when bad things occur.

Once a crime has been committed, it is important to note that, especially in the current generation and for individuals from low-resource areas, a diagnosis of ASD may not pre-exist legal proceedings. It is imperative that legal staff (or at least one person involved in the proceedings) has some knowledge of ASD and can recommend further evaluation. Although autistic individuals are not believed to commit crimes at a higher rate than their neurotypical peers, they likely comprise a larger percentage of the incarcerated population due to social naivete, strict adherence to rules, or social expectations that result in aggression when violated, and the pursuit of restricted interests beyond appropriate boundaries (Howlin, 2004).

In short, clear explanations of the process and expected behavior should be consistently made available to autistic defendants. For legal professionals involved in a case, detailed information about autism generally and then for the particular defendant should be provided by a medical professional, and ideally, one who has a long history of knowing the defendant, as well as speciality training in autism. As it stands, the system and sentencing results have not been adapted to fit autistic profiles and thus we must work with the resources we have as we continue to advocate for improvements. In the meantime, pursuit of educational opportunities to share information about autism with individuals in the criminal justice system, police force, and service agencies can help proactively manage these pieces.

To support change and awareness on a larger scale, those with knowledge of autism and the legal process should be proactive about connecting with local criminal system representatives, police force, and service agencies to share information about autism. The integration of autistic advocates into the police system in the United Kingdom should serve as an example for other systems. Specifically, training for individuals at any points of the legal system (police, judges, prison staff) on autism and autism representatives can improve accessibility.

Future Directions

Researchers and clinicians alike should mindfully pursue research opportunities, especially in collaboration with advocacy organizations and representatives of the criminal justice system, that measure how autism impacts the experience of the criminal justice system, and what modifications can improve it. Much work in this area would be helped immensely with clearer information about autistic people who are incarcerated, to inform the design and implementation of supportive systems in collaboration with autistic adults. Since too often the individuals with knowledge of ASD and those who understand the legal process are distinct groups, we recommend seeking out conferences and journals that are related to the legal system and legal advocacy if you are on the clinical side, or on autism and developmental disabilities if your work relates to criminal justice or legal advocacy.

References

Allely, C. S., & Cooper, P. (2017). Jurors' and judges' evaluation of defendants with Autism and the impact on sentencing: A systematic preferred reporting items for systematic reviews and meta-analyses (PRISMA) review of Autism spectrum disorder in the courtroom. *Journal of Law and Medicine, 25*(1), 105–123.

Baron-Cohen, S., O'Riordan, M., Stone, V., Jones, R., & Plaisted, K. (1999). Recognition of faux pas by normally developing children and children with Asperger syndrome or high-functioning autism. *Journal of Autism and Developmental Disorders, 29*(5), 407–418. https://doi.org/10.1023/a:1023035012436.

Baron-Cohen, S. (1988). Social and pragmatic deficits in autism: Cognitive or affective? *Journal of Autism and Developmental Disorders, 18*(3), 379–402. https://doi.org/10.1007/BF02212194.

Bolling, D. Z., Pitskel, N. B., Deen, B., Crowley, M. J., McPartland, J. C., Kaiser, M. D., Vander Wyk, B. C., Wu, J., Mayes, L. C., & Pelphrey, K. A. (2011). Enhanced neural responses to rule violation in children with autism: A comparison to social exclusion. *Developmental Cognitive Neuroscience, 1*(3), 280–294. https://doi.org/10.1016/j.dcn.2011.02.002.

Bonnie, R. J. (1990). The competence of criminal defendants with mental retardation to participate in their own defense. *The Journal of Criminal Law and Criminology (1973–), 81*(3), 419. https://doi.org/10.2307/1143845.

Browning, A., & Caulfield, L. (2011). The prevalence and treatment of people with Asperger's syndrome in the criminal justice system. *Criminology & Criminal Justice, 11*(2), 165–180. https://doi.org/10.1177/1748895811398455.

Chamberlain, P. D., Rodgers, J., Crowley, M. J., White, S. E., Freeston, M. H., & South, M. (2013). A potentiated startle study of uncertainty and contextual anxiety in adolescents diagnosed with autism spectrum disorder. *Molecular Autism, 4*(1), 31. https://doi.org/10.1186/2040-2392-4-31.

Chebuhar, A., McCarthy, A. M., Bosch, J., & Baker, S. (2013). Using picture schedules in medical settings for patients with an Autism spectrum disorder. *Journal of Pediatric Nursing, 28*(2), 125–134. https://doi.org/10.1016/j.pedn.2012.05.004.

Council, N. R. (2001). *Crime victims with developmental disabilities: Report of a workshop.* https://doi.org/10.17226/10042.

Crane, L., Wilcock, R., Maras, K. L., Chui, W., Marti-Sanchez, C., & Henry, L. A. (2018). Mock Juror perceptions of child witnesses on the Autism spectrum: The impact of providing diagnostic labels and information about Autism. *Journal of Autism and Developmental Disorders.* https://doi.org/10.1007/s10803-018-3700-0.

Dettmer, S., Simpson, R. L., Myles, B. S., & Ganz, J. B. (2000). The use of visual supports to facilitate transitions of students with Autism. *Focus on Autism and Other Developmental Disabilities, 15*(3), 163–169. https://doi.org/10.1177/108835760001500307.

Eales, M. J. (1993). Pragmatic impairments in adults with childhood diagnoses of autism or developmental receptive language disorder. *Journal of Autism and Developmental Disorders, 23*(4), 593–617. https://doi.org/10.1007/bf01046104.

Fullerton, A., & Coyne, P. (1999). Developing skills and concepts for self-determination in young adults with Autism. *Focus on Autism and Other Developmental Disabilities, 14*(1), 42–52. https://doi.org/10.1177/108835769901400106.

Gillott, A., & Standen, P. J. (2007). Levels of anxiety and sources of stress in adults with autism. *Journal of Intellectual Disabilities, 11*(4), 359–370. https://doi.org/10.1177/1744629507083585.

Hare, D. J., Mellor, C., & Azmi, S. (2007). Episodic memory in adults with autistic spectrum disorders: Recall for self-versus other-experienced events. *Research in Developmental Disabilities, 28*(3), 317–329. https://doi.org/10.1016/j.ridd.2006.03.003.

Hobson, R. P. (2012). Autism, literal language and concrete thinking: Some developmental considerations. *Metaphor and Symbol, 27*(1), 4–21. https://doi.org/10.1080/10926488.2012.638814.

Howlin, P. (2004). *Autism: Preparing for adulthood* (2nd ed.). London: Routledge.

Johnson, J. L., Goodman, G. S., & Mundy, P. C. (2018). *The Wiley handbook of memory, Autism spectrum disorder, and the law*. Wiley.

Kenworthy, L., Yerys, B. E., Weinblatt, R., Abrams, D. N., & Wallace, G. L. (2013). Motor demands impact speed of information processing in Autism spectrum disorders. *Neuropsychology, 27*(5), 529–536. https://doi.org/10.1037/a0033599.

King, C., & Murphy, G. H. (2014). A systematic review of people with Autism spectrum disorder and the criminal justice system. *Journal of Autism and Developmental Disorders, 44*(11), 2717–2733. https://doi.org/10.1007/s10803-014-2046-5.

Lewin, M. R., McNeil, D. W., & Lipson, J. M. (1996). Enduring without avoiding: Pauses and verbal dysfluencies in public speaking fear. *Journal of Psychopathology and Behavioral Assessment, 18*(4), 387–402. https://doi.org/10.1007/BF02229142.

Lytle, R., & Todd, T. (2009). Stress and the student with Autism spectrum disorders: Strategies for stress reduction and enhanced learning. *Teaching Exceptional Children, 41*(4), 36–42. https://doi.org/10.1177/004005990904100404.

Mansell, S., Sobsey, D., & Moskal, R. (1998). Clinical findings among sexually abused children with and without developmental disabilities. *Mental Retardation, 36*(1), 12–22. https://doi.org/10.1352/0047-6765(1998)036%3c0012:CFASAC%3e2.0.CO;2.

Maras, K. L., & Bowler, D. M. (2014). Eyewitness testimony in Autism spectrum disorder: A review. *Journal of Autism and Developmental Disorders, 44*(11), 2682–2697. https://doi.org/10.1007/s10803-012-1502-3.

Mayes, T. A. (2003). Persons with Autism and criminal justice: Core concepts and leading cases. *Journal of Positive Behavior Interventions, 5*(2), 92–100. https://doi.org/10.1177/10983007030050020401.

Müller, E., Schuler, A., & Yates, G. B. (2008). Social challenges and supports from the perspective of individuals with Asperger syndrome and other autism spectrum disabilities. *Autism, 12*(2), 173–190. https://doi.org/10.1177/1362361307086664.

Murrie, D. C., Warren, J. I., Kristiansson, M., & Dietz, P. E. (2002). Asperger's syndrome in forensic settings. *International Journal of Forensic Mental Health, 1*(1), 59–70. https://doi.org/10.1080/14999013.2002.10471161.

Myles, B. S., Grossman, B. G., Aspy, R., Henry, S. A., & Coffin, A. B. (2007). Planning a comprehensive program for students with Autism spectrum disorders using evidence-based practices. *Education and Training in Developmental Disabilities, 42*(4), 398–409. Retrieved from JSTOR.

O'Brien, G. (2002). Dual diagnosis in offenders with intellectual disability: Setting research priorities: A review of research findings concerning psychiatric disorder (excluding personality disorder) among offenders with intellectual disability. *Journal of Intellectual Disability Research, 46*(1), 21–30.

Paterson, P. (2008). How well do young offenders with Asperger syndrome cope in custody?*British Journal of Learning Disabilities—Wiley Online Library*. https://onlinelibrary.wiley.com/doi/full/10.1111/j.1468-3156.2007.00466.x.

Phipps, C. A., & Ells, M. L. (1995). Facilitated communication: Novel scientific evidence or novel communication? *Nebraska Law Review, 74*, 58.

Rainville, C. (2013, April). Prosecuting cases for children on the autism spectrum. *Child Law Practice Newsletter, 32*(4), 49. Retrieved from Academic OneFile.

Randi, J., Newman, T., & Grigorenko, E. L. (2010). Teaching children with Autism to read for meaning: Challenges and possibilities. *Journal of Autism and Developmental Disorders, 40*(7), 890–902. https://doi.org/10.1007/s10803-010-0938-6.

Rispoli, M., Neely, L., Lang, R., & Ganz, J. (2011). Training paraprofessionals to implement interventions for people autism spectrum disorders: A systematic review. *Developmental Neurorehabilitation, 14*(6), 378–388. https://doi.org/10.3109/17518423.2011.620577.
Rodgers, J., Glod, M., Connolly, B., & McConachie, H. (2012). The relationship between anxiety and repetitive behaviours in Autism spectrum disorder. *Journal of Autism and Developmental Disorders, 42*, 2404–2409. https://doi.org/10.1007/s10803-012-1531-y.
Sasson, N. J., & Morrison, K. E. (2019). First impressions of adults with autism improve with diagnostic disclosure and increased autism knowledge of peers. *Autism, 23*(1), 50–59. https://doi.org/10.1177/1362361317729526.
Smith, K. R. M., & Matson, J. L. (2010). Behavior problems: Differences among intellectually disabled adults with co-morbid autism spectrum disorders and epilepsy. *Research in Developmental Disabilities, 31*(5), 1062–1069. https://doi.org/10.1016/j.ridd.2010.04.003.
Vermeulen, P. (2015). Context blindness in Autism spectrum disorder: Not using the forest to see the trees as trees. *Focus on Autism and Other Developmental Disabilities, 30*(3). https://journals.sagepub.com/doi/full/10.1177/1088357614528799.
Vicker, B. (n.d.). *Social communication and language characteristics associated with high functioning, verbal children and adults with ASD*. Retrieved July 25, 2019, from Indiana Resource Center for Autism website: https://www.iidc.indiana.edu/pages/Social-Communication-and-Language-Characteristics-Associated-with-High-Functioning-Verbal-Children-and-Adults-with-ASD.
Weiss, J. A., Wingsiong, A., & Lunsky, Y. (2014). Defining crisis in families of individuals with autism spectrum disorders. *Autism, 18*(8), 985–995. https://doi.org/10.1177/1362361313508024
White, S. W., Oswald, D., Ollendick, T., & Scahill, L. (2009). Anxiety in children and adolescents with autism spectrum disorders. *Clinical Psychology Review, 29*(3), 216–229. https://doi.org/10.1016/j.cpr.2009.01.003.
Woodbury-Smith, M., & Dein, K. (2014). Autism spectrum disorder (ASD) and unlawful behaviour: Where do we go from here? *Journal of Autism and Developmental Disorders, 44*(11), 2734–2741. https://doi.org/10.1007/s10803-014-2216-5.

Dr. Eileen T. Crehan is a Clinical Psychologist who specializes in autism spectrum disorder in adolescents and adulthood. In collaboration with an Autism Community Advisory Board, she leads a research lab at Tufts University which focuses on improving access to care, especially sexuality and relationship education, for autistic people across the lifespan. She consults with schools, medical providers, and care professionals on best practices for supporting and promoting healthy outcomes for and with autistic individuals. Prior to joining the faculty at Tufts, she was the Associate Clinic Director at the Autism Assessment, Research, and Treatment Services Center at Rush University Medical Center.

Frederic S. Ury is a Founding Partner of the law firm of Ury & Moskow, LLC located in Fairfield, Connecticut and Washington, DC. Fred has been practicing law for 44 years. Ury & Moskow is a small boutique trial firm handling major civil, criminal, and mass tort cases throughout the State of Connecticut and the United States. Fred is a member of the Connecticut Bar where he was the President of the State Bar in 2004–2005. He has been a member of the ABA for 43 years. He was the past President of the National Conference of Bar Presidents from 2011–2012. Presently, he is the Chair of the Co-ordinating Council of the ABA Center for Professional Responsibility.

Chapter 7
Obtaining Testimony from Autistic People

Katie Maras

Background

Language, Social Communication and Narrative Ability in ASD

Police interviews are, by definition, formal social interactions that require narrative communication of past personally experienced events. Autism spectrum disorder (ASD) is a lifelong neurodevelopmental disorder that is characterised by persistent deficits in social communication alongside restricted and repetitive behaviours and interests (American Psychiatric Association, 2013). While language ability per se can vary wildly among individuals on the autism spectrum—from an individual who has never acquired language to a highly fluent, articulate individual—and everything else in between, an impaired ability to use language effectively to *communicate* (particularly in regard to pragmatics) is a core feature of ASD, regardless of an individual's level of intellectual functioning (Boucher, 2012; Tager-Flusberg, 2000). However, since expressive language is often better than receptive language ability in ASD (Boucher, 2012) such difficulties are not always immediately apparent, and a formidable vocabulary and good structural language ability—particularly among very intellectually able individuals—can initially mask an individual's broader vulnerabilities and the level of support and adaptations they require (see Crane et al., 2016; Maras et al., 2018).

Even autistic individuals with good expressive language will usually experience some degree of impairment in their ability to construct and relate a coherent narrative (Tager-Flusberg et al., 2005). While autistic people generally do not differ from language-matched typically developing (TD) individuals on some basic and global

K. Maras (✉)
University of Bath, Bath, UK
e-mail: K.L.Maras@bath.ac.uk

F. R. Volkmar et al. (eds.), *Handbook of Autism Spectrum Disorder and the Law*,
https://doi.org/10.1007/978-3-030-70913-6_7

aspects of the narrative, such as the identification of the main characters and settings of an event (Beaumont & Newcombe, 2006; Capps et al., 2000; Henry et al., 2020; Hilvert et al., 2016; Hogan-Brown et al., 2013; Losh & Capps, 2003; Tager-Flusberg & Sullivan, 1995), their stories often tend to lack causation and coherence, particularly with regard to temporality and the causal connection of plot points (e.g., Capps et al., 2000; Diehl et al., 2006; Hilvert et al., 2016; King et al., 2014; Kuijper et al., 2017; Lee et al., 2018; Losh & Capps, 2003, 2006; Losh & Gordon, 2014; McCabe et al., 2013; Tager-Flusberg, 2000). They can also show difficulties in using appropriate personal pronouns and referential expressions to convey who the character is at different points in a story (Colle et al., 2008; Norbury & Bishop, 2003).

It has been suggested that these difficulties in providing appropriate structure and content to narratives, and impaired use of cohesive linguistic devices may be explained in part by difficulties in considering the needs and perspectives of the listener (e.g., Baron-Cohen, 1988; Colle et al., 2008; Bruner & Feldman, 1993; Goldman, 2008; Hilvert et al., 2016; Tager-Flusberg, 1995; Tager-Flusberg & Sullivan, 1995), as well as broader difficulties in executive functioning and the ability to extract global meaning (e.g., Barnes & Baron-Cohen, 2012; Diehl et al., 2006; King et al., 2014; Losh & Capps, 2003). For example, executive functioning issues may result in difficulties generating, strategically planning and organizing one's recall of an event in the first instance (Barnes & Baron-Cohen, 2012). Moreover, while a tendency to focus on local over global detail may, on the one hand, appear to be useful in obtaining investigative important finer detail, difficulties in higher order processing and linking ideas together may further diminish the coherence, meaning and causality of accounts, making it more difficult for a listener to decipher and contextualise the narrative. Finally, a lack of appreciation of the listener's perspective in terms of what they already know and what they want to know impedes the production and organisation of an appropriately detailed, coherent, causal and relevant account (Colle et al., 2008).

Indeed, it has been suggested that individuals with ASD perform poorly on some cognitive tasks simply due to mentalising impairments leading to difficulties forming an implicit understanding of the experimenter's expectations for the task (e.g., Kenworthy et al., 2008; White, 2013; White et al., 2009). Specifically, White (2013) has argued that open-ended test situations where task instructions do not provide the individual with an explicit understanding of the task result in autistic individuals imposing their own task demands or arbitrary rules of the test situation. Thus, autistic individuals' performance usually becomes more impeded relative to TD individuals the more open-ended the task becomes. For example, Losh and Gordon (2014) found that autistic participants performed more poorly than TD participants on a semi-structured conversation narrative recall task; producing more off-topic and irrelevant remarks, departing from the main stories' themes and producing more incoherent stories. These differences in performance were diminished, however, on a structured story task that involved narrating from a wordless picture book, indicating that the provision of cues can reduce the ambiguity of what is required, and help to control attention and facilitate the organisation of language production (Losh & Gordon, 2014).

These issues should be borne in mind when interviewing an autistic person as difficulties in executive function, central coherence, social communication and implicit mentalising (e.g., Brunsdon et al., 2015) will only become further encumbered without appropriate adaptations and support. There is a need for further research to empirically test the efficacy of various types of support for autistic people to construct a coherent and appropriate narrative account, but such techniques might involve reducing and explicating the parameters, and providing non-leading prompts in order to alleviate cognitive load and minimise implicit task demands (see also memory section below and the discussion of intermediaries later in this chapter).

Memory in ASD

Memory for an event and the quality of the subsequent narrative account of it are of course inextricably linked, and there is more underlying the impoverished recall of past events than reduced narrative ability alone (Lind et al., 2014). Evidence suggests that autistic individuals may interpret, organise and extract meaning from events differently—both in terms of making sense of the event at the encoding stage and in how the event is processed relation to oneself, which in turn can impact how the memory is recalled (e.g., Berna et al., 2016; Brown, Morris, et al., 2012; Crane et al., 2009, 2010; Losh & Capps, 2006; Loveland et al., 1990; Southwick et al., 2011; Williams et al., 2006; Zalla et al., 2013). For example, Zalla et al. (2013) reported that autistic participants were less accurate at detecting an event's natural segmentation into meaningful units of activity than TD individuals, which was subsequently associated with diminished event recall and poorer memory for event sequences. Research also suggests that autistic individuals may extract less personal meaning from their experiences; for example, Crane et al. (2009) reported that, unlike TD individuals, autistic adults were less likely to retrieve more specific memories in relation to personal goal-related cues, and Crane et al. (2010) reported that autistic adults' autobiographical narratives contained less 'meaning making' in the form of lessons learnt from their experiences compared to TD individuals. It is important to note, however, that the task instructions employed by Crane et al. (2010) only asked participants to describe their memory—there was no explicit requirement to report instances of meaning-making, which relates back to the notion that autistic individuals may perform differently on certain tasks due to difficulties appreciating the implicit task requirements (e.g., White, 2013).

The pattern of memory functioning in ASD is distinct. *Semantic memory*—that is, general knowledge of timeless facts about oneself and others and extended memories lasting longer than a day (e.g., 'last year we went on holiday to France') tends to be intact, while *episodic memory* (i.e., of specific events that are bound in time, place, space and other contextual details) is typically reduced (e.g., Ben Shalom, 2003; Bowler et al., 2000; Crane & Goddard, 2008; Crane, Lind, et al., 2013; Gaigg et al., 2014; Goddard et al., 2007; Klein et al., 1999; Tanweer et al., 2010; and see Crane &

Maras, 2018; Gaigg & Bowler, 2018). For example, utilising semi-structured interviews and an autobiographical fluency task (asking participants to generate memories in response to particular lifetime periods), Crane and Goddard (2008) found that autistic adults recalled fewer specific episodic memories (i.e., of particular instances) from their past, but had no apparent difficulties in reporting general semantic autobiographical knowledge (such as the name of their first teacher at school). Moreover, the memories reported by autistic individuals, while lacking specific and contextual episodic details, contained more general and factual information than those without ASD (Crane & Goddard, 2008).

Autonoetic Awareness and Self-Related Processing

The distinct memory profile observed in ASD is argued to be associated with a reduction in *autonoetic awareness*, which is compensated for by an increase in *noetic awareness* (Bowler et al., 2007; Gardiner, 2001; Tanweer et al., 2010; see also Lind & Bowler, 2008). Autonoetic awareness refers to the conscious re-experiencing of a specific past event with its contextual details, while noetic awareness is an awareness of information in the absence of recollecting and re-experiencing contextual details that signal the acquisition of that knowledge (Tulving, 1983). The diminished autonoetic awareness observed in ASD has been posited to be underpinned by reduced self-awareness, leading to a reduced sense of agency in experiences, a reduction in the organisation and processing of memories in relation to the self, and thus a weakened phenomenological experience of recollection (e.g., Crane et al., 2009; Lind, 2010; see also Lind et al., 2018). This has led to the suggestion that autistic individuals do not preferentially encode self-relevant information at a deeper level (as TD individuals do), with some support for this notion reported in studies showing that autistic individuals fail to demonstrate enhanced recall of adjectives that they were previously instructed to consider in relation to their self- versus another person (e.g., Henderson et al., 2009; Lombardo et al., 2007; Toichi et al., 2002; see also Grisdale et al., 2014). This has potential consequences when recalling instances of victimisation and experiences in which the individual was an active participant. However, other studies examining the 'self-enactment effect' in ASD, whereby (in TD individuals) *actions* that are self-performed are better remembered than actions that are observed being performed by another person, have produced mixed findings. While some studies have reported a diminished or absent self-enactment effect in ASD (e.g., Dunphy-Lelii & Wellman, 2012; Farrant et al., 1998; Hare et al., 2007; Millward et al., 2000; Russell & Jarrold, 1999; Wojcik et al. 2011), others have reported that autistic individuals do recall more of their own actions than those of another person (e.g., Grainger et al., 2014; Hare et al. 2007; Lind & Bowler, 2009; Maras et al., 2013; Summers & Craik, 1994; Williams & Happé, 2009; Zalla et al., 2010; and see also Lind, 2010; and Lind et al., 2014).

These discrepant findings are often related to the methodologies employed, and in particular to the level of task support provided. For example, the reduced or absent self-enactment effect found on tests of free recall does not appear to extend to tests of recognition or cued recall (Hare et al., 2007; Lind & Bowler, 2009; Lind et al., 2019; Zalla et al., 2010). Moreover, Maras et al. (2013) found that while autistic adults recalled more self- than other-performed actions both on a test of free recall and in cued follow-up questions, the autistic group erroneously attributed more self-performed actions as being performed by someone else in their free recall, but these errors were diminished in responses to the cued questions. Taken together, these findings indicate that self-performed actions are at least processed at a deeper level than other-performed actions by both autistic and TD individuals, and that the degree to which they recall this information often depends largely on the conditions in which they come to retrieve them. This has important implications for ensuring optimal interviewing procedures when an autistic person is providing testimony regarding their personal experiences in the CJS.

Source Monitoring, Relational Processing and the Task Support Hypothesis

As is starting to become clear, the memory impairments in ASD are particularly marked on tasks requiring a free narrative account of experienced events (Adler et al., 2010; Bowler et al., 1997, 2008; Chaput et al., 2013; Crane & Goddard, 2008; Crane et al., 2009, 2010, 2012; Crane, Lind, et al., 2013; Goddard et al., 2007; Smith et al., 2007; Tanweer et al., 2010). Episodic events comprise a number of relational elements comprising the *who, when, where, what* and other detailed information including perceptual, temporal, spatial, semantic and affective contextual information. The relations among these items need to be bound together at encoding and organised effectively (analogous to a jigsaw) in order to form contextually rich representations that make that episode distinct from other episodes and enable an individual to mentally travel back in time (Tulving, 2001) to freely recall all elements of the experience at retrieval (Johnson et al., 1993; Schacter et al., 1998). If these features are not sufficiently bound then source monitoring failures can occur, where one aspect or feature of the episode is retrieved but without the context of the rest of the episode. Thus, the individual may recall an element of the experience but cannot recall which experience it was from (e.g., Squire, 1995). Source monitoring failures can also occur when the features of an episode are bound at encoding but there is not enough information to pinpoint the source of the feature at retrieval. For instance, it is often difficult to identify a specific episode of a repeated event, such as a commute to work, which shares many of the same features of other episodes (Renoult et al., 2012).

There is now robust evidence showing that, on unsupported test procedures, autistic people have difficulty in monitoring the source of their memories; for example, recalling when, where or with whom a detail occurred (e.g., Bennetto et al., 1996; Bowler et al., 2004, 2008; Cooper et al., 2016; Lind & Bowler, 2009; Maras et al., 2013). However, these differences are largely eliminated when support for source is provided at test, for example with the use of cued recall or recognition tests (e.g., Bennetto et al., 1996; Bowler et al., 1997, 2004, 2008, 2015). For example, Bowler et al. (2004) presented autistic and TD participants with words to learn that were presented in various contexts (e.g., at the top of bottom of the screen, or in a male or female voice) before asking them to recall each of the words and the format in which it was presented. When participants were given 'support' at test (e.g., with the modes of presentations as options) they performed similarly to the TD group. By contrast, in the 'unsupported' condition, where participants were simply asked to freely recall the context in which each word was presented, they performed significantly worse than the TD group. Such findings have led Bowler and colleagues to propose the task support hypothesis (Bowler et al., 1997, 2004), which states that memory performance in ASD is enhanced on tasks that provide more support for the to-be-remembered material at test.

This pattern of memory performance in ASD suggests that difficulties are related to retrieval, rather than encoding mechanisms (e.g., Cooper et al., 2017), and specifically in re-constructing the spatio-temporal features of the recollected episode (see Bowler et al., 2011). Difficulty in processing the *relations* among items of experience has been suggested to underlie this (see, e.g., Bowler et al., 2011, 2014; Gaigg & Bowler, 2018; Gaigg et al., 2008, 2015). For example, autistic individuals' performance is usually unimpaired when freely recalling lists of unrelated words or items, but when the to-be-remembered items can be categorised into semantically meaningful categories (such as items of fruit, animals, furniture, etc.) they do not utilise the semantic relations among items to bolster their recall (e.g., Boucher & Warrington, 1976; Bowler et al., 1997, 2008, 2009, 2010; Gaigg et al., 2008, 2015; Hermelin & O'Connor, 1967; Minshew & Goldstein, 1993; Renner et al., 2000; Tager-Flusberg, 1991). Autistic participants also make more familiarity-based recognition judgements (which can be mediated on the basis of available item-specific information alone) and fewer autonoetic recollective-based responses, which require drawing on context and the relations among contextual details to aid remembering (e.g., Bowler et al., 2000, 2004, 2007, 2008; Cooper et al., 2016; Lind & Bowler, 2010; Meyer et al., 2014; Tanweer et al., 2010). Critically, autistic individuals can, however, utilise contextual details and the relations among items when the task is structured in a manner that enables the person to organise their responses (e.g., Bowler et al., 1997, 2000, 2008; Hermelin & O'Connor, 1970; Tager-Flusberg, 1991). Again, this is important for the provision of testimony; however, broader difficulties experienced by autistic people in time-related processing such as serial recall (Poirier et al., 2011), temporal estimation (Martin et al., 2010) and time perception (Allman et al., 2011) appear to be more robust and resistant to task support (Bowler et al., 2015). More research is needed, but this does tentatively suggest that autistic witnesses may need particular support in recalling temporal detail.

As well as providing specific support for relational processing, cued recall and recognition tests may also be particularly effective in supporting an autistic person's retrieval difficulties by reducing demands on executive functions and freeing up cognitive resources required to elicit an appropriate search strategy and generate a response. Evidence suggests that autistic individuals rely on effortful executive resources as a compensatory mechanism for relational memory difficulties in order to retrieve episodic and relational memories (Goddard et al., 2014; Maister et al., 2013), yet they also experience broad difficulties in executive functioning (see Demetriou et al., 2018). Moreover, returning to the hypothesis that a failure in 'implicit mentalising' means that autistic difficulties are greatest in open-ended test situations in which the inherent requirements of a task must be garnered via the socially mediated expectations of the experimenter, more directive prompting also serves to diminish the implicit social demands and 'open-endedness' of the task (Kenworthy et al., 2008; Ozonoff, 1995; White, 2013; White et al., 2009).

Eyewitness Testimony in ASD—Evidence to Date

In sum, findings from studies of memory in ASD suggest that the retrieval of specific episodic memories can be difficult (resulting in deployment of more effortful strategies), but that more support at test usually alleviates these differences. To date, studies specifically examining eyewitness memory in children and adults with ASD have largely mirrored these findings of diminished memory performance under free recall conditions, either in terms of fewer correct details reported (e.g., Almeida et al., 2019; Bruck et al., 2007; Henry, Messer, et al., 2017; Henry et al., 2020; Maras & Bowler, 2011, 2012a; Maras et al., 2012, 2013; Maras, Dando, et al., 2020; Mattison et al., 2015; McCrory et al., 2007), or increased errors/reduced accuracy (Maras & Bowler, 2010, 2011, 2012a; Maras et al., 2012, 2013; Mattison et al., 2015). When details are coded for type, this tends to be at the expense of information about people and/or actions (Henry et al., 2017a; Maras & Bowler, 2010, 2012a; Mattison et al., 2015), whereas reporting of surrounding and object information is more likely to undiminished or even enhanced (Maras & Bowler, 2010, 2012a; but see Henry, Messer, et al., 2017; Mattison et al., 2015). Only one study to date has looked at the narrative coherence of autistic witnesses' accounts. Henry et al. (2020) applied a story grammar framework to code autistic and TD children's testimony and found that, while the autistic children recalled fewer event details, they did not differ from TD children on narrative coherence, narrative length, or semantic diversity.

Interview Techniques

In terms of the effectiveness of different interviewing techniques to support testimony by autistic witnesses, however, findings are more mixed. In the first investigation of retrieval support for autistic witnesses, Maras and Bowler (2010) tested the Cognitive interview (CI; Fisher & Geiselman, 1992)—a widely used, evidence-based police interviewing model that has been shown to increase the amount of correct information that adult witnesses recall without a concomitant increase in errors (for a meta-analysis, see Memon, Meissner, et al., 2010). In addition to social communication techniques such as rapport building and transferring control of the interview to the witness, the CI contains various cognitive mnemonics, including instructions from the interviewer to mentally reinstate the context that was experienced during encoding, as well as varied retrieval attempts such as recalling the details in a different order, or changing the perspective of recall (see Dando et al., 2015). Based on the task support hypothesis (Bowler et al., 1997, 2004), it was predicted that the CI would offer useful retrieval support for autistic mock witnesses in recalling a previously viewed video of a stabbing. However, Maras and Bowler (2010) found that the CI had a detrimental effect on autistic adults' recall. Not only did it fail to elicit more correct details from autistic witnesses compared to a structured comparison interview (which had the same number of retrieval attempts and follow-up questions, but without the cognitive mnemonics), it also resulted in significantly more errors and so reduced the overall accuracy of the information they recalled compared to TD witnesses.

The procedure to elicit reinstatement of encoding context in particular was ineffective, which could be related to one of two possibilities. Either autistic individuals failed to encode contextual details during the encoding of an event (in which reinstating the context during retrieval would never be effective), or they experienced difficulty in retrieving the context under the standard verbal interview instructions. To test whether this was more of an encoding or retrieval issue Maras and Bowler (2012a) interviewed autistic and TD adults with the context reinstatement instructions either in a different room from which they witnessed the event (as is usual for this type of eyewitness paradigm) or in the same room, to physically reinstate the context. When interviewed in a different room, the context reinstatement instructions once again resulted in diminished performance by autistic witnesses in terms of both the quantity (number of correct details recalled) and quality (overall accuracy) of recall relative to the TD comparison group. Physically returning to the encoding context at retrieval, however, resulted in better more complete and accurate recall by the autistic group, to the extent that there was no difference between groups in the amount or accuracy of details reported. These findings support the notion that the difficulties autistic people experience in utilising context to enhance their recall are related to retrieval, rather than encoding issues.

Needless to say, returning to the scene of a crime in real life will rarely be practically possible or theoretically appropriate (for instance, if the crime scene has significantly changed or there is risk of post-event misinformation). There is therefore a need for alternative methods of interview-based support to elicit more detailed and accurate recall from autistic witnesses. The Self-Administered Interview (SAI) is a pen and paper evidence-based interview developed by Gabbert et al. (2009) to obtain an early, quality retrieval from witnesses in real-life instances where there are multiple witnesses but limited police resources to interview each witness immediately. Crucially, the SAI contains some of the cognitive mnemonics of the CI, including context reinstatement, but being self-administered removes the social communication techniques. This lack of social element may be pertinent for autistic witnesses given the core social communication difficulties that characterise ASD. Moreover, previous research has found no difference between autistic and TD participants' recall when personal episodic memory tasks are presented in written (Crane, Lind, et al., 2013) and online formats (Zamoscik et al., 2016). As such, the SAI offers potential for autistic witnesses, who may otherwise struggle with the inherently social nature of a police interview (see also White, 2013; White et al., 2009). Maras et al. (2014) tested the effectiveness of the SAI for autistic witnesses. Whereas the context reinstatement instructions remained ineffective in eliciting more detail (compared to a standard control written free recall test), the 'varied retrieval' component, whereby witnesses generated a sketch of the scene, increased recall, indicating that drawing may be a promising avenue to support retrieval by autistic witnesses.

Sketching to reinstate the context (Sketch-RC) is another recently developed variant of the CI which has been found to support witnesses from various populations (including TD adults, older adults and TD children) to recall more information without concomitant increases in errors, and in some cases with significantly reduced errors (e.g., Dando, 2013; Dando et al., 2009). The Sketch-RC supports witnesses to construct a narrative by asking them to sketch what reminds them of the event while verbally describing what they are drawing (see Dando, 2013). Mattison and colleagues (Mattison et al., 2015, 2018) found that sketching significantly improved recall accuracy of an episodic event in autistic children and adolescents versus a matched group who were unsupported. However, despite improved levels of accuracy that put them on a par with their TD peers, autistic participants still recalled less information, in both the free narrative and questioning that followed, indicating a need for research to explore further techniques.

Given the wide heterogeneity in ASD in terms of language, social communication, memory and key other abilities for recalling an event in a police interview, it is likely that autistic individuals need tailored, *individualised* support. Throughout England and Wales, all vulnerable witnesses are eligible for provision of a Registered Intermediary (RI) at police interview and throughout trial (with similar schemes recently introduced in Northern Ireland and New South Wales, Australia; see Cooper & Mattison, 2017). An intermediary's role includes conducting an assessment of the person's communication needs, and providing person-specific recommendations and strategies for (i) how police and the court can communicate information and questions effectively and appropriately (prior to and during questioning); (ii) how best to communicate when preparing the person for the various stages of the criminal justice process; (iii) how to monitor and manage anxiety associated with giving evidence where it impacts upon communication; and (iv) how to appropriately use communication aids and/or devices to support communication such as body diagrams and drawings ('props'). Portrayals of the utility of intermediaries have been positive for use with all vulnerable witnesses (Cooper & Mattison, 2017; Henderson, 2015; O'Mahony et al., 2011) including children (e.g., Marchant, 2013), witnesses with learning disability (O'Mahony, 2010), and autistic witnesses (Cooper & Allely, 2017; Maras et al., 2017), however until recently there have been no empirical investigations of their effectiveness in eliciting more detailed evidence.

Henry, Crane, et al. (2017) examined the efficacy of intermediaries against a standard Best Practice (control) interview and two further supportive interview techniques in a large study of 71 autistic and 199 TD children, aged 6–11 years. Autistic and TD child witnesses viewed (either live or via video) a staged event involving a theft before being immediately interviewed with a 'brief interview' of what they saw (as may be carried out by response officer at the scene; but see Dando et al.,

2018). They were then interviewed again with a full investigative interview one week later, in one of four interview conditions: (i) a Best Practice police interview, based on Achieving Best Evidence (Home Office, 2011), which involved the usual rapport building, background, explaining aims and free recall followed by questioning based on what the child had previously recalled; (ii) a 'Verbal Labels' procedure which differed only in that following free recall, children received 'tell me more' prompts specifically in relation to people, settings, objects, actions and conversations (see Brown & Pipe, 2003); (iii) a Sketch-RC condition, whereby witnesses were instructed to think about the event and draw whatever reminded them about it whilst narrating to the interviewer about what they were sketching, before then engaging in a full free recall attempt; and (iv) a RI condition. Here, children were individually assessed by practising RI in terms of their individual needs (e.g., their language and communication abilities, and their requirement for visual and concrete aids, etc.) prior to the interview, and the RI was then present during the interview to facilitate communication between the witness and interviewer.

For the TD children, the RI and Verbal Labels conditions resulted in significantly more correct details being reported than both Sketch-RC and Best Practice (control) interviews, which did not differ from one another. For the autistic witness group, in contrast, there was no significant difference in the amount of correct details they recalled between any of the conditions. Overall, the autistic children recalled significantly fewer correct details than the TD children (although there was no difference in accuracy), and further analyses indicated that these differences were only statistically significant in the RI condition, indicating that Verbal Labels, Sketch-RC and standard Best Practice interviews were all, on the face of it, effective in eliciting as many correct details from autistic and TD witnesses (Henry, Crane, et al., 2017). However, it is worth noting that the autistic group still recalled around a third fewer correct details ($M = 20.06$ details, $SD = 15.11$) than the TD group ($M = 30.04$ details, $SD = 18.03$) with the Best Practice interviews, suggesting that additional prompting in the form of Verbal Labels ($M = 32.00$ details, $SD = 16.56$) and sketching techniques ($M = 27.17$ details, $SD = 24.11$) are the most useful for autistic witnesses. A recent study examining the effectiveness of a variation of Verbal Labels, which had the addition of a visual pie chart cueing witnesses to recall detail about who, what, where etc. (termed Visual-Verbal Prompting, or V-VP), was also particularly effective in improving the specificity of autistic adults' responses and may prove a useful tool in eliciting specific information from autistic interviewees (Norris et al., 2020).

It is potentially critical that the interview techniques tested by Henry, Crane, et al. (Henry, Crane, et al., 2017) were done so in isolation; in real life they may be carried out in combination—for example, an RI may suggest the use of sketching and Verbal Labels-type prompts during interviews. There are also further methodological imitations in using RIs for the purposes of a large experimental study which may have limited their utility in this context; for example one of only two intermediaries worked with all the children in the RI condition, and there was a significant difference in the amount of information elicited by each of them (see Dando et al., 2018; Henry et al., 2018 for a full and lively discussion of the complexities and potential limitations of this study). Nevertheless, it is important to acknowledge that even with these limitations, the RIs still elicited a similar number of correct details from the autistic group as the current standard Best Practice interviewing protocol in England and Wales; thus, even at worst they still do not have a detrimental effect on recall performance and are likely to have positive effects in other ways, such as whether a witness can be called to give evidence at all (Henry, Crane, et al., 2017; Plotnikoff & Woolfson, 2015).

The Need for Parameters

The prevalent approach for interviewing witnesses in England and Wales is to use a phased approach that commences with a free narrative account of what has occurred, followed by a series of more probing questions concerning topics that were mentioned during free recall (e.g., Milne & Bull, 1999; Ministry of Justice, 2011). Standard open-ended prompts, such as '*report all information, no matter how small or trivial it may seem*' to elicit an exhaustive free narrative account followed by further open questions (e.g., '*Tell me about...*') are, appropriately, ubiquitous within a gold standard police interview (Home Office, 2011). However, as the pattern of findings above indicates, an initial unbounded comprehensive free account may be suboptimal for an autistic witness who may struggle to gauge the demands of the task (how much to report? Does this include what they had for breakfast?) and generate an efficient search strategy (e.g., Maister et al., 2013). Moreover, while limited work to date has examined the *relevance* of details reported by autistic witnesses, findings from the narrative literature indicate that they may make more irrelevant and off-topic intrusions in their accounts when the task is unstructured (e.g., Bruck et al. 2007; Diehl et al., 2006; Losh & Gordon, 2014).

One of the likely reasons why sketching is effective in improving the accuracy (albeit not the completeness) of autistic witnesses' accounts (Mattison et al., 2015, 2018) is that it somewhat reduces the parameters of the to-be-recalled information and alleviates cognitive load from an already burdened retrieval process. Similarly, limited findings tentatively suggest that cued questioning may also be effective in providing direct, target-specific cues that support autistic witnesses to retrieve information (Maras et al., 2012, 2013, 2014; Mattison et al., 2018; McCrory et al., 2007; Millward et al., 2000; Norris et al., 2020). For example, in a personally experienced 'live' eyewitness experiment, Maras et al. (2013) found that, although adults with ASD recalled more self- than other-performed actions on a test of free recall (demonstrating an intact self-enactment effect), they also erroneously attributed more self-performed actions as being performed by someone else in their free recall, but these errors were diminished when cued follow-up questions were used. Research with autistic children also indicates that they require a higher number of prompts during their recall (Almeida et al., 2019; Bruck et al., 2007; Henry, Messer, et al., 2017; see also Goddard et al., 2014). These findings are unsurprising given the robust findings from a now substantial body of laboratory-based experimental work with more basic stimuli showing that memory impairments in ASD are attenuated with task support (e.g., Bowler et al., 2004, 2008, 2015; Hare et al., 2007; Yamamoto & Masumoto, 2018; Zalla et al., 2010; for reviews see Boucher & Bowler, 2008; Boucher et al., 2012).

Most of the current best-practice methods such as the CI, and also the Sketch-RC technique, all rely on free recall from the outset in order to elicit an uncontaminated witness-led account that forms the basis for subsequent probing (Milne & Bull, 1999), yet these techniques, in their current form, are ineffective in improving the completeness of autistic witnesses' accounts. The importance of a quality initial recall attempt cannot be overstated in preserving the integrity and completeness of subsequent retrievals (e.g., Gabbert et al., 2009, 2012; Memon, Zaragoza, et al., 2010; Shaw et al., 1995). Thus, if free recall is suboptimal for autistic witnesses then this may have a knock-on effect in limiting their successive retrieval attempts even with the provision of questions. However, while the use of cued recall, closed, directed and recognition recall techniques can be effective for supporting autistic witnesses to recall more information or more accurately in laboratory settings, for the criminal justice system the use of questions that are not preceded by some form of witness-led free account is highly problematic for several reasons. First, the questions would be solely guided by what information the interviewer *knows* at the time (e.g., from other witnesses, crime reports, etc.) and, relatedly, what the interviewer *thinks* is important. Second, TD individuals tend to produce less information in response to more specific questions as opposed to free recall prompts (e.g., Fisher & Geiselman, 1992; Milne & Bull, 1999). Third, specific questions are also known to reduce accuracy generally (Brown & Lamb, 2015), and may introduce leading and demand characteristics in an autistic witness (Chander et al., 2018; North et al., 2008). Finally, eliciting recall that is not initially witness-driven may result in the evidence obtained being inadmissible in court (Walker, 2002).

Thus, witness-led recall, in response to some form of an 'open' prompt, is necessary to commence the interview and scaffold the questioning that follows, in order to ensure that memory for the event is uninfluenced by the interviewer and is compatible within legally and theoretically based frameworks. As noted by Oxburgh et al. (2010), however, the classification of different question types and what defines an 'open' question is a grey area. For example, while the focus is often on how a question is phrased, with wide agreement that TED questions ('Tell', 'Explain', 'Describe') are usually more appropriate at the outset of an interview than 5WH (commencing with 'who', 'what', 'when', 'where' and 'why') and specific closed questions, others have argued that the function of the question is more important, for instance, in terms of the *breadth* or *depth* of answer that it aims to elicit (Powell & Snow, 2007; see also Grant et al., 2015; Griffiths & Milne, 2006).

Based on the pattern of findings from the ASD literature discussed thus far, from narratives to memory to the effectiveness of interviewing techniques, it is tempting to suggest that autistic individuals may need more scaffolding to support the depth of information they provide, while tapering the breadth that is required at any one time. Ultimately, autistic witnesses may require 'open' recall invitations that nevertheless include more specific guidance regarding where the parameters lie and breaking recall into smaller units of information—for example, '*tell me everything that happened yesterday in the park*'. Indeed, Almeida et al. (2019) recently provided empirical evidence that cued invitations that focus the witness's recall (e.g., 'tell me more about that') elicits more details from both autistic and TD witnesses compared to both very open invitations (e.g., 'tell me everything that happened') and to more closed forms of questioning (e.g., 'what colour was it?'). Cued invitations are a distinctive feature of the National Institute of Child Health and Human Development (NICHD) Investigative Interview Protocol for interviewing children (see Lamb et al., 2007), and maybe particularly helpful for autistic witnesses. Encouragingly, a survey of police officers in England and Wales indicated that police officers themselves recognised the importance of narrowing the parameters in their questioning (Crane et al., 2016), for instance by specifying the time frame, place or event that the witness should focus on.

Preliminary findings testing a recently developed novel interviewing technique designed specifically to support the aforementioned difficulties experienced by autistic individuals within a legally appropriate framework appear promising (Maras, Dando, et al., 2020). In the Witness-Directed First Account (WAFA), the witness self-segments their memory of an event into their own discrete parameter-bound 'topic boxes' at the outset, before engaging in an exhaustive free recall retrieval attempt (followed by interviewer probing) within the parameters of each topic box in turn. Here, the interviewer will encourage the witness to section their memory of the event with the instruction, '*in just a few words or a couple of sentences, what was the most important thing that you saw in the video*'. The witness might indicate that they saw two men having a fight. The interviewer will then ask them again to recall in just a few words or a couple of sentences something else that they saw happen, and so forth until the witness indicates they have segmented the entire event. The interviewer notes each of these topics on a post-it note and displays it on the wall for both interviewer and interviewee to see as they go. Next, the witness engages in an exhaustive free recall retrieval attempt (followed by interviewer probing) within the parameters of each topic box in turn. Thus, the witness still self-directs their recall, as would happen during a typical free narrative account, but rather than having a free flow verbalisation of the entire event—which is difficult for autistic individuals and so they inevitably underperform—they provide their own segmentation of the event. Displaying the topic boxes on post-it notes serves as a reminder of the structure of the event and reduces the amount of event information that they have to hold 'online', which may reduce demands on executive functions and working memory, freeing up cognitive resources and allowing the witness to focus their search and retrieval strategies within individual segments. Findings indicate that the WAFA interview elicits more detailed and accurate recall from both autistic and TD witnesses than a standard best practice interview. The WAFA technique may be a useful tool to improve autistic (and indeed TD) witnesses' accounts within a legally appropriate, non-leading framework.

Suggestibility and Compliance

As discussed, while autistic witnesses may need more focused prompts to reduce social and cognitive demands, they should nevertheless be open in order to elicit longer and more detailed and accurate responses and to avoid leading and contaminating the witness' recall (see Ridley et al., 2012). Based on the pattern of memory findings discussed earlier in this chapter (particularly regarding source monitoring), it would seem reasonable to suggest that autistic individuals may be more likely to confuse the source of their memories, accept misinformation and yield to leading questions. To date, five studies have examined susceptibility to suggestive questions and misinformation in individuals ASD, two with children (Bruck et al., 2007; McCrory et al., 2007) and three with adults (), and none have found evidence of heightened suggestibility. Indeed, across a range of paradigms from live events with or without personal involvement followed by misleading questions (Bruck et al., 2007; McCrory et al., 2007), to a standardised suggestibility scale (the Gudjonsson Suggestibility Scale; Gudjonsson, 1997) involving recall of an audio narrative with leading questions and negative feedback from the interviewer (Maras & Bowler, 2012b; North et al., 2008), to post-event 'schema-typical' misinformation presented in a newspaper report about a previously viewed slide sequence of a bank robbery, autistic witnesses are no more—or less—suggestible than their TD peers. However, it is worth noting that Bruck et al. (2007) found that while autistic children resisted misleading questions and incorporated suggested information into their reports to the same extent as TD children, they were more likely to assent to questions about 'silly' questions such 'Have you ever helped a lady find a monkey in the park?'

A key point here is that all of these studies included relatively cognitively able individuals (that is, without accompanying intellectual impairment). Nevertheless, these findings indicate that intellectually able autistic individuals are *not* more likely to come to accept suggestions from an interviewer's questions or misinformation from say a co-witness than TD individuals are. Nor, however, are they any *less* likely to do so. Thus, an interviewer's questions must always be unbiased.

Whereas suggestibility refers to the extent to which an individual is genuinely misled about information, to the extent that they come to accept as true (Gudjonsson & Clark, 1986), compliance, on the other hand, refers to an individual's tendency to carry out the requests or demands of others or being led, manipulated or pressured into agreeing to a statement or falsely confessing for some immediate instrumental gain such as terminating the interview earlier (Gudjonsson, 1989, 2003). Using an informant-reported version of a standardised measure of compliance—the Gudjonsson Compliance Scale (GCS, Gudjonsson, 1997), North et al. (2008) reported that autistic individuals were more compliant than TD adults. However, using a self-report version of the same scale, Maras and Bowler (2012b) reported no difference between autistic and TD participants. These discrepant findings might be related to the different samples recruited by each study which, although comparable in terms of age and gender, may have differed with respect to self-esteem, anxiety and other predisposing factors (e.g., Carter-Sowell et al., 2008; Gudjonsson et al.,

2002). For example, North et al. (2008) sampled inpatients on a specialist unit for people with autism, while Maras and Bowler (2012b) recruited participants from an existing research database, suggesting potential subtle differences in vulnerability between samples. Moreover, difficulties in self-reflection are reported in ASD (e.g., Ben Shalom et al., 2006; Mazefsky et al., 2011), with some evidence that autistic individuals under-report their difficulties (Findon et al., 2016). Thus, the self-reported version of the GCS utilised by Maras and Bowler (2012b) may have resulted in an under-estimation of compliance. Using self-report measures may have further shortcomings: conceptually, the GCS measures compliance globally, rather than in response to a specific situation. This is problematic, as people may be more or less compliant in different situations, based on who they are with and what is being asked of them (Gudjonsson et al., 2004).

To examine this further, Chandler et al. (2019) administered the GCS alongside a behavioural measure of compliance, the 'door in the face' task (Cialdini et al., 1975), which is based on the notion that a request made to others is more likely to be agreed to if it is preceded by the offer and refusal of a more expensive request (Pascual & Guéguen, 2005). Here, participants completed questionnaires as part of their planned research participation session. In the end, when they expected to leave, they were asked to complete an additional two hours' worth of tasks for no additional reimbursement of their time. Most TD individuals rejected this original costly request, instead agreeing to a subsequent smaller 'target' request of 20 min of their time. Chandler et al. (2019), however, found that that autistic individuals were more likely to agree to the highly unreasonable request in the first instance. The autistic group also self-reported higher compliance on the CGS, which appeared to be driven by lower self-esteem. These findings highlight that extreme caution is warranted by criminal justice professionals to ensure that autistic witnesses, victims and suspects are not unduly influenced to being led while giving evidence.

Interview Format

It is important to consider the setting and format in which the questions are asked; for example, whether in a social situation (such as a traditional face-to-face interview) or non-socially (e.g., via pen and paper, email or an online questionnaire). As noted earlier, autistic people's abilities may often be under-estimated because their difficulties understanding others' intentions and needs can make it difficult for them to know what is required of them. Indeed, when more explicit instructions are provided, or when computerised tasks are used, autistic people's difficulties are often reduced (Kenworthy et al., 2008; White, 2013; White et al., 2009).

Hsu and Teoh (2017) examined the potential utility of a computer avatar interviewing aid to reduce the social demands of an interview. Autistic and TD children participated in a target event before being interviewed by either an avatar or a human using the NICHD Investigative Interview Protocol (see Lamb et al., 2007), which was followed by six misleading questions. Initial analyses indicated no effect of being interviewed by the avatar vs. human for either recall completeness or resistance to misleading questions by either group. However, a subsequent Bayesian analysis (which is less impacted by issues with sample size) indicated that, for the autistic children only, the avatar interviewer was more likely to elicit details about the event with higher accuracy than the human interviewer. Moreover, when interviewed by the computer avatar, the autistic group children actually gave more information and were more accurate than the TD children. However, the avatar interviewer resulted in less accurate responses to misleading questions by both groups, warranting caution in its broader practical utility. Nevertheless, the preliminary finding that avatar-based interviewing elicits more correct details from autistic witnesses is potentially promising.

Maras, Norris, et al. (2020) recently examined the impact of social (face-to-face questions) vs. non-social (an online questionnaire) interview format on the informativeness and accuracy of autistic and TD witnesses' memory reports. Contrary to predictions, delivering the questions socially improved overall accuracy rates for both groups compared to online delivery. However, the autistic group nevertheless showed poorer metacognitive control in their reporting decisions (in terms of optimising both accuracy and informativeness) compared to TD witnesses under social, but not online, reporting conditions. Thus, it seems that while autistic individuals may be as motivated as TD individuals to enhance their accuracy under social reporting conditions, underlying social cognitive difficulties may over-burden autistic individuals' executive resources in contexts involving social interaction, limiting their ability to make optimal reporting decisions (see also Dichter & Belger, 2007). Maras, Norris, et al. (2020) also included a condition explicitly instructing witnesses to maximise accuracy over informativeness, which improved both autistic and TD witnesses' reporting accuracy similarly and substantially. This is consistent with the contention that autistic individuals' performance is more impaired the greater the degree of open-endedness of the test situation (e.g., Ciesielski & Harris, 1997; Van Eylen et al., 2011; White, 2013; White et al., 2009), and has implications for the instructions they receive about the importance of accuracy when providing eyewitness testimony.

These findings have a number of important practical implications for obtaining eyewitness testimony from autistic individuals. First and foremost, autistic witnesses can provide as detailed and accurate testimony as non-autistic witnesses when specific and cued questions are used. Further, while both autistic and TD witnesses are sometimes more accurate in their recall of events when questions are delivered socially, autistic witnesses appear to have subtle difficulties in reporting control under social conditions, indicating that social situations may be motivating but nevertheless more cognitively burdensome for autistic witnesses. Further research is needed, but tentatively this suggests that interview situations which are fundamentally social (e.g., where questions are delivered by an interviewer) but in which social complexities and ambiguities have been minimised (e.g., avoiding the pressure for eye contact, using more direct language, etc.) may optimise recall from autistic witnesses.

Intellectual Disability and Co-occurring Conditions

Research indicates that between around one-third (Christensen et al., 2016) to over half of all autistic individuals (Baird et al., 2006) also have accompanying intellectual impairment, which can in itself pose (not insurmountable) challenges for obtaining evidence (e.g., Brown, Lewis, et al., 2012; Henry & Gudjonsson, 2007; see Milne & Bull, 2006). There is a paucity of research examining eyewitness recall by autistic individuals who also have intellectual impairment, however general intellectual disability more broadly tends to be associated with free recall that is less complete (e.g., Agnew & Powell, 2004; Cederborg et al., 2012; Henry & Gudjonsson, 2007; Perlman et al., 1994), but not necessarily less accurate (e.g., Agnew & Powell, 2004; Henry & Gudjonsson, 2003; see also Bull, 2010; Henry et al., 2011). However, less complete free recall in the first instance can also lead an interviewer to relying on more specific and closed forms of questioning to elicit more details (e.g., Cederborg & Lamb, 2008; Kebbell et al., 2004). A weakened memory trace in combination with specific questions can result in a lower accuracy reporting threshold and, accordingly, heightened suggestibility (see Maras & Wilcock, 2012). Cognitive limitations can also lead to difficulties in understanding questions unless communication is appropriately modified (see O'Mahony et al., 2015). While this brief overview paints a relatively negative picture, individuals with intellectual disability can and do provide important, detailed and good quality evidence (e.g., Agnew & Powell, 2004). Indeed, though an autistic person's overall level of cognitive functioning and language ability are significant factors in the level of support they require in order to provide a comprehensive account, even severe impairments do not necessarily preclude an individual's ability to provide detailed key investigative information—as long as they supported appropriately. Even witnesses as young as 22-months have been documented to provide key evidence with appropriate professional support such as with a Registered Intermediary (Marchant, 2016; O'Mahony et al., 2015).

ASD is also associated with a high rate of co-occurring psychiatric disorders including depression, anxiety, attention-deficit/hyperactivity disorder (ADHD), bipolar disorder, obsessive–compulsive disorder and schizophrenia (e.g., Croen et al., 2015; Russell et al., 2016; Simonoff et al., 2008; Wigham et al., 2017). Each of these conditions can present its own challenges for memory encoding and retrieval processes. For example, ADHD poses obvious issues in maintaining attention during an interview (see Alderson et al., 2013), while depression is associated with attenuated retrieval of specific memories (e.g., Dalgleish et al., 2007). Co-occurring anxiety, which is particularly exacerbated in new and unpredictable situations, can also make an interview process extremely difficult for an autistic person (Wigham et al., 2015).

Police Suspects

A police suspect interview is a complex social situation that can vacillate between information gathering and confrontational (Soukara et al., 2009). Most detecting deception techniques are designed to impose additional mental effort on a suspect, on the basis that lying requires more mental resources than truth telling (see Vrij et al., 2008). For example, an interviewer may reveal evidence in a tactical manner, forcing the interviewee to respond to challenges without an opportunity to rehearse a response (see Bull, 2014). An individual who has impaired insight into others' intentions and finds it difficult to predict their responses will naturally be at a disadvantage in such a context. Indeed, regardless of whether they are telling the truth or not, core impairments in social communication impairments and behavioural inflexibility (American Psychiatric Association, 2013), together with executive function impairments (Demetriou et al., 2018), difficulties in seeing information in context (Happé & Frith, 2006) and considering the knowledge and beliefs held by the interviewer (Baron-Cohen et al., 1985) may all make a police suspect interview extremely difficult for an autistic person. No research to date has examined how autistic individuals fare under a police suspect interview, but the heightened cognitive complexities imposed by a police interviewer, shifting social demands, and the stress of being interviewed as a police suspect (Vrij et al., 2006, 2017) are only likely to heighten these impairments.

The prevalent approach to interviewing suspects in the US and some parts of Canada is the controversial Reid Technique of interviewing and interrogation (Inbau et al., 2013), which is guilt-presumptive and seeks hypothesis confirmation through the coercion and manipulation of a suspect (Gudjonsson, 2003; Vrij, 2008). It is associated with a high rate of false confessions even in TD populations (see Gudjonsson & Pearse, 2011) and would without a doubt be particularly perilous with an autistic suspect who has social communication difficulties and a greater tendency towards compliance (Chandler et al., 2019; North et al., 2008).

In contrast, when suspects are interviewed in England and Wales, the 'PEACE' model of investigative interviewing (an acronym for: Preparation and Planning; Engage and Explain; Account, Clarify and Challenge; Closure) is employed where the focus is on *information gathering* and hypothesis *testing* (Home Office, 2017). This model promotes the use of the cognitive interview (CI) and/or conversation management approach for interviews with police suspects (Clarke & Milne, 2001). Although the PEACE model and specific techniques within it, such as the strategic or tactical disclosure of evidence, are evidence-based in eliciting more key evidence and true confessions, together with fewer false confessions from the general population (Bull, 2010; Meissner et al., 2014; Soukara et al., 2009), their utility with autistic suspects remains to be tested. Evidence shows that the CI is ineffective for interviewing autistic witnesses (Maras & Bowler, 2010, 2012a; Maras et al., 2014; Mattison et al., 2015, 2018), and it thus seems unlikely that it would be effective for autistic suspects. Moreover, while asking for detailed explanations of behaviours and using unpredictable questioning strategies are often effective in triggering 'neurotypical' behavioural indicators of deception such as speech hesitations and errors, as well as leakage of information that could not be known by a truth teller (e.g., Ormerod & Dando, 2015; Porter & Brinke, 2010; Vrij et al., 2009), such techniques may have an unduly negative impact on the perceived credibility of an autistic suspect (see also Maras et al., 2019). Autistic individuals already display manifestations that others may consider indicative of dishonesty (see DePaulo et al., 2003), such as atypical eye contact (Neumann et al., 2006; Senju & Johnson, 2009), stereotyped body movements and gestures (de Marchena & Eigsti, 2010; Gritti et al., 2003), atypical speech characteristics and prosody (Peppé et al., 2007), and unusual expression of emotion (Loveland et al., 1994). These behaviours are likely to be exacerbated further during the stress and social cognitive complexity of a police suspect interview (e.g., Boulter et al., 2014; Rodgers et al., 2012).

Police interviewers are provided with very little guidance on how to interview vulnerable suspects (O'Mahony et al., 2012, 2015). Although Registered Intermediaries (RIs) are mandatory at police interviews and court for vulnerable witnesses in England and Wales, suspects are only permitted a (non-registered) intermediary at court. Nevertheless, the provision of an Appropriate Adult (AA) is required for all vulnerable suspects in England and Wales (Home Office, 2011). The AA maybe a friend, family member or professional, and their role is to support, advise and assist the detainee to ensure they understand what is happening at the police station during the interview and investigative stages. They may also facilitate communication between the detainee and police. The AA must be present during interviews and may intervene if they feel it necessary to improve communication, advise that a break is needed, or recommend that the detainee should seek legal advice. Previous research indicates some negativity by police in the use of AAs (Leggett et al., 2007; Oxburgh et al., 2016). While they often remain passive and have been found to interact inappropriately at times, the mere presence of an AA may have a positive impact on police interviewing practice (Medford et al., 2003).

Richards and Milne (2020) recently explored the ability of AAs to recognise and support the specific needs of an autistic suspect at interview. They found that while many of the AAs they surveyed had basic knowledge of the key features of autism, they generally had little awareness of the potential impact that these might have upon custody and interviewing procedures. Richards and Milne warn that general knowledge of autism is not enough in this context, and that a failure to acknowledge how the consequences of autism may impact their performance in a suspect interview will limit their ability as their AA to support them. Given the mandatory status of AAs and the confusion some police officers demonstrate regarding their role (Maras et al., 2018), there is an urgent need for future research to empirically examine their utility for interviews with suspects with autism.

At Court

While police witness interviews are constrained to the use of non-leading, witness-led styles of questioning with the aim of eliciting a detailed and accurate portrayal of what happened, the aim of cross-examination in court is to discredit the witness (Stone, 1988). The use of suggestive (e.g., '*he was wearing a red hat, wasn't he?*'), leading (e.g., '*did he have a knife?*'), multiple part (e.g., '*did you leave the house and was this before or after you received the phone call?*'), complex (e.g., '*Is it not the case that when you saw John his demeanour was shifty which led to you to believe that his must have done something untoward?*'), negative and double negative (e.g., '*is it not the case that he did not go outside?*') and tag questions (e.g., '*you got the bus here, didn't you?*') is widespread, even though research has shown that even TD adults are susceptible to the negative effects of cross-examination and become less, rather than more, accurate (e.g., Ellison & Wheatcroft, 2010; Kebbell et al., 2010; Wheatcroft & Ellison, 2012). For example, laboratory studies show that adults are just as likely to change a correct answer as they are an incorrect one (Valentine & Maras, 2011), and the impact of cross-examination on the testimony of children is, unsurprisingly, deleterious (e.g., Zajac & Hayne, 2003, 2006). Thus, the effect of the sort of adversarial, leading, negative and complex questions favoured by barristers on individuals with intellectual disability and social communication impairments is also likely to be particularly dismal (see Gudjonsson, 2003; Henderson et al., 2015; Kebbell & Hatton, 1999). Worryingly, Kebbell et al. (2004) showed that lawyers do not change their style of questioning for witnesses with intellectual disability. No research to date has examined how autistic individuals fare under cross-examination in court, but given the core social communication difficulties it is unlikely to be favourably, neither in terms of the quality of the information that they provide nor for how credible they are perceived to be by others (see Crane et al., 2018; Maras et al., 2019).

The 1999 Youth Justice and Criminal Evidence Act in England and Wales enables a range of 'Special Measures' to be used to assist the provision of testimony from vulnerable witnesses and victims. These include the use of screens in court (so that the witness cannot see the defendant), evidence via live video link to the courtroom, video-recorded evidence-in-chief (e.g., the previously video recorded investigative interview with the police, if appropriate), the use of a RI (both at court or during the police interview to assist communication), and communication aids (usually with the assistance of a skilled communication expert such as an RI)—to enable a vulnerable witness to give their best evidence (see Bull, 2010; O'Mahony et al., 2015). The presence of an RI may be key in both facilitating communications as well as improving perceptions. Although no research has examined the impact of an RI's presence on perceptions of autistic witnesses, Collins et al. (2017) recently reported that child witnesses' behaviour and communication was rated more positively when an RI was present, as was the quality of the cross-examination more generally (see also Ridley et al., 2015).

It has been argued that the Special Measures that are available to vulnerable witnesses in England and Wales should also be offered to vulnerable suspects (Jacobson, 2008; O'Mahony et al., 2015), and recent development in England and Wales is that defendants will now be eligible for the provision of an intermediary to support them in giving evidence at court. The effect of their presence on both a defendant's provision of evidence and their perceived credibility awaits empirical scrutiny in future research.

Although the focus of this chapter has been on obtaining testimony in criminal cases, many of the underlying principles will also apply to the family courts and civil cases. The family justice system in particular is a largely overlooked but critically important area that can have huge repercussions on an individual's life. George et al. (2018) reported that legal professionals have low levels of confidence working with autistic individuals in the family justice system. Legal practitioners were particularly concerned about communication—both in terms of how an autistic person is able to communicate effectively with others but also how they should adopt their own communication styles. George et al. (2018) provide a number of useful recommendations including the use of clear, unambiguous language, visual aids such as a written agenda to remind the person of the structure and content of the proceedings (e.g., with photographs and names of the people involved in the case), and pretrial familiarisation visits so that the individual is more relaxed in giving evidence on the day.

The Advocate's Gateway (www.theadvocatesgateway.org) also provides practical guidance on vulnerable witnesses and defendants, including a range of toolkits that provide general good practice guidance across the criminal, family and civil courts when preparing for trial in cases involving a witness or defendant who is vulnerable (including two specifically on ASD).

Stress, Sensory Sensitivities and Other Practical Issues

Before concluding this chapter, it is imperative to mention sensory issues and other potential precursors that can cause sometimes debilitating levels of stress for an autistic person. Restricted and repetitive behaviours and an insistence on sameness are core features of the disorder (American Psychiatric Association, 2013), and high rates of clinical levels of anxiety (Russell et al., 2016; Simonoff et al., 2008) together difficulties in coping with change, anticipation and unpleasant events will only be compounded in a new and highly stressful social environment such as a police interview (Gillot & Standen, 2007).

Sensory sensitivities are also common in ASD (e.g., Ben-Sasson et al., 2009; Liss et al., 2006). For example, many autistic people are hypersensitive, meaning that they find sensory information such as lighting or noises almost painful and can have difficulty screening them out (Rogers & Ozonoff, 2005). Again, this is often worsened under new or anxiety-provoking situations, such as a police interview (Neil et al., 2016). Police environments and courtrooms are often loud, brightly lit (e.g., with florescent strip lighting) and sometimes strong-smelling environments. It is therefore necessary to consider how the environment might be adapted to minimise potential sources of sensory discomfort for an autistic interviewee, while also bearing in mind that no two also autistic individuals are the same—one person may be extremely sensitive to touch, for example, while others have little notion of personal space (e.g., Kennedy & Adolphs, 2014). Thus, it is important to consult the individual and/or those who know them well regarding what particular sensitivities, triggers and other stressors they may experience and where possible the timing and location of the interview should be planned around these. This may be as simple as removing a ticking clock from the wall of the interview room, but other times it will be necessary to interview the person in a familiar environment such as their own home in order to elicit the best evidence (see Maras et al., 2018). A witness who feels more relaxed and comfortable can provide more detailed and accurate evidence (Geiselman et al., 1984).

It is also worth noting that 'stimming', a self-stimulatory behaviour common in ASD (usually involving repetitive movements such as flapping the arms or flicking the hands, rubbing fingers together, or making faces), is often used as a soothing mechanism and a way of regulating sensory input in ASD (Sinha et al., 2014). It is important that an interviewer does not try to stop an individual from stimming, nor take away any objects they may have (e.g., a fidget spinner), as this can cause extreme anxiety, damaging rapport and trust and ultimately evidence quality.

Practical Recommendations

- Potential sensory issues should be considered. An alternative interview location in a more familiar and comfortable environment may be more appropriate. If not, modifications to the existing setting may be necessary.
- Disruption to routine, a new environment and lack of predictability are all inherently stressful for an autistic person, so it is important that the interview is planned, and the individual is given detailed information about this in advance, so they know what will happen and when.
- The aim of the interview (and particular questions that are not obviously related to the incident in question) should be clearly outlined to the individual at the outset.
- An autistic person may be less likely to engage with/understand the point of rapport building (see Vallano & Schreiber Compo, 2015) at the start of the interview. When rapport building, it may be helpful to find out the person's interests and avoid small talk.
- An interviewer should be clear, direct and unambiguous. Metaphors, sarcasm, non-literal questions and questions that are posed as statements should be avoided. Information that is implied by an interviewer's facial expressions or body language but is not supported by their speech may also go unrecognised.

- An autistic person's expressive (spoken) language may be better than their receptive (comprehending and understanding) language ability, and they may therefore need more time to process questions before answering.
- Relatedly, holding and considering multiple sources of information 'online' can be difficult some autistic people, so it is important that questions do not exacerbate this by being overly complex, long, or multiple part. They also should only be asked one question at a time.
- Some autistic people confuse pronouns (e.g., saying 'her mum' when talking about a *male's* mother or *their own* mother). If in doubt, the person they are referring to should be checked.
- An autistic person may repeat certain phrases, words, or sounds over and over (termed 'Echolalia') or may repeat back something the interviewer has just said (see Boucher, 2012). This should not be confused with rudeness, a lack of understanding, compliance, or their genuine answer to your question (e.g., Q: '*Did you go to the hospital last Tuesday?*' A: '*hospital last Tuesday*').
- Autistic people often have difficulty generating a coherent narrative of events in response to a single prompt, but they may have excellent recall when asked specific *non-leading* questions (e.g., '*tell me about what happened in the car park*').
- An autistic person may be more compliant to false confessions to stop conversation, or to conform to suggestions without realising the consequences of this. As with all witnesses, leading and suggestive questions should be avoided.

Summary and Conclusion

A police interview is an anxiety-provoking situation for most people but especially those with ASD, and core difficulties in social communication coupled with specific memory difficulties can be particularly exacerbated by stress. Constructing an exhaustive free narrative requires retrieving a specific past event and generating, monitoring and controlling output while understanding the listener's perspective and bigger picture in order to produce an appropriately detailed, coherent, causal and relevant account. These are all areas of difficulty for an autistic person. Accordingly, although free recall is widely accepted in both psychology and policing as the gold standard to produce the most accurate, uncontaminated witness recall (Home Office, 2011), autistic people may need more guided and focused retrieval from the outset to: (a) support their memory retrieval; (b) reduce implicit social demands regarding what is relevant for recall; and (c) minimise cognitive load and demands on 'executive resources'.

Rather than unbounded free recall instructions, autistic individuals may require more focused prompts that specify the parameters or breadth of information to be recalled, but questions should remain open-ended in the sense of eliciting depth of detail; closed and forced-choice questions should be avoided where possible. Several studies have investigated different techniques for supporting autistic witnesses, but there remains a need to examine further techniques that increase the completeness and accuracy of their recall. There is also an urgent need for empirical investigations of obtaining testimony from autistic individuals in court and from autistic suspects. Nevertheless, *all* autistic individuals should be treated as vulnerable regardless of their level of intellectual functioning. Even autistic individuals with very high intelligence have difficulty with social interaction and communication. Where available, an RI should always be appointed at the earliest possible stage.

In sum, interviewing techniques should support autistic people's individual processing style while utilising parameter-bound retrieval methods that reduce cognitive load and implicit task demands. They must also be compatible with both practical frameworks (e.g., *Achieving Best Evidence* guidance; Home Office, 2011) and theoretical understanding of the importance of witness-compatible retrieval (see Fisher & Geiselman, 1992). Across the studies reviewed in this chapter, it is pertinent to note the large heterogeneity in performance within the autistic groups. Indeed, as Henry, Crane, et al. (2017) note, the most effective interventions for autistic witnesses tend to be individualised; what does not work for one autistic witness is effective for another. It is therefore important that interviewing techniques are used flexibly, based on an individual witness' needs and abilities.

References

Adler, N., Nadler, B., Eviatar, Z., & Shamay-Tsoory, S. G. (2010). The relationship between theory of mind and autobiographical memory in high-functioning autism and Asperger syndrome. *Psychiatry Research, 178*, 214–216. https://doi.org/10.1016/j.psychres.2009.11.015.

Agnew, S. E., & Powell, M. B. (2004). The effect of intellectual disability on children's recall of an event across different question types. *Law and Human Behavior, 28*(3), 273–294.

Alderson, R. M., Kasper, L. J., Hudec, K. L., & Patros, C. H. G. (2013). Attention-Deficit/Hyperactivity Disorder (ADHD) and working memory in adults: A meta-analytic review. *Association, 27*(3), 287–302. https://doi.org/10.1037/a0032371.

Allman, M. J., DeLeon, I. G., & Wearden, J. H. (2011). Psychophysical assessment of timing in individuals with autism. *American Journal of Intellectual and Developmental Disabilities, 116*, 165–178.

Almeida, T. S., Lamb, M. E., & Weisblatt, E. J. (2019). Effects of delay, question type, and socioemotional support on episodic memory retrieval by children with autism spectrum disorder. *Journal of Autism and Developmental Disorders, 49*, 1111–1130. https://doi.org/10.1007/s10803-018-3815-3.

American Psychiatric Association (2013). *Diagnostic and statistical manual of mental disorders* (5th ed). Arlington: VA: American Psychiatric Publishing.

Baird, G., Simonoff, E., Pickles, A., Chandler, S., Loucas, T., Meldrum, D., & Charman, T. (2006). Prevalence of disorders of the autism spectrum in a population cohort of children in South Thames: The Special Needs and Autism Project (SNAP). *Lancet, 368*, 210–215. https://doi.org/10.1016/S0140-6736(06)69041-7.

Barnes, J. L., & Baron-Cohen, S. (2012). The big picture: Storytelling ability in adults with autism spectrum conditions. *Journal of Autism and Developmental Disorders, 42*, 1557–1565. https://doi.org/10.1007/s10803-011-1388-5.

Baron-Cohen, S. (1988). Social and pragmatic deficits in autism: Cognitive or affective? *Journal of Autism and Developmental Disorders, 18*(3), 379–402.

Baron-Cohen, S., Leslie, A. M., & Frith, U. (1985). Does the autistic child have a theory of mind? *Cognition, 21*, 37–46.

Beaumont, R., & Newcombe, P. (2006). Theory of mind and central coherence in adults with high-functioning autism or Asperger syndrome. *Autism, 10*(4), 365–382.

Bennetto, L., Pennington, B. F., & Rogers, S. J. (1996). Intact and impaired memory functions in autism. *Child Development, 67*, 1816–1835. https://doi.org/10.2307/1131734.

Berna, F., Göritz, A. S., Schröder, J., Coutelle, R., Danion, J.-M., Cuervo-Lombard, C. V., & Moritz, S. (2016). Self-disorders in individuals with autistic traits: Contribution of reduced autobiographical reasoning capacities. *Journal of Autism and Developmental Disorders, 46*, 2587–2598. https://doi.org/10.1007/s10803-016-2797-2.

Ben-Sasson, A., Hen, L., Fluss, R., Cermak, S. A., Engel-Yeger, B., & Gal, E. (2009). A meta-analysis of sensory modulation symptoms in individuals with autism spectrum disorders. *Journal of Autism and Developmental Disorders, 39*, 1–11. https://doi.org/10.1007/s10803-008-0593-3.

Ben Shalom, D. (2003). Memory in autism: Review and synthesis. *Cortex, 39*(4–5), 1129–1138.

Ben Shalom, D., Mostofsky, S. H., Hazlett, R. L., Goldberg, M. C., Landa, R. J., Faran, Y., et al. (2006). Normal physiological emotions but differences in expression of conscious feelings in children with high-functioning autism. *Journal of Autism and Developmental Disorders, 36*(3), 395–400.

Boucher, J. (2012). Research review: Structural language in autistic spectrum disorder–characteristics and causes. *Journal of Child Psychology and Psychiatry, 53*(3), 219–233.

Boucher, J., & Bowler, D. M. (Eds.). (2008). *Memory in autism.* Cambridge University Press.

Boucher, J., Mayes, A., & Bigham, S. (2012). Memory in autistic spectrum disorder. *Psychological Bulletin, 138*, 458–496. https://doi.org/10.1037/a0026869.

Boucher, J., & Warrington, E. K. (1976). Memory deficits in early infantile autism: Some similarities to the amnesic syndrome. *British Journal of Psychology, 67*, 73–87. https://doi.org/10.1111/j.2044-8295.1976.tb01499.x.

Boulter, C., Freeston, M., South, M., & Rodgers, J. (2014). Intolerance of uncertainty as a framework for understanding anxiety in children and adolescents with autism spectrum disorders. *Journal of Autism and Developmental Disorders, 44*, 1391–1402. https://doi.org/10.1007/s10803-013-2001-x.

Bowler, D. M., Gaigg, S. B., & Gardiner, J. M. (2008). Effects of related and unrelated context on recall and recognition by adults with high-functioning autism spectrum disorder. *Neuropsychologia, 46*(4), 993–999. https://doi.org/10.1007/s10803-007-0366-4.

Bowler, D. M., Gaigg, S. B., & Gardiner, J. M. (2009). Free recall learning of hierarchically organised lists by adults with Asperger's syndrome: Additional evidence for diminished relational processing. *Journal of Autism and Developmental Disorders, 39*, 589–595. https://doi.org/10.1007/s10803-007-0366-4.

Bowler, D. M., Gaigg, S. B., & Gardiner, J. M. (2010). Multiple list learning in adults with autism spectrum disorder: Parallels with frontal lobe damage or further evidence of diminished relational processing? *Journal of Autism and Developmental Disorders, 40*, 179–187. https://doi.org/10.1007/s10803-009-0845-x.

Bowler, D. M., Gaigg, S. B., & Gardiner, J. M. (2014). Binding of multiple features in memory by high-functioning adults with autism spectrum disorder. *Journal of Autism and Developmental Disorders, 44*, 2355–2362. https://doi.org/10.1007/s10803-014-2105-y.

Bowler, D. M., Gaigg, S. B., & Gardiner, J. M. (2015). Brief report: The role of task support in the spatial and temporal source memory of adults with autism spectrum disorder. *Journal of Autism and Developmental Disorders, 45*, 2613–2617. https://doi.org/10.1007/s10803-015-2378-9.

Bowler, D. M., Gaigg, S. B., & Lind, S. (2011). Memory in autism: Binding, self and brain. In I. Roth & P. Rezaie (Eds.), *Researching the autism spectrum: Contemporary perspectives* (pp. 316–346). Cambridge University Press. ISBN 9780521736862.

Bowler, D. M., Gardiner, J. M., & Berthollier, N. (2004). Source memory in adolescents and adults with Asperger's syndrome. *Journal of Autism and Developmental Disorders, 34*, 533–542. https://doi.org/10.1007/s10803-004-2548-7.

Bowler, D. M., Gardiner, J. M., & Gaigg, S. B. (2007). *Factors Affecting Conscious Awareness in the Recollective Experience of Adults with Asperger's Syndrome., 16*, 124–143. https://doi.org/10.1016/j.concog.2005.12.001.

Bowler, D. M., Gardiner, J. M., & Grice, S. J. (2000). Episodic memory and remembering in adults with Asperger syndrome. *Journal of Autism and Developmental Disorders, 30*, 295–304. https://doi.org/10.1023/A:1005575216176.

Bowler, D. M., Matthews, N. J., & Gardiner, J. M. (1997). Asperger's syndrome and memory: Similarity to autism but not amnesia. *Neuropsychologia, 35*, 65–70. https://doi.org/10.1016/S0028-3932(96)00054-1.

Brown, B. T., Morris, G., Nida, R. E., & Baker-Ward, L. (2012). Brief report: Making experience personal: Internal states language in the memory narratives of children with and without Asperger's disorder. *Journal of Autism and Developmental Disorders, 42*, 441–446. https://doi.org/10.1007/s10803-011-1246-5.

Brown, D. A., Lewis, C. N., Lamb, M. E., & Stephens, E. (2012). The influences of delay and severity of intellectual disability on event memory in children. *Journal of Consulting and Clinical Psychology, 80*, 829–841. https://doi.org/10.1037/a0029388.

Brown, D., & Pipe, M.-E. (2003). Individual differences in children's event memory reports and the narrative elaboration technique. *Journal of Applied Psychology, 88*, 195–206. https://doi.org/10.1037/0021-9010.88.2.195.

Brown, D. A., & Lamb, M. E. (2015). Can children be useful witnesses? It depends how they are questioned. *Child Development Perspectives, 9*(4), 250–255. https://doi.org/10.1111/cdep.12142.

Brown-Lavoie, S. M., Viecili, M. A., & Weiss, J. A. (2014). Sexual knowledge and victimization in adults with autism spectrum disorders. *Journal of Autism and Developmental Disorders, 44*, 2185–2196. https://doi.org/10.1007/s10803-014-2093-y.

Bruck, M., London, K., Landa, R., & Goodman, J. (2007). Autobiographical memory and suggestibility in children with autism spectrum disorder. *Development and Psychopathology, 19*, 73–95. https://doi.org/10.1017/s0954579407070058.

Bruner, J., & Feldman, C. (1993). Theories of mind and the problem of autism. In S. Baron-Cohen, H. Tager-Flusberg, & D. J. Cohen (Eds.), U*nderstanding other minds: Perspectives from autism.* Oxford University Press.

Brunsdon, V. E., Colvert, E., Ames, C., Garnett, T., Gillan, N., Hallett, V., ... Happé, F. (2015). Exploring the cognitive features in children with autism spectrum disorder, their co-twins, and typically developing children within a population-based sample. *Journal of Child Psychology and Psychiatry, 56*(8), 893–902.

Bull, R. (2010). The investigative interviewing of children and other vulnerable witnesses: Psychological research and working/professional practice. *Legal and Criminological Psychology, 15*, 5–23. https://doi.org/10.1348/014466509X440160.

Bull, R. (2014). When in interviews to disclose information to suspects and to challenge them? In *Investigative interviewing* (pp. 167–181). Springer New York. https://doi.org/10.1007/978-1-4614-9642-7_9.

Capps, L., Losh, M., & Thurber, C. (2000). '"The frog ate the bug and made his mouth sad"': Narrative competence in children with autism. *Journal of Abnormal Child Psychology, 28*(2), 193–204.

Carter-Sowell, A. R., Chen, Z., & Williams, K. D. (2008). Ostracism increases social susceptibility. *Social Influence, 3*(3), 143–153.

Cederborg, A. C., Hultman, E., & La Rooy, D. (2012). The quality of details when children and youths with intellectual disabilities are interviewed about their abuse experiences. *Scandinavian Journal of Disability Research, 14*, 113–125.
Cederborg, A. C., & Lamb, M. (2008). Interviewing alleged victims with intellectual disabilities. *Journal of Intellectual Disability Research, 52*, 49–58. https://doi.org/10.1111/j.1365-2788.2007.00976.x.
Chandler, R. J., Russell, A., & Maras, K. L. (2019). Compliance in autism: Self-report in action. *Autism, 23*(4). https://doi.org/10.1177/1362361318795479.
Chaplin, E., & Mukhopadhyay, S. (2018). Autism spectrum disorder and hate crime. *Advances in Autism, 4*, 30–36. https://doi.org/10.1108/AIA-08-2017-0015.
Chaput, V., Amsellem, F., Urdapilleta, I., Chaste, P., Leboyer, M., Delorme, R., & Goussé, V. (2013). Episodic memory and self-awareness in Asperger syndrome: Analysis of memory narratives. *Research in Autism Spectrum Disorders, 7*, 1062–1067. https://doi.org/10.1016/j.rasd.2013.05.005.
Christensen, D. L., Bilder, D. A., Zahorodny, W., Pettygrove, S., Durkin, M. S., Fitzgerald, R. T., ... Yeargin-Allsopp, M. (2016). Prevalence and characteristics of autism spectrum disorder among 4-year-old children in the autism and developmental disabilities monitoring network. *Journal of Developmental & Behavioral Pediatrics, 37*(1), 1–8.
Cialdini, R. B., Vincent, J. E., Lewis, S. K., Catalan, J., Wheeler, D., & Darby, B. L. (1975). Reciprocal concessions procedure for inducing compliance: The door-in-the- face technique. *Journal of Personality and Social Psychology, 31*, 206–215.
Ciesielski, K. T., & Harris, R. J. (1997). Factors related to performance failure on executive tasks in autism. *Child Neuropsychology, 3*(1), 1–12.
Clarke, C., & Milne, R. (2001). *National evaluation of the PEACE investigative interviewing course. In Police research award scheme*. Home Office.
Colle, L., Baron-Cohen, S., Wheelwright, S., & van der Lely, H. K. J. (2008). Narrative discourse in adults with high-functioning autism or Asperger syndrome. *Journal of Autism and Developmental Disorders, 38*, 28–40. https://doi.org/10.1007/s10803-007-0357-5.
Collins, K., Harker, N., & Antonopoulos, G. A. (2017). The impact of the registered intermediary on adults' perceptions of child witnesses: evidence from a Mock cross examination. *European Journal on Criminal Policy and Research, 23*, 211–225. https://doi.org/10.1007/s10610-016-9314-1.
Cooper, P., & Allely, C. S. (2017). You can't judge a book by its cover: Evolving professional responsibilities, liabilities and 'judgecraft' when a party has Asperger's syndrome. *Northern Ireland Legal Quarterly, 68*, 35–58.
Cooper, P., & Mattison, M. (2017). Intermediaries, vulnerable people and the quality of evidence. *The International Journal of Evidence & Proof, 21*, 351–370. https://doi.org/10.1177/1365712717725534.
Cooper, R. A., Plaisted-Grant, K. C., Baron-Cohen, S., & Simons, J. S. (2016). Reality monitoring and metamemory in adults with autism spectrum conditions. *Journal of Autism and Developmental Disorders, 46*, 2186–2198. https://doi.org/10.1007/s10803-016-2749-x.
Cooper, R. A., Plaisted-Grant, K. C., Baron-Cohen, S., & Simons, J. S. (2017). Eye movements reveal a dissociation between memory encoding and retrieval in adults with autism. *Cognition, 159*, 127–138. https://doi.org/10.1016/J.COGNITION.2016.11.013.
Crane, L., & Goddard, L. (2008). Episodic and semantic autobiographical memory in adults with autism spectrum disorders. *Journal of Autism and Developmental Disorders, 38*, 498–506. https://doi.org/10.1007/s10803-007-0420-2.
Crane, L., Goddard, L., & Pring, L. (2009). Specific and general autobiographical knowledge in adults with autism spectrum disorders: The role of personal goals. *Memory, 17*, 557–576. https://doi.org/10.1080/09658210902960211.
Crane, L., Goddard, L., & Pring, L. (2010). Brief report: Self-defining and everyday autobiographical memories in adults with autism spectrum disorders. *Journal of Autism and Developmental Disorders, 40*, 383–391. https://doi.org/10.1007/s10803-009-0875-4.

Crane, L., Goddard, L., & Pring, L. (2013). Autobiographical memory in adults with autism spectrum disorder: the role of depressed mood, rumination, working memory and theory of mind. *Autism, 17*, 205–219. https://doi.org/10.1177/1362361311418690.
Crane, L., Lind, S. E., & Bowler, D. M. (2013). Remembering the past and imagining the future in autism spectrum disorder. *Memory, 21*, 157–166. https://doi.org/10.1080/09658211.2012.712976.
Crane, L., & Maras, K. (2018). General memory abilities for autobiographical events in adults with autism spectrum disorder. In *The Wiley handbook of memory, autism spectrum disorder, and the law* (pp. 146–178). https://doi.org/10.1002/9781119158431.ch8.
Crane, L., Maras, K. L., Hawken, T., Mulcahy, S., & Memon, A. (2016). Experiences of autism spectrum disorder and policing in England and Wales: Surveying police and the autism community. *Journal of Autism and Developmental Disorders, 46*, 2028–2041. https://doi.org/10.1007/s10803-016-2729-1.
Crane, L., Pring, L., Jukes, K., & Goddard, L. (2012). Patterns of autobiographical memory in adults with autism spectrum disorder. *Journal of Autism and Developmental Disorders, 42*, 2100–2112. https://doi.org/10.1007/s10803-012-1459-2.
Crane, L., Wilcock, R., Maras, K. L., Chui, W., Marti-Sanchez, C., & Henry, L. A. (2018). Mock juror perceptions of child witnesses on the autism spectrum: The impact of providing diagnostic labels and information about autism. *Journal of Autism and Developmental Disorders*, 1–11. https://doi.org/10.1007/s10803-018-3700-0.
Croen, L. A., Zerbo, O., Qian, Y., Massolo, M. L., Rich, S., Sidney, S., & Kripke, C. (2015). The health status of adults on the autism spectrum. *Autism, 19*, 814–823. https://doi.org/10.1177/1362361315577517.
Dalgleish, T., Williams, J. M. G., Golden, A.-M. J., Perkins, N., Barrett, L. F., Barnard, P. J., … Watkins, E. (2007). Reduced specificity of autobiographical memory and depression: the role of executive control. *Journal of Experimental Psychology. General, 136*, 23–42. https://doi.org/10.1037/0096-3445.136.1.23.
Dando, C. J. (2013). Drawing to remember: external support of older adults' eyewitness performance. *PLoS ONE, 8*, e69937. https://doi.org/10.1371/journal.pone.0069937.
Dando, C. J., Geiselman, R. E., MacLeod, N., & Griffiths, A. (2015). Interviewing adult witnesses and victims. In *Communication in investigative and legal contexts* (pp. 79–106). Wiley. https://doi.org/10.1002/9781118769133.ch5.
Dando, C. J., Ormerod, T. C., Cooper, P., Marchant, R., Mattison, M., Milne, R., & Bull, R. (2018). No evidence against sketch reinstatement of context, verbal labels or the use of registered intermediaries for children with autism spectrum disorder: Response to Henry et al. (2017). *Journal of Autism and Developmental Disorders, 48*, 2593–2596. https://doi.org/10.1007/s10803-018-3479-z.
Dando, C. J., Wilcock, R., Milne, R., & Henry, L. (2009). An adapted cognitive Interview procedure for frontline police investigators. *Applied Cognitive Psychology, 23*, 698–716.
de Marchena, A., & Eigsti, I. M. (2010). Conversational gestures in autism spectrum disorders: Asynchrony but not decreased frequency. *Autism Research, 3*, 311–322. https://doi.org/10.1002/aur.159.
Demetriou, E. A., Lampit, A., Quintana, D. S., Naismith, S. L., Song, Y. J. C., Pye, J. E., … Guastella, A. J. (2018). Autism spectrum disorders: a meta-analysis of executive function. *Molecular Psychiatry, 23*, 1198–1204. https://doi.org/10.1038/mp.2017.75.
DePaulo, B. M., Lindsay, J. J., Malone, B. E., Muhlenbruck, L., Charlton, K., & Cooper, H. (2003). Cues to deception. *Psychological Bulletin, 129*, 74–118. https://doi.org/10.1037/0033-2909.129.1.74.
Dichter, G. S., & Belger, A. (2007). Social stimuli interfere with cognitive control in autism. *Neuroimage, 35*(3), 1219–1230.
Diehl, J. J., Bennetto, L., & Young, E. C. (2006). Story recall and narrative coherence of high-functioning children with autism spectrum disorders. *Journal of Abnormal Child Psychology, 34*, 83–98. https://doi.org/10.1007/s10802-005-9003-x.

Dunphy-Lelii, S., & Wellman, H. M. (2012). Delayed self recognition in autism: A unique difficulty? *Research in Autism Spectrum Disorders, 6*, 212–223. https://doi.org/10.1016/j.rasd.2011.05.002.
Ellison, L., & Wheatcroft, J. (2010). Could you ask me that in a different way please? Exploring the impact of courtroom questioning and witness familiarisation on adult witness accuracy. *Criminal Law Review, 11*, 823–839.
Farrant, A., Blades, M., & Boucher, J. (1998). Source monitoring by children with autism. *Journal of Autism and Developmental Disorders, 28*(1), 43–50. https://doi.org/10.1023/A:1026010919219.
Findon, J., Cadman, T., Stewart, C. S., Woodhouse, E., Eklund, H., Hayward, H., … McEwen, F. S. (2016). Screening for co-occurring conditions in adults with autism spectrum disorder using the strengths and difficulties questionnaire: A pilot study. *Autism Research, 9*, 1353–1363. https://doi.org/10.1002/aur.1625.
Fisher, R. P., & Geiselman, R. E. (1992). *Memory-enhancing techniques for investigative interviewing: The cognitive interview*. Charles C Thomas.
Gabbert, F., Hope, L., & Fisher, R. P. (2009). Protecting eyewitness evidence: Examining the efficacy of a self-administered interview tool. *Law and Human Behavior, 33*, 298–307. https://doi.org/10.1007/s10979-008-9146-8.
Gabbert, F., Hope, L., Fisher, R. P., & Jamieson, K. (2012). Protecting against misleading post-event information with a self-administered interview. *Applied Cognitive Psychology, 26*, 568–575. https://doi.org/10.1002/acp.2828.
Gaigg, S. B., & Bowler, D. M. (2018). A relational processing framework of memory in autism spectrum disorder. In *The Wiley handbook of memory, autism spectrum disorder, and the law* (pp. 9–26). Wiley. https://doi.org/10.1002/9781119158431.ch1.
Gaigg, S. B., Bowler, D. M., Ecker, C., Calvo-Merino, B., & Murphy, D. G. (2015). Episodic recollection difficulties in ASD result from atypical relational encoding: Behavioral and neural evidence. *Autism Research, 8*, 317–327. https://doi.org/10.1002/aur.1448.
Gaigg, S. B., Bowler, D. M., & Gardiner, J. M. (2014). Episodic but not semantic order memory difficulties in autism spectrum disorder: Evidence from the Historical Figures Task. *Memory, 22*(6), 669–678.
Gaigg, S. B., Gardiner, J. M., & Bowler, D. M. (2008). Free recall in autism spectrum disorder: The role of relational and item-specific encoding. *Neuropsychologia, 46*, 983–992. https://doi.org/10.1016/j.neuropsychologia.2007.11.011.
Gardiner, J. M. (2001). Episodic memory and autonoetic consciousness: A first-person approach. *Philosophical Transactions of the Royal Society of London. Series B, Biological Sciences, 356*, 1351–1361. https://doi.org/10.1098/rstb.2001.0955.
Geiselman, R. E., Fisher, R. P., Firstenberg, I., Hutton, L., Sullivam, S. J., Avetissian, I. V., & Prosk, A. (1984). Enhancement of eyewitness memory: An empirical evaluation of the cognitive interview. *Journal of Police Science & Administration, 12*(1), 74–80.
George, R., Crane, L., Bingham, A., Pophale, C., & Remington, A. (2018). Legal professionals' knowledge and experience of autistic adults in the family justice system. *Journal of Social Welfare and Family Law, 40*, 78–97. https://doi.org/10.1080/09649069.2018.1414381.
Gillot, A., & Standen, P. J. (2007). Levels of anxiety and sources of stress in adults with autism. *Journal of Intellectual Disabilities, 11*(4), 359–370.
Goddard, L., Dritschel, B., Robinson, S., & Howlin, P. (2014). Development of autobiographical memory in children with an autism spectrum disorder: Deficits, gains and predictors of performance. *Development and Psychopathology, 26*(1), 215–228.
Goddard, L., Howlin, P., Dritschel, B., & Patel, T. (2007). Autobiographical memory and social problem-solving in Asperger syndrome. *Journal of Autism and Developmental Disorders, 37*(2), 291–300. https://doi.org/10.1007/s10803-006-0168-0.
Goldman, S. (2008). Brief report: Narratives of personal events in children with autism and developmental language disorders: Unshared memories. *Journal of Autism and Developmental Disorders, 38*, 1982–1988. https://doi.org/10.1007/s10803-008-0588-0.

Grainger, C., Williams, D. M., & Lind, S. E. (2014). Online action monitoring and memory for self-performed actions in autism spectrum disorder. *Journal of Autism & Developmental Disorders*, 1–14. https://doi.org/10.1007/s10803-013-1987-4.

Grant, T., Taylor, J., Oxburgh, G., & Myklebust, T. (2015). Exploring types and functions of questions in police interviews. In G. Oxburgh, T. Myklebust, T. Grant, & R. Milne (eds.) *Communication in investigative and legal contexts*. Wiley. https://doi.org/10.1002/9781118769133.ch2.

Griffiths, A., & Milne, R. (2006) Will it all end in tiers? Police interviews with suspects in Britain. In T. A. Williamson (Ed.) *Investigative interviewing: Rights, research, regulation* (pp. 167–189). Willan.

Grisdale, E., Lind, S. E., Eacott, M. J., & Williams, D. M. (2014). Self-referential memory in autism spectrum disorder and typical development: Exploring the ownership effect. *Consciousness and Cognition, 30*, 133–141.

Gritti, A., Bove, D., Di Sarno, A. M., D'Addio, A. A., Chiapparo, S., & Bove, R. M. (2003). Stereotyped movements in a group of autistic children. *Functional Neurology, 18*(2), 89–94.

Gudjonsson, G. H. (1989). Compliance in an interrogative situation—A new scale. *Personality and Individual Differences, 10*(5), 535–540.

Gudjonsson, G. H. (1997). *The Gudjonsson Suggestibility Scales manual*. Psychology Press.

Gudjonsson, G. H. (2003). *The psychology of interrogations and confessions: A handbook*. John Wiley.

Gudjonsson, G. H., & Pearse, J. (2011). Suspect interviews and false confessions. *Current Directions in Psychological Science, 20*, 33–37. https://doi.org/10.1177/0963721410396824.

Gudjonsson, G. H., Sigurdsson, J. F., Bragason, O., Einarsson, E., & Valdimarsdottir, E. B. (2004). Compliance and personality: The vulnerability of the unstable introvert. *European Journal of Personality, 18*, 435–443. https://doi.org/10.1002/per.514.

Gudjonsson, G. H., Sigurdsson, J. F., Brynjólfsdóttir, B., & Hreinsdóttir, H. (2002). The relationship of compliance with anxiety, self-esteem, paranoid thinking and anger. *Psychology, Crime & Law, 8*(2), 145–153.

Happé, F., & Frith, U. (2006). The weak coherence account: Detail-focused cognitive style in autism spectrum disorders. *Journal of Autism and Developmental Disorders, 36*(1), 5–25.

Hare, D. J., Mellor, C., & Azmi, S. (2007). Episodic memory in adults with autistic spectrum disorders: Recall for self- versus other-experienced events. *Research in Developmental Disabilities, 28*, 317–329. https://doi.org/10.1016/j.ridd.2006.03.003.

Heeramun, R., Magnusson, C., Gumpert, C. H., Granath, S., Lundberg, M., Dalman, C., & Rai, D. (2017). Autism and convictions for violent crimes: Population-based cohort study in Sweden. *Journal of the American Academy of Child & Adolescent Psychiatry, 56*, 491-497.e2. https://doi.org/10.1016/j.jaac.2017.03.011.

Henderson, E. (2015). "A very valuable tool": Judges, advocates and intermediaries discuss the intermediary system in England and Wales. *The International Journal of Evidence & Proof, 19*, 154–171. https://doi.org/10.1177/1365712715580535.

Henderson, E., Heffer, C., & Kebbell, M. (2015). Courtroom questioning and discourse. In G. Oxburgh, T. Myklebust, T. Grant, & R. Milne (eds.) *Communication in investigative and legal contexts*. Wiley. https://doi.org/10.1002/9781118769133.ch9.

Henderson, H. A., Zahka, N. E., Kojkowski, N. M., Inge, A. P., Schwartz, C. B., Hileman, C. M., … Mundy, P. C. (2009). Self-referenced memory, social cognition, and symptom presentation in autism. *Journal of Child Psychology and Psychiatry, 50*(7), 853–61. https://doi.org/10.1111/j.1469-7610.2008.02059.x.

Henry, L. A., Bettenay, C., & Carney, D. P. J. (2011). Children with intellectual disabilities and developmental disorders. In *Children's testimony* (pp. 251–283). Wiley. https://doi.org/10.1002/9781119998495.ch13..

Henry, L. A., Crane, L., Fesser, E., Harvey, A., Palmer, L., & Wilcock, R. (2020). The narrative coherence of witness transcripts in children on the autism spectrum. *Research in Developmental Disabilities, 96*. https://doi.org/10.1016/j.ridd.2019.103518.

Henry, L. A., Crane, L., Nash, G., Hobson, Z., Kirke-Smith, M., & Wilcock, R. (2017). Verbal, visual, and intermediary support for child witnesses with autism during investigative interviews. *Journal of Autism and Developmental Disorders, 47*(8), 2348–2362. https://doi.org/10.1007/s10803-017-3142-0.

Henry, L. A., Crane, L., Nash, G., Hobson, Z., Kirke-Smith, M., & Wilcock, R. (2018). Response to "No Evidence Against Sketch Reinstatement of Context, Verbal Labels or Registered Intermediaries." *Journal of Autism and Developmental Disorders, 48*, 2597–2599. https://doi.org/10.1007/s10803-018-3496-y.

Henry, L. A., & Gudjonsson, G. H. (2003). Eyewitness memory, suggestibility and repeated recall sessions in children with mild and moderate intellectual disabilities. *Law and Human Behavior, 27*(5), 481–505.

Henry, L. A., & Gudjonsson, G. H. (2007). Individual and developmental differences in eyewitness recall and suggestibility in children with intellectual disabilities. *Applied Cognitive Psychology, 21*(3), 361–381.

Henry, L. A., Messer, D. J., Wilcock, R., Nash, G., Kirke-Smith, M., Hobson, Z., & Crane, L. (2017). Do measures of memory, language, and attention predict eyewitness memory in children with and without autism? *Autism & Developmental Language Impairments, 2*, 239694151772213. https://doi.org/10.1177/2396941517722139.

Hermelin, B., & O'Connor, N. (1967). Remembering of words by psychotic and subnormal children. *British Journal of Psychology, 58*, 213–218. https://doi.org/10.1111/j.2044-8295.1967.tb01075.x.

Hermelin, B., & O'Connor, N. (1970). *Psychological experiments with autistic children: Psychological experiments with autistic children.* Pergamon Press.

Hilvert, E., Davidson, D., & Gámez, P. B. (2016). Examination of script and non-script based narrative retellings in children with autism spectrum disorders. *Research in Autism Spectrum Disorders, 29–30*, 79–92. https://doi.org/10.1016/J.RASD.2016.06.002.

Hogan-Brown, A. L., Losh, M., Martin, G. E., & Mueffelmann, D. J. (2013). An investigation of narrative ability in boys with autism and fragile X syndrome. *American Journal on Intellectual and Developmental Disabilities, 118*(2), 77–94.

Home Office. (2011). *Achieving best evidence in criminal proceedings: Guidance on interviewing victims and witnesses, and using special measures.* London: Her Majesty's Stationary Office.

Home Office. (2017). *Interviewing suspects.* Her Majesty's Stationary Office.

Hsu, C.-W., & Teoh, Y.-S. (2017). Investigating event memory in children with autism spectrum disorder: Effects of a computer-mediated interview. *Journal of Autism and Developmental Disorders, 47*, 359–372. https://doi.org/10.1007/s10803-016-2959-2.

Inbau, F. E., Reid, J. E., Buckley, J. P., & Jayne, B. C. (2013). *Essentials of the Reid technique.* Jones & Bartlett Publishers.

Jacobson, J. (2008). No One Knows: Police responses to suspects with learning disabilities and learning difficulties: A review.

Johnson, M. K., Hashtroudi, S., & Lindsay, D. S. (1993). Source monitoring. *Psychological Bulletin, 114*(1), 3–28.

Kebbell, M. R., Evans, L., & Johnson, S. D. (2010). The influence of lawyers' questions on witness accuracy, confidence, and reaction times and on mock jurors' interpretation of witness accuracy. *Journal of Investigative Psychology and Offender Profiling, 7*, 262–272. https://doi.org/10.1002/jip.125.

Kebbell, M. R., & Hatton, C. (1999). People with mental retardation as witnesses in court: A review. *Mental Retardation, 37*(3), 179–187. https://doi.org/10.1352/0047-6765(1999)037%3C0179:PWMRAW%3E2.0.CO;2.

Kebbell, M. R., Hatton, C., & Johnson, S. D. (2004). Witnesses with intellectual disabilities in court: What questions are asked and what influence do they have? *Legal and Criminological Psychology, 9*, 23–35.

Kennedy, D. P., & Adolphs, R. (2014). Violations of personal space by individuals with autism spectrum disorder. *PLoS ONE, 9*, e103369. https://doi.org/10.1371/journal.pone.0103369.

Kenworthy, L., Yerys, B. E., Anthony, L. G., & Wallace, G. L. (2008). Understanding executive control in autism spectrum disorders in the lab and in the real world. *Neuropsychology Review, 18*, 320–338. https://doi.org/10.1007/s11065-008-9077-7.

King, D., Dockrell, J., & Stuart, M. (2014). Constructing fictional stories: A study of story narratives by children with autistic spectrum disorder. *Research in Developmental Disabilities, 35*, 2438–2449. https://doi.org/10.1016/J.RIDD.2014.06.015.

Klein, S. B., Chan, R. L., & Loftus, J. (1999). Independence of episodic and semantic self-knowledge: The case from autism. *Social Cognition, 17*, 413–436. https://doi.org/10.1521/soco.1999.17.4.413.

Kuijper, S. J. M., Hartman, C. A., Bogaerds-Hazenberg, S. T. M., & Hendriks, P. (2017). Narrative production in children with autism spectrum disorder (ASD) and children with attention-deficit/hyperactivity disorder (ADHD): Similarities and differences. *Journal of Abnormal Psychology, 126*(1), 63–75. https://doi.org/10.1037/abn0000231.

Lamb, M. E., Orbach, Y., Hershkowitz, I., Esplin, P. W., & Horowitz, D. (2007). A structured forensic interview protocol improves the quality and informativeness of investigative interviews with children: A review of research using the NICHD investigative interview protocol. *Child Abuse & Neglect, 31*(11–12), 1201–1231.

Lee, M., Martin, G. E., Hogan, A., Hano, D., Gordon, P. C., & Losh, M. (2018). What's the story? A computational analysis of narrative competence in autism. *Autism, 22*, 335–344. https://doi.org/10.1177/1362361316677957.

Leggett, J., Goodman, W., & Dinani, S. (2007). People with learning disabilities? Experiences of being interviewed by the police. *British Journal of Learning Disabilities, 35*, 168–173. https://doi.org/10.1111/j.1468-3156.2007.00458.x.

Lind, S. E. (2010). Memory and the self in autism: A review and theoretical framework. *Autism, 14*, 430–456. https://doi.org/10.1177/1362361309358700.

Lind, S., & Bowler, D. (2008). Episodic memory and autonoetic consciousness in autistic spectrum disorders: The roles of self-awareness, representational abilities and temporal cognition. In J. Boucher & D. Bowler (Eds.), *Memory in autism: Theory and evidence.* (pp. 166–187). Cambridge University Press.

Lind, S. E., & Bowler, D. M. (2009). Recognition memory, self-other source memory, and theory-of-mind in children with autism spectrum disorder. *Journal of Autism and Developmental Disorders, 39*, 1231–1239. https://doi.org/10.1007/s10803-009-0735-2.

Lind, S. E., & Bowler, D. M. (2010). Episodic memory and episodic future thinking in adults with autism. *Journal of Abnormal Psychology, 119*, 896–905. https://doi.org/10.1037/a0020631.

Lind, S. E., Williams, D. M., Bowler, D. M., & Peel, A. (2014). Episodic memory and episodic future thinking impairments in high-functioning autism spectrum disorder: An underlying difficulty with scene construction or self-projection? *Neuropsychology, 28*, 55–67. https://doi.org/10.1037/neu0000005.

Lind, S. E., Williams, D. M., Grainger, C., & Landsiedel, J. (2018). The self in autism and its relation to memory. In *The Wiley handbook of memory, autism spectrum disorder, and the law* (pp. 70–91). Wiley. https://doi.org/10.1002/9781119158431.ch4..

Lind, S. E., Williams, D. M., Nicholson, T., Grainger, C., & Carruthers, P. (2019). The self-reference effect on memory is not diminished in autism: Three studies of incidental and explicit self-referential recognition memory in autistic and neurotypical adults and adolescents. *Journal of Abnormal Psychology*. https://doi.org/10.1037/abn0000467.

Lindblad, F., & Lainpelto, K. (2011). Sexual abuse allegations by children with neuropsychiatric disorders. *Journal of Child Sexual Abuse, 20*, 182–195. https://doi.org/10.1080/10538712.2011.554339.

Liss, M., Saulnier, C., Fein, D., & Kinsbourne, M. (2006). Sensory and attention abnormalities in autistic spectrum disorders. *Autism, 10*, 155–172. https://doi.org/10.1177/1362361306062021.

Lombardo, M. V., Barnes, J. L., Wheelwright, S. J., & Baron-Cohen, S. (2007). Self-referential cognition and empathy in autism. *PLoS ONE, 2*, e883.

Loveland, K. A., Tunali-Kotoski, B., Pearson, D. A., Brelsford, K. A., Ortegon, J., & Chen, R. (1994). Imitation and expression of facial affect in autism. *Development and Psychopathology, 6*, 433. https://doi.org/10.1017/S0954579400006039.
Losh, M., & Capps, L. (2003). Narrative ability in high-functioning children with autism or Asperger's syndrome. *Journal of Autism and Developmental Disorders, 33*, 239–251. https://doi.org/10.1023/A:1024446215446.
Losh, M., & Capps, L. (2006). Understanding of emotional experience in autism: Insights from the personal accounts of high- functioning children with autism. *Developmental Psychology, 42*(5), 809–818.
Losh, M., & Gordon, P. C. (2014). Quantifying narrative ability in autism spectrum disorder: A computational linguistic analysis of narrative coherence. *Journal of Autism and Developmental Disorders, 44*, 3016–3025. https://doi.org/10.1007/s10803-014-2158-y.
Loveland, K. A., McEvoy, R. E., & Tunali, B. (1990). Narrative story telling in autism and Down's syndrome. *British Journal of Developmental Psychology, 8*, 9–23. https://doi.org/10.1111/j.2044-835X.1990.tb00818.x.
Maister, L., Simons, J. S., & Plaisted-Grant, K. (2013). Executive functions are employed to process episodic and relational memories in children with autism spectrum disorders. *Neuropsychology, 27*(6), 615–627. https://doi.org/10.1037/a0034492.
Maras, K. L., & Bowler, D. M. (2010). The cognitive interview for eyewitnesses with autism spectrum disorder. *Journal of Autism and Developmental Disorders, 40*, 1350–1360. https://doi.org/10.1007/s10803-010-0997-8.
Maras, K., & Bowler, D. M. (2011). Brief report: Schema consistent misinformation effects in eyewitnesses with autism spectrum disorder. *Journal of Autism and Developmental Disorders, 41*, 815–820. https://doi.org/10.1007/s10803-010-1089-5.
Maras, K. L., & Bowler, D. M. (2012a). Context reinstatement effects on eyewitness memory in autism spectrum disorder. *British Journal of Psychology, 103*, 330–342. https://doi.org/10.1111/j.2044-8295.2011.02077.x.
Maras, K. L., & Bowler, D. M. (2012b). Brief report: Suggestibility, compliance and psychological traits in high-functioning adults with autism spectrum disorder. *Research in Autism Spectrum Disorders, 6*, 1168–1175. https://doi.org/10.1016/j.rasd.2012.03.013.
Maras, K. L., Crane, L., Mulcahy, S., Hawken, T., Cooper, P., Wurtzel, D., & Memon, A. (2017). Brief report: Autism in the courtroom: experiences of legal professionals and the autism community. *Journal of Autism and Developmental Disorders, 47*, 2610–2620. https://doi.org/10.1007/s10803-017-3162-9.
Maras, K., Dando, C., Stephenson, H., Lambrechts, A., Anns, S., & Gaigg, S. (2020). The Witness-Aimed First Account (WAFA): A new technique for interviewing autistic witnesses and victims. *Autism*. https://doi.org/10.1177/1362361320908986.
Maras, K. L., Gaigg, S. B., & Bowler, D. M. (2012). Memory for emotionally arousing events over time in Autism Spectrum Disorder. *Emotion, 12*, 1118–1128. https://doi.org/10.1037/a0026679.
Maras, K. L., Marshall, I., & Sands, C. (2019). Mock Juror perceptions of credibility and culpability in an autistic defendant. *Journal of Autism and Developmental Disorders, 49*(3), 996–1010. https://doi.org/10.1007/s10803-018-3803-7.
Maras, K. L., Memon, A., Lambrechts, A., & Bowler, D. M. (2013). Recall of a live and personally experienced eyewitness event by adults with autism spectrum disorder. *Journal of Autism and Developmental Disorders, 43*, 1798–1810. https://doi.org/10.1007/s10803-012-1729-z.
Maras, K., Mulcahy, S., Crane, L., Hawken, T., & Memon, A. (2018). Obtaining best evidence from the autistic interviewee: Police-reported challenges, legal requirements and psychological research-based recommendations. *Investigative Interviewing Research and Practice, 9*(1), 52–60.
Maras, K. L., Mulcahy, S., Memon, A., Picariello, F., & Bowler, D. M. (2014). Evaluating the effectiveness of the self-administered interview© for witnesses with autism spectrum disorder. *Applied Cognitive Psychology, 28*(5), 693–701. https://doi.org/10.1002/acp.3055.

Maras, K., Norris, J. E., & Brewer, N. (2020). Metacognitive monitoring and control of eyewitness memory reports in autism. *Autism Research*. https://doi.org/10.5255/UKDA-SN-854140.

Maras, K. L., & Wilcock, R. (2012). Suggestibility in vulnerable groups: witnesses with intellectual disability, autism spectrum disorder, and older people. In *Suggestibility in Legal Contexts: Psychological Research and Forensic Implications*, 49–170. https://doi.org/10.1002/9781118432907.ch8.

Marchant, R. (2013). How young is too young? The evidence of children under five in the English criminal justice system. *Child Abuse Review, 22*, 432–445. https://doi.org/10.1002/car.2273.

Marchant, R. (2016). Age is not determinative': The evidence of very young children in the English justice system. *Criminal Law and Justice Weekly, 180* (12 & 13).

Martin, J. S., Poirier, M., & Bowler, D. M. (2010). Brief report: Impaired temporal reproduction performance in adults with autism spectrum disorder. *Journal of Autism and Developmental Disorders, 40*, 640–646. https://doi.org/10.1007/s10803-009-0904-3.

Mattison, M. L. A., Dando, C. J., & Ormerod, T. C. (2015). Sketching to remember: Episodic free recall task support for child witnesses and victims with autism spectrum disorder. *Journal of Autism and Developmental Disorders, 45*, 1751–1765. https://doi.org/10.1007/s10803-014-2335-z.

Mattison, M., Dando, C. J., & Ormerod, T. C. (2018). Drawing the answers: Sketching to support free and probed recall by child witnesses and victims with autism spectrum disorder. *Autism, 22*, 181–194. https://doi.org/10.1177/1362361316669088.

Mazefsky, C. A., Kao, J., & Oswald, D. P. (2011). Preliminary evidence suggesting caution in the use of psychiatric self-report measures with adolescents with high-functioning autism spectrum disorders. *Research in Autism Spectrum Disorders, 5*, 164–174. https://doi.org/10.1016/j.rasd.2010.03.006.

McCabe, A., Hillier, A., & Shapiro, C. (2013). Brief report: Structure of personal narratives of adults with autism spectrum disorder. *Journal of Autism and Developmental Disorders, 43*, 733–738. https://doi.org/10.1007/s10803-012-1585-x.

McCrory, E., Henry, L., & Happé, F. (2007). Eye-witness memory and suggestibility in children with Asperger syndrome. *Journal of Child Psychology and Psychiatry, 48*, 482–489. https://doi.org/10.1111/j.1469-7610.2006.01715.x.

Meissner, C. A., Redlich, A. D., Michael, S. W., Evans, J. R., Camilletti, C. R., Bhatt, S., & Brandon, S. (2014). Accusatorial and information-gathering interrogation methods and their effects on true and false confessions: A meta-analytic review. *Journal of Experimental Criminology, 10*(4), 459–486. https://doi.org/10.1007/s11292-014-9207-6.

Medford, S., Gudjonsson, G. H., & Pearse, J. (2003). The efficacy of the appropriate adult safeguard during police interviewing. *Legal and Criminological Psychology, 8*, 253–266. https://doi.org/10.1348/135532503322363022.

Memon, A., Meissner, C. A., & Fraser, J. (2010). The cognitive interview: A meta-analytic review and study space analysis of the past 25 years. *Psychology, Public Policy, and Law, 16*, 340–372. https://doi.org/10.1037/a0020518.

Memon, A., Zaragoza, M., Clifford, B. R., & Kidd, L. (2010). Inoculation or antidote? The effects of cognitive interview timing on false memory for forcibly fabricated events. *Law and Human Behavior, 34*, 105–117. https://doi.org/10.1007/s10979-008-9172-6.

Meyer, B. J., Gardiner, J. M., & Bowler, D. M. (2014). Directed forgetting in high-functioning adults with autism spectrum disorders. *Journal of Autism and Developmental Disorders, 44*, 2514–2524. https://doi.org/10.1007/s10803-014-2121-y.

Millward, C., Powell, S., Messer, D., & Jordan, R. (2000). Recall for self and other in autism: Children's memory for events experienced by themselves and their peers. *Journal of Autism and Developmental Disorders, 30*, 15–28. https://doi.org/10.1023/A:1005455926727.

Milne, R., & Bull, R. (1999). *Investigative interviewing: Psychology and practice*. Wiley.

Milne, R., & Bull, R. (2006). Interviewing victims of crime, including children and people with intellectual disabilities. In M. Kebbell & G. Davies (Eds.) *Practical psychology for forensic investigations and prosecutions*. Wiley.

Ministry of Justice. (2011). *Achieving best evidence in criminal proceedings guidance on interviewing victims and witnesses, and guidance on using special measures*. Home Office.

Minshew, N. J., & Goldstein, G. (1993). Is autism an amnesic disorder? Evidence from the California Verbal Learning Test. *Neuropsychology, 7*(2), 209–216.

Neil, L., Olsson, N. C., & Pellicano, E. (2016). The Relationship Between Intolerance of uncertainty, sensory sensitivities, and anxiety in autistic and typically developing children. *Journal of Autism and Developmental Disorders, 46*, 1962–1973. https://doi.org/10.1007/s10803-016-2721-9.

Neumann, D., Spezio, M. L., Piven, J., & Adolphs, R. (2006). Looking you in the mouth: abnormal gaze in autism resulting from impaired top-down modulation of visual attention. *Social Cognitive and Affective Neuroscience, 1*, 194–202. https://doi.org/10.1093/scan/nsl030.

Norbury, C. F., & Bishop, D. V. M. (2003). Narrative skills of children with communication impairments. *International Journal of Language & Communication Disorders, 38*, 287–313. https://doi.org/10.1080/1368203100001O8133.

Norris, J. E., Crane, L., & Maras, K. (2020). Interviewing autistic adults: Adaptations to support recall in police, employment, and healthcare interviews. *Autism*. https://doi.org/10.1177/1362361320909174.

North, A., Russell, A., & Gudjonsson, G. (2008). High functioning autism spectrum disorders: an investigation of psychological vulnerabilities during interrogative interview. *Journal of Forensic Psychiatry & Psychology, 19*, 323–334. https://doi.org/10.1080/14789940701871621.

O'Mahony, B. M. (2010). The emerging role of the registered intermediary with the vulnerable witness and offender: Facilitating communication with the police and members of the judiciary. *British Journal of Learning Disabilities, 38*, 232–237. https://doi.org/10.1111/j.1468-3156.2009.00600.x.

O'Mahony, B. M., Marchant, R., & Fadden, L. (2015). Vulnerable Individuals, Intermediaries and Justice. In G. Oxburgh, T. Myklebust, T. Grant, & R. Milne (Eds.) *Communication in investigative and legal contexts*. Wiley. https://doi.org/10.1002/9781118769133.ch13.

O'Mahony, B. M., Milne, B., & Grant, T. (2012). To Challenge, or not to challenge? Best practice when interviewing vulnerable suspects. *Policing, 6*, 301–313. https://doi.org/10.1093/police/pas027.

O'Mahony, B. M., Smith, K., & Milne, B. (2011). The early identification of vulnerable witnesses prior to an investigative interview. *The British Journal of Forensic Practice, 13*(2), 114–123.

Ormerod, T. C., & Dando, C. J. (2015). Finding a needle in a haystack: Toward a psychologically informed method for aviation security screening. *Journal of Experimental Psychology: General, 144*, 76–84. https://doi.org/10.1037/xge0000030.

Oxburgh, G. E., Myklebust, T., & Grant, T. (2010). The question of question types in police interviews: A review of the literature from a psychological and linguistic perspective. *International Journal of Speech, Language & the Law, 17*(1).

Oxburgh, L., Gabbert, F., Milne, R., & Cherryman, J. (2016). Police officers' perceptions and experiences with mentally disordered suspects. *International Journal of Law and Psychiatry, 49*, 138–146. https://doi.org/10.1016/j.ijlp.2016.08.008.

Ozonoff, S. (1995). Reliability and validity of the Wisconsin Card Sorting Test in studies of autism. *Neuropsychology, 9*, 491–500. https://doi.org/10.1037/0894-4105.9.4.491.

Pascual, A., & Guéguen, N. (2005). Foot-in-the-door and door-in-the-face: A comparative meta-analytic study. *Psychological Reports, 96*, 122–128. https://doi.org/10.2466/pr0.96.1.122-128.

Peppé, S., McCann, J., Gibbon, F., O'Hare, A., & Rutherford, M. (2007). Receptive and expressive prosodic ability in children with high-functioning autism. *Journal of Speech Language and Hearing Research, 50*, 1015. https://doi.org/10.1044/1092-4388(2007/071).

Perlman, N. B., Ericson, K. I., Esses, V. M., & Isaacs, B. J. (1994). The developmentally handicapped witness: Competency as a function of question format. *Law and Human Behavior, 18*(2), 171–187.

Plotnikoff, J., & Woolfson, R. (2015). *Intermediaries in the criminal justice system: Improving communication for vulnerable witnesses and defendants*. Policy Press.
Poirier, M., Martin, J. S., Gaigg, S. B., & Bowler, D. M. (2011). Short-term memory in autism spectrum disorder. *Journal of Abnormal Psychology, 120*, 247–252.
Porter, S., & Brinke, L. (2010). The truth about lies: What works in detecting high-stakes deception? *Legal and Criminological Psychology, 15*, 57–75. https://doi.org/10.1348/135532509X433151.
Powell, M. B., & Snow, P. C. (2007). Guide to questioning children during the free-narrative phase of an investigative interview. *Australian Psychologist, 42*(1), 57–65.
Rava, J., Shattuck, P., Rast, J., & Roux, A. (2017). The Prevalence and correlates of involvement in the criminal justice system among youth on the autism spectrum. *Journal of Autism and Developmental Disorders, 47*, 340–346. https://doi.org/10.1007/s10803-016-2958-3.
Renner, P., Klinger, L. G., & Klinger, M. R. (2000). Implicit and explicit memory in autism: Is autism an amnesic disorder? *Journal of Autism and Developmental Disorders, 30*(1), 3–14.
Renoult, L., Davidson, P. S. R., Palombo, D. J., Moscovitch, M., & Levine, B. (2012). Personal semantics: at the crossroads of semantic and episodic memory. *Trends in Cognitive Sciences, 16*, 550–558. https://doi.org/10.1016/J.TICS.2012.09.003.
Richards, J., & Milne, R. (2020). Appropriate adults, their experiences and understanding of autism spectrum disorder. *Research in Developmental Disabilities*. https://doi.org/10.1016/j.ridd.2020.103675.
Ridley, A. M., Gabbert, F., & La Rooy, D. J. (2012). *Suggestibility in legal contexts: psychological research and forensic implications*. Wiley-Blackwell.
Ridley, A. M., Van Rheede, V., & Wilcock, R. (2015). Interviews, intermediaries and interventions: Mock-jurors', police officers' and barristers' perceptions of a child witness interview. *Investigative Interviewing: Research and Practice, 7*(1), 21–35.
Rodgers, J., Glod, M., Connolly, B., & McConachie, H. (2012). The relationship between anxiety and repetitive behaviours in autism spectrum disorder. *Journal of Autism and Developmental Disorders, 42*, 2404–2409. https://doi.org/10.1007/s10803-012-1531-y.
Rogers, S. J., & Ozonoff, S. (2005). Annotation: What do we know about sensory dysfunction in autism? A critical review of the empirical evidence. *Journal of Child Psychology and Psychiatry, and Allied Disciplines, 46*(12), 1255–1268. https://doi.org/10.1111/j.1469-7610.2005.01431.x.
Russell, A. J., Murphy, C. M., Wilson, E., Gillan, N., Brown, C., Robertson, D. M., ... Murphy, D. G. (2016). The mental health of individuals referred for assessment of autism spectrum disorder in adulthood: A clinic report. *Autism, 20*, 623–627. https://doi.org/10.1177/1362361315604271.
Russell, J., & Jarrold, C. (1999). Memory for actions in children with autism: Self versus other. *Cognitive Neuropsychiatry, 4*, 303–331. https://doi.org/10.1080/135468099395855.
Schacter, D. L., Norman, K. A., & Koutstaal, W. (1998). The cognitive neuroscience of constructive memory. *Annual Review of Psychology, 49*, 289–318.
Senju, A., & Johnson, M. H. (2009). Atypical eye contact in autism: Models, mechanisms and development. *Neuroscience and Biobehavioral Reviews, 33*, 1204–1214. https://doi.org/10.1016/j.neubiorev.2009.06.001.
Shaw, J. S., & III., Bjork, R. A., & Handal, A.. (1995). Retrieval-induced forgetting in an eyewitness-memory paradigm. *Psychonomic Bulletin & Review, 2*, 249–253. https://doi.org/10.3758/BF03210965.
Simonoff, E., Pickles, A., Charman, T., Chandler, S., Loucas, T., & Baird, G. (2008). Psychiatric disorders in children with autism spectrum disorders: Prevalence, comorbidity, and associated factors in a population-derived sample. *Journal of the American Academy of Child and Adolescent Psychiatry, 47*(8), 921–929. https://doi.org/10.1097/CHI.0b013e318179964f.
Sinha et al., 2014.Sinha, P., Kjelgaard, M. M., Gandhi, T. K., Tsourides, K., Cardinaux, A. L., Pantazis, D., ... Held, R. M. (2014). Autism as a disorder of prediction. *Proceedings of the National Academy of Sciences, 111*(42), 15220-15225.
Smith, B. J., Gardiner, J. M., & Bowler, D. M. (2007). Deficits in free recall persist in Asperger's syndrome despite training in the use of list-appropriate learning strategies. *Journal of Autism and Developmental Disorders, 37*, 445–454. https://doi.org/10.1007/s10803-006-0180-4.

Soukara, S., Bull, R., Vrij, A., Turner, M., & Cherryman, J. (2009). What really happens in police interviews of suspects? Tactics and confessions. *Psychology, Crime & Law, 15*, 493–506. https://doi.org/10.1080/10683160802201827.
Southwick, J. S., Bigler, E. D., Froehlich, A., Dubray, M. B., Alexander, A. L., Lange, N., & Lainhart, J. E. (2011). Memory functioning in children and adolescents with autism. *Neuropsychology, 25*, 702. https://doi.org/10.1037/a0024935.
Squire, L. R. (1995). Biological foundations of accuracy and inaccuracy in memory. In D. L. Schacter (Ed.), *Memory distortions: How minds, brains, and societies reconstruct the past.* (pp. 197–225). Harvard University Press.
Stone, M. (1988). *Cross-examination in criminal trials.* Butterworths.
Summers, J. A., & Craik, F. I. M. (1994). The effects of subject-performed tasks on the memory performance of verbal autistic children. *Journal of Autism and Developmental Disorders, 24*, 773–783. https://doi.org/10.1007/BF02172285.
Tager-Flusberg, H. (1991). Semantic processing in the free recall of autistic children—Further evidence for a cognitive deficit. *British Journal of Developmental Psychology, 9*, 417–430.
Tager-Flusberg, H. (1995). 'Once upon a ribbit': Stories narrated by autistic children. *British Journal of Developmental Psychology, 13*(1), 45–59.
Tager-Flusberg, H. (2000). Language and understanding other minds: Connections in autism. In S. Baron-Cohen, H. Tager-Flusberg, & D. Cohen (Eds.), *Understanding other minds.* (2nd ed., pp. 124–149). OUP.
Tager-Flusberg, H., Paul, R., & Lord, C. (2005). Language and communication in autism. In F. Volkmar, R. Paul, & A. Klin (Eds.), *Handbook on autism and pervasive developmental disorders.* (3rd ed., pp. 335–364). Wiley.
Tager-Flusberg, H., & Sullivan, K. (1995). Attributing mental states to story characters: A comparison of narratives produced by autistic and mentally retarded individuals. *Applied Psycholinguistics, 16*(3), 241–256.
Tanweer, T., Rathbone, C. J., & Souchay, C. (2010). Autobiographical memory, autonoetic consciousness, and identity in Asperger syndrome. *Neuropsychologia, 48*, 900–908. https://doi.org/10.1016/j.neuropsychologia.2009.11.007.
Tint, A., Palucka, A. M., Bradley, E., Weiss, J. A., & Lunsky, Y. (2017). Correlates of police involvement among adolescents and adults with autism spectrum disorder. *Journal of Autism and Developmental Disorders, 47*, 2639–2647. https://doi.org/10.1007/s10803-017-3182-5.
Toichi, M., Kamio, Y., Okada, T., Sakihama, M., Youngstrom, E. A., Findling, R. L., & Yamamoto, K. (2002). A lack of self-consciousness in autism. *The American Journal of Psychiatry, 159*(8), 1422–1424.
Tulving, E. (1983). *Elements of episodic memory*. Oxford University Press.
Tulving, E. (2001). Episodic memory and common sense: How far apart? *Philosophical Transactions of the Royal Society, B, 356*, 1505–1515.
Valentine, T., & Maras, K. L. (2011). The effect of cross-examination on the accuracy of adult eyewitness testimony. *Applied Cognitive Psychology, 25*, 554–561. https://doi.org/10.1002/acp.1768.
Vallano, J. P., & Schreiber Compo, N. (2015). Rapport-building with cooperative witnesses and criminal suspects: A theoretical and empirical review. *Psychology, Public Policy, and Law, 21*(1), 85.
Van Eylen, L., Boets, B., Steyaert, J., Evers, K., Wagemans, J., & Noens, I. (2011). Cognitive flexibility in autism spectrum disorder: Explaining the inconsistencies? *Research in Autism Spectrum Disorders, 5*, 1390–1401. https://doi.org/10.1016/j.rasd.2011.01.025.
Vrij, A. (2008). Nonverbal dominance versus verbal accuracy in lie detection: A plea to change police practice. *Criminal Justice and Behavior, 35*(10), 1323–1336.
Vrij, A., Fisher, R. P., & Blank, H. (2017). A cognitive approach to lie detection: A meta-analysis. *Legal and Criminological Psychology, 22*, 1–21. https://doi.org/10.1111/lcrp.12088.
Vrij, A., Fisher, R., Mann, S., & Leal, S. (2006). Detecting deception by manipulating cognitive load. *Trends in Cognitive Sciences, 10*, 141–142. https://doi.org/10.1016/j.tics.2006.02.003.

Vrij, A., Fisher, R., Mann, S., & Leal, S. (2008). A cognitive load approach to lie detection. *Journal of Investigative Psychology and Offender Profiling, 5*, 39–43. https://doi.org/10.1002/jip.82.
Vrij, A., Leal, S., Granhag, P. A., Mann, S., Fisher, R. P., Hillman, J., & Sperry, K. (2009). Outsmarting the liars: The benefit of asking unanticipated questions. *Law and Human Behavior, 33*, 159–166. https://doi.org/10.1007/s10979-008-9143-y.
Walker, N. E. (2002). Forensic interviews of children: The components of scientific validity and legal admissibility. *Law and Contemporary Problems, 65*(1), 149–178.
Weiss, J. A., & Fardella, M. A. (2018). Victimization and perpetration experiences of adults with autism. *Frontiers in Psychiatry, 9*, 203. https://doi.org/10.3389/fpsyt.2018.00203.
Wheatcroft, J. M., & Ellison, L. E. (2012). Evidence in court: Witness preparation and cross-examination style effects on adult witness accuracy. *Behavioral Sciences & the Law, 30*, 821–840. https://doi.org/10.1002/bsl.2031.
White, S. J. (2013). The Triple I Hypothesis: taking another('s) perspective on executive dysfunction in autism. *Journal of Autism and Developmental Disorders, 43*, 114–121. https://doi.org/10.1007/s10803-012-1550-8.
White, S. J., Burgess, P. W., & Hill, E. L. (2009). Impairments on "open-ended" executive function tests in autism. *Autism Research, 2*, 138–147. https://doi.org/10.1002/aur.78.
Wigham, S., Barton, S., Parr, J. R., & Rodgers, J. (2017). A systematic review of the rates of depression in children and adults with high-functioning autism spectrum disorder. *Journal of Mental Health Research in Intellectual Disabilities, 10*, 267–287. https://doi.org/10.1080/19315864.2017.1299267.
Wigham, S., Rodgers, J., South, M., McConachie, H., & Freeston, M. (2015). The interplay between sensory processing abnormalities, intolerance of uncertainty, anxiety and restricted and repetitive behaviours in autism spectrum disorder. *Journal of Autism and Developmental Disorders, 45*, 943–952. https://doi.org/10.1007/s10803-014-2248-x.
Williams, D., & Happé, F. (2009). Pre-conceptual aspects of self-awareness in autism spectrum disorder: The case of action-monitoring. *Journal of Autism and Developmental Disorders, 39*, 251–259. https://doi.org/10.1007/s10803-008-0619-x.
Williams, D. L., Goldstein, G., & Minshew, N. J. (2006). The profile of memory function in children with autism. *Neuropsychology, 20*, 21–29. https://doi.org/10.1037/0894-4105.20.1.21.
Wojcik, D. Z., Allen, R. J., Brown, C., & Souchay, C. (2011). Memory for actions in autism spectrum disorder. *Memory, 19*, 549–558. https://doi.org/10.1080/09658211.2011.590506.
Yamamoto, K., & Masumoto, K. (2018). Brief report: Memory for self-performed actions in adults with autism spectrum disorder: Why does memory of self decline in ASD? *Journal of Autism and Developmental Disorders*, 1–7. https://doi.org/10.1007/s10803-018-3559-0.
Zajac, R., & Hayne, H. (2003). I don't think that's what really happened: The effect of cross-examination on the accuracy of children's reports. *Journal of Experimental Psychology: Applied, 9*, 187–195. https://doi.org/10.1037/1076-898X.9.3.187.
Zajac, R., & Hayne, H. (2006). The negative effect of cross-examination style questioning on children's accuracy: Older children are not immune. *Applied Cognitive Psychology, 20*, 3–16. https://doi.org/10.1002/acp.1169.
Zalla, T., Daprati, E., Sav, A.-M., Chaste, P., Nico, D., & Leboyer, M. (2010). Memory for self-performed actions in individuals with Asperger syndrome. *PLoS ONE, 5*, e13370. https://doi.org/10.1371/journal.pone.0013370.
Zalla, T., Labruyère, N., & Georgieff, N. (2013). Perceiving goals and actions in individuals with autism spectrum disorders. *Journal of Autism and Developmental Disorders, 43*, 2353–2365. https://doi.org/10.1007/s10803-013-1784-0.
Zamoscik, V., Mier, D., Schmidt, S. N. L., & Kirsch, P. (2016). Early memories of individuals on the autism spectrum assessed using online self-reports. *Frontiers in Psychiatry, 7*, 79. https://doi.org/10.3389/fpsyt.2016.00079.

Dr Katie Maras is a Senior Lecturer in Psychology and Deputy Director of the Centre for Applied Autism Research at the University of Bath. The main focus of Katie's research is on autistic people's experiences within the Criminal Justice System and the adaptations that police and other professionals can make to accommodate their differences. Katie works with police and other legal professionals to provide evidence-based policy, guidance and training when working with autistic people, and has particular expertise regarding police interviewing techniques.

Chapter 8
ASD and Unlawful Behaviour: Background

Marc Woodbury-Smith

Introduction

In his published case series from 1943, Hans Asperger drew attention to a group of children with a fundamental difficulty relating to others, most notably their peers, and among whom aggressive behaviour towards these others was often observed (Asperger, 1944/1991). This description, and its similarities to those children described earlier by Leo Kanner (Kanner, 1943), formed the basis for the subsequent operationalization of autism as a spectrum, although the potential for aggressive interpersonal behaviour was never foregrounded. Nonetheless, since the recognition of this continuum, and the subsequent inclusion of cognitively more able individuals in its definition, a body of research has existed that describes unlawful behaviour, including aggression, among people with ASD (Dein & Woodbury-Smith, 2010; Woodbury-Smith & Dein, 2014). Subsequent chapters in this current volume will examine this literature in some detail. Consequently, to avoid repetition, this introductory chapter will merely present a framework for the interpretation of the texts that follows, as well as how this framework might best be applied in the future.

ASD and Criminal Justice System: History of the Literature

Wing drew attention to the cases first described by Asperger in her 1981 paper by presenting a series of brief case descriptions with similar phenomenology (Wing, 1981). She drew parallels with the social impairments of Kanner's cases, broadened the list of secondary features, and de-emphasized any differences, thereby laying the

M. Woodbury-Smith (✉)
Biosciences Institute, Newcastle University, Newcastle upon Tyne, UK
e-mail: marc.woodbury-smith@newcastle.ac.uk

F. R. Volkmar et al. (eds.), *Handbook of Autism Spectrum Disorder and the Law*,
https://doi.org/10.1007/978-3-030-70913-6_8

foundation for a diagnostic 'spectrum'. The idea of a spectrum often suggests a two-dimensional construct, but of course, spectra can be multidimensional. In the case of ASD this is certainly true; Wing and others since have pointed out variation across individuals with ASD in terms of cognitive ability, social skills, communicative abilities, and a range of other disorder-related factors. One such factor was the "small minority [who] have a history of bizarre antisocial acts, perhaps because of their lack of empathy" (Wing, 1981: 116). Indeed, Asperger himself had described 'autistic malice' in seven out of 46 children seen in his clinic (15%) (Hippler & Klicpera, 2003). These children presented 'with malicious pleasure and apparent pride in what they had done. Some of the children were said to experiment on others, that is, they seemed to do things on purpose to see how others reacted to provoke a certain reaction' (Hippler & Klicpera, 2003: 294). The possibility, therefore, that not only might some children with this syndrome engage in violent behaviour, but also that it might in some way be related to the core phenotype, has been of interest to the clinical and scientific community since the birth of the concept of ASD itself.

The early literature comprised case descriptions of principally adults who were seen by mental health services in the context of alleged unlawful behaviour (Dein & Woodbury-Smith, 2010, and references therein). Diagnosis often post-dated service involvement, i.e. the possibility of ASD had not been raised during their earlier years. This may simply reflect the fact that, at the time, ASD was extremely rare and thereby unlikely to be on diagnosticians' radars, with little availability within clinical services of the necessary diagnostic expertise. This notwithstanding, these case descriptions, were meticulous in their account of phenotype, providing little doubt that these cases resembled those of Wing and Asperger.

These single case studies and case series set the stage for a substantial body of research over a period of 30 years that has evolved very slowly, and meandered through, but largely failed to answer, various fundamental questions. These include: (i) are people with ASD over-represented in incarcerated populations? (ii) is unlawful behaviour higher among those with ASD than others in the community? and (iii) if there is indeed an increased prevalence of unlawful behaviour, how might we understand the nature of the relationship to ASD? Unfortunately, as will be discussed subsequently, even the most basic of questions remain poorly understood, demanding a more robust approach to studying this population, which may itself be very difficult to achieve.

At the outset, I must provide some clarification on terminology. This can sometimes be a little sloppy in the scientific literature, making it difficult to adjudicate the data within. The terms 'unlawful behavior' and 'illegal behavior' are used synonymously to refer to any transgression of a legally defined construct in the particular jurisdiction. This does lead to possible inconsistency, if, for example, countries define what is and isn't a transgression differently. However, for our purposes this is largely uncontroversial as the focus is on more serious transgressions that are likely to be defined similarly wherever it has taken place. Indeed, much of the literature is from Western Europe, Australasia and North America, where criminal law is comparable. The terms 'offending' and 'criminal behavior' also generally refer to the same type of transgression, and so these, too, must be considered synonymous. However, it is worth bearing in mind that not all behaviour that is illegal results in a conviction, as people with mental disorders, including developmental disorders such as ASD, will often be 'diverted' into treatment programmes at healthcare facilities using appropriate legislation, such as the 1983 Mental Health Act in the UK. Others may be similarly diverted, but not until after their conviction. Others too many be deemed Not Guilty by Reason of Insanity. It quickly becomes apparent that the pathways from alleged offence to outcome are numerous, with many influencing factors, as discussed throughout this volume.

Diagnosis also needs some clarification. The term Asperger Syndrome is no longer used in clinical practice, but it is reasonable to assume that such cases will be captured by the more general term ASD, as was the original intention. However, this is not to say that what we now understand as ASD is synonymous with the continuum as articulated by Wing in the 1980s. Consideration of prevalence trajectories alone is enough evidence to support that conjecture: prevalence has ballooned in the last decade. In the absence of a reasonable biological explanation, the assumption is that this is due to a broadening of the concept of ASD (Baio et al., 2018). In turn, Wing's own cases will differ in certain ways from Kanner's and Asperger's. These shifting nosological sands, although by no means peculiar to ASD alone, do undermine researchers' attempts to study them, and, indeed, clinicians' attempts to keep up with and make sense of the literature. Without labouring the point too much, a critical reader will bear this in mind when reading the text that follows.

How Many People with ASD Engage in Unlawful Behaviour?

The prevalence of ASD among offender populations has been very well studied, principally in Europe and the USA (King & Murphy, 2014). For example, in the 1990s attempts were made to estimate the prevalence of ASD in maximum secure psychiatric hospitals in England, with the results supporting a raised prevalence based on contemporaneous population estimates (Hare et al., 1999; Scragg & Shah, 1994). A similar pattern was observed in a Swedish hospital population (Mouridsen et al., 2008). Other studies have looked at prevalence among convicted offenders referred for psychiatric evaluation (Siponmaa et al., 2001; Soderstrom et al., 2004), and in a male prison population (Underwood et al., 2016). The rates vary depending on the year of publication, the population studied and ascertainment methods employed. Moreover, because of changes in diagnostic criteria over time it is also very difficult to conflate studies to give an overall median. Indeed, the figure may be as low as 3%, or as high as 27%, shedding light on the need to examine what factors might underlie such a large variation.

Examining place of incarceration does offer some consistency. For example, two large prison studies conducted within the last 8 years, one in Scotland (Robinson et al., 2012) and the other in the USA (Fazio et al., 2012) found 4 and 4.4% screened positively for ASD respectively. Interestingly, none of the screen-positives from the 2,458 prisoners (predominantly male) surveyed in Scottish prisons met the diagnostic criteria for ASD. Unfortunately, in the US study Fazio and colleagues were unable to follow up their screening assessment with an interview to determine diagnosis more definitively. There may be several reasons to cast some doubt as to whether 4.4% is a realistic figure. Those who agreed to take part are self-selected, and little is known about those who did not take part. For example, those who are aloof and withdrawn, both potential indicators of ASD, may be less likely to become involved in research. Furthermore, the screening questionnaires used have been developed to differentiate those with ASD from their non-ASD counterparts *in the community*. Simply transferring or modifying them for use in the offender population may not be robust. For, as a group, people detained in prisons harbour a disproportionate burden for mental health diagnoses and personality disorders (Fazel & Danesh, 2002; Fazel et al., 2016). Moreover, this population includes individuals with a range of interpersonal difficulties, including attachment disorders and other psychodynamically driven pathological patterns of relatedness to others (Farrington et al., 2017; Ogilvie et al., 2014). This may be particularly true among violent offenders. ASD focussed screening questionnaires have little ability to capture the complexity of interpersonal behaviour in psychodynamic aetiological terms. This is also true of diagnostic assessments, something I will return to later.

The prevalence of ASD in maximum secure psychiatric hospitals in the UK is in the region of 2.5%, perhaps as many as 5% if 'possible' cases are also considered (Hare et al., 1999; Scragg & Shah, 1994). These studies were conducted in the 1990s using non-standardized diagnostic criteria. Even by today's standards, with a population prevalence of 1.5% or more (Van Naarden Braun et al., 2015), this still reflects a raised prevalence. Of course, all the caveats described with reference to studying the prison population are also true in this setting. While these figures are in line at least with the prison estimates, data from Scandinavia concerning prevalence among convicted offenders referred for psychiatric evaluation support a much higher value. For example, Soderstrom (Soderstrom et al., 2004) identified that 3, 5, and 10% of this population met the diagnostic criteria for Autism, Asperger Syndrome and Autism Spectrum Disorder NOS respectively. Consecutive referrals to forensic psychiatric services over a five-year period were studied by Siponmaa and colleagues (2001), who identified Pervasive Developmental Disorder in 27% (Siponmaa et al., 2001). This higher figure may represent national or local policy, whereby diversion from the criminal justice system is mandated as a way to protect this potentially vulnerable population, who may then subsequently end up in less secure provisions or serving a community-based probation. This figure may also reflect crime recording: it is not safe to assume that these will be defined in a consistent manner from one jurisdiction to another, particularly among crimes at the less severe end of the spectrum.

A more robust approach to examining the prevalence of criminality among people with ASD is by way of an epidemiological community-based study. Indeed, if Siponmaa and Soderstrom's figures are to be accepted, then the prevalence of such behaviour in the community should also be proportionately higher. However, this is not the case. Cheely et al. (2012) examined figures for all young people aged 11–18 years registered as part of the Carolina Autism and Developmental Disabilities Monitoring Project. Among the 609 identified with ASD, 32 had contact with the

Department for Juvenile Justice. This figure of 5.24% is by no means low, but when compared with other mental health groups, it is certainly no higher, and as such may simply be a reflection of a variety of factors relevant to all those with neuropsychiatric disorders. Indeed, Heeramun et al. (2017) analysed data from the Stockholm Youth Cohort, comprising 295,734 individuals of whom 5,739 were diagnosed with ASD. Although the risk of violent offending was estimated to be higher in this group (adjusted relative risk 1.39, 95% CI 1.23–1.58), this was markedly attenuated after taking certain comorbidities into consideration, specifically comorbidity with ADHD or Conduct Disorder.

For the time being, at least, it may be difficult to argue definitely for an increased risk of offending in this population. Nevertheless, despite the variance in figures, the research *seems* to point to this conclusion, and it is on this basis that the questions described in the following sections are of importance.

What Is the Nature of the Vulnerability to Unlawful Behaviour in ASD?

It would be nice to offer some conclusion from all these data, but unfortunately, as the reader will have no doubt observed, the picture is complicated. It is reasonable to expect that some people with ASD may come into contact with the criminal justice system following alleged unlawful behaviour, but what is the nature of their vulnerability? In part it may be a reflection of comorbidity with conduct disorder or ADHD. It is now recognized that the prevalence of ADHD is significantly higher in ASD than their non-ASD peers, with a population-based Birth Register study identifying almost half of all individuals with ASD as also having an ADHD diagnosis (48%, Ghirardi et al., 2018). This is striking, particularly so as ADHD itself is strongly associated with offending. Notably, between 20 and 40% of convicted prisoners (as opposed to those on remand) have a diagnosis of ADHD, perhaps related to ADHD's strong association with conduct disorder and impulsive behaviour (Ginsberg et al., 2010; Moore et al., 2016). Of course, impulsivity and otherwise dysexecutive cognition may also lead to a greater chance of being apprehended. However, as the figures are so high this seems unlikely. It is worth noting that independently of an ADHD diagnosis, Farrington and West's longitudinal Study of Delinquent Development in Cambridge, UK, provided evidence for an association between traits of impulsivity and inattention with a later risk of arrest (Farrington, 2003). Of course, what has not been similarly investigated is whether the association of ADHD with offending is actually mediated by its strong association with ASD. As unlikely as this sounds, until longitudinal epidemiological data are available, we can never be certain.

The relationship of ASD to conduct disorder and psychopathy also needs careful consideration. This is particularly true given (i) the association of ASD with ADHD, and, in turn, ADHD's own association with conduct disorder, and (ii) the psychopathy literature which describes a number of socio-emotional vulnerabilities at the cognitive level that appear to overlap with those of ASD (Blair, 2013; Salekin, 2017). These include the ability to recognize the emotional valence of stimuli such as facial expression, vocalization and gestures; physiological arousal to distressing and/or otherwise disturbing images; and, appreciating the mental states of others (i.e. theory of mind), a cognitive domain which mediates a person's beliefs and attitudes. There is a large body of scientific literature examining these cognitive domains in adults with psychopathy, as well as adolescents at risk of psychopathy (Blair, 1997, 2003; Blair et al., 1997; Salekin, 2017). This largely supports impairments in the ability to recognize and elicit a physiological response to distress, with imaging studies also supporting a role for the amygdala and its temporofrontal connections (Blair, 2003; Raine, 2002). In contrast, whether or not people with psychopathy have impaired theory of mind is not clear (Blair et al., 1996; Richell et al., 2003). However, people with ASD also have difficulty processing emotionally laden stimuli, and some have a cognitive profile that overlaps with psychopathy (Woodbury-Smith et al., 2005; Rogers et al., 2006). In one study, for example, a group of adults with ASD who had a history of offending were shown to have a superior Theory of Mind but specific impairment in the recognition of fear, i.e. an identical cognitive profile to psychopathy (Woodbury-Smith et al., 2005). What was striking about this study is that the clinical phenotype among this ASD-offending subgroup showed no features of conduct disorder or psychopathy. Indeed, they were much the same as their non-offending ASD counterparts (Woodbury-Smith et al., 2005).

If functioning at the cognitive level does little to predict clinical phenotype then our objective neuropsychological tests, some of which are used adjunctly in diagnosis, could be incorrectly interpreted. Conversely, it may point to the need to use these cognitive tests more frequently in diagnostic assessment, to fully capture a person's areas of vulnerability and potential risk, irrespective of what diagnosis they may have clinically. From the point of view of this current discussion, however, this does indicate that it may not be the ASD per se that is most strongly associated with risk; instead, the risk may be the comorbidity, and this comorbidity may only be at the level of endophenotype rather than clinical phenotype. In the future, therefore, research will need to more closely examine the relationship between ASD and other clinical phenotypes, *and* the underlying vulnerabilities at the brain (endophenotype) level.

Having considered comorbidity, what, if any, contribution may be deemed the direct impact of the ASD itself? For example, in clinical terms the intensity and/or focus of some people's 'circumscribed interests' may be of concern (Helverschou et al., 2015). There are case studies in the literature of people with ASD whose offences were, for different reasons, related to their interest. This includes interests that are potentially violent in nature, such as an interest in weapons, and illegal behaviour in the pursuit of an interest (Woodbury-Smith et al., 2010). Importantly, interests that have violence as a theme, such as an obsession with weapons or with an infamous historical figure, may not necessarily be driven by any intent to harm. A 'fascination' with weapons, Hitler or atrocities in general may be detached from the inherent reality of suffering and pain, particularly if the ability to empathize with others is impacted. However, these interests will be red flags, and may in and of themselves result in contact with the criminal justice system (CJS) due to *perceived* risk, even in the absence of any unlawful behaviour. In contrast, a benign interest, such as collecting Pokémon cards, may also result in contact with the CJS if the financial means for the acquisition of a desired object is unavailable, and the person chooses instead to acquire illegally. Clearly in all such cases knowledge of diagnosis will be crucial in any consideration of motivation and risk.

The tendency for certain individuals with ASD to develop fixations, whether in the pursuit of an interest or due to having a fairly strong and rigid moral compass, is also relevant, as is the 'black and white' style of thinking that is often described among such individuals. While the motivation for holding extremist views is complicated (Kruglanski et al., 2014), it is certainly possible that the fixed, black and white beliefs in ASD may develop into views that are politicized and associated with negative emotions towards particular groups (Palermo, 2013). Of course, many people hold beliefs that are extreme, even fundamental, but without necessarily having violent intent. Nonetheless, holding extremist views may clearly spiral into violence, although this has not been studied specifically among those with ASD who have extremist views.

Beyond holding extremist views, consideration also needs to be given to risk of radicalization. Those individuals who are marginalized or otherwise socially isolated and searching for a sense of belonging are at a particularly high risk (Kruglanski et al., 2014); numbered among such people may be some with ASD, who may be additionally vulnerable due to their own suggestibility and acquiescence (Maras & Bowler, 2012 and references therein for background on suggestibility). Communication by way of the internet also provides the opportunity to meet others without the challenge of interaction—itself an avenue for their recruitment, perhaps unbeknownst to them.

Stalking may also be a consequence of the tendency for fixation (Stokes et al., 2007). It has been well documented that although some people with ASD may be aloof, for most there is a wish for romantic relationships, albeit oftentimes without the capacity to initiate and maintain such relationships (Post et al., 2014). Consequently, attempts to engage with another may be clumsy or inappropriate. In some situations, such approaches may have been 'learnt' through studying the behaviour of others; there may be a lack of appreciation that in some of these observed situations the individuals involved may already be on intimate terms. For others, however, anxiety buffers their ability to actually make contact, and so they may watch and follow another but never approach them. Over time they may send letters or emails and despite lack of reciprocity they may persist, particularly if, for them, rejection is the norm. Importantly, with perspective-taking difficulties, they may not appreciate the annoyance or distress experienced by their victim. Such stalking behaviour in ASD has been well documented (Post et al., 2014; Stokes & Newton, 2004; Stokes et al., 2007) and once again, an understanding of the underlying ASD and its associated impairments is vital in any consideration of motivation and risk.

Considering the Diagnosis of Social Vulnerabilities in the Forensic and Prison Populations

The prison population represents a sector of society that has experienced a disproportionate amount of mental health morbidity and childhood trauma, including neglect and abuse. Moreover, educational attainment is lower than the general population, and many incarcerated individuals will have experienced social disadvantage. These factors will invariably impact on social development, and so untangling this from ASD may be a challenging task. Indeed, in this population, confidence in diagnosis may be confounded.

Using gold standard assessments such as the ADI-R and ADOS should theoretically ensure that diagnoses are robust. However, there may be reasons to doubt the validity of the algorithmic classification offered by these assessments. It is certainly the case that if administered according to recommended protocol, these assessments can facilitate the acquisition of useful information regarding social and communicative development, play and other behaviours. However, among older adolescents and adults much of the information concerning earlier development is based on parental or carer recall, which may be unreliable (e.g., Ozonoff et al., 2018). It is for this reason that less established measures are often used in this age group, although, of course, it should not be assumed that circumventing semi-structured assessment in favour of clinical interviewing is less robust.

Consideration does need to be given to differential diagnosis given that ASD-specific assessments do not explore other conditions that may exist comorbidly with ASD. This may be easily addressed by merely adding additional measures, or otherwise expanding on the clinical assessment. However, there is also a risk that merely focussing on diagnostic 'labelling' may undermine the true aim of clinical evaluation, which is an understanding of the pathway to outcome, and the factors that comprise this pathway and their inter-relationship, diagnostic and otherwise. In failing to consider other possible factors in the development of social and communication and other behavioural vulnerabilities, we limit the opportunities for treatment.

By way of example, abnormal attachment in early infancy can have a major impact on the subsequent development of social interaction and communication (Ogilvie et al., 2014; Sroufe et al., 1999). The most severe examples have been articulated by Rutter and colleagues in their description of Romanian orphans (Hoksbergen et al., 2005). Strikingly, a large number demonstrated autistic traits, inattention and hyperactivity and behaviour problems even 5 years post-adoption. Although this clearly represents an extreme sample in terms of experiences of major early neglect, the fact that early environment can have a lasting impact on social and communication functioning is of major importance for treatment; classifying as ASD may be inappropriate given that their treatment needs may be different. However, a study of early attachment does not form a part of contemporary developmental assessment. This may be particularly important among those who are in the CJS as this population has experienced a disproportionate amount of early trauma and neglect (Duke et al., 2010; Hughes et al., 2017; Im, 2016).

Beyond attachment, other aspects of personality may present with a primary difficulty forming and maintaining relationships with others. For example, schizoid personality disorder remains nosologically distinct from ASD, and its differentiation from Asperger Syndrome was well described by Sula Wolff in her description of loners followed longitudinally through childhood and early adulthood (Wolff, 1991; Wolff et al., 1991). Whether or not this is a distinct disorder remains unknown, but for the time being at least, while remaining separate, it may be considered from the point of personality development and managed accordingly. Indeed, other disorders of personality development may equally impact on interpersonal behaviour (Dell'Osso et al., 2018).

A comprehensive assessment that takes into consideration all these dimensions is not straightforward in the CJS setting. Developmental trajectory is important, and a reliable informant is required to capture this longitudinal rather than cross-sectional history. Of course, a parent or guardian could certainly fulfil this role, but recall of important information may be unreliable. The assessee themselves may also be unreliable, particularly in relation to an objective account of their childhood experiences. The very process of self-reflection is complex, and even in the absence of ASD, the task of reflecting on one's interactions with others is difficult to achieve. These various elements of diagnostic interviewing need to be carefully considered in the interpretation of provided information.

Considering the Limitations in the Research

I have already alluded to the voluminous nature of research focussing on the interface between ASD and the criminal justice system, as well as some of the limitations that may reduce the generalizability of the results this research has generated. Factors such as small sample size are inherent in the type of research being conducted, be it case study or case series. Nonetheless, even case studies can be useful to illustrate a novel association between a diagnosis, its characteristics and outcome. They provide neither 'proof' nor 'evidence' of an association, although unfortunately that is still sometimes how they are interpreted.

Studies of a specific population such as prison or secure hospital are also likely to be impacted by small sample size unless conducted using a multicentre approach. The difficulties of conducting a multi-centre study are evident: the co-ordination required between people from a variety of different backgrounds, not to mention studying populations that may move around geographically from one institution to another on a regular basis is a formidable task. Indeed, perhaps the biggest concern in this area of research is diagnostic clarification. The availability of an informant who knows the person during their formative years, who can recall information in an unbiased manner, and who may be willing—and can commit the time—to be interviewed (ideally) face to face may be unrealistic.

One final consideration that potentially undermines all research is the stability of the diagnostic construct of ASD itself. The concept of 'autism' has evolved over time, considerably so in the last 25 years. This poses a real difficulty: how can policy ever be developed if the underlying concept is so unstable and thereby amorphous? If the ICD and DSM were developed to encourage a better understanding of the concepts described through creating research criteria, it is unfortunate that these criteria have continued to change so rapidly and *not necessarily in response to the scientific data.* Consequently, to undertake longitudinal research of a nature similar to Farrington and West's (Farrington, 2003) or Loeber's (Loeber & Burke, 2011) will be problematic if the concepts we are trying to measure continue to change into less clearly defined entities. As emphasized above, this will be compounded if there is also a failure to take into consideration the more complex 'non-diagnostic' elements of a person's interpersonal behaviour.

Conclusion

A lot has been learnt from research that has attempted to understand criminal behaviour among people with ASD, as attested by the chapters in this book that highlight the most robust data so far. Unfortunately, research has been confounded by a number of methodological limitations and other biases, often outwith the control of the researchers. The pathway to criminal behaviour is complex, and its full realization will require collaboration between researchers from different backgrounds, bringing with them multiple perspectives and unique expertise. Moreover, the availability of longitudinal data will be crucial, as well as data that capture interpersonal behaviour beyond simple diagnostic categorization. Finally, research agnostic to diagnosis, but which instead captures the same vulnerabilities in dimensional terms, may help overcome some of the difficulties inherent in our nosological shifting sands.

References

Asperger, H. (1944). Die "autistichen Psychopathen" im Kindersalter. *Archive fur psychiatrie und Nervenkrankheiten, 117,* 76–136. Translated in Uta Frith, ed. (1991). *Autism and Asperger Syndrome.* Cambridge University Press.

Baio, J., Wiggins, L., Christensen, D. L., Maenner, M. J., Daniels, J., Warren, Z., ... Dowling, N. F. (2018). Prevalence of autism spectrum disorder among children aged 8 years—Autism and developmental disabilities monitoring network, 11 sites, United States, 2014. *MMWR Surveillance Summaries, 67*(6), 1–23.

Blair, R. J. (1997). Moral reasoning and the child with psychopathic tendencies. *Personality and Individual Differences, 22*(5), 731–739.

Blair, R. J. (2003). Neurobiological basis of psychopathy. *British Journal of Psychiatry, 182,* 5–7.

Blair, R. J. R. (2013). Psychopathy: Cognitive and neural dysfunction. *Dialogues in Clinical Neuroscience, 15*(2), 181–190.

Blair, R. J., Jones, L., Clark, F., & Smith, M. (1997). The psychopathic individual: A lack of responsiveness to distress cues? *Psychophysiology, 34*(2), 192–198.

Blair, R. J., Sellers, C., Strickland, I., Clark, F., Williams, A., Smith, M., & Jones, L. (1996). Theory of mind in the psychopath. *The Journal of Forensic Psychiatry, 7*(1), 15–25.
Cheely, C. A., Carpenter, L. A., Letourneau, E. J., Nicholas, J. S., Charles, J., & King, L. B. (2012). The prevalence of youth with autism spectrum disorders in the criminal justice system. *Journal of Autism and Developmental Disorders, 42*(9), 1856–1862.
Dein, K., & Woodbury-Smith, M. (2010). Asperger syndomre and criminal behaviour. *Advances in Psychiatric Treatment, 16,* 37–43.
Dell'Osso, L., Cremone, I. M., Carpita, B., Fagiolini, A., Massimetti, G., Bossini, L., … Gesi, C. (2018). Correlates of autistic traits among patients with borderline personality disorder. *Comprehensive Psychiatry, 83,* 7–11.
Duke, N. N., Pettingell, S. L., McMorris, B. J., & Borowsky, I. W. (2010). Adolescent violence perpetration: Associations with multiple types of adverse childhood experiences. *Pediatrics, 125*(4), e778–786.
Farrington, D. (2003). Developmental and life course criminology: Key theoretical and clinical issues. *Criminology, 41,* 201–235.
Farrington, D. P., Gaffney, H., & Ttofi, M. M. (2017). Systematic reviews of explanatory risk factors for violence, offending, and delinquency. *Aggression and Violent Behavior, 33,* 24–36.
Fazel, S., & Danesh, J. (2002). Serious mental disorder in 23,000 prisoners: A systematic review of 62 surveys. *Lancet, 359,* 545–550.
Fazel, S., Hayes, A. J., Bartellas, K., Clerici, M., & Trestman, R. (2016). Mental health of prisoners: Prevalence, adverse outcomes, and interventions. *Lancet Psychiatry, 3*(9), 871–881.
Fazio, R. L., Pietz, C. A., & Denney, R. L. (2012). An estimate of the prevalence of autsm spectrum disorders in an incarcerated population. *Open Access Journal of Forensic Psychology*, 69–80.
Ghirardi, L., Brikell, I., Kuja-Halkola, R., Freitag, C. M., Franke, B., Asherson, P., … Larsson, H. (2018). The familial co-aggregation of ASD and ADHD: A register-based cohort study. *Molecular Psychiatry, 23*(2), 257–262.
Ginsberg, Y., Hirvikoski, T., & Lindefors, N. (2010). Attention Deficit Hyperactivity Disorder (ADHD) among longer-term prison inmates is a prevalent, persistent and disabling disorder. *BMC Psychiatry, 10,* 112.
Hare, D. J., Gould, J., Mills, R., & Wing, L. (1999). *A preliminary study of individuals with autistic spectrum disorders in three special hospitals in England*. National Autistic Society.
Heeramun, R., Magnusson, C., Gumpert, C. H., Granath, S., Lundberg, M., Dalman, C., & Rai, D. (2017). Autism and convictions for violent crimes: Population-based cohort Study in Sweden. *Journal of the American Academy of Child & Adolescent Psychiatry, 56*(6), 491–497, e492.
Helverschou, S. B., Rasmussen, K., Steindal, K., Sondanaa, E., Nilsson, B., & Nottestad, J. A. (2015). Offending profiles of individuals with autism spectrum disorder: A study of all individuals with autism spectrum disorder examined by the forensic psychiatric service in Norway between 2000 and 2010. *Autism, 19*(7), 850–858.
Hippler, K., & Klicpera, C. (2003). A retrospective analysis of the clinical case records of 'autistic psychopaths' diagnosed by Hans Asperger and his team at the University Children's Hospital, Vienna. *Philosophical Transactions of the Royal Society of London, 358,* 291–301.
Hoksbergen, R., ter Laak, J., Rijk, K., van Dijkum, C., & Stoutjesdijk, F. (2005). Post-institutional autistic syndrome in romanian adoptees. *Journal of Autism and Developmental Disorders, 35*(5), 615–623.
Hughes, K., Bellis, M. A., Hardcastle, K. A., Sethi, D., Butchart, A., Mikton, C., … Dunne, M. P. (2017). The effect of multiple adverse childhood experiences on health: A systematic review and meta-analysis. *Lancet Public Health, 2*(8), e356–e366.
Im, D. S. (2016). Trauma as a contributor to violence in autism spectrum disorder. *The Journal of the American Academy of Psychiatry and the Law, 44*(2), 184–192.
Kanner, L. (1943). Autistic disturbances of affective contact. *Nervous Child, 2,* 217–250.
King, C., & Murphy, G. H. (2014). A systematic review of people with autism spectrum disorder and the criminal justice system. *Journal of Autism and Developmental Disorders, 44*(11), 2717–2733.

Kruglanski, A., Gelfand, M., Belanger, J., Sheveland, A., Hetiarachchi, M., & Gunaratna, R. (2014). The psychology of radicalization and deradicalization: How significance quest impacts violent extremism. *Advances in Political Psychology, 35*(Suppl. 1), 69–93.

Loeber, R., & Burke, J. D. (2011). Developmental pathways in juvenile externalizing and internalizing problems. *Journal of Research on Adolescence, 21*(1), 34–46.

Maras, K. L., & Bowler, D. M. (2012). Brief report: Suggestibility, compiance and psychological traits in high-functioning adults with autism spectrum disorder. *Research in Autism Spectrum Disorders, 6*(3), 1168–1175.

Moore, E., Sunjic, S., Kaye, S., Archer, V., & Indig, D. (2016). Adult ADHD among NSW prisoners: Prevalence and psychiatric comorbidity. *Journal of Attention Disorders, 20*(11), 958–967.

Mouridsen, S. E., Rich, B., Isager, T., & Nedergaard, N. J. (2008). Pervasive developmental disorders and criminal behaviour: A case control study. *International Journal of Offender Therapy and Comparative Criminology, 52*(2), 196–205.

Ogilvie, C. A., Newman, E., Todd, L., & Peck, D. (2014). Attachment & violent offending: A meta-analysis. *Aggression and Violent Behavior, 19*(4), 322–339.

Ozonoff, S., Li, D., Deprey, L., Hanzel, E. P., & Iosif, A. M. (2018). Reliability of parent recall of symptom onset and timing in autism spectrum disorder. *Autism, 22*(7), 891–896.

Palermo, M. T. (2013). Developmental disorders and political extremism: A case of Asperger Syndrome and the neo-nazi subculture. *Journal of Forensic Psychology Practice, 13*(4), 341–354.

Post, M., Haymes, L., Storey, K., Loughrey, T., & Campbell, C. (2014). Understanding stalking behaviors by individuals with Autism Spectrum Disorders and recommended prevention strategies for school settings. *Journal of Autism and Developmental Disorders, 44*(11), 2698–2706.

Raine, A. (2002). Annotation: The role of prefrontal deficits, low autonomic arousal, and early health factors in the development of antisocial and aggressive behavior in children. *Journal of Child Psychology and Psychiatry, 43*(4), 417–434.

Richell, R. A., Mitchell, D. G. V., Newman, C., Leonard, A., Baron-Cohen, S., & Blair, R. J. R. (2003). Theory of mind and psychopathy: Can psychopathic individuals read the 'language of the eyes'? *Neuropsychologia, 41,* 523–526.

Robinson, L., Spencer, M. D., Thomson, L. D., Stanfield, A. C., Owens, D. G., Hall, J., & Johnstone, E. C. (2012). Evaluation of a screening instrument for autism spectrum disorders in prisoners. *PLoS One, 7*(5), e36078.

Rogers, J., Viding, E., Blair, R. J., Frith, U., & Happe, F. (2006). Autism spectrum disorder and psychopathy: Shared cognitive underpinnings or double hit? *Psychological Medicine, 36*(12), 1789–1798.

Salekin, R. T. (2017). Research review: What do we know about psychopathic traits in children? *Journal of Child Psychology and Psychiatry, 58*(11), 1180–1200.

Scragg, P., & Shah, A. (1994). Prevalence of Asperger's syndrome in a secure hospital. *British Journal of Psychiatry, 165*(5), 679–682.

Siponmaa, L., Kristiansson, M., Jonson, C., Nyden, A., & Gillberg, C. (2001). Juvenile and young adult mentally disordered offenders: The role of child neuropsychiatric disorders. *Journal of the American Academy of Psychiatry and the Law, 29*(4), 420–426.

Soderstrom, H., Sjodin, A.-K., Carlstedt, A., & Forsman, A. (2004). Adult psychopathic personality with childhood onset hyperactivity and conduct disorder: A central problem constellation in forensic psychiatry. *Psychiatry Research, 121,* 271–280.

Sroufe, L. A., Carlson, E. A., Levy, A. K., & Egeland, B. (1999). Implications of attachment theory for developmental psychopathology. *Development and Psychopathology, 11*(1), 1–13.

Stokes, M., & Newton, N. (2004). Autism spectrum disorders and stalking. *Autism, 8*(3), 337–339.

Stokes, M., Newton, N., & Kaur, A. (2007). Stalking, and social and romantic functioning among adolescents and adults with autism spectrum disorder. *Journal of Autism and Developmental Disorders, 37*(10), 1969–1986.

Underwood, L., McCarthy, J., Chaplin, E., Forrester, E., Mills, R., & Murphy, D. (2016). Autism spectrum disorder traits among prisoners. *Advances in Autism, 2*(3), 106–117.

Van Naarden Braun, K., Christensen, D., Doernberg, N., Schieve, L., Rice, C., Wiggins, L., ... Yeargin-Allsopp, M. (2015). Trends in the prevalence of autism spectrum disorder, cerebral palsy, hearing loss, intellectual disability, and vision impairment, metropolitan atlanta, 1991–2010. *PLoS One, 10*(4), e0124120.

Wing, L. (1981). Asperger's syndrome: A clinical account. *Psychological Medicine, 11*(1), 115–129.

Wolff, S. (1991). 'Schizoid' personality in childhood and adult life. I: The vagaries of diagnostic labelling. *The British Journal of Psychiatry, 159,* 615–620, 634–615.

Wolff, S., Townshend, R., McGuire, R. J., & Weeks, D. J. (1991). 'Schizoid' personality in childhood and adult life. II: Adult adjustment and the continuity with schizotypal personality disorder. *British Journal of Psychiatry, 159,* 620–629.

Woodbury-Smith, M., Clare, I. C. H., Holland, A. J., Kearns, A., Staufenberg, E., & Watson, P. (2005). A case-control study of offenders with high functioning autistic spectrum disorders. *The Journal of Forensic Psychiatry & Psychology, 16*(4), 747–763.

Woodbury-Smith, M., Clare, I. C., Holland, A., Kearns, A., Staufenberg, E., & Watson, P. (2010). Circumscribed interests among offenders with autistic spectrum disorders: A case-control study. *Journal of Forensic Psychiatry and Psychology, 21*(3), 366–377.

Woodbury-Smith, M., & Dein, K. (2014). Autism spectrum disorder (ASD) and unlawful behaviour: Where do we go from here? *Journal of Autism and Developmental Disorders, 44*(11), 2734–2741.

Marc Woodbury-Smith is a Clinical Senior Lecturer in the Biosciences Institute at Newcastle University, UK and an Honorary Consultant Psychiatrist. He is also an Associate Investigator at the Centre for Applied Genomics at the Hospital for Sick Children in Toronto, Canada. He trained in psychiatry in Cambridge, UK and at the Yale Child Study Center, USA. As a psychiatrist specializing in developmental disabilities, he has worked clinically with children and adults with autism spectrum disorder (ASD) for more than 20 years, and has published widely on both basic sciences (genetics) and legal aspects of ASD. He is currently an Associate Editor of the Journal of Autism and Developmental Disorders.

Chapter 9
Bullying & Autism and Related Disorders

Fred R. Volkmar and Brian Pete

The term bullying has its origins in the mid-sixteenth century from the Dutch word 'buele,' which was a term of endearment in a relationship but, over time, the meaning evolved to involve aspects of aggression and protection. By the seventeenth century the word, in English, become similar to how we know it today (Rivara & Le Menestrel, 2016).

In this chapter, we review some aspects of bullying in general (how it is defined, characteristics of the bully and bullied, consequence of bullying, and epidemiology) before turning to the smaller literature on autism per se. The latter discussion is divided by age into bullying in children of elementary school to high school age and then bullying in adults (notably, workplace bullying). We have a somewhat separate discussion of cyberbullying for two reasons: (1) this is a rather different kind of bullying and (2) it is a special problem for individuals on the autism spectrum. We review some of the laws on bullying (this varies considerably from state to state) and discuss bullying in the workplace before closing with a brief summary on intervention programs. As noted, while bullying laws exist in all 50 states these laws, rules, and regulations are notably varied. And while we discuss some legal aspects of bullying, it is also important to note that, effectively, nondisclosure agreements mean that we know very little of how bullying cases are decided in the courts—with a few notable exceptions.

F. R. Volkmar (✉)
Yale Child Study Center and Autism Center of Excellence, Yale University and Southern Conn. State University, New Haven, USA
e-mail: fred.volkmar@yale.edu

B. Pete
Lewis Brisbois Bisgaard & Smith LLP, New York, NY, USA
e-mail: Brian.Pete@lewisbrisbois.com

F. R. Volkmar et al. (eds.), *Handbook of Autism Spectrum Disorder and the Law*,
https://doi.org/10.1007/978-3-030-70913-6_9

Definitions

There is not a simple definition of bullying, but it is generally agreed to refer to a person (or group of persons) who use power, strength, or some kind of dominant position to intimidate a person or persons who are perceived (often correctly) as being more vulnerable and weaker (Juvonen & Graham, 2014). It is this inequality that differentiates bullying from other conflicts where the 'standing' is more equal. Bullying can include a range of behaviors and various types of bullying have been proposed. Bullying might be verbal (threat, ridicule, harassment), physical (aggression or physical coercion), emotional (abusive and belittling language), or computer/online related (cyberbullying). The latter (cyberbullying) has some important differences from other forms of bullying and we discuss this separately in this chapter (see Rivara & Le Menestrel, 2016, for a helpful overview of bullying in general). Text Box 1 summarizes the usual distinctions made in types of bullying. Note that many forms of aggressive behavior fall outside the usual definitions of bullying, e.g., fighting between peers, child abuse, workplace violence. Direct bullying consists of physical and verbal aggression, whereas indirect bullying involves relational aggression. Cyberbullying is an emerging problem that may be more difficult to identify and intervene with than traditional bullying.

Text Box 1
Types of Bullying

- **Physical**—hitting, tripping, shoving, etc.
  - Sometimes this entails theft or damage to property of the bullied
- **Verbal**—oral or written taunting, name calling, etc.
- **Emotional/Social**—taunting, rumor spreading, or other behaviors designed to ostracize or isolate the individual being bullied
- **Cyberbullying**—use of internet, social media, doctored pictures, etc.

The Center for Disease Control has its own definition of bullying:

> *Bullying is a form of youth violence. CDC defines bullying as any unwanted aggressive behavior(s) by another youth or group of youths, who are not siblings or current dating partners that involves an observed or perceived power imbalance and is repeated multiple times or is highly likely to be repeated. Bullying may inflict harm or distress on the targeted youth including physical, psychological, social, or educational harm.*
>
> *Bullying can include aggression that is physical (hitting, tripping), verbal (name calling, teasing), or relational/social (spreading rumors, leaving out of group). Bullying can also occur through technology and is called electronic bullying or cyberbullying. A young person can be a perpetrator, a victim, or both (also known as "bully/victim").* (Gladden et al., 2014)

This definition has limitations, however. It specifically excludes siblings from being bullies even though this is observed, including in siblings of individuals with autism (Toseeb et al., 2018). The CDC's definition also is not so clearly applicable to cyberbullying (Tokunaga, 2010). The issues of repetitive bullying for the individual person are complex (DeNigris et al., 2018; Lund & Ross, 2017). Bullying can be part of a much broader general culture (e.g., as in the behavior of Nazis in Germany) or it can be part of highly specific situations, e.g., hazing in sports or fraternities, and remains common in college—even in college classrooms (DeNigris et al., 2018; Heil, 2016; Lund & Ross, 2017).

Text Box 2
A college student with Asperger's who was very interested in physics reported to his therapist that the students and professor in his classroom were making fun of him in the class. With the permission of the stsudent and professor the therapist sat in on the class and verified that this was true. The student always had his hand up to ask questions or comment and other students and professor made jokes about him openly in the classroom with the professor making derogatory comments or sarcastic asides like "why don't you teach the class." After the class was over the therapist spoke with the professor and pointed out that his behavior was inappropriate and verged on bullying, particularly for a student who did not always understand and whose enthusiasm for the materials ought to be channeled rather than made fun of. With the agreement of the student and professor the student was able to ask exactly two questions during the class but then had 5 minutes with the professor after class. This was a mutually satisfactory solution on all sides. The professor had not been aware of the student's social disability (even though it had been disclosed to the learning supports office).

With all these caveats it is clear that bullying can occur in dyadic contests (i.e., the bully and his or her victim) or it can be carried out by a group of individuals against a victim. Unfortunately, it is often under recognized. Bullying can start as early as pre-school, and seems to peak in middle childhood and early adolescence (Rivara & Le Menestrel, 2016), but can persist into adulthood and the workplace (Bartlett & Bartlett, 2011). This may not be true, however, for cyberbullying, reflecting a host of factors including the increasingly sophisticated technology, the phenomenon of more or less constant online access, the rise of various social media format, etc. Cyberbullying is, probably predictably, more likely done outside school (Rivara & Le Menestrel, 2016). Boys are more likely to engage in direct aggressive bullying whereas for girls' indirect methods (gossip, social media) are more likely. Bullying can sometimes be subtle and at other times rather overt. Bullying can be an isolated incident or a recurrent pattern of behavior both for the bully and the target (Rivara & Le Menestrel, 2016).

Bullying among children is a significant public health problem world wide. In the U.S., studies suggest that about 20% of children are involved in bullying. Bullies, victims, and bully victims are at risk for negative short-and long-term consequences such as depression, anxiety, low self-esteem, and delinquency. Various individual, parental, and peer factors increase the risk for involvement in bullying. Anti-bullying interventions are predominantly school-based and demonstrate variable results. Healthcare providers can intervene in bullying by identifying potential bullies or victims, screening them for comorbidities, providing counseling and resources, and advocating for bullying prevention (Shetgiri, 2013).

Risk Factors: Characteristics of Victims and Perpetrators

A host of factors have been identified in bullying, e.g., based on race, ethnicity, social class, gender and gender identification, learning differences, and disability, physical disabilities and physical size, and so forth (see Berger & Rodkin, 2009; Fisher, 2013; Rivara & Le Menestrel, 2016; Vitoroulis & Vaillancourt, 2015). Individuals with Autism/Asperger's are at special risk (Zablotsky et al., 2014). Sexual minorities and LGBTQ youth are also at special risk. Children who have been maltreated within their families may also be significantly more likely to be bullied (Shields & Cicchetti, 2001); it presents various challenges in providing care for the bullied child (Abreu et al., 2016).

Type of bullying can vary with age and development. In one study of those who bully (Shetgiri, 2013), a large sample was obtained from the National Survey of Children's Health. In this study, the parent-reported bullying measure found that parent-reported anger, maternal mental health problems, and a range of emotional/developmental/behavioral problems were associated with greater risk for bullying. Parents more involved in the child's life (e.g., knowing the child's friends) were less likely to report bullying in the child.

Several meta-analytic studies (studies that synthesize the results of multiple studies) have examined predictors of bullying behavior as well as the risk for being bullied (and sometimes both). Cook and colleagues (Cook et al., 2010) analyzed data from a large group of studies and found that the most powerful predictors of bullying were externalizing problems (e.g., problems in conduct, aggression) and cognitive problems, while social status, peer friendships, and social competence were the strongest predictors of being bullied. Bully-victims (i.e., children who were in both groups) had lower social competence, low to poor academic and social competence skills, and low self-esteem. A study of adolescents (Kljakovic & Hunt, 2016) analyzed papers from 1985 until July 2014 related to adolescent bullying. Predictors of bullying were found (across studies) to include four major factors: prior victimization, conduct issues and problems, social difficulties, and "internalizing" problems (the latter referent to another range of difficulties like anxiety and depression). The authors emphasized the need for more and better research, but did emphasize that social difficulties and conduct problems seemed the most robust predictors of bullying behavior and, thus, the potential focus for future interventions.

Bullying can have some superficially adaptive function for the child, e.g., increasing social status (van Dijk et al., 2017) both inside and outside the classroom setting. In contrast those bullied are less likely to have friends and may be less actively involved with peers in the classroom setting. Bullying can occur within the classroom but is clearly most frequent in less supervised school settings—gym, recess, bus, and cafeteria.

The child who is both a bully and is (or has been) bullied presents some complex issues (Camodeca, 2003; Gasser & Keller, 2009). In this group, associated mental health problems (both concurrent and future) are more common. These can include a range of difficulties that persists past childhood. The onset and course of bullying perpetration are influenced by individual as well as systemic factors.

Consequences of Bullying

The immediate consequences of bullying on the victim can be both more and less oblivious, e.g., unexplained physical injuries of bruises, missing money or electronics, school avoidance or refusal, and so forth. Sometimes witnesses will have reported bullying. Less obvious signs can be increased anxiety or depression, and even suicidal ideation, or a range of physical symptoms or school avoidance. At other times effects can be less obvious. For example, Sansone and Sansone (2008) reported that less obvious signs can include social difficulties, increased anxiety or depression, even suicidal ideation or a range of physical symptoms or school avoidance (Ttofi et al., 2011). There can be a host of negative longer term effects of bullying relating to both physical and mental health issues, longer term interpersonal relations, and employment (Pozzoli & Gini, 2013; Saintil, 2018; Wolke et al., 2013). For bullying that is continuous over a period of time, the effects of stress may cause endocrine changes and the possibility of brain changes has also been suggested. Mental health issues can include both more internalizing problems (anxiety, depression, etc.) as well as externalizing problems (aggression, conduct issues). Risk for substance abuse later in development may also be increased (Sanchez et al., 2017).

Adverse effects can also be seen in those who engage in bullying (Cowie & Colliety, 2018). Children who engage in bullying do so for many reasons—some already have emotional difficulties, others seek higher social status (Vaillancourt et al., 2003). This difference complicates interpretation of studies conducted on the consequence of bullying but, those who bully are at risk for various psychiatric problems including psychosomatic problems (Gini & Pozzoli, 2009) and for later onset psychotic disorders (Wolke & Lereya, 2014). Occasionally, of course, the bullying backfires and the negative reaction understandably leads to public shaming and social ostracism.

Cyberbullying

This form of bullying differs in important ways from others and poses special risk for children, youth, and adults with ASD given their often strong interest and involvement in the internet. In this form of bullying an individual (or group of individuals) harass others over the internet, often using social media. This form of bullying, particularly frequent among teenagers, can involve posting negative or derogatory comments, rumors, threats, sexual remarks, or even invasion of the individual's personal information that, in turn, can be used to further engage in harassment. Risk is increased given the frequent involvement of individuals with ASD in online gaming and the internet in general making them ready targets for cyberbullying

In one review and meta-analysis, Gardella et al. (2017) note that in adolescence the ready availability and lack of supervision make the internet a particularly fertile environment for bullying and victimization and their associations with school attendance and other problems. For individuals with ASD, technology, in general, and the internet, in particular, provide a life line with information that can be readily obtained, is typically free of much adult supervision, and plays to many of the strengths of individuals with ASD while minimizing the direct social interaction that can be such a major source of difficulty. Cyberbullying can lead to further social isolation of the individual with autism and further decrease self-esteem in a population already at risk for anxiety and depression (Wright, 2018). Cyberbullying is associated with increased rates of suicidality (Gini & Espelage, 2014; Saleh et al., 2014). Youth who are LGBTQ are at increased risk and also have higher rates of suicidality; given the sometimes fluid gender identity of those with autism this would presumably further increase the risk for those in the LGBTQ community with ASD (Potts, 2018; van Schalkwyk et al., 2015). Please see Chap. 10 for more information about cybercrimes.

Bullying in the Workplace

Bullying in the workplace can take many forms, e.g., physical abuse, psychological intimidation, social isolation, and so forth. It can also be either verbal or nonverbal or can even take the form of cyberbullying. The phenomenon first came to general attention in 1992 (Adams, 1992). It is now well recognized in the workplace.

This type of bullying differs in many ways from that which occurs in schools, notably because it occurs within the context of a unique workplace with its own culture, history, and structure. While bullying by superiors is probably the most common form, but bullying can also happen between employees who are essentially peers or even by subordinates (Rayner & Cooper, 2006).

In their review of the topic, Bartlett and Bartlett (2011) noted several important obstacles to document and understanding workplace bullying including the lack of overarching federal legislation and the wide range of forms of bullying, with potentially serious problems for the individuals involved as well as the workplace as a whole. For the organization, the negative impact could be seen in cost, productivity, and reputation as well, of course, in the costs of litigation.

Unfortunately, there is still not a generally accepted definition of bullying in the workplace, but laws like the American with Disabilities Act (ADA, 1990) may cover acts that target people with disabilities. The impact of bullying in the workplace can, of course, be more widespread than on only the individual per se. The bullying can be quite obvious and overt (aggressive acts) or subtle and covert (spreading rumors, social isolation). As with a school setting, bullying can be a more isolated or more systemic phenomenon. In the workplace, some additional aspects of bullying can arise, e.g., through blocked progress for promotions, incessant criticism, persistent derogatory comments, and so forth.

Information on workplace bullying is available if somewhat inconsistent in coverage. The experience of being bullied in the workplace is fairly common; in one national survey of the U.S. (NHIS-OHS, 2015), the rate was nearly 10%. One recent meta-analysis (McCord et al., 2018) of workplace mistreatment found that women were more likely to perceive more sex-based mistreatment, although other forms of mistreatment did not have strong gender differences. Similarly, members of racial minority groups were more likely to perceive race-based mistreatment in the workplace but strong effects from other forms of mistreatment based on race were not striking. A study from Sweden of employed persons (Persson et al., 2009) specifically examined issues of personality and emotional stability of those who are bullied at work and found that those bullied were more likely to have higher levels of irritability and personality traits related to the three major dimensions of neuroticism, extraversion, and aggressiveness. Bullied persons had higher scores on all six scales within the neuroticism dimension as well as higher irritability and mistrust.

Workers with disabilities are at increased risk for losing their jobs even before the impact of bullying is considered. Van Wieren and colleagues (2008) found that persons with autism were found to be more likely to make charges of discrimination against retail industry employers. Claims were more frequently made by younger individuals and a claim was more likely to success in larger volume employees and in-service industries.

Epidemiology and International Perspectives

Some countries, e.g., Canada and Norway, have had a strong interest in bullying prevention and consequently have some of the lowest rates in the world. There is a large body of international on the topic with some excellent treatment programs as well as on correlates of bullying/victimization and longer term outcome (Farrington et al., 2017). The U.S. ranks in the middle of the world with reported bullying rates of about 18%, while other countries have much higher rates—around 30%.

Within the U.S., several studies have attempted to examine rates of bullying in nationally representative samples (see NRC report for a summary and discussion of study limitations; Rivara & Le Menestrel, 2016). Rates can vary dramatically depending on definitions used, methods of survey and assessments (Rivara & Le Menestrel, 2016). But essentially, survey data from the CDC has shown that about 19% of children between 14 and 18 years of age report being bullied and nearly 15% report being cyberbullied (Gladden et al., 2014). It should be noted that this data reveals considerable state to state variation. The Health Behavior Survey study noted that within the sample of U.S. children (10–16 years of age) about 30% of children reported being bullied at school and nearly 15% reported some form of cyberbullying experience. This study also had data on reported rates of bullying and noted that about 32% of children reported being bullied during the prior month and 14% reported cyberbullying other children (Iannotti, 2012, 2013; Perlus et al., 2014). The issue of whether rates of bullying are changing over time is controversial, although cyberbullying does appear to be increasing in frequency (Rivara & Le Menestrel, 2016) and presents special problems for detection and intervention.

ASD and Bullying

The child/individual with ASD, both lower and higher cognitively functioning, is a particular target. Variable factors all contribute to this risk (Sreckovic et al., 2014). For example, individuals with autism are less socially able and as a result are frequently more isolated and at the periphery. They are less socially attuned, may dress in unusual ways, and are rigid about change and this can contribute to their 'standing out' as targets. Similarly, unusual and idiosyncratic interests not typical of age mates can lead to bullying (Sreckovic et al., 2014; Zablotsky et al., 2014). Many children with autism don't immediately appear disabled so their difficulties with social interaction can be readily misinterpreted. Similarly, in Autism and related conditions difficulties with social nuance and aspects of communication like figurative language, sarcasm, or irony make it frequent they case they are laughed at (without appreciating they've made a joke) or are so literal they don't understand when something else is meant. Even when they attempt to make social contact/friendships with peers, their unusual social style may be further isolating. See Text Box 3 for a summary.

Text Box 3

Factors increasing risk for bullying in autism:

- Don't appreciate subtle interaction or nuance
- Generally, less socially capable
- May appear, dress, or otherwise appear differently
- Don't fit in with usual interests (may have odd interest)
- Lack of social network/status in social hierarchy

It is important to understand how frequent bullying is for children with autism. In the U.S. among children and adolescents with ASD, rates range from 30 to 75% (van Roekel et al., 2010), i.e., double or triple the rate for the population at large. It does appear that the presence of additional problems in addition to autism, e.g., anxiety, further increases the risk (Essique, 2018).

Contextual and individual factors in ASD also contribute to increased risk. In one review of 21 studies, Sreckovic et al. (2014) observed both that features of autism increased risk (e.g., social isolation, vulnerability, behavioral problems) as did context (school setting, bus, family problems, social supports). Sadly, within the family, children with ASD are more likely to be abused by their siblings than typically developing children (as noted previously some definitions of bullying do NOT encompass sibling bullying) (Menesini et al., 2010; Toseeb et al., 2018). Furthermore, the experience of being bullied further increases the risk for the student with ASD to develop other problems (Toseeb et al., 2019).

Within the classroom there may be complex interactions of the features of ASD with behavior and bullying risk, e.g., the child with ASD may need to be placed closer to the teacher, away from distractions, and so forth. Efforts must be made to help the child with ASD focus and learn most effectively. But these futher make the child stand out. Unusual behaviors and interests can, of course, also lead to the 'targeting' of the child with ASD. As noted previously, the less 'structured' settings in school are often the places where bullying is more frequent, e.g., recess, cafeteria, and gym. Problems with social interaction and motor skills often impact the student in organized sports activities leading to further social isolation and risk for negative comments and bullying. And bullying can, of course, be increased in sport activities in general (Heil, 2016). Ashburner et al. (2018) observed that students who also had anxiety were at increased risk for face-to-face victimization, and those with depression were more likely to report cyberbullying. Parents understandably are frequently concerned about school safety, attendance, self-esteem, mental health, social participation, academic performance, and behavior.

For students with ASD, the experience of being bullied remains common in high school and continues into college (McLeod et al., 2019). Self-reporting of adolescents with autism who have been bullied suggests that both verbal bullying and, to a lesser extent, cyberbullying are more common (Leaf, 2017) and can have a major negative impact on inhibiting social interaction and inclusion.

Intervention Programs

With the growing awareness of bullying as a problem, a number of interventions have been developed (although it is important to note that often well-controlled evaluations are lacking). In addition, all 50 states now require some form of teacher training (Hatzenbuehler et al., 2015; Stuart-Cassel et al., 2011). As noted by Rivara and colleagues, there are essentially three groups of intervention programs: universal (school/community wide), more selective preventive interventions (targeting individuals at risk), and therapeutic interventions.

Universal programs aim to expose the entire population to information on bullying and to reduce the risk for bullying by increasing awareness and providing strategies for students (and staff) in preventing and dealing with bullying. These can include specific lessons/curricula within the classroom with explicit teaching of strategies for responding to or reporting of bullying. Several such programs have not been evaluated in rigorous research (e.g. Ttofi & Farrington, 2011; Jimenez-Barbero et al., 2016). These programs have been noted to have important benefits for students and teachers alike (Domitrovich et al., 2016).

In contrast selective preventive interventions specifically target youth at risk (for bullying or being bullied). These can include more specific training in issues of anger management, coping, effective de-escalation procedures, and so forth. These programs can meet the need of youth who have not responded to the more universal approaches noted above. Obviously, they do not impact the school or community as a whole. Preventive interventions can have an impact for individuals with positive risk factors (Espelage & Horne, 2008). This form of intervention may involve more individuals in schools and the community as supporters and teachers. Compared to the universally focused programs, these selective intervention prevention programs have been much less extensively researched in terms of their efficacy (Swearer et al., 2008). There are a few important exceptions, e.g., the effectiveness of gay-straight alliance programs in school has been noted to be effective in one large meta-analysis (Marx & Kettrey, 2016). Often some aspects of these three approaches must be integrated, i.e., the school should have a general prevention policy, but also be able to address students at risk or already involved in bullying activities.

In their rigorous and comprehensive review of all the available data on effective prevention practice around the world, Ttofi and Farrington (2011) observed an overall significant reduction in bullying and in being bullied occurred (around 20% for both). It remains unclear which aspects of comprehensive programs are most critical and Tofti and Farring also emphasized the importance of a broader context, i.e., of good playground supervision, parental involvement, information dissemination along with good classroom management and disciplinary practices. The 'whole school' approach (i.e., rather than teacher training only) seems to be more effective (Vreeman & Carroll, 2007). It should be noted, however, that the available data also suggests that such programs are somewhat more effective outside the U.S., perhaps because of greater cultural homogeneity, less time devoted to standardized testing, and greater commitment on the part of school staff (Evans et al., 2014).

There is, of course, some overlap of these programs with other programs intending to decrease school violence and encourage more effective anger management and coping. Several good resources for parents and students are available, e.g. (Dubin, 2007; Heinrichs, 2003; Hinduja & Patchin, 2015; Lonie, 2015). For children with autism, all of these approaches may be useful, but more specific intervention strategies are also clearly needed. Various steps can be helpful in preventing bullying. These include more general approaches, e.g., in developing effective peer support networks (Sreckovic et al., 2017) and effective social skills teaching; Laugeson, 2017). Other interventions have been directed specifically for the ASD population (Berreman, 2018).

For students with sexual identity issues (including many individuals with ASD (Hissle-Groman et al., 2019), gay-straight alliances (GSAs) organizations may be helpful. Other programs have focused on including persons who are LGBTQ (and see also Fisher & Komosa-Hawkins, 2013).

Legal Aspects of Bullying

All 50 U.S. States now have anti-bullying laws—these vary in terms of coverage, focus, etc. There are no specific federal laws on bullying although, as we note below, some court decisions and aspects of federal law can apply in either school (children and adolescents) or work (adult) settings. Laws and regulations focused on discrimination may apply, e.g., when bullying is based on protected classes under the discrimination laws such as race, gender, sexual orientation, and gender identity (depending on the state), disability, and so forth. If such behavior is not addressed, or is tolerated or encouraged, schools or employers can be found liable, i.e., both schools and workplaces should maintain environments that prevent and discourage harassment and bullying. Federal recommendations for state and local laws and regulations typically play an important role in the development of state statutes (Rivara & Le Menestrel, 2016). However, it must be noted that state and local laws have now drastically expanded the scope of protections under federal law especially where sexual orientation and gender identity are concerned.

In the vast majority of instances cyberbullying will fall under the ambit of federal and state laws on bullying. Often, local school districts are allowed some flexibility in the development and implementation of policies related to bullying (Rivara & Le Menestrel, 2016).

The U.S. Department of Education (2010a, 2010b) noted a series of important issues to be considered in state and federal law and regulations relative to bullying. These included the following: purpose of the law/regulation, scope, nature of prohibited conduct, identification of those groups at risk, implementation of local education authority procedures/policies, provision for review of school programs and policies as well as their content, procedures for communication of policies to students parents, teacher/school staff, training, monitoring and the explicit statement that individuals continue do have rights to redress (US Dept. of Ed, 2016). Despite this attempt to introduce uniformity, such uniformity does not, in fact, exist. States vary significantly in their laws and policies related to bullying. For example in some states, a single incident may suffice whereas in others there must be an ongoing pattern of bullying (Rivara & Le Menestrel, 2016). It is also important to note that definitions used often do not correspond to those used in research or in the development of anti-bullying programs, further complicating the task for researchers. Similar issues arise relative to cyberbullying, e.g., some states specifically refer to 'cyberbullying,' while others refer to 'electronic communication' more generally. Awareness of cyberbullying has increased in the U.S. over the last decade and a few states have now passed laws in an attempt to criminalize this behavior. At the Federal level, 18 U.S.C. § 875(c) has criminalized threats made over the internet.

The definition of bullying adopted by Massachusetts is one of the more comprehensive and especially addresses issues of perceived identities as a potential aspect of the cyberbullying. Other differences between state laws relate to the ways in which specific groups (i.e., those at risk) are or are not enumerated as well as in terms of specific locations where the bullying activity takes place (e.g., on or off school grounds). States also differ in the degree to which they manage school personnel training and in procedures for reporting bullying or safeguarding students. Unfortunately, mandates for school training and prevention may not always be funded.

The study of litigations relative to bullying, in theory, provides some way to shed light on bullying in a range of contexts and to highlight factors and circumstances associated with outcomes. Unfortunately, research on this topic is fairly limited. In one review, Holben and Zirkel (2016) noted that litigation had increased over time particularly when schools were unresponsive to complaints. Their study quantified frequency and outcomes for bullying cases in over 200 court decisions over a period of two decades.

In this review the student characteristics associated with increased frequency of claims for judicial redress included middle school students, those with claims related to gender-based claims, and bullying that was physical or verbal in nature. The authors emphasized the importance of prevention in schools in preventing claims. If schools do not create policies and procedures regarding bullying they will have difficulty in proving that students failed to adhere to certain standards of conduct.

Claims by plaintiffs are often made based on the Title IX Civil Rights act of 1964, as well as on the 14th amendment's due process and equal protection provisions. Often federal, rather than state law, is used perhaps reflecting attempts to avoid immunities in certain state laws, e.g., the barring of claims against state municipalities in state courts. Private employers on the other hand will be subject to suit in federal court as well as state court under both federal and local laws. Other reasons may reflect the lack of provisions in state bullying laws for redress relative to sovereign immunity preventing suit. Finally, decisions of state administrative bodies such as state departments of educations are more difficult to find than state and federal court cases. Variations in state definitions of bullying are placating complicating factors as well (Russell, 2017).

As noted previously, individuals with autism are at increased risk for bullying—this is true both for the more and less verbal and cognitively able. For the more able individuals, after effects can be pronounced and are often readily identified and related to bullying, e.g., ongoing school refusal, anxiety, specific fears, depression, and PTSD A small literature exists on the latter topic (Capaccioli, 2010; DaSilva & Keeler, 2017; de Albuquerque & de Albuquerque Williams, 2015). Given unusual communication patterns or sometimes limited verbal abilities, an experienced clinician is often needed in the assessment of less verbal or nonverbal individuals. It is important to note, and under score, even very low cognitively functioning individuals may be damaged by bullying—particularly if this is prolonged and crosses the line from bullying to outright abuse. The latter, of course, should be reported to state authorities, when it occurs. In the experience of the first author, chronic abuse can lead to marked difficulties in less cognitively able individuals. The occasional assumption on the parts of defending attorneys that the individual is 'too low functioning' to be damaged is not at all true. However, this argument will remain commonplace because it can impact monetary damages awarded by a court or jury.

Bullying in the workplace raises somewhat different issues than bullying in schools. Most anti-bullying laws do not apply in the workplace and bullying is not as generally accepted as a problem in the adult workplace. However, actions that amount to bullying—teasing, physical conduct, etc.,—can constitute hostile work environments under federal and state anti-discrimination laws if based on a protected activity. For example, an employee with Tourette Syndrome may experience random verbal and motor tics that are not really under the individual's control. This can lead to mocking and teasing by coworkers—this is especially likely in workplaces that employ teens and young adults such as retail stores. This conduct can potentially constitute a hostile work environment for which employers are liable.

In their review of litigated cases, Martin and LaVan (2010) examined a random sample of nearly 50 cases within the U.S. Most of these had been adjudicated in district courts. About 20% involved physical violence and in most cases the supervisor was the alleged perpetrator. In only one-third of these cases was a workplace policy specifically addressing bullying in place. This is unfortunate given how common the problem is (Marx & Kettrey, 2016) and given that specific intervention programs have been developed (Rikleen, 2019). Employers typically only enact policies they are legally required to or that are recommended by legal counsel. Anti-bullying policies in the workplace have only recently become something that employers are adopting.

Summary

Bullying is a frequent experience for children, youth, and adults with ASD (Zeedyk et al., 2014). Individuals with ASD are clearly at increased risk for many reasons—social isolation, differences in dress, speech, interests. They are 'easy targets' for both individual and group bullying. For children, bullying is likelier to occur in less supervised parts of the school day. Bullying can have a host of adverse effects. It can also occur in adulthood in college or work environments and have serious adverse consequences for the individual as well as the organization or company in which it occurs.

This risk for bullying in this population is clearly increased and bullying can have lasting negative impacts both on those bullied as well as those bullying. The available data suggests that prevention is a key factor in reducing rates of bullying—i.e., in terms of developing a climate in the school or workplace where bullying is not tolerated.

All 50 U.S. States now have anti-bullying laws—these vary in terms of coverage, focus, etc. Laws and regulations focused on discrimination may apply, e.g., when bullying is based on discrimination, race, gender, and so forth. The various states vary significantly in their laws and policies related to bullying. For example, in some states a single incident may suffice whereas in others there must be an ongoing pattern of bullying (Rivara & Le Menestrel, 2016). It is also important to note that definitions used in the legal system often do not correspond to those used in research or in the development of anti-bullying programs, further complicating the task for researchers. Similar issues arise relative to cyberbullying, e.g., some states specifically refer to 'cyberbullying' while others refer to 'electronic communication' more generally. The definition adopted by Massachusetts is one of the more comprehensive and especially addresses issues of assuming false identities as a potential aspect of cyberbullying. Others state differences relate to the ways in which specific groups (i.e., those at risk) are or are not enumerated, as well as in terms of specific locations where the activity takes place (e.g., on or off school grounds). States also differ in the degree to which they manage school personnel training and in procedures for reporting bullying or safeguarding students. Unfortunately mandates for school training and prevention may not always be funded ones.

It is important to note, and under score, even very low cognitively functioning individuals may be damaged by bullying. The occasional assumption on the parts of defending attorneys that the individual is 'too low functioning' to be damaged is not at all true. Attorneys asked to consult on cases will, of course, need to be aware of their own state laws and regulations as well as federal laws that may apply, e.g., the Americans with Disabilities Act and U.S. Department of Education, and the specific circumstances unique to each case.

References

Abreu, R. L., Black, W. W., Mosley, D. V., & Fedewa, A. L. (2016). LGBTQ youth bullying experiences in schools: The role of school counselors within a system of oppression. *Journal of Creativity in Mental Health, 11*(3–4), 325–342.

Adams, A. (1992). *Bullying at work: How to confront and overcome it.* Viarago/Little Brown.

Ashburner, J., Saggers, B., Campbell, M. A., Dillon-Wallace, J. A., Hwang, Y.-S., Carrington, S., & Bobir, N. (2018). How are students on the autism spectrum affected by bullying? Perspectives of students and parents. *Journal of Research in Special Educational Needs*, No Pagination Specified. http://dx.doi.org/10.1111/1471-3802.12421.

Bartlett, J. E., II, & Bartlett, M. E. (2011). Workplace bullying: An integrative literature review. *Advances in Developing Human Resources, 13*(1), 69–84.

Berger, C., & Rodkin, P. C. (2009). Male and female victims of male bullies: Social status differences by gender and informant source. *Sex Roles: A Journal of Research, 61*(1–2), 72–84. https://doi.org/10.1007/s11199-009-9605-9.

Berreman, L. (2018). A bullying prevention and treatment program for children with autism spectrum disorder in mainstream schools. *Dissertation Abstracts International: Section B: The Sciences and Engineering, 79*(8-B(E)), No Pagination Specified.

Camodeca, M. (2003). Bullying and victimization at school (Amsterdam, PI Research/Free University).

Capaccioli, K. (2010). An examination of the relationship between sibling and peer victimization and subsequent prediction of PTSD symptomology. *Dissertation Abstracts International: Section B: The Sciences and Engineering, 70*(9-B), 5810.

Cook, C. R., Williams, K. R., Guerra, N. G., Kim, T. E., & Sadek, S. (2010). Predictors of bullying and victimization in childhood and adolescence: A meta-analytic investigation. *School Psychology Quarterly, 25*(2), 65–83.

Cowie, H., & Colliety, P. (2018). Addressing the mental health and emotional needs of children who bully. In *School bullying and mental health: Risks, intervention and prevention* (pp. 90–100). Routledge/Taylor & Francis Group.
DaSilva, S. M., & Keeler, C. (2017). Adolescent peer victimization and PTSD risk. *Adolescent Psychiatry, 7*(1), 25–43. https://doi.org/10.2174/2210676606666161121103635.
de Albuquerque, P. P., & de Albuquerque Williams, L. C. (2015). Predictor variables of PTSD symptoms in school victimization: A retrospective study with college students. *Journal of Aggression, Maltreatment & Trauma, 24*(10), 1067–1085. https://doi.org/10.1080/10926771.2015.1079281.
DeNigris, D., Brooks, P. J., Obeid, R., Alarcon, M., Shane-Simpson, C., & Gillespie-Lynch, K. (2018). Bullying and identity development: Insights from autistic and non-autistic college students. *Journal of Autism and Developmental Disorders, 48*(3), 666–678. https://doi.org/10.1007/s10803-017-3383-y.
Domitrovich, C. E., Bradshaw, C. P., Berg, J. K., Pas, E. T., Becker, K. D., Musci, R., Embry, D. D., & Ialongo, N. (2016). How do school-based prevention programs impact teachers? Findings from a randomized trial of an integrated classroom management and social-emotional program. *Prevention Science, 17*(3), 325–337. https://doi.org/10.1007/s11121-015-0618-z.
Dubin, N. (2007). *Asperger syndrome and bullying: Strategies and solutions.* Jessica Kingsley Publishers.
Education, U. S. D. o. (2016). *Student reports of bullying: Results from the 2015 school crime supplement to the national crime victimization survey.* Retrieved from https://nces.ed.gov/pubs2017/2017015.pdf.
Espelage, D. L., & Horne, A. M. (2008). School violence and bullying prevention: From research-based explanations to empirically based solutions. In S. D. Brown & R. W. Lent (Eds.), *Handbook of counseling psychology* (pp. 588–598). John Wiley & Sons, Inc.
Essique, T. J. (2018). Gaining a better understanding of bullying behavior and peer victimization: An analysis of personality characteristics of adolescents with an autism spectrum disorder. *Dissertation Abstracts International: Section B: The Sciences and Engineering, 78*(9-B(E)), No Pagination Specified.
Evans, C., Fraser, M., & Cotter, K. (2014). The effectiveness of school-based bullying prevention programs: A systemic review. *Aggression and Violent Behavior, 19*(5), 532–544. https://doi.org/10.1016/j.avb.2014.07.004.
Farrington, D. P., Gaffney, H., Losel, F., & Ttofi, M. M. (2017). Systematic reviews of the effectiveness of developmental prevention programs in reducing delinquency, aggression, and bullying. *Aggression and Violent Behavior, 33*, 91–106. https://doi.org/10.1016/j.avb.2016.11.003.
Fisher, E. S. (2013). Supporting lesbian, gay, bisexual, transgender, and questioning students and families. In *Creating safe and supportive learning environments: A guide for working with lesbian, gay, bisexual, transgender, and questioning youth and families* (pp. 3–9). Routledge/Taylor & Francis Group.
Fisher, E. S., & Komosa-Hawkins, K. (2013). Creating safe and supportive learning environments: A guide for working with lesbian, gay, bisexual, transgender, and questioning youth and families. In *Creating safe and supportive learning environments: A guide for working with lesbian, gay, bisexual, transgender, and questioning youth and families* (pp. xi, 265). Routledge/Taylor & Francis Group.
Gardella, J. H., Fisher, B. W., & Teurbe-Tolon, A. R. (2017). A systematic review and meta-analysis of cyber-victimization and educational outcomes for adolescents. *Review of Educational Research, 87*(2), 283–308.
Gasser, L., & Keller, M. (2009). Are the competent the morally good? Perspective taking and moral motivation of children involved in bullying. *Social Development,* 18: 798–816. https://doi.org/10.1111/j.1467-9507.2008.00516.x.
Gini, G., & Espelage, D. L. (2014). Peer victimization, cyberbullying, and suicide risk in children and adolescents. *JAMA: Journal of the American Medical Association, 312*(5): 545–546.
Gini, G., & Pozzoli, T. (2009). Association between bullying and psychosomatic problems: a meta-analysis. *Pediatrics, 123*(3), 1059–1065. https://doi.org/10.1542/peds.2008-1215.

Gladden, R. M., Vivolo-Kantor, A. M., Hamburger, M. D., & Lumpkin, C. D. (2014). *Bullying Surveillance among Youths: Uniform definition for public health and recommend data elements.* Centers for Disease Control and Prevention U.S. Department of Education.
Hatzenbuehler, M. L., Schwab-Reese, L., Ranapurwala, S. I., Hertz, M. F., & Ramirez, M. R. (2015). Associations between antibullying policies and bullying in 25 states. *JAMA pediatrics, 169*(10), e152411. https://doi.org/10.1001/jamapediatrics.2015.2411.
Heil, J. (2016). Sport advocacy: Challenge, controversy, ethics, and action. *Sport, Exercise, and Performance Psychology, 5*(4), 281–295. https://doi.org/10.1037/spy0000078.
Heinrichs, R. (2003). *Perfect targets: Asperger syndrome and bullying—Practical solutions for surviving the social world.* Shawnee Mission, Kansas, Autism Asperger Publishing Company.
Hinduja, S., & Patchin, J. W. (2015). *Bullying beyond the schoolyard: Preventing and responding to cyber bullying.* Corwin.
Hissle-Groman, E., Landis, C. A., Sussi, A., Shvey, N., Gorman, G., et al. (2019). Gender Dysphoria in Children with Autism Spectrum Disorder. *LBGT Health, 6*(3), 95–99. https://doi.org/10.1089/lgbt.2018.0252.
Holben, D. M., & Zirkel, P. A. (2016). School bullying case law: Frequency and outcomes for school level, protected status, and bullying actions. *Ethical Human Psychology and Psychiatry: An International Journal of Critical Inquiry, 18*(2), 111–133. https://doi.org/10.1891/1559-4343.18.2.111.
Iannotti, R. J. (2012). *Health behavior in school-aged children (HBSC), 2005–2006.* Inter-university Consortium for Political and Social Research.
Iannotti, R. J. (2013). *Health behavior in school-aged children (HBSC), 2009–2010.* Inter-university Consortium for Political and Social Research.
Jimenez-Barbero, J. A., Ruiz-Hernandez, J. A., Llor-Zaragoza, L., Perez-Garcia, M., & Llor-Esteban, B. (2016, Feb). Effectiveness of anti-bullying school programs: A meta-analysis [Meta Analysis]. *Children and Youth Services Review, 61*, 165–175. https://doi.org/10.1016/j.childyouth.2015.12.015.
Juvonen, J., & Graham, S. (2014). Bullying in schools: The power of bullies and the plight of victims. *Annual Review of Psychology, 65*, 158–184. https://doi.org/10.1146/annurev-psych-010213-115030. PMID 23937767.
Kljakovic, M., & Hunt, C. (2016). A meta-analysis of predictors of bullying and victimisation in adolescence. *Journal of Adolescence, 49,* 134–145.
Laugeson, E. A. (2017). *PEERS for young adults: Social skills training for adults with autism spectrum disorder and other social challenges.* Routledge/Taylor & Francis Group.
Leaf, J. B. (2017). Handbook of social skills and autism spectrum disorder: Assessment, curricula, and intervention. In *Handbook of social skills and autism spectrum disorder: Assessment, curricula, and intervention* (xvii, 445 pp). Springer International Publishing.
Lonie, N. (2015). *Online safety for children and teens on the autism spectrum: A parent's and carer's guide.* Jessica Kingsley.
Lund, E. M., & Ross, S. W. (2017). Bullying perpetration, victimization, and demographic differences in college students: A review of the literature. *Trauma, Violence, & Abuse, 18*(3), 348–360. https://doi.org/10.1177/1524838015620818.
Martin, W., & LaVan, H. (2010). Workplace bullying: A review of litigated cases. *Employee Responsibilities and Rights Journal, 22*(3), 175–194. https://doi.org/10.1007/s10672-009-9140-4.
Marx, R. A., & Kettrey, H. H. (2016). Gay-straight alliances are associated with lower levels of school-based victimization of LGBTQ+ youth: A systematic review and meta-analysis. *Journal of Youth and Adolescence, 45*(7), 1269–1282. https://doi.org/10.1007/s10964-016-0501-7.
McCord, M. A., Joseph, D. L., Dhanani, L. Y., & Beus, J. M. (2018). A meta-analysis of sex and race differences in perceived workplace mistreatment. *Journal of Applied Psychology, 103*(2), 137–163. https://doi.org/10.1037/apl0000250.
McLeod, J. D., Meanwell, E., & Hawbaker, A. (2019). The experiences of college students on the autism spectrum: A comparison to their neurotypical peers. *Journal of Autism and Developmental Disorders, No Pagination Specified.* https://doi.org/10.1007/s10803-019-03910-8.

Menesini, E., Camodeca, M., & Nocentini, A. (2010). Bullying among siblings: The role of personality and relational variables. *British Journal of Developmental Psychology, 28*(4), 921–939. https://doi.org/10.1348/026151009X479402.

National Health Interview Survey– Occupatiponal Health Supplement (2015). https://www.cdc.gov.

Perlus, J. G., Brooks-Russell, A., Wang, J., & Iannotti, R. J. (2014). Trends in bullying, physical fighting, and weapon carrying among 6th- through 10th-grade students from 1998 to 2010: findings from a national study. *American Journal of Public Health, 104*(6), 1100–1106. https://doi.org/10.2105/AJPH.2013.301761.

Persson, R., Hogh, A., Hansen, A.-M., Nordander, C., Ohlsson, K., Balogh, I., Österberg, K., & Orbaek, P. (2009). Personality trait scores among occupationally active bullied persons and witnesses to bullying. *Motivation and Emotion, 33*(4), 387–399. http://dx.doi.org/10.1007/s11031-009-9132-6.

Potts, L. C. (2018). The influence of social media use on male college students' gender identity and gendered performance. *Dissertation Abstracts International Section A: Humanities and Social Sciences, 78*(12-A(E)): No Pagination Specified.

Pozzoli, T., & Gini, G. (2013). Why do bystanders of bullying help or not? A multidimensional model. *The Journal of Early Adolescence, 33*(3), 315–340.

Rayner, C., & Cooper, C. L. (2006). Workplace Bullying. In E. Kelloway, J. Barling, & J. Hurrell, Jr. (Eds.), *Handbook of workplace violence.* Sage.

Rikleen, L. S. (2019). *The shield of silence: How power perpetuates a culture of harassment and bullying in the workplace.* American Bar Association.

Rivara, F. P., & Le Menestrel, S. M, et al. (2016). *Preventing bullying through science policy and practice* (F. P. Rivara & S. M. Le Menestrel, Eds.). National Academy Press.

Russell, S. T., Horn, S. S., Moody, R. L., Fields, A., & Tilley, E. (2017). Enumerated U.S. state laws: Evidence from policy advocacy. In *Sexual orientation, gender identity, and schooling: The nexus of research, practice, and policy* (pp. 255–271). Oxford University Press: US. https://ovidsp.ovid.com/ovidweb.cgi?T=JS&CSC=Y&NEWS=N&PAGE=fulltext&D=psyc14&AN=2017-30970-015.

Saintil, M. (2018). Long-term effects of peer victimization: Examining the link among early experiences with victimization, social support, and current well-being in honors college students. *Dissertation Abstracts International: Section B: The Sciences and Engineering, 78*(11-B(E)).

Saleh, F. M., Feldman, B. N., Grudzinskas, A. J., Jr., Ravven, S. E., & Cody, R. (2014). Cybersexual harassment and suicide. In *Adolescent sexual behavior in the digital age: Considerations for clinicians, legal professionals, and educators* (pp. 139–160). Oxford University Press.

Sanchez, F. C., Navarro-Zaragoza, J., Ruiz-Cabello, A. L., Romero, M. F., & Maldonado, A. L. (2017). Association between bullying victimization and substance use among college students in Spain. *Adicciones, 29*(1), 22–32.

Sansone, R. A., & Sansone, L. A. (2008). Bully victims: Psychological and somatic aftermaths. *Psychiatry, 5*(6), 62–64.

Shetgiri, R. (2013). Bullying and victimization among children. *Advances in Pediatrics, 60*(1), 33–51. https://doi.org/10.1016/j.yapd.2013.04.004.

Shields, A., & Cicchetti, D. (2001). Parental maltreatment and emotion dysregulation as risk factors for bullying and victimization in middle childhood. *Journal of Clinical Child Psychology, 30*(3), 349–363. https://doi.org/10.1207/S15374424JCCP3003_7.

Sreckovic, M. A., Brunsting, N. C., & Able, H. (2014). Victimization of students with autism spectrum disorder: A review of prevalence and risk factors. *Research in Autism Spectrum Disorders, 8*(9), 1155–1172. https://doi.org/10.1016/j.rasd.2014.06.004.

Sreckovic, M. A., Hume, K., & Able, H. (2017). Examining the efficacy of peer network interventions on the social interactions of high school students with autism spectrum disorder. *Journal of Autism and Developmental Disorders, 47*(8), 2556–2574. https://doi.org/10.1007/s10803-017-3171-8.

Stuart-Cassel, V., Bell, A., Springer, J. F. (2011). Analysis of State Bullying Laws and Policies. *Office of Planning, Evaluation and Policy Development, US Department of Education*. https://eric.ed.gov/?id=ED527524.

Swearer, S. M., Turner, R. K. J. . Givens, E. & Pollack W. S. (2008). "You're so gay!": Do different forms of bullying matter for adolescent males? *School psychology review, 37*(2), 160–173. https://doi.org/10.1080/02796015.2008.12087891.

The Americans with Disabilities Act of 1990 or ADA (42 U.S.C. § 12101).

Tokunaga, R. S. (2010). Following you home from school: A critical review and synthesis of research on cyberbullying victimization. *Computers in Human Behavior, 26*(3), 277–287. https://doi.org/10.1016/j.chb.2009.11.014.

Toseeb, U., McChesney, G., Oldfield, J., & Wolke, D. (2019). Sibling bullying in middle childhood is associated with psychosocial difficulties in early adolescence: The case of individuals with autism spectrum disorder. *Journal of Autism and Developmental Disorders, No Pagination Specified*. https://doi.org/10.1007/s10803-019-04116-8.

Toseeb, U., McChesney, G., & Wolke, D. (2018). The prevalence and psychopathological correlates of sibling bullying in children with and without autism spectrum disorder. *Journal of Autism and Developmental Disorders, 48*(7), 2308–2318. https://doi.org/10.1007/s10803-018-3484-2.

Ttofi, M. M., & Farrington, D. P. (2011, Mar). Effectiveness of school-based programs to reduce bullying: A systematic and meta-analytic review [Literature Review; Systematic Review; Meta Analysis]. *Journal of Experimental Criminology, 7*(1), 27–56. https://doi.org/10.1007/s11292-010-9109-1.

Ttofi, M. M., Farrington, D. P., Lösel, F., & Loeber, R. (2011). The predictive efficiency of school bullying versus later offending: a systematic/meta-analytic review of longitudinal studies. *Criminal behaviour and mental health: CBMH, 21*(2), 80–89. https://doi.org/10.1002/cbm.808.

U.S. Dept. Education (2010a). Dear Colleauges – Letter. https://www2.ed.gov/about/offices/list/ocr/letters/colleague-201010.html.

U.S. Dept. Education (2010b). Guidance Targeting Harassment Outlines Local and Federal Responsibility, *Office of Planning, Evaluation, and Policy Development*, https://www2.ed.gov/about/offices/list/opepd/ppss/reports.html#safe.

Vaillancourt, T., Hymel, S., & McDougall, P. (2003). Bullying is power: Implications for school-based intervention strategies. *Journal of Applied School Psychology, 19*(2), 157–176. https://doi.org/10.1300/J008v19n02_10.

van Dijk, A., Poorthuis, A., & Malti, T. (2017). Psychological processes in young bullies versus bully-victims. *Aggressive Behavior, 43*(5), 430–439. https://doi.org/10.1002/ab.21701.

van Roekel, E., Scholte, R. H., & Didden, R. (2010). Bullying among adolescents with autism spectrum disorders: Prevalence and perception. *Journal of Autism and Developmental Disorders, 40*(1), 63–73. https://doi.org/10.1007/s10803-009-0832-2.

van Schalkwyk, G. I., Klingensmith, K., & Volkmar, F. R. (2015). Gender identity and autism spectrum disorders. *Yale Journal of Biology & Medicine, 88*(1), 81–83.

Van Wieren, T. A., Reid, C. A., & McMahon, B. T. (2008). Workplace discrimination and autism spectrum disorders: The National EEOC Americans with Disabilities Act Research project [Empirical Study; Quantitative Study]. *Work: Journal of Prevention, Assessment & Rehabilitation, 31*(3), 299–308. https://ovidsp.ovid.com/ovidweb.cgi?T=JS&CSC=Y&NEWS=N&PAGE=fulltext&D=psyc6&AN=2008-17035-004.

Vitoroulis, I., & Vaillancourt, T. (2015). Meta-analytic results of ethnic group differences in peer victimization. *Aggressive Behavior, 41*(2), 149–170.

Vreeman, R. C., & Carroll, A. E. (2007). A systematic review of school-based interventions to prevent bullying. *Archives of pediatrics & adolescent medicine, 161*(1), 78–88. https://doi.org/10.1001/archpedi.161.1.78.

Wolke, D., & Lereya, S. T. (2014). Bullying and parasomnias: a longitudinal cohort study. *Pediatrics, 134*(4), e1040–e1048. https://doi.org/10.1542/peds.2014-1295.

Wolke, D., Copeland, W. E., Angold, A., & Costello, E. J. (2013). Impact of bullying in childhood on adult health, wealth, crime, and social outcomes. *Psychol Sci, 24*(10), 1958–1970. https://doi.org/10.1177/0956797613481608.

Wright, M. F. (2018). Cyber victimization and depression among adolescents with autism spectrum disorder: The buffering effects of parental mediation and social support. *Journal of Child & Adolescent Trauma, 11*(1), 17–25.

Zablotsky, B., Bradshaw, C. P., Anderson, C. M., & Law, P. (2014). Risk factors for bullying among children with autism spectrum disorders. *Autism, 18*(4), 419–427. https://doi.org/10.1177/1362361313477920.

Zeedyk, S., Rodriguez, G., Tipton, L., Baker, B., & Blacher, J. (2014). Bullying of youth with autism spectrum disorder, intellectual disability, or typical development: Victim and parent perspectives. *Research in Autism Spectrum Disorders, 8*(9), 1173–1183. https://doi.org/10.1016/j.rasd.2014.06.001.

Fred R. Volkmar M.D. is the Irving B. Harris Professor of Child Psychiatry, Pediatrics, and Psychology at the Yale Child Study Center, Yale University School of Medicine and the Dorothy Goodwin Family Chair in Special Education at Southern Connecticut State University. An international authority on Asperger's disorder and autism, Dr. Volkmar was the primary author of the DSM-IV autism and pervasive developmental disorders section. He has authored several hundred scientific papers and has co-edited numerous books, including Asperger Syndrome, Healthcare for Children on the Autism Spectrum: A Guide to Medical, Nutritional, and Behavioral Issues, and the recently released third edition of The Handbook of Autism and Pervasive Developmental Disorders. He serves as an Associate Editor of the Journal of Autism, the Journal of Child Psychology and Psychiatry, and the American Journal of Psychiatry. He also serves as a Co-Chairperson of the autism/MR committee of the American Academy of Child and Adolescent Psychiatry. Since 2007 he has served as the Editor of the Journal of Autism and more recently of the Encyclopedia of Autism.

Brian Pete J.D. is a graduate of New York University School of Law. He is a Labor & Employment partner in the New York office of Lewis Brisbois Bisgaard & Smith LLP and was formerly outside counsel to New Jersey public school districts.

Chapter 10
Cyber-Dependent Crime, Autism, and Autistic-Like Traits

Mark Brosnan

Cyber-Dependent Crime

Ledingham and Mills (2015) define cybercrime as 'The illegal use of computers and the internet or crime committed by means of computers and the internet'. How cybercrime is defined legally will be discussed within a UK context, though many countries have similar legislation (e.g. the USA, Australia, New Zealand, Germany, the Netherlands, Denmark; Ledingham & Mills, 2015). In the Serious and Organised Crime Strategy (Home Office, 2013), the UK Government highlighted a central distinction between 2 types of cybercriminal activity:

1. Cyber-dependent crimes: Those which can only be committed using computers, computer networks, or other forms of information communication technology (ICT). They include the creation and spread of malware for financial gain, hacking to steal important personal or industry data, and denial of service (DDoS) attacks to cause reputational damage (p. 22).
2. Cyber-enabled crimes: Those which can be conducted on or offline, but online may take place at unprecedented scale and speed (p. 22).

A crime such as online fraud would be considered to be a cyber-enabled crime. Fraud has been committed for millennia, and the online aspect is simply a new format of a traditional crime. Perpetrators of such activities would be prosecuted for fraud. Cyber-dependent crimes, however, are a new form of crime that did not exist before the advent of ICT and are also referred to as 'pure' cybercrime (NCA, 2017). In 2015 the Crime Survey for England and Wales included cybercrime in its statistics for the first time and the crime rate more than doubled as a consequence (NCA, 2016). 20% of all crime in the UK is cyber-dependent crime (ONS, 2017), which is an offence

M. Brosnan (✉)
Centre for Applied Autism Research (CAAR), University of Bath, Bath, UK
e-mail: M.J.Brosnan@bath.ac.uk

F. R. Volkmar et al. (eds.), *Handbook of Autism Spectrum Disorder and the Law*,
https://doi.org/10.1007/978-3-030-70913-6_10

under the Computer Misuse Act (1990), which outlined three offences (amended twice, by the Police and Justice Act 2006 and by the Serious Crime Act 2015):

1. Unauthorised access to computer material (*up to 2 years imprisonment*).
2. Unauthorised access with intent to commit or facilitate commission of further offences (*up to 5 years imprisonment*).
3. Unauthorised acts with intent to impair, or with recklessness as to impairing, operation of computer, etc. (*up to 10 years imprisonment*).

   Unauthorised acts causing, or creating risk of, serious damage (*up to life imprisonment*).
   Making, supplying or obtaining articles for use in offences 1 or 3 above (*up to 2 years imprisonment*).

Cyber-dependent crime is therefore computer misuse covering any unauthorized access to computer material as defined above. This is not limited to desk or laptop computers and can include any device using operating software accessible online, for example, games consoles, smart phones, and smart TVs. In the year up to March 2018 there were 1,239,000 reported cases of computer misuse in England and Wales (ONS, 2018). Over a third of adult internet users are estimated to have experienced some form of cyber-dependent criminal activity, predominantly virus attacks (Home Office, 2013). There is some evidence that this number may be decreasing—as anti-malware software develops or is used more, it seems this has an impact upon the number of people reporting incidents of computer misuse. In addition, many incidents go unreported, and consequently attempts to quantify cyber-dependent crime specifically have resulted in dramatically varied numbers, highlighting the difficulty of trying to establish the scale, cost, and impact of cyber-dependent attacks. Furnell et al. (2015) proposed that it is more important to understand the impact of cyber-dependent incidents and how to prevent them, than to focus on metrics. Consistent with this, whilst the available metrics for cyber-dependent crime are high, there are relatively few prosecutions under the Computer Misuse Act. For example, 88 people were sentenced in total between 2007 and 2012 in the UK (Home Office, 2013). This is not due to lack of evidence, as typically the evidence is very strong and if a decision is made to proceed with a prosecution, sentencing is highly likely. Rather it is the profile of some of the people who engage in cybercrime that presents a challenge for the legal system.

Initial analysis of cyber-dependent criminals suggests that their motivations may not always be for personal financial gain or to harm others. Rather the motivation for cyber-dependent crimescan be self-satisfaction from the challenge of hacking into a computer system, or the attention, recognition, or adulation this may confer from other hackers (Ledingham & Mills, 2015). This is because cyber-dependent crime requires an advanced level of cyber skills such as: Understanding architecture, administration, and management of operating systems, networking, and virtualization software; General programming/software development concepts and software analytical skills; Proficiency in programming in Java, C/C++, disassemblers, and assembly language and programming knowledge of two or more scripting languages

(PHP, Python, Perl, or shell); Understanding of how the different type of firewalls and network load balancers work; A deep understanding of how network routers and switches work; and evaluating systems and network architectures (Insights, 2018). Clearly such skills are also essential for cyber security, and law enforcement agencies (such as the NCA and Europol, Interpol) explicitly promote the application of such skills to cyber security rather than cybercrime.

The UK's National Crime Agency (NCA) has a National Cybercrime Unit which focuses upon cyber-dependent crime. In 2015, the average age of those arrested for cybercrime was 17, the vast majority of whom were male (for comparison, the average age of those arrested for economic crime is 39: NCA, 2017). However, the NCA also notes that around two-thirds of those arrested had begun cyber-dependent criminal activity before the age of 16. The high proportion of children (legally speaking) engaging in cyber-dependent criminal activity is one of the challenges faced by the law enforcement agencies. As an example, a 17-year old was convicted of perpetrating a 'significant and sustained' cyber-attack on telecoms giant TalkTalk, which the company estimates cost it £42 m. As a child, the perpetrator cannot be named for legal reasons. He told magistrates 'I was just showing off to my mates', and there was no evidence of any personal financial gain. The serious nature of this crime could warrant a 10 year to life prison sentence (see above) for an adult perpetrator seeking to gain financially or cause serious damage. The 17-year old was given a 12-month youth rehabilitation order, had his smartphone and computer hard drive confiscated, and was told 'Your IT skills will always be there—just use them legally in the future' (Guardian, 2016).

Having interviewed these cyber-dependent criminals, the NCA's intelligence assessment (2017) identifies the perceived state of affairs as:

- A number of UK teenagers who we assess are unlikely to be involved in traditional crime are becoming involved in cybercrime.
- To date there has been no socio-demographic bias amongst offenders or those on the periphery of criminality.
- Availability of low-level hacking tools encourages criminal behaviour.
- Autism spectrum disorder (ASD) appears to be more prevalent amongst cyber criminals than the general populace though this remains unproven.
- Offenders begin to participate in gaming cheat websites and 'modding' (game modification) forums and progress to criminal hacking forums without considering consequences.
- Financial gain is not necessarily a priority for young offenders.
- Completing the challenge, sense of accomplishment, proving oneself to peers is a key motivation for those involved in cyber criminality.
- Offenders perceive the likelihood of encountering law enforcement as low.
- Cybercrime is not solitary and anti-social. Social relationships, albeit online, are key. Forum interaction and building of reputation drives young cyber criminals.
- Positive opportunities, role models, mentors can deter young people away from cybercrime.

- Targeted interventions at an early stage can steer pathways towards positive outcomes.

The fourth point above concerning autism is based on anecdotal accounts from the NCA that they are breaking down doors and seizing computers from bemused, young teenage males who thought it would be funny to DDoS their friends, or a challenge to hack into a major corporation—and who could be looking at up to 10 years imprisonment for their first offence. Again anecdotally, the NCA reports that these cyber-dependent criminals do not have a history of the increasing criminality that is more typical of criminals facing a 10-year prison sentence. Rather they tend to find socially awkward young males who are 'nice kids' and freely divulge all the incriminating evidence of their illegal activities. Again, it is anecdotal that the NCA has speculated whether there are autism-like issues amongst such cyber-dependent criminals. For example, one suspect said 'I just got a bee in my bonnet trying to understand how things work' (NCA, 2017) which may relate to aspects of autism (see below).

Autism and Cyber-Dependent Crime

So why might there be an association between autism and cyber-dependent crime? This has two associated questions—is autism related to crime and is autism related to cyber dependency?

Is There a Relationship Between Autism and Crime?

As cyber-dependent crime is relatively new and under researched, we need to look briefly at the broader literature. This has indicated that crimes committed by autistic people may be more directed against a person than against property (e.g. Cheeley et al., 2012; Kumagami & Matsuura, 2009; see Gunasekaran & Chaplin, 2012, for review). However, a large body of research has suggested that autistic people are generally law abiding with low rates of criminality (Blackmore et al., 2017; Ghaziuddin et al., 1991; Howlin, 2007; Murrie et al., 2002; Wing, 1981; Woodbury-Smith et al., 2006). In a Swedish population-based cohort study containing 5739 autistic people, Heeramun et al. (2017) report that autism was a risk factor associated with violent crime. However, this was found to be attributable to comorbid ADHD. Indeed, when accounting for ADHD, autism was a protective factor against criminality (see also Blackmore et al., 2017). Thus from the general literature on autism and crime we would not predict a strong relationship between autism and cyber-dependent crime. [See chapters in this book for a fuller account.]

Is There a Relationship Between Autism and Cyber Dependency?

Within autism research and practice, autism is often characterized as a relative weakness in social processing (with other humans) and relative strengths in non-social processing (how things work in the physical world: e.g. Baron-Cohen, 2002, 2009; Baron-Cohen et al., 2005; Klin et al., 2009). In 'Autism and the Technical Mind', Baron-Cohen (2012) speculates: 'Silicon Valley and other tech-savvy communities report exceptionally high rates of autism. These trends might reflect a link between genes that contribute to autism and genes behind technical aptitude'. This speculation is consistent with the autistic author Temple Grandin, who has written that her mind works like a computer and has also written about an autistic computer programmer who visualizes the entire program tree in his mind and then just fills in the code (Grandin, 1990, 1995). Importantly, such speculation and anecdotal accounts do not suggest that all autistic people are tech-savvy nor that all tech-savvy people are autistic. No one has suggested, for example, that most children born in Silicon Valley or most computer science students are autistic. This is significant as an advanced level of cyber skills is required to commit cyber-dependent crime—and most people with advanced cyber skills are not autistic (and most autistic people do not have advanced cyber skills). The autistic author Damion Milton (2018) argues that comparing the autistic mind to a computer can be dehumanizing, casting autistic people as 'only capable of compiling and broadcasting strings of information'.

One pathway into cyber-dependent crime is through gaming (online, video, etc.) and autistic people have been found to particularly enjoy gaming, typically playing for twice as long as non-autistic peers (Mazurek & Engelhardt, 2013a, 2013b). However, Mazurek and Engelhardt also found that those with ADHD engaged in gaming in similar quantities to autistic people, and it is not time spent gaming per se that relates to cyber-dependent crime but rather the development of the cyber skills needed to modify games (called 'modding'). As an example, Minecraft is an open-ended virtual world with no particular goals or play requirements that is popular with some autistic children who 'mod' the Minecraft system to support self-regulation and community engagement (Ringland et al., 2016). Modding Minecraft is perfectly legal, which is explicitly stated in the Minecraft licence agreement. Thus, as with the speculation concerning a 'technical mind', autistic people developing (legal) modding skills which can be a precursor to engaging in (illegal) cyber-dependent crime, does not necessarily imply that autistic people are more likely to engage in cyber-dependent crime. In the event of an autistic person having a circumscribed interest in technology or gaming, it does not follow that this would relate to the nature of any criminality (Woodbury-Smith et al., 2010). Indeed, should the findings above of autism being a protective factor against engaging in traditional crimes extend to cybercrimes, some autistic people may be characterized by an advanced level of cyber skills combined with a reduced likelihood of engaging in cybercrime—the exact profile the law enforcement agencies are attempting to encourage into cyber security.

There is also evidence that autistic people can perform better on assessments when they are computer-mediated. For example, autistic people can improve on theory of mind when assessment is computer-based (Swettenham, 1996), do not show deficits in executive functioning when assessment is computer-based (Ozonoff, 1995), and can show enhanced emotion recognition in animated faces, compared to human faces (Brosnan et al., 2015). Autistic people can also demonstrate relatively greater social communication when using social media (Brosnan & Gavin, 2015; Ward et al., 2018) or talking to social robots compared to humans (Kim et al., 2018). Thus, digital technology may ameliorate some issues experienced by some autistic people, but does this constitute cyber dependency? A 2018 Pew (which is well-regarded research centre) survey of teens in the USA found that 45% reported that they were 'online almost constantly' (and 44% online several times a day; Anderson & Jiang, 2018). Any concerns over compulsive use of digital technology are comparable between autistic and non-autistic people (Shane-Simpson et al., 2016). Thus any orientation towards digital technology would seem to be fairly universal rather than autism-specific.

Autistic-Like Traits

Autistic-like traits are argued to vary continuously across the general population, with autism residing at the extreme end of this continuum (Baron-Cohen et al., 2001, 2006; Constantino & Todd, 2003; Kanne et al., 2012; Plomin et al., 2009; Posserud et al., 2006; Skuse et al., 2009; see also Bölte et al., 2011; Gernsbacher et al., 2017; Ronald & Hoekstra, 2011; Ruzich et al., 2015a for meta-analysis). Autistic-like traits refer to behavioural traits such as social imperviousness, directness in conversation, lack of imagination, affinity for solitude, and difficulty displaying emotions (Gernsbacher et al., 2017). These are typically assessed through self-report measures such as the Autism Spectrum Quotient (AQ: Baron-Cohen et al., 2001; see also Baghdadli et al., 2017). Ruzich et al.'s (2015a) meta-analysis of responses to the AQ from almost 7,000 non-autistic and 2,000 autistic respondents identified that non-autistic males had significantly higher levels of autistic-like traits than non-autistic females, and that autistic people had significantly higher levels of autistic-like traits compared to the non-autistic males (with no sex difference within the autistic sample). The AQ comprises 50 questions, made up of 10 questions assessing 5 different areas, including 3 social subscales of social skills, communication and imagination, and 2 non-social subscales of attention switching and attention to detail. Baron-Cohen et al. (2001) report that autistic people self-report significantly poorer scores on the social subscales (resulting in a higher score, indicating higher autistic-like traits). Autistic people also score higher on the non-social subscales, indicating significantly stronger attention to detail and focus of attention. Whilst a higher score on the non-social subscales of the AQ can be considered a relative strength associated with autistic-like traits, a stronger focus of attention could also be described as poorer attention switching.

Comparing autistic and non-autistic people with identical levels of autistic-like traits, Lundqvist and Lindner (2017) found they were similar on 45 items of the AQ. Of the remaining five items, three items were endorsed more by the autistic group ('I would rather go to a library than a party'; 'I am fascinated by numbers'; 'I find it hard to make new friends') and two items were endorsed more by the non-autistic group ('I find making up stories easy, I enjoy social occasions'). This is consistent with arguments of overlapping genetic and biological aetiology underlying autism and autistic-like population traits (Bralten et al., 2018; Focquaert & Vanneste, 2015). Importantly, however, other authors have argued that autism is not simply high levels of autistic-like traits but rather a qualitative difference. Frith (2014), for example, argues that 'people with autism really have a very different mind and different brain'. Thus there maybe two different groups with high levels of autistic-like traits (e.g. above a cut off of 26; Woodbury-Smith et al., 2005): Those who have autism and those who do not. The anecdotal evidence of apparent autism-like behaviours in cyber-dependent criminals may therefore reflect people with high levels of autistic-like traits who do not have a diagnosis of autism.

Autistic-Like Traits and Cybercrime

Baron-Cohen et al. (2001, see also Billington et al., 2007) and Ruzich et al. (2015b) found that science students and employees, including computer science students and ICT-related employees, were relatively high in autistic-like traits Thus, whilst it was noted above that most computer scientists are not autistic, they do have higher levels of autistic-like traits. The relationship between computer science and autistic-like traits is potentially important as cyber-dependent criminal activity requires an advanced level of cyber skills.

Assessing the relationship between autistic-like traits and cyber deviancy in a sample of college students, Seigfried-Spellar et al. (2015) found that of 296 university students, 179 (60%) engaged in some form of cyber deviant behaviour and the AQ distinguished between those who did and those who did not self-report some kinds of cyber deviant behaviour, but not other kinds of cyber deviant behaviour. This is why the definition of cyber-dependent crime is significant. In this study, cyber deviant behaviour included cyber-enabled crimes such as cyberbullying and identity theft, and cyber-dependent crimes such as hacking and virus writing. Those who engaged in all forms of cybercrime scored higher on the AQ than those who engaged in some types of cybercrime—but which types of cybercrime were not specified. The authors also report that if they used a cut-off score on the AQ of 26 to indicate high levels of autistic-like traits associated with autism, then 7% of the computer non-deviants and 6% of the computer deviants scored in this range. The authors conclude that 'based on these findings alone, there is no evidence of a significant link between clinical levels of [autism] and computer deviance in the current sample. However, the current study did find evidence for computer deviants reporting more autistic-like traits, according to the AQ, compared to computer non-deviants'. There may be important differences in the relationship between autistic-like traits and cyber-dependent crime compared with cyber-enabled crime. In future work a specific focus upon cyber-dependent crime may be particularly beneficial for understanding the role of autistic-like traits, as cyber-dependent crime is sometimes called 'pure' cybercrime, whereas cyber-enabled crime may have a greater role for the offline factors associated with the fraud or identity theft (for example). Recently, Payne et al. (2019) found that greater levels of autistic-like traits related to an increased risk of committing cyber-dependent crime. Importantly, a diagnosis of autism related to a decreased risk of committing cyber-dependent crime. This is early research, but the evidence may be suggesting that higher autistic-like traits, not autism, relate to cyber-dependent crime.

Future Work

Cyber-dependent crime can be extremely serious and the skills and sophistication of international crime groups make them the most competent and dangerous criminals targeting the UK (NCA, 2016). In addition, there are large numbers of teenage males engaging in cyber-dependent crime which is not for personal gain or to cause harm to others. Higher levels of autistic-like traits may be present in this latter group. It may be that non-social strengths such as attention to detail support the development of cyber skills and relatively compromised social skills result in greater involvement with online forums. Such online forums may engender an environment within which cyber skills enabling cyber-dependent crime are shared and reputations are enhanced by undertaking cyber-dependent crime.

Autistic people have higher levels of autistic-like traits than the general population. In addition, however, it has often been found that autistic people tend to be law-abiding. Whilst highlighting that an activity is illegal may not be preventative for young people generally, it may be that such a strategy would be more effective for this group. Whilst a clear message that cyber-dependent crime is illegal can only be beneficial, hacking represents a cyber-dependent crime that is not so black-and-white (literally). Hackers can be described in different ways, and some use the terms 'black hats' (violate systems often for illegal purposes), 'white hats' (skilled but use skills to collaborate with the establishment), and 'grey hats' (ethical hackers hack because they perceive it is justified; Ledingham & Mills, 2015). It is possible to study for an undergraduate degree at university majoring in Ethical Hacking (Abertay, 2018), for example, highlighting the potential complexity in developing a clear message concerning 'what is right and what is wrong'.

Ethical Hacking in the university context represents an 'accredited programme for cyber security' where students can learn 'the process of hacking attacks and how to stop them'. As noted above, a combination of possessing advanced cyber skills and a predisposition to be law-abiding would represent an ideal skill set for the cyber security industry. The NCA (2018) has developed a 'digital defender' package to encourage young people into cyber security. Given many from the autistic community take issue with the term 'Disorder' (Kenny et al., 2016) within this context, ASD could be developed in terms of 'Autism Spectrum Defender' to highlight the positive attributes autism can bring to cyber security. The term 'autism' embraces a wide array of capabilities and preferences and it is important to reiterate how heterogeneous the autistic community is, and it will undoubtedly have members who have no interest in cyber security. The point is not to suggest that all autistic people will have advanced cyber skills (or have computer-like brains), rather that some might have a desirable skill set and may be a real asset if given the opportunity to apply these skills.

It is possible that the study of cyber-dependent crime may also be able to contribute to the debate concerning the relationship between autism and autistic-like traits (Abu-Akel et al., 2019; Brosnan, 2020). Having a diagnosis of autism can be used by defence lawyers to avoid a prison sentence, or indeed extradition (as mentioned in the opening paragraph). Within the legal context of being arrested for cyber-dependent crime, there could be perceived benefits to getting a diagnosis of autism and lawyers forwarding an 'autism defence' (Kushner, 2011). Thus future research teasing out the relative influence of autism and autistic-like traits upon cyber-dependent crime is essential (Payne et al., 2019). However discerning appropriate samples will be challenging, not least because those who are identified as cyber-dependent criminals (e.g. by law enforcement agencies) will represent a subset of potential participants—namely those who have been caught.

To date there is one research paper exploring autism and cybercrime and two papers exploring autistic-like traits and cybercrime. The NCA, Barclays Bank, and Research Autism are working with the University of Bath to explore the relationship between autism, autistic-like traits, and cyber-dependent crime. The research is ongoing and explores the role of advanced cyber skills in any potential relationships. There are additional research questions, for example—where are the females? Given the sex differences identified in autistic-like traits (above, as well as autism), we may anticipate fewer females committing cybercrime. However, it could also be the case that females are better at not getting caught. Given the male domination of the cyber security industry (86%: Govtech, 2018) and of computer science courses (87%: Computerworlduk, 2018) at university (that both also require advanced levels of cyber skills), it may be the case that there are much fewer female cyber-dependent criminals (as there are fewer female traditional criminals).

References

Abertay. (2018). https://www.abertay.ac.uk/course-search/undergraduate/ethical-hacking/.

Abu-Akel, A., Allison, C., Baron-Cohen, S., & Heinke, D. (2019). The distribution of autistic traits across the autism spectrum: Evidence for discontinuous dimensional subpopulations underlying the autism continuum. *Molecular Autism, 10*(1), 24.

Anderson, M., & Jiang, J. (2018). *Teens, social media & technology 2018*. Pew Internet & American Life Project. Retrieved June 3, 2018.

Baghdadli, A., Russet, F., & Mottron, L. (2017). Measurement properties of screening and diagnostic tools for autism spectrum adults of mean normal intelligence: A systematic review. *European Psychiatry, 44*, 104–124.

Baron-Cohen, S. (2002). The extreme male brain theory of autism. *Trends in Cognitive Sciences, 6*(6), 248–254.
Baron-Cohen, S. (2009). Autism: The empathizing–systemizing (E-S) theory. *Annals of the New York Academy of Sciences, 1156*(1), 68–80.
Baron-Cohen, S. (2012). Autism and the technical mind. *Scientific American, 307*(5), 72–75.
Baron-Cohen, S., Hoekstra, R. A., Knickmeyer, R., & Wheelwright, S. (2006). The Autism-Spectrum Quotient (AQ)—Adolescent version. *Journal of Autism and Developmental Disorders, 36*, 343–350
Baron-Cohen, S., Knickmeyer, R. C., & Belmonte, M. K. (2005). Sex differences in the brain: Implications for explaining autism. *Science, 310*(5749), 819–823.
Baron-Cohen, S., Wheewright, S., Skinner, R., Martin, J., & Clubley, E. (2001). The Autism-Spectrum Quotient (AQ): Evidence from Asperger syndrome/high functioning autism, males and females, scientists and mathematicians. *Journal of Autism and Developmental Disorders, 31*, 5–17.
Billington, J., Baron-Cohen, S., & Wheelwright, S. (2007). Cognitive style predicts entry into physical sciences and humanities: Questionnaire and performance tests of empathy and systemizing. *Learn Individ Differ, 17*, 260–268.
Blackmore, C. et al. (2017). *Adults with autism spectrum disorder and the criminal justice system: An investigation of prevalence of ofending, risk factors and gender differences*. Paper presented at INSAR, May 11, San Francisco.
Bölte, S., Westerwald, E., Holtmann, M., Freitag, C., & Poustka, F. (2011). Autistic traits and autism spectrum disorders: The clinical validity of two measures presuming a continuum of social communication skills. *Journal of Autism and Developmental Disorders, 41*(1), 66–72.
Bralten, J., Van Hulzen, K. J., Martens, M. B., Galesloot, T. E., Vasquez, A. A., Kiemeney, L. A., Buitelaar, J. K., Muntjewerff, J. W., Franke, B., & Poelmans, G. (2018). Autism spectrum disorders and autistic traits share genetics and biology. *Molecular Psychiatry, 23*(5), 1205–1212
Brosnan, M. (2020). An exploratory study of a dimensional assessment of the diagnostic criteria for autism. *Journal of Autism and Developmental Disorders*, 1–7.
Brosnan, M., & Gavin, J. (2015). Why those with an autism spectrum disorder (ASD) thrive in online cultures but suffer in offline cultures. *The Wiley Handbook of Psychology, Technology, and Society* (p. 250).
Brosnan, M., Johnson, H., Grawmeyer, B., Chapman, E., & Benton, L. (2015). Emotion recognition in animated compared to human stimuli in adolescents with autism spectrum disorder. *Journal of Autism and Developmental Disorders, 45*(6), 1785–1796.
Charlton, J. (2011). Crime of the times. *Information Today, 28*(8), 14–15
Cheeley, C. A., Carpenter, L. A., Letourneau, E. J., Nicholas, J. S., Charles, J., & King, L. B. (2012). The prevalence of youth with autism spectrum disorders in the criminal justice system. *Journal of Autism and Developmental Disorders, 42*, 1856–1862
CSIS. (2018). https://ia.acs.org.au/article/2018/cost-of-cybercrime-soars.html.
Computerworlduk. (2018). https://www.computerworlduk.com/careers/women-studying-computer-science-in-uk-universities-is-declining-3621040/.
Constantino, J. N., & Todd, R. D. (2003). Autistic traits in the general population: A twin study. *Archives of General Psychiatry, 60*, 524–530
Focquaert, F., & Vanneste, S. (2015). Autism spectrum traits in normal individuals: A preliminary VBM analysis. *Frontiers in Human Neuroscience, 9*, 264
Furnell, S., Emm, D., & Papadaki, M. (2015). The challenge of measuring cyber-dependent crimes. *Computer Fraud & Security, 2015*(10), 5–12
Frith, U. (2014). Autism-are we any closer to explaining the enigma? *Psychologist, 27*(10), 744–745
Gernsbacher, M. A., Stevenson, J. L., & Dern, S. (2017). Specificity, contexts, and reference groups matter when assessing autistic traits. *PLoS ONE, 12*(2), e0171931
Ghaziuddin, M., Tsai, L., & Ghaziuddin, N. (1991). Brief report: Violence in Asperger syndrome, a critique. *Journal of Autism and Developmental Disorders, 21*(3), 349–354

Govtech. (2018). https://www.govtech.com/workforce/Why-Are-So-Few-Women-in-Cybersecurity.html
Grandin, T. (1990). Needs of high functioning teenagers and adults with autism (Tips from a recovered autistic). *Focus on Autistic Behavior, 5*(1), 1–16
Grandin, T. (1995). How people with autism think. In *Learning and cognition in autism* (pp. 137–156). Springer.
Guardian. (2016). https://www.theguardian.com/business/2016/dec/13/teenager-who-hacked-talktalk-website-given-rehabilitation-order.
Gunasekaran, S., & Chaplin, E. (2012). Autism spectrum disorders and offending. *Advances in Mental Health and Intellectual Disabilities, 6*(6), 308–313.
Heeramun, R., Magnusson, C., Gumpert, C. H., Granath, S., Lundberg, M., Dalman, C., & Rai, D. (2017). Autism and convictions for violent crimes: Population-based cohort study in Sweden. *Journal of the American Academy of Child & Adolescent Psychiatry, 56*(6), 491–497
Home Office. (2013). https://assets.publishing.service.gov.uk/government/uploads/system/uploads/attachment_data/file/246751/horr75-chap1.pdf.
Howlin, P. (2007). The outcome in adult life for people with ASD. *Autism and Pervasive Developmental Disorders*, 269–306.
Insights. (2018). https://insights.dice.com/cybersecurity-skills/4/.
Kanne, S. M., Wang, J., & Christ, S. E. (2012). The Subthreshold Autism Trait Questionnaire (SATQ): Development of a brief self-report measure of subthreshold autism traits. *Journal of Autism and Developmental Disorders, 42,* 769–780
Kenny, L., Hattersley, C., Molins, B., Buckley, C., Povey, C., & Pellicano, E. (2016). Which terms should be used to describe autism? Perspectives from the UK autism community. *Autism, 20,* 442–4662.
Kim, M., Kwon, T., & Kim, K. (2018). Can human-robot interaction promote the same depth of social information processing as human-human interaction? *International Journal of Social Robotics, 10*(1), 33–42
Klin, A., Lin, D. J., Gorrindo, P., Ramsay, G., & Jones, W. (2009). Two-year-olds with autism orient to non-social contingencies rather than biological motion. *Nature, 459*(7244), 257
Kumagami, T., & Matsuura, N. (2009). Prevalence of pervasive developmental disorder in juvenile court cases in Japan. *The Journal of Forensic Psychiatry and Psychology, 20,* 974–987
Kushner, D. (2011). The autism defense. *Spectrum, IEEE, 48*(7), 32–37.
Ledingham, R., & Mills, R. (2015). A preliminary study of autism and cybercrime in the context of international law enforcement. *Advances in Autism, 1*(1), 2–11
Lundqvist, L. O., & Lindner, H. (2017). Is the autism-spectrum quotient a valid measure of traits associated with the autism spectrum? A Rasch validation in adults with and without autism spectrum disorders. *Journal of Autism and Developmental Disorders, 47*(7), 2080–2091
Mazurek, M. O., & Engelhardt, C. R. (2013a). Video game use in boys with autism spectrum disorder, ADHD, or typical development. *Pediatrics*, peds-2012.
Mazurek, M. O., & Engelhardt, C. R. (2013b). Video game use and problem behaviors in boys with autism spectrum disorders. *Research in Autism Spectrum Disorders, 7*(2), 316–324
McCoogan, C. (2016). The full story of Lauri Love's fight against extradition. *The Telegraph.*
Murrie, D. C., Warren, J. I., Kristiansson, M., & Dietz, P. E. (2002). Asperger's syndrome in forensic settings. *International Journal of Forensic Mental Health, 1*(1), 59–70
Milton, D. (2018). cited in: https://www.wired.co.uk/article/autisim-children-treatment-robots.
NCA. (2016). https://www.nationalcrimeagency.gov.uk/publications/709-cyber-crime-assessment-2016/file.
NCA. (2017). https://www.nationalcrimeagency.gov.uk/crime-threats/cyber-crime/cyber-crime-preventing-young-people-from-getting-involved.
NCA. (2018). https://www.nationalcrimeagency.gov.uk/publications/759-the-digital-defenders-your-future-fighting-cyber-crime/file.
ONS. (2017). Office for National Statistics. (2017). Crime in England and Wales: Year ending June 2017. Retrieved 19th December 2017 from https://www.ons.gov.uk/peoplepopulationandco

mmunity/crimeandjustice/bulletins/crimeinenglandandwales/june2017#latest-violent-crime-figures-continue-to-present-acomplex-picture.
ONS. (2018). Crime in England and Wales: Year ending March 2018. https://www.ons.gov.uk/peoplepopulationandcommunity/crimeandjustice/bulletins/crimeinenglandandwales/yearendingmarch2018.
Ozonoff, S. (1995). Reliability and validity of the Wisconsin Card Sorting Test in studies of autism. *Neuropsychology, 9*(4), 491
Payne, K. L., Russell, A., Mills, R., Maras, K., Rai, D., & Brosnan, M. (2019). Is there a relationship between cyber-dependent crime, autistic-like traits and autism? *Journal of Autism and Developmental Disorders, 49*(10), 4159–4169
Plomin, R., Haworth, C. M. A., & Davis, O. S. P. (2009). Common disorders are quantitative traits. *Nature Reviews Genetics, 10,* 872–878.
Posserud, M. B., Lundervold, A. J., & Gillberg, C. (2006). Autistic features in a total population of 7–9-year-old children assessed by the ASSQ (Autism Spectrum Screening Questionnaire). *Journal of Child Psychology and Psychiatry, 47,* 167–175.
Ringland, K. E., Wolf, C. T., Boyd, L. E., Baldwin, M. S., & Hayes, G. R. (2016, October). Would you be mine: Appropriating minecraft as an assistive technology for youth with autism. In *Proceedings of the 18th International ACM SIGACCESS Conference on Computers and Accessibility* (pp. 33–41). ACM.
Ronald, A., & Hoekstra, R. A. (2011). Autism spectrum disorders and autistic traits: a decade of new twin studies. *American Journal of Medical Genetics Part B: Neuropsychiatric Genetics, 156*(3), 255–274
Ruzich, E., Allison, C., Smith, P., Watson, P., Auyeung, B., Ring, H., & Baron-Cohen, S. (2015a). Measuring autistic traits in the general population: A systematic review of the Autism-Spectrum Quotient (AQ) in a nonclinical population sample of 6,900 typical adult males and females. *Molecular Autism, 6,* 2.
Ruzich, E., Allison, C., Chakrabarti, B., Smith, P., Musto, H., Ring, H., et al. (2015b). Sex and STEM occupation predict Autism-Spectrum Quotient (AQ) scores in half a million people. *PLoS ONE, 10,* e0141229.
Seigfried-Spellar, K. C., O'Quinn, C. L., & Treadway, K. N. (2015). Assessing the relationship between autistic traits and cyberdeviancy in a sample of college students. *Behaviour & Information Technology, 34*(5), 533–542.
Shane-Simpson, C., Brooks, P. J., Obeid, R., Denton, E. G., & Gillespie-Lynch, K. (2016). Associations between compulsive internet use and the autism spectrum. *Research in Autism Spectrum Disorders, 23,* 152–165.
Sharp, J. (2013). *Saving Gary McKinnon: A Mother's Story*. Biteback Publishing.
Skuse, D., Mandy, W., Steer, C., Miller, L., Goodman, R., Lawrence, K., et al. (2009). Social communication competence and functional adaptation in a general population of children: Preliminary evidence for sex-by-verbal IQ differential risk. *Journal of the American Academy of Child and Adolescent Psychiatry, 48,* 128–137.
Swettenham, J. (1996). Can children with autism be taught to understand false belief using computers? *Journal of Child Psychology and Psychiatry, 37*(2), 157–165.
Ward, D. M., Dill-Shackleford, K. E., & Mazurek, M. O. (2018). Social media use and happiness in adults with autism spectrum disorder. *Cyberpsychology, Behavior, and Social Networking, 21*(3), 205-209.
Wing, L. (1981). Asperger's syndrome. *A Clinical Account Psychological Medicine, 11*(1), 115–129.
Woodbury-Smith, M., Clare, I. C., Holland, A., & Kearns, A. (2006). High functioning autistic spectrum disorder offending and other law breaking: findings from a community sample. *The Journal of Forensic Psychiatry and Psychology, 17*(1), 108–120.
Woodbury-Smith, M. R., Clare, I. C. H., Holland, A. J., Watson, P. C., Bambrick, M., Kearns, A., & Staufenberg, E. (2010). Circumscribed interests and 'offenders' with autism spectrum disorders: a case-control study. *Journal of Forensic Psychiatry & Psychology, 21*(3), 366–377.

Woodbury-Smith, M. R., Robinson, J., Wheelwright, S., & Baron-Cohen, S. (2005). Screening adults for Asperger syndrome using the AQ: A preliminary study of its diagnostic validity in clinical practice. *Journal of Autism and Developmental Disorders, 35*(3), 331–335.

Mark Brosnan is Professor of Psychology at the University of Bath (in the UK) and Director of the Centre for Applied Autism Research (CAAR: go.bath.ac.uk/caar). I have 20 years' experience working with members of the autistic community. Together we have co-designed and co-developed a range of digital technologies to help support the autism community. These include the Stories Online For Autism app (sofa-app.org) and Building Evidence for Technology and Autism project (BETA-project.org). This chapter emerged from a Cybercrime Project sponsored by Barclays Bank and the National Crime Agency, collaborating with Research Autism. The other researchers were Katy-Louise Payne, Ailsa Russell, Richard Mills, Katie Maras and Dheeraj Rai. I am a Chartered Psychologist with the British Psychological Society, a member of the Scientific Review Panel of the charity Autistica and a trustee of the charity Autism Wessex.

Chapter 11
Violent Behavior in Autism and Asperger's Disorder

Clare S. Allely

Violent Behavior in Autism and Asperger's Disorder

Media reports of violent crime committed by individuals with ASD and some academic studies have led to the idea that there is a relationship between ASD and violent behavior (Allen et al., 2008; Brewer et al., 2017; Maras et al., 2015; Mukaddes & Topcu, 2006; Murphy, 2010). It has also been suggested that the prevalence of ASD in the prison population is greater than that found in the general population (Scragg & Shah, 1994). However, numerous follow-up studies have argued that, compared to the general population, individuals with ASD are no more likely to engage in violent criminal behavior (Ghaziuddin et al., 1991; Hippler et al., 2010; Wing, 1981) and some studies have even suggested that they may be *less* likely (Lundström et al., 2014; Mouridsen et al., 2008; Woodbury-Smith et al., 2006). It is important to note here that much of the earlier research looking at violent behavior and autism focused on individuals with Asperger's disorder specifically (e.g., Baron-Cohen, 1988). However, the current conceptualization of ASD includes autistic disorder, Asperger's disorder, childhood disintegrative disorder, or the catch-all diagnosis of pervasive developmental disorder not otherwise specified. Individuals with developmental disabilities (e.g., ASD) have also been found to be more likely to be the victims of crime rather than the perpetrator (Modell & Mak, 2008; Sobsey et al., 1995). There is no empirical support for the idea that there exists an association between ASD and criminality (in particular violent crime) (Ghaziuddin et al., 1991; Howlin, 2004; Murrie et al., 2002).

Dr. Clare S. Allely, Reader in Forensic Psychology, School of Health and Society, University of Salford, Manchester, England and affiliate member of the Gillberg Neuropsychiatry Centre, Sahlgrenska Academy, University of Gothenburg, Gothenburg, Sweden.

C. S. Allely (✉)
School of Health and Society, University of Salford, Salford, England
e-mail: c.s.allely@salford.ac.uk

F. R. Volkmar et al. (eds.), *Handbook of Autism Spectrum Disorder and the Law*,
https://doi.org/10.1007/978-3-030-70913-6_11

In their landmark study, Hippler et al. (2010) carried out an investigation of penal register data regarding Hans Asperger's original group of 177 patients. In the case records spanning 22 years and 33 convictions, there were only three cases of bodily injury, one case of robbery and one case of violent and threatening behavior. Their investigation found that the rate and nature of offenses committed by individuals with ASD did not differ from that found in the general population (Hippler et al., 2010). From their systematic review examining in detail the literature on ASD in the criminal justice system, King and Murphy (2014) concluded that the notion that individuals with ASD are disproportionately overrepresented in the criminal justice system is not supported by evidence in the literature. The review also emphasized the limited evidence in support of the long-held notion that for certain crime types there is an over-representation of individuals with ASD. In order to avoid stigmatizing an already vulnerable group, it is imperative that such findings are stressed in any dissemination of research looking at neurodevelopmental disorders and violent offending behavior (e.g., Allely et al., 2017). Although most individuals with ASD are law-abiding (Frith, 1991; Tantam, 1991), a small subgroup does become involved with the criminal justice system (Murrie et al., 2002).

Helverschou et al. (2017) have highlighted that the studies which have investigated the association between criminality and ASD has predominantly looked at prevalence, types of crimes committed and the characteristics of ASD offenders. However, the findings have not been consistent across the studies (e.g., Mouridsen et al., 2008). Some studies have indicated that there are increased rates of offending behavior in individuals with ASD (even more so in those with Asperger's syndrome). Other studies have found that individuals with ASD are less likely to offend (Bjørkly, 2009; Cashin & Newman, 2009; King & Murphy, 2014). Moreover, individuals with ASD have been suggested to be less likely to commit certain types of offenses like probation violations and property offenses (e.g., Cheely et al., 2012; Kumagami & Matsuura, 2009) and more likely to commit other types of crime such as arson (e.g., Hare et al., 1999; Haskins & Silva, 2006; Mouridsen, 2012; Mouridsen et al., 2008), sexual offenses (e.g., Cheely et al., 2012; Kumagami & Matsuura, 2009) or assault and robbery (e.g., Cheely et al., 2012). Methodological limitations (e.g., small sample sizes; no control/comparison groups; inadequate methods for diagnosing ASD in adults) in some of the studies may explain the contradictions in findings (King & Murphy, 2014; Underwood et al., 2013) and means that any conclusions surrounding the association between offending behavior and ASD need to be interpreted with extreme caution (King & Murphy, 2014).

Case Studies

The literature has been dominated by single case reports or small case series describing individuals with an ASD who have committed violent offenses (e.g., Baron-Cohen, 1988; Barry-Walsh & Mullen, 2004; Chen et al., 2003; Chesterman & Rutter, 1993; Cooper et al., 1993; Hall & Bernal, 1995; Hollander et al., 2001; Kohn et al., 1998; Kumar et al., 2017; Mawson et al., 1985; Milton et al., 2002; Murrie et al., 2002; Silva et al., 2002a, 2002b, 2003b, 2003c, 2004; Simblett & Wilson, 1993; Tantam, 1988a, 1988b) or studies investigating the small samples of males and females detained in high secure psychiatric hospitals (Hare et al., 1999; Scragg & Shah, 1994). In one of the earliest published case studies of violence in an individual with an ASD, Baron-Cohen (1988) outlined the assessment of violence in a 21-year-old man, John, who had a diagnosis of Asperger's syndrome. When he was 17-years-old, he was sent to a remand home following his arrest for stealing. Upon leaving the remand home, he went to live with his aunt (his father's sister). During a visit from his father, he used a hammer to 'smash up' his father's car and motorbike. At 19-years of age, he was sent to a probation hostel where he was reported to have exhibited bizarre behaviors (e.g., gazing continuously into the mirror, smearing fecal matter on the walls, etc.). John then went back to stay with his aunt but shortly thereafter went to live with a friend of hers, Betty, a 71-year-old lady who he referred to as his girlfriend. During the four years they lived together, John repeatedly attacked her, resulting in him being admitted twice to his local psychiatric hospital. It was hypothesized by Baron-Cohen that an inability to appreciate the mental states of his victims (impaired theory of mind) was the factor contributing to John's violent behavior. Baron-Cohen carried out a psychometric assessment (WAIS-R) and a series of semi-structured interviews with John, his father, and Betty. Findings from these assessments and interviews supported Baron-Cohen's hypothesis that feelings and behaviors associated with the clinical features of Asperger's syndrome were the antecedents to John's violent aggression toward Betty.

Another case study was described by Mawson et al. (1985) of a man who reported having violent fantasies and an extensive interest in poisons. He also would assault women for 'idiosyncratic reasons'. For instance, striking one woman using a saw blade because she was wearing shorts, and using a screw driver to stab a woman because he disliked women drivers. Mawson and colleagues (1985) also report the case of a man who spoke openly about his attacks on people and admitted to having an extreme distaste for high-pitched sounds (in particular, soprano voices). The patient was unable and expressed no desire to restrain his impulses to attack infants and women on some occasions, particularly when they made sounds which he found distasteful (e.g., a crying baby). He was admitted to Broadmoor Hospital on a hospital order with restrictions after having attacked a baby who had been crying in a supermarket. During his time in Broadmoor, he would sometimes have sudden attacks on sources of high-pitched sound. For instance, there had been occasions where he had attacked a television or radio (Mawson et al., 1985).

Empirical Studies

The majority of the case studies reviewed above are descriptive and there are methodological limitations in some of the studies (Howlin, 2004). Further, very broad definitions of violence (including agitation, non-violent anger, damage to property, etc.) were used in some of these case studies (Bjørkly, 2009). However, there is relatively little empirical research examining offenders with ASD (Browning & Caulfield, 2011; Dein & Woodbury-Smith, 2010). Some studies have investigated the prevalence of offending behavior among patients with ASD who received treatment in a psychiatric care system or have been hospitalized (e.g., Långström et al., 2009). Other studies have examined the prevalence of ASD among people who committed crime and came in contact with the criminal justice system (e.g., Fazel et al., 2008; Siponmaa et al., 2001). A number of empirical studies, discussed below, found no evidence to support the notion that individuals with ASD are more at risk of engaging in criminal behavior (Cederlund et al., 2008; Lundström et al., 2014; Mouridsen et al., 2008; Woodbury-Smith et al., 2006).

A retrospective study of the prevalence of child neuropsychiatric disorders in young offenders (15–22 years, $n = 126$) who were consecutively referred for presentencing forensic psychiatric investigation (FPI) in Stockholm, Sweden was carried out by Siponmaa and colleagues (2001). In the sample of juvenile offenders, 15% had pervasive developmental disorder (PDD), including 12% PDD not otherwise specified (PDD-NOS) and 3% fulfilled the diagnostic criteria for Asperger's syndrome (Siponmaa et al., 2001). Compared to other prevalence studies (e.g., Scragg & Shah, 1994 based on an adult forensic population), this rate is higher and may indicate the existence of a 'true developmental difference'. Specifically, that there is an increased risk of offending behavior in individuals with ASD who are younger. Alternatively, it could simply be a reflection of the challenges in an adult being appropriately diagnosed with ASD or at all (Sevlever et al., 2013). A large Swedish epidemiological study found elevated rates of offending behavior in adolescents and adults with ASD (Fazel et al., 2008). Fazel and colleagues (2008) investigated rates of psychiatric disorders among adolescent and young adult "serious offenders" who had been referred to pre-sentence forensic psychiatric services during 1997–2001. This resulted in 3,058 individuals (90% male, mean age = 35.3 years). Patterns of psychiatric disorders in this group were compared to a group of individuals who were adult forensic referrals and age-matched general psychiatric inpatients. It is worthy to note here that criminal offenders can be referred for an extensive court-ordered presentence inpatient forensic psychiatric assessment in Sweden. Fazel and colleagues investigated the DSM-IV psychiatric diagnoses across three age categories in the criminal offenders: 15–17 years ($n = 60$), 18–21 years ($n = 300$) and 22 years and older ($n = 2{,}698$). The same age categories were applied to the individuals admitted to general psychiatric hospitals. A diagnosis of ASD was found for 8.3% ($n = 5$) of the 15–17 year-olds, 7.4% ($n = 22$) of the 18–21 year-olds and 2.6% ($n = 70$) of individuals 22 years and older (Fazel et al., 2008).

In a consecutive cohort study of young adult male offenders ($n = 270$, age 18–25 years) who had received a sentence for "hands-on" violent offences and were serving time in a Swedish prison, Billstedt and colleagues (2017) found that from the 71% who met inclusion criteria to participate, 10% fulfilled the diagnostic criteria (based on the DSM-IV) for ASD (Billstedt et al., 2017).

There has also been a number of empirical studies which have found no evidence to support the notion that individuals with ASD are more at risk of being violent or engaging in criminal behavior compared to the general population (Cederlund et al., 2008; Lundström et al., 2014; Mouridsen et al., 2008; Woodbury-Smith et al., 2006). The prevalence and pattern of criminal behavior in a population of 313 former child psychiatric in-patients with pervasive developmental disorders were studied. Mouridsen and colleagues (2008) divided patients into three subgroups (childhood autism, atypical autism and Asperger's syndrome) and compared with 933 matched controls from the general population. Age at follow-up was between 25 and 59 years. An account of convictions in the nationwide Danish Register of Criminality was used as a measure of criminal behavior. Among 113 cases with childhood autism, 0.9% had been convicted. In atypical autism ($n = 86$) and Asperger's syndrome ($n = 114$) the percentages were 8.1 and 18.4%, respectively. The corresponding rate of convictions in the comparison groups was 18.9, 14.7, and 19.6% respectively (Mouridsen et al., 2008). This finding of a lower rate of offending behavior across all three ASD groups in the study by Mouridsen and colleagues (2008) is consistent with a study published the same year.

In a prospective follow-up study of 70 males with Asperger's syndrome and 70 males with autism more than five years after original diagnosis, Cederlund and colleagues (2008) found that rates of criminal acts were not very high. However, in some cases, the offending behaviors were considered odd and reflected a lack of common sense. The majority of individuals in the Asperger's syndrome study group were extremely law-abiding. However, based on data from parental reports, seven males with Asperger's syndrome (10%) had been involved with the criminal justice system for various acts of crime, namely, (fraud ($n = 1$), harassment of police officer ($n = 1$), harassment of young woman ($n = 1$), stealing ($n = 1$), assault ($n = 1$), sexual abuse ($n = 1$) and unknown in one case). A criminality rate of 10% in this age group in Sweden is not considered unusual. However, in several cases it was noted that the criminal behaviors carried out by some of the men with Asperger's syndrome were particularly "severe" and highlighted issues surrounding perspective taking and understanding the impact and consequences of their offense, consistent with the findings from a previous study (Cederlund et al., 2008; Murphy, 2003).

Additionally, based on the population-based registers of all child and adolescent mental health services in Stockholm, Lundström and colleagues (2014) identified 3,391 children who were born between 1984 and 1994 and had a neurodevelopmental disorder. This group was compared to matched controls in relation to the risk for violent offending. Individuals with ASD were not found to be at increased risk of committing violent crime. Therefore, ASD was not found to be a risk factor for subsequent violent crime (Lundström et al., 2014). Another study found that the rate of offending behavior was even lower than that found in a well-controlled control group of individuals with no ASD diagnosis. In this study, Woodbury-Smith et al. (2006) examined the illegal behaviors of a small sample ($n = 25$) of individuals with ASD. Both self-report and "official" data suggested that the rate of offending behavior was significantly less compared to a comparison group of individuals without ASD ($n = 20$). In the ASD group, 12 (48%) reported having ever engaged in the illegal behaviors which were in the self-report schedule. However, in the comparison group this was significantly higher with 16 (80%) reporting having ever engaged in the illegal behaviors which were in the self-report schedule. Only two (8%) individuals in the ASD group were listed on the Offenders Index which supports the low level of self-reported offending. Both of the offenses were not included in the self-report questionnaire (conviction for arson and conviction for an assault on a female aged less than sixteen years). Interestingly, participants with ASD were significantly less likely to report engaging in illicit drug taking (three, 11% versus 11, 55%) but were significantly more likely to report activities which could be categorized as 'criminal damage' (five, 19%, versus none of the individuals in the control group). They were also more likely to have a greater history of violent behaviors (Woodbury-Smith et al., 2006).

There have been a number of empirical studies which have highlighted the crucial involvement of psychiatric comorbidities and other disorders such as substance use disorder in offending behavior in individuals with ASD, thus supporting the importance of the appropriate and timely assessment and management of psychiatric comorbidities in individuals with ASD to decrease the risk of violent behavior (Långström et al., 2009). For instance, over a 10-year duration in Norway, Søndenaa and colleagues (2014) investigated all forensic examination reports where there was a charge of either a violent ($n = 21$) or a sexual ($n = 12$) offense and the individual had an ASD diagnosis. Findings revealed that compared to the sex offenders, there were more severe mental health problems and less intellectual problems in the violent offenders (Søndenaa et al., 2014).

Additionally, in their study, Långström and colleagues (2009) utilized data from Swedish longitudinal registers for 422 individuals (317 with a diagnosis of autism and 105 with a diagnosis of AS) hospitalized with autistic disorder or Asperger syndrome during 1988–2000. In this sample of 422 individuals, Långström and colleagues compared those who had committed violent or sexual offenses with those who had committed no such offenses. Findings showed that two individuals with ASD had committed a sexual offense and 31 (7%) had committed a violent non-sexual crime. When autistic disorder and Asperger's syndrome are analyzed individually, 3.2% ($n = 10$) were found to have been convicted of a violent crime in the autistic disorder group. In the Asperger's syndrome group, the convictions for a violent crime were significantly higher, with 20.0% ($n = 21$) found to have committed such an offense. Consistent with the literature, comorbid psychotic and substance use disorders were found to be related to violent offending. Findings showed that in the individuals with ASD, 7% (31/422) offended violently. However, 19% (12/62) of individuals with any psychiatric comorbidity offended violently and corresponding percentages were 18% (8/44) for comorbid schizophrenia, 33% (3/9) for personality disorder and 71% (5/7) for substance misuse. Consistent with previous studies (e.g., Palermo,

2004), this study would seem to support the theory that the same sociodemographic and psychiatric disorders that are consistently found in violent offenders with no diagnosis of ASD are also found in those violent offenders with ASD (Långström et al., 2009). The data were obtained retrospectively, therefore it is possible that forensic cases of ASD were not diagnosed or misdiagnosed in the criminal registry (Sevlever et al., 2013).

Factors Which May Increase the Risk of Offending Among Individuals with ASD

Comorbid Psychopathology

When individuals with ASD commit violent or criminal acts, research indicates strongly that comorbidity is a likely factor (Im, 2016a; Newman & Ghaziuddin, 2008; Wachtel & Shorter, 2013). Some of the comorbidities commonly found in individuals with ASD include: mood disorders including anxiety and depression (e.g., Bruggink et al., 2016; Ghaziuddin et al., 2002; Hammond & Hoffman, 2014; Maddox & White, 2015; Matson & Williams, 2014; Moss et al., 2015) and behavioral disorders including attention-deficit/hyperactivity disorder (ADHD) (e.g., Antshel et al., 2016; Chen et al., 2015; Taylor et al., 2015).

Newman and Ghaziuddin (2008) carried out a review to investigate the role that psychiatric factors play in contributing to criminal behavior in individuals with ASD. The majority of the 17 publications identified in the review which met the inclusion criteria were single case reports. In the 17 publications, there was a total of 37 cases. At the time of the offense, a definite psychiatric disorder was found in 11 of these cases (29.7%) and a probable psychiatric disorder was found in 20 cases (54%). They found that the majority of the literature on violent offenders with ASD shows that these individuals also had numerous psychiatric comorbidities (e.g., conduct disorder, depression, schizoaffective disorder). These psychiatric disorders (conduct disorder being a notable exception) by themselves do not cause a substantial additional risk of violent offending behavior. The presence of psychiatric comorbidities in individuals with ASD (and the relationship between the two) who offend needs more investigation (Newman & Ghaziuddin, 2008).

Numerous studies have found a significantly higher prevalence of psychiatric disorders in individuals with ASD compared to the general population (see Helverschou et al., 2011). Studies have found that comorbid psychiatric disorders (such as psychotic, personality, substance abuse) may increase the risk of violent behavior in individuals with ASD (Lazaratou et al., 2016; Newman & Ghaziuddin, 2008). In offenders with ASD, studies have found a history of psychiatric comorbidities to be common (e.g., Ghaziuddin et al., 1998; Gillberg & Billstedt, 2000; Tantam, 2003; Wing, 1981), with the most frequent comorbidities being depression, schizophrenia and anxiety (Allen et al., 2008).

Acknowledging that individuals with ASD are no more likely to engage in violent behavior compared to individuals without ASD, Wachtel and Shorter (2013) have argued that in some of the tragic cases of mass murder ASD in addition to psychosis were involved. They detail three issues related to the notion of individuals with comorbid ASD and psychosis who commit violent offending. First, studies have shown that there is an increased risk of psychiatric comorbidity (such as psychosis) which was found to be associated with violent behavior. In a study based on 122 adults with normal-intelligence-ASD recruited from Swedish and Parisian expert diagnostic centers, mood disorders were identified as the most common comorbidity (with 53% of the 122 adults experiencing this). Additionally, psychotic illness was found in 12% (Hofvander et al., 2009). This increased prevalence is consistent with the findings from other studies (e.g., Nylander et al., 2008; Skokauskas & Gallagher, 2010). Second, in the last few decades, the content of psychotic ideation has become significantly more violent and lethal (Junginger, 1990, 1996). Third, it may be the case that there is a greater propensity to act on psychotic impulses compared to those without ASD. This possibility needs to be explored further. In sum, Wachtel and Shorter (2013) advocate the importance of recognizing the increased susceptibility of individuals with ASD to psychotic illness in order to raise the chance that they can be identified and appropriate intervention can be delivered in order to try and reduce potential violent outcomes.

Haw et al. (2013) based on a sample of 51 individuals with ASD and 43 controls with no ASD diagnosis, found that nearly 75% of the individuals with ASD had a comorbid psychiatric disorder (the most common being schizophrenia). However, uncommon in this group were personality disorder and drug and alcohol disorders which was not the case with the control group. Lifetime sexually inappropriate behavior and physical violence and medication non-compliance were also less common in the ASD group. However, a lifetime history of physical violence was found in 78% and a third had been convicted for grievous bodily harm (GBH) or homicide. Haw and colleagues also report that sometimes the offending behavior was atypical in nature and some received convictions for unusual offending behaviors including harassment and stalking (Haw et al., 2013).

In his study, Murphy (2003) has a group of 13 male adult patients with ASD and compared this group with two comparison groups of matched male patients with schizophrenia and personality disorder, respectively, in a special hospital. He found reduced rates of previous violence, substance abuse and less violent index offenses in the group of patients with ASD compared to the two other patient groups. Woodbury-Smith and colleagues (2005) investigated whether there is any relationship between the vulnerability to engage in offending behavior and cognitive impairments in individuals with ASD. To investigate this question, they had a group of 21 adults with ASD and a history of offending, a group of 23 adults with ASD and no offending history, and a general population group of 23 people with no diagnosis of ASD. Findings showed that the ASD offenders exhibited a significantly increased impairment in recognition of emotional expressions of fear (but no difference in theory of mind, executive function, and recognition of facial expressions of sadness) when compared with their non-offending peers (Woodbury-Smith et al., 2005).

Heeramun and colleagues (2017) examined data from the Stockholm Youth Cohort which is a total population-based record-linkage cohort based in Stockholm County in Sweden. It consists of 295,734 individuals followed up between the ages of 15 and 27 years. A recorded ASD diagnosis was found in 5,739 individuals of the cohort. Convictions for violent crimes were identified based on data from the Swedish National Crime Register which was the main outcome measure. Initially, it appeared that individuals with ASD were at increased risk of violent offending, particularly those individuals with ASD with no intellectual disability. However, after the comorbidities, namely, attention-deficit/hyperactivity disorder (ADHD) or conduct disorder (CD) were controlled for, these associations significantly reduced. The strongest predictors of violent criminality in individuals with ASD included: male sex; psychiatric conditions; parental criminal; psychiatric history and socioeconomic characteristics. Therefore, the association which was initially found between ASD and violent crimes at a population level was explained by comorbid psychiatric disorders, namely, ADHD and conduct disorder. It is also important to note here that someone with ASD under trial may be more likely to be convicted due to being more adherent to the truth, for example (see Maras & Bowler, 2012; Maras et al., 2017; Woodbury-Smith & Dein, 2014) which may introduce a degree of 'differential outcome misclassification bias'. Moreover, in the cohort, a diagnosis of attention-deficit/hyperactivity disorder (ADHD) or conduct disorder (CD) was identified in more than one-fourth of the individuals with ASD. Additionally, and perhaps most importantly, the co-existence of these disorders with ASD significantly influenced convictions for violent criminality. Indeed, it has been well-established in the literature that there is an increased risk of antisocial and violent behavior in children diagnosed with ADHD or CD (e.g., Norén Selinus et al., 2015; Satterfield et al., 2007). Lastly, this study found that, when compared to those with no autism diagnosis, there was a reduced risk of convictions in individuals with an autism diagnosis (Heeramun et al., 2017).

How Certain Diagnostically Relevant Traits Among Individuals with ASD May Contribute to Their Offending

It is crucial to consider how the unique features of ASD may contribute to violence. There are a number of case studies in the literature of young adults which have outlined the way in which unique features of ASD (e.g., impaired social understanding and restricted empathy; lack of perspective taking; social naivety; pursuit of special circumscribed interests, especially when these involve morbid fascination with violence) may result in violent offending behavior in some kinds of provocative circumstances (e.g., Baron-Cohen, 1988; Barry-Walsh & Mullen, 2004; Haskins & Silva, 2006; Kohn et al., 1998; Lazaratou et al., 2016; Murrie et al., 2002). Surprisingly, the association between circumscribed interests in individuals with ASD and violence is not well understood.

However, a number of case reports indicate a direct relationship. Everall and LeCouteur (1990), Hare and colleagues (1999) and Barry-Walsh and Mullen (2004) all report case studies involving individuals whose offending escalated from an interest and preoccupation with fire to arson. Hare and colleagues (1999) also report the case where the individual had an interest in knives and was convicted of unlawful wounding. The relationship between the interest and the offending behavior has in other cases appeared to be not as strong. For instance, Tantam (1988a, 1988b) reported a case of a person who was fascinated with National Socialism and put on a Nazi uniform before he assaulted a soldier. Case reports also describe individuals where the content of the circumscribed interest does not appear to be relevant and what is important and problematic in these cases is the *intensity* with which the interest is pursued irrespective of impact or potential consequences (Woodbury-Smith et al., 2010). An example of this would be the case presented by Chen and colleagues (2003) of repeated stealing and the collecting behaviors in a 21-year-old male patient who developed this obstinate stealing behavior when he was 17-years-old. He would collect objects such as paper, boxes, cups and plastic bags. The objects he had stolen or collected were hoarded in his living room. Chen and colleagues highlight that he would act under obsessive impulses when committing theft and collecting. Moreover, when these acts were prohibited, he would exhibit aggressive attitudes and would also be easily annoyed if others touched his collections (Chen et al., 2003).

Woodbury-Smith and colleagues (2010) compared the circumscribed interests of a group of 21 intellectually able 'offenders' with a diagnosis of ASD (18 males and three females; mean age: 35.4 years, SD: 11.6) to those of 23 individuals with no 'offending' history (20 males and three females; mean age: 29.7, SD: 7.9). 'Offenders' were found to be significantly more likely to report interests rated as having a 'violent' content. The 'index offense' appeared to be related to his or her interest(s) in 29% of the sample. Woodbury-Smith and colleagues' study supports the theory that a circumscribed interest which has a violent content (involving threat or harm to others) raises the risk of the individuals with ASD engaging in offending behavior. Additionally, some of the participants described how their circumscribed interests began in childhood (remaining unchanged into adulthood) which indicate the importance of the early identification of individuals with 'violent' interests so that timely support and intervention can be given (Woodbury-Smith et al., 2010).

Medical Factors

To date, there has been little research focus on the medical factors that may contribute to violence in some individuals with ASD (Ghaziuddin, 2005).

History of Psychological Trauma

One potential contributory factor to violence in individuals with ASD which has been relatively unexplored is a history of psychological trauma (Im, 2016b). To date, there have been just a few published reports which have investigated the possible contributory role of this factor (e.g., Kawakami et al., 2012; Mandell et al., 2005; Mehtar & Mukaddes, 2011). Im (2016b) investigated the mechanisms that may underlie the association between violence and a history of trauma in individuals with ASD and puts forward the suggestion that individuals with ASD may "possess sensitized prefrontal-cortical-limbic networks that are overloaded in the face of trauma, leading to unchecked limbic output that produces violent behavior, and/or cognitive dysfunction (including deficits in theory of mind, central coherence, and executive function) that impacts trauma processing in ways that portend violence" (p. 184). Future research is needed to investigate the possibility of individuals with ASD having sensitized prefrontal-cortical-limbic networks that are overloaded in the face of trauma and to study if there is an increased risk of violent behavior as a result of trauma in individuals with ASD. In order to study this, Im (2016b) recommends that when evaluating all individuals (as well as those with ASD) clinical and forensic professionals should obtain a trauma history.

Summary

There is some degree of inconsistency in the findings in terms of whether there is an association between ASD and violent offending. One explanation for the inconsistency in findings across all the prevalence studies could be the different methodological or diagnostic approaches used (Haskins & Silva, 2006). However, research indicates "the presence of at least some extant relationship that should be considered, although further research with large representative samples to validate the risk remains necessary" (Lerner et al., 2012: 179). In order to investigate whether individuals with ASD are more violent, research studies should adopt a prospective, community-based design. It also needs to comprise of two groups: individuals with ASD and those without ASD (those without ASD needs to be matched on a number of factors including age; sex; comorbidities; education attainment, etc.) (Im, 2016a).

Single and Multiple Homicide in Autism and Asperger's Disorder

ASD and Single Homicide

This chapter has so far considered all types of criminal behavior. However, there is also more specific concern that people with ASD may be involved in more serious crimes, including single and multiple homicide. Murphy (2010) outlines a case study of a young man (AB) with a diagnosis of ASD who was convicted of manslaughter and subsequently admitted to high-security psychiatric care (HSPC). When AB was assessed within the HSPC, he was 21 years old, on remand following a charge of murder. He was later convicted of manslaughter and received a discretionary life sentence. Several independent professionals suspected that AB may have an ASD while he was on remand. However, the diagnosis of ASD was only made during his admissions assessment to HSPC. ASD was the primary diagnosis. However, during times of stress, there was also the presence of psychotic symptoms. The victim was AB's work supervisor. A group of teenage girls who had been eating in the restaurant which AB was cleaning had apparently begun to taunt him, using straws to blow pieces of carrot at him, for instance. This made AB angry and anxious as his job was to keep the restaurant clean, particularly as restaurant inspectors were due to make an inspection that day. AB also reported significant levels of anxiety due to changes in break times. AB was apparently unable to handle the girls appropriately and ended up punching one of them in the face which was witnessed by his supervisor. AB was later dismissed from his job. He was tearful, blaming his supervisor for giving out free food to the girls, and said that he would kill her. AB then left the restaurant and bought a knife from a local hardware store, returned to the restaurant and stabbed his supervisor several times. AB felt he was justified in his assault of the girl, stating that he was "protecting company property." He blamed his supervisor for giving out free food which was "against company rules," failing to appreciate that this "free food" was part of the restaurant's healthy eating campaign. AB was considered fit to plead using the conventional Pritchard criteria. However, his competence to stand trial was called in to question due to the number of aspects of his limited decision-making (MacKay, 2007). Significant cognitive difficulties (e.g., with perspective taking, cognitive rigidity, ability to prioritize information; separate relevant from irrelevant information) were clearly evident in this case. AB knew that it was wrong to kill, however he failed to appreciate the consequences of his actions. He also felt justified in having killed his victim (Murphy, 2010).

A case study was described of a 10-year-old girl (OG) with a diagnosis of Autistic Disorder (also a history of epilepsy), who threw her 6-month-old sister out of a fifth-floor window, killing her (Mukaddes & Topcu, 2006). OG was the product of an unwanted and unplanned pregnancy. In their paper, Mukaddes and Topcu (2006) outlined a number of potential risk factors in this case which may be related to OG's violence. For instance, she was raised in a disorganized family environment. Her parents, particularly her mother, had negative feelings toward her, were often physically abusive, failed to protect her from physical abuse from others and delayed seeking help from mental health professionals. Her parents never provided her with appropriate supervision and did not go to any treatment program for her. She was referred to the authors' Child Psychiatry Department by her aunts. Mukaddes and Topcu (2006) reported that there was a persistent pattern in the aggressive-impulsive behavior exhibited by OG. Hostility directed to her 6-month-old sister began one month before she killed her. First, she started to hit her sister frequently. The mother, being aware of this, would watch them carefully. When the younger sister was by herself, their mother would shut the door in order to prevent the autistic child from going into her room. The one time that their mother forgot to close the door, OG went into her little sister's room and threw her out of the fifth-floor window. The fact that OG's aggression toward her baby sister commenced one month before she killed her suddenly and with little planning led the authors to consider this case to be a "homicide" rather than due to stereotypical behavior (Mukaddes & Topcu, 2006). However, it is important to note here that both may well have contributed to varying degrees to the homicide.

Schwartz-Watts (2005) described three defendants charged with homicide who also had Asperger's disorder. In all three cases, the diagnosis was speculated to be related to the charge. A prior diagnosis of an ASD (specifically, pervasive developmental disorder) was only found in one of the defendants. In the other two cases, the forensic psychiatrist was the first professional to make the diagnosis. The first case described by Schwartz-Watts (2005) involved a 22-year-old Hispanic male who was charged with the murder of an eight-year-old boy. The defendant had a diagnosis of an ASD (specifically, pervasive developmental disorder) beginning at the age of five years. His family was in the military and they frequently had to move to location. In each new school, his teachers sent him for evaluation due to his impaired functioning. None of the recommended treatments were followed up by his parents. When he was in school he attended special education classes and was frequently bullied. The defendant's intelligence was within the normal range. He was hospitalized following a Tylenol overdose, three months before his offense. His parents would not let him return home and he then slept in their tool shed (without their knowledge). On the day of the incident he had left work at the local sandwich shop and purchased beer at the local grocery store. He drank the beer then, as he walked to a place he was going to spend the evening, an eight-year-old on a bicycle approached him and asked him about Game Boy games. He reported asking the boy to leave him alone and that the boy ran over his foot with his bicycle. He recalled taking out his gun and shooting the boy. In this case, the court-ordered forensic psychiatrist and the retained forensic psychiatrist was in agreement that the defendant's diagnosis was a contributory factor relating to his charge. Directly preceding his attack, the defendant had experienced "tactile defensiveness." Following neurological examination, it was established that the defendant had an oversensitivity to touch on both his hands and feet. Consistent with his stereotyped interests, the defendant also had a fascination with and collection of guns and swords. The defendant was sentenced to life in prison rather than given the death penalty. He has since had a fair adjustment to incarceration and is housed in a unit with other mentally disordered inmates (Schwartz-Watts, 2005).

The second case was a 35-year-old Pakistani male (with no prior ASD diagnosis) charged with the murder of a neighbor who entered his apartment while the defendant was on the telephone to a friend. The defendant tried to reason with the neighbor, who was alleging the defendant owed him money for a grill. The victim struck the defendant about the face, hitting his glasses. The defendant then made his way to his bedroom where he kept guns and the victim followed him. The defendant repeatedly shot the victim. He then retrieved another gun from his bedroom and fired another shot into the victim's head. In this case, an ASD diagnosis was only made during the court proceedings. Specifically, the diagnosis of Asperger's disorder was based on interviews conducted with the defendant and also his family, neuropsychological testing and a consultation from a Neurologist who had significant experience in diagnosing autism. The defendant reported his oversensitivity when someone touched his glasses. Additionally, he failed to appreciate the nature of "overkill" (overkill being the excessive use of force or action that goes further than what is necessary to achieve the goal) of his victim. Specifically, his response when asked why he retrieved the second gun to shoot the victim in the head (the "overkill"), was that he had watched an episode of "America's Most Wanted," in which someone was shot a number of times but was still alive. Also, the defendant had reported having watched numerous horror movies involving someone being shot and then being able to get up and attack after. The judge directed a verdict of self-defense during the jury trial and the defendant was subsequently acquitted of all charges (Schwartz-Watts, 2005). The paper does not detail exactly what were considered in this case to be the mitigating factors.

The third case involved a 20-year-old Hispanic man (with no prior diagnosis of ASD) who was charged with murdering the father of his girlfriend. Before the murder, the father had phoned the defendant asking him to collect some personal belongings in his car which was at his daughter's beach house. During the court proceedings, the defendant stated that he had forgotten to give the father one item (a belt) and the father had then walked to his car to get it. As he approached the car, the defendant removed a shotgun from the trunk of his car and shot the father as he approached. The defendant had an impaired ability to recognize the facial expression (as well as the non-verbal behaviors) of his victim, which is a common feature in individuals with ASD (e.g., Griffiths et al., 2017; Pelphrey et al., 2002; Serra et al., 2003; Song & Hakoda, 2017). He consistently maintained that he was defending himself stating that his victim looked as if he was going to cause him harm. He was given a conviction for murder and was sentenced to life in prison. Interestingly, a psychiatric testimony during his trial was not permitted by the Judge. He was subsequently housed in a unit for mentally disordered offenders (Schwartz-Watts, 2005).

Lazaratou et al. (2016) review a case of a 17-year-old boy (X) with Asperger's syndrome charged with matricide. He had no history of aggression and violent behavior or an established history of comorbid disorder. Based on accounts from the father of X, X's mother had never accepted her son's diagnosis and throughout childhood and adolescence (and leading up to the national university entrance exams that X's mother wanted him to take and pass) had put a lot of pressure on X to achieve academically. If he did not complete his homework or comply with what she wanted she would get angry and harsh with X (also making threats and derogatory statements regarding his abilities as well as depriving him of things he enjoyed doing such as his play station). Although not agreeing with the harsh approach his wife took, X's father never intervened. During grade 12, X started to develop an interest in sex and would spend hours online on sites relating to sex and gender identity themes. X was reported by his father to have difficulties in managing and controlling the impulses arising from his increased and unsatisfied sexual drive. He demonstrated little understanding of social codes. On one occasion he touched his teacher in a sexually inappropriate manner and did not appear to understand the need to apologize to his teacher for this behavior. A few times, he also asked his father to find him a woman or would make remarks which were inappropriate (e.g., his sexual desires could be satisfied by his mother). At this time, X's relationship with his mother took on some sexual overtones. On one occasion, X lifted up his mother's skirt to "feel her up." X was noted to have become increasingly withdrawn in the five months preceding his crime. He was also more irritable, and prone to outbursts of anger and aggression toward his mother. There were isolated incidents where X would push his mother. X's alleged act of matricide is suggested by Lazaratou and colleagues to be due to a confrontational attack (the concept "confrontational attack" is not defined in their paper) coupled with an accumulation of stressful events over time. It has been posited that aggression exhibited by individuals with ASD is due to "time slip" (Tochimoto et al., 2011), whereby individuals re-experience (with the emotions) trivial events that have occurred in their past as if they were taking place in the present—which, it was suggested, was true for X. Given the difficulties in understanding the intentions of others, it is possible that X misinterpreted the intention of his mother's behavior, perceiving it as highly threatening (Newman & Ghaziuddin, 2008). The case illustrates the importance of understanding that ASD-related vulnerabilities can be compounded by cumulative stress leading to potentially negative outcomes (Lazaratou et al., 2016).

ASD and Multiple Homicide

There is a very small subgroup of individuals with ASD who exhibit extreme violent offending (such as mass violence) and it has been suggested that other factors, such as adverse childhood experiences, are important contributory factors toward the extreme violence (Allely et al., 2014). Silva et al. (2004) suggest that there may be an association between ASD and serial homicidal behavior. Previous published case study reports by the same group indicated that there is a close association between autism spectrum psychopathology and violent behavior in a subgroup of serial killers (e.g., Silva et al., 2002a, 2002b; 2003a). These papers indicate that there may be some behavioral characteristics associated with ASD that may contribute to the risk of serial homicide. Additionally, Silva and colleagues argue that the high heritability of ASD (e.g., Colvert et al., 2015; Sandin et al., 2014; Santangelo & Folstein, 1999; Tick et al., 2016) and well-established neuropsychiatric nature of ASD (Povinelli & Preuss, 1995; Schultz et al., 2000) provide some support to the notion of "the possibility that autistic psychopathology may represent a complex set of biological markers of value in the study of sexual serial homicide" (Silva et al., 2004: 788).

Fitzgerald (2015) has argued that it is not uncommon for school shootings and mass killings to be carried out by individuals with neurodevelopmental disorders, who often displayed warning indicators in the weeks, months or years leading up to their attack. In order to investigate this, Allely et al. (2017) used the 73 mass shooting events identified by Mother Jones (motherjones.com) in their database for potential features of ASD. There are 73 mass shooting events but this included two mass shooting events which involved two perpetrators which meant that 75 mass shooter cases were studied. Of the total 75 mass shooter cases, information was found for six cases (8%) that referred to a formal diagnosis of an ASD or strong suggestions of possible ASD was made by family and friends (Chris Harper Mercer; Adam Lanza; James Holmes; Ian Stawicki; Seung Hui Cho, and Dean Allen Mellberg). This is significantly higher than the prevalence found in the general population (of approximately 1.5%). An additional 16 cases (21% of the total sample) where there were some indications of traits of ASD (according to the authors based on reports of the individual) were identified (Pedro Vargas; Andrew Engeldinger; Wade Michael Page; Jared Loughner; Nidal Malik Hasan; Jiverly Wong; Steven Kazmierczak; Kyle Aaron Huff; Jeffrey Weise; Terry Michael Ratzmann; Michael McDermott; Larry Gene Ashbrook; Eric Harris; Gang Lu; George Hennard and Dylan Klebold). However, it is important that these findings are treated with caution as they are only potential traits of ASD and, therefore, do not equate with a diagnosis. It is important that it is highlighted that this study is not advancing the notion that individuals with ASD are more likely to be mass shooters or engage in extreme acts of violence. However, it does suggest that there may be a very small subgroup of individuals with ASD who are more likely to become serious offenders.

What Allely and colleagues described in a very small subgroup of individuals with ASD has also been considered by Faccini (2016) in his theoretical paper where he applied two different models to understand the pathway to intended mass violence in the case of Adam Lanza. The three factors of autism-based deficits, psychopathology and deficient psychosocial development were integrated into the "Path to Intended Violence" model in order to attempt to understand the pathway to mass shooting in the minority of individuals with ASD who perpetrate such attacks. According to Calhoun and Weston (2003), The "Path to Violence" model comprises six behavioral stages. These six behavioral stages include: holding a grievance (e.g., due to a perceived sense of injustice, a threat or loss, a need for fame, or revenge), ideation (believing violence to be the only option, sharing one's thoughts with others, or modeling oneself after other assailants—such as high profile mass shooters), research and planning (obtaining information on one's target, or stalking the target), preparations (obtaining one's costume, weapon(s), equipment, transportation, or engaging in "final act" behaviors), breach (assessing levels of security, devising "sneaky or covert approach") and, lastly, attack (Allely et al., 2017; Faccini, 2010).

In order to show how combining the two models can be applied to try to understand the process which leads to someone carrying out a mass shooting attack, Faccini (2016) used the case of the serial murderer, Adam Lanza, as exemplification. He showed how Lanza experienced a sense of a threatening world due to the presence of a variety of comorbid problems such as sensory processing difficulties, contamination rituals, anxiety and exaggerated fears. Lanza's arrival at the first stage of the path to intended violence (grievance) was his perception of a threatening world which was "exacerbated by progressive losses." In Lanza's case "the nexus of the two models occurred when autistic restricted interests in death and violence, combined with depression and suicidal ideation, progressed into a fascination and restricted interest in mass shootings and shooters" (Faccini, 2016: 1). Consistent with the second of six stages ("ideation") in the Path to Violence model, Lanza had a fascination with weapons and mass murderers which subsequently lead to the mass shooting in Newtown. Faccini (2016) argues that this model "presents with substantial face validity when applied to the mass shooting" (p. 1). This model has also recently been applied to a number of other contemporary mass shooters (see: Allely & Faccini, 2017, 2019; Faccini & Allely, 2016a, 2016b).

Conclusion

It is crucial that we develop an increased understanding about some of the factors which contributed to different types of offending behavior in individuals with ASD in order to inform preventative measures and develop more effective services for those who do become involved in the criminal justice system (Helverschou et al., 2017). In their systematic review, Melvin and colleagues (2017) highlighted the need for more robust research to investigate the effectiveness and outcomes of offending behavior treatment programs for individuals with ASD. The majority of the studies they identified in their review recognized the challenges in delivering effective treatment for offenders with ASD (e.g., no ASD-specific interventions being available and some current treatments not being appropriate for those with ASD) (Melvin et al., 2017). Given that a small subgroup of individuals with ASD do come into contact with the criminal justice system (North et al., 2008), specific legal education delivered to all children and adolescents with ASD may be useful. This legal education would give specific scenarios of situations that individuals might find themselves in. These examples would be developed and informed by the findings from published forensic literature on ASD. This education could also be delivered in a variety of domains (e.g., public schooling, special education and vocational rehabilitation programs for adults) (Lerner et al., 2012). Bjørkly (2009) has recommended that future studies investigating ASD and offending behaviors (e.g., sexual offending; arson; homicide, etc.) adopt a prospective design. There also needs to be more sensitive and reliable measurement and analysis of the relative contribution of the various features of ASD symptomology, and also use of differentiated measures and analysis in relation to severity levels of violence. It would also be useful to study the association between types of aggressive behavior (e.g., physical, psychological and sexual violence) and ASD (Bjørkly, 2009).

Recommended Resources

The Advocate's Gateway is hosted by the Inns of Court College of Advocacy (ICCA, formerly the ATC). See www.theadvocatesgateway.org. The website's guidance has been widely endorsed by the senior judiciary both in England and Wales and in Northern Ireland, for example, see R v Lubemba [2014] EWCA Crim 2064 and The Right Honourable Lord Justice Gillen/The Review Group, Review of Civil and Family Justice: The Review Group's Draft Report on Civil Justice (JSB 2016) 199, para 14.75.

References

Allely, C. S., & Faccini, L. (2017). "Path to intended violence" model to understand mass violence in the case of Elliot Rodger. *Aggression and Violent Behavior, 37,* 201–209.

Allely, C. S., & Faccini, L. (2019). Clinical profile, risk, and critical factors and the application of the "path toward intended violence" model in the case of mass shooter Dylann Roof. *Deviant Behavior, 40*(6), 672–689.

Allely, C. S., Minnis, H., Thompson, L., Wilson, P., & Gillberg, C. (2014). Neurodevelopmental and psychosocial risk factors in serial killers and mass murderers. *Aggression and Violent Behavior, 19*(3), 288–301.

Allely, C. S., Wilson, P., Minnis, H., Thompson, L., Yaksic, E., & Gillberg, C. (2017). Violence is rare in autism: When it does occur, is it sometimes extreme? *The Journal of Psychology, 151*(1), 49–68.

Allen, D., Evans, C., Hider, A., Hawkins, S., Peckett, H., & Morgan, H. (2008). Offending behaviour in adults with Asperger syndrome. *Journal of Autism and Developmental Disorders, 38*(4), 748–758.

Antshel, K. M., Zhang-James, Y., Wagner, K., Ledesma, A., & Faraone, S. V. (2016). An update on the comorbidity of ASD and ADHD: A focus on clinical management. *Expert Review of Neurotherapeutics, 16*(3), 279–293.

Baron-Cohen, S. (1988). An assessment of violence in a young man with Asperger's syndrome. *Journal of Child Psychology and Psychiatry, 29*(3), 351–360.

Barry-Walsh, J. B., & Mullen, P. E. (2004). Forensic aspects of Asperger's Syndrome. *Journal of Forensic Psychiatry and Psychology, 15*(1), 96–107.

Billstedt, E., Anckarsäter, H., Wallinius, M., & Hofvander, B. (2017). Neurodevelopmental disorders in young violent offenders: Overlap and background characteristics. *Psychiatry Research, 252,* 234–241.

Bjørkly, S. (2009). Risk and dynamics of violence in Asperger's syndrome: A systematic review of the literature. *Aggression and Violent Behavior, 14*(5), 306–312.

Brewer, N., Zoanetti, J., & Young, R. L. (2017). The influence of media suggestions about links between criminality and autism spectrum disorder. *Autism, 21*(1), 117–121.

Browning, A., & Caulfield, L. (2011). The prevalence and treatment of people with Asperger's Syndrome in the criminal justice system. *Criminology and Criminal Justice, 11*(2), 165–180.

Bruggink, A., Huisman, S., Vuijk, R., Kraaij, V., & Garnefski, N. (2016). Cognitive emotion regulation, anxiety and depression in adults with autism spectrum disorder. *Research in Autism Spectrum Disorders, 22,* 34–44.

Calhoun, F. S., & Weston, S. W. (2003). *Contemporary threat management: A practical guide for identifying, assessing, and managing individuals of violent intent.* Specialized Training Services.

Cashin, A., & Newman, C. (2009). Autism in the criminal justice detention system: A review of the literature. *Journal of Forensic Nursing, 5*(2), 70–75.

Cederlund, M., Hagberg, B., Billstedt, E., Gillberg, I. C., & Gillberg, C. (2008). Asperger syndrome and autism: A comparative longitudinal follow-up study more than 5 years after original diagnosis. *Journal of Autism and Developmental Disorders, 38*(1), 72–85.

Cheely, C. A., Carpenter, L. A., Letourneau, E. J., Nicholas, J. S., Charles, J., King, L. B. (2012). The prevalence of youth with autism spectrum disorders in the criminal justice system. *Journal of Autism and Developmental Disorders, 42*(9), 1856–1862.

Chen, M. H., Wei, H. T., Chen, L. C., Su, T. P., Bai, Y. M., Hsu, J. W., & Chen, Y. S. (2015). Autistic spectrum disorder, attention deficit hyperactivity disorder, and psychiatric comorbidities: A nationwide study. *Research in Autism Spectrum Disorders, 10,* 1–6.

Chen, P. S., Chen, S. J., Yang, Y. K., Yeh, T. L., Chen, C. C., & Lo, H. Y. (2003). Asperger's disorder: A case report of repeated stealing and the collecting behaviours of an adolescent patient. *Acta Psychiatrica Scandinavica, 107*(1), 73–76.

Chesterman, P., & Rutter, S. C. (1993). Case report: Asperger's syndrome and sexual offending. *The Journal of Forensic Psychiatry, 4*(3), 555–562.

Colvert, E., Tick, B., McEwen, F., Stewart, C., Curran, S. R., Woodhouse, E., Gillan, N., Hallett, V., Lietz, S., Garnett, T., Ronald, A., Plomin, R., Rijsdijk, F., Happé, F., & Bolton, P. (2015). Heritability of autism spectrum disorder in a UK population-based twin sample. *JAMA Psychiatry, 72*(5), 415–423.

Cooper, S. A., Mohamed, W. N., & Collacott, R. A. (1993). Possible Asperger's syndrome in a mentally handicapped transvestite offender. *Journal of Intellectual Disability Research, 37*(2), 189–194.

Dein, K., & Woodbury-Smith, M. (2010). Asperger syndrome and criminal behaviour. *Advances in Psychiatric Treatment, 16*(1), 37–43.

Everall, I. P., & Lecouteur, A. (1990). Firesetting in an adolescent boy with Asperger's syndrome. *The British Journal of Psychiatry, 157*(2), 284–287.

Faccini, L. (2010). The man who howled wolf: Diagnostic and treatment considerations for a person with ASD and impersonal repetitive fire, bomb and presidential threats. *American Journal of Forensic Psychiatry, 31*(4), 47.

Faccini, L. (2016). The application of the models of autism, psychopathology and deficient Eriksonian development and the path of intended violence to understand the Newtown shooting. *Archives of Forensic Psychology, 1*(3), 1–13.

Faccini, L., & Allely, C. S. (2016a). Mass violence in individuals with Autism Spectrum Disorder and Narcissistic Personality Disorder: A case analysis of Anders Breivik using the "Path to Intended and Terroristic Violence" model. *Aggression and Violent Behavior, 31,* 229–236.

Faccini, L., & Allely, C. S. (2016b). Mass violence in an individual with an autism spectrum disorder: A case analysis of Dean Allen Mellberg using the "Path to Intended Violence" model. *International Journal of Psychological Research, 11*(1), 1–18.

Fazel, M., Långström, N., Grann, M., & Fazel, S. (2008). Psychopathology in adolescent and young adult criminal offenders (15–21 years) in Sweden. *Social Psychiatry and Psychiatric Epidemiology, 43*(4), 319.

Fitzgerald, M. (2015). Autism and school shootings—Overlap of autism (Asperger's Syndrome) and general psychopathy. In *Autism spectrum disorder-recent advances.* InTech.

Frith, U. (1991). Asperger and his syndrome. In U. Frith (Ed.), *Autism and Asperger syndrome.* (pp. 1–36). Cambridge University Press.

Ghaziuddin, M. (2005). Violence in Autism and Asperger syndrome. In M. Ghaziuddin (Ed.), *Mental health aspects of autism and Asperger syndrome* (pp. 214–232). Jessica Kingsley Publishers.
Ghaziuddin, M., Ghaziuddin, N., & Greden, J. (2002). Depression in persons with autism: Implications for research and clinical care. *Journal of Autism and Developmental Disorders, 32*(4), 299–306.
Ghaziuddin, M., Tsai, L., & Ghaziuddin, N. (1991). Brief report: violence in Asperger syndrome, a critique. *Journal of Autism and Developmental Disorders, 21*(3), 349–354.
Ghaziuddin, M., Weidmer-Mikhail, E., & Ghaziuddin, N. (1998). Comorbidity of Asperger syndrome: A preliminary report. *Journal of Intellectual Disability Research, 42,* 279–283.
Gillberg, C., & Billstedt, E. (2000). Autism and Asperger syndrome: Coexistence with other clinical disorders. *Acta Psychiatrica Scandinavica, 102,* 321–330.
Griffiths, S., Jarrold, C., Penton-Voak, I. S., Woods, A. T., Skinner, A. L., & Munafò, M. R. (2017). Impaired recognition of basic emotions from facial expressions in young people with autism spectrum disorder: Assessing the importance of expression intensity. *Journal of Autism and Developmental Disorders, 49*(7), 1–11.
Hall, I., & Bernal, J. (1995). Asperger's syndrome and violence. *The British Journal of Psychiatry, 166*(2), 262–262.
Hammond, R. K., & Hoffman, J. M. (2014). Adolescents with high-functioning autism: An investigation of comorbid anxiety and depression. *Journal of Mental Health Research in Intellectual Disabilities, 7*(3), 246–263.
Hare, D. J., Gould, J., Mills, R., & Wing, L. (1999). *A preliminary study of individuals with autistic spectrum disorders in three special hospitals in England*. National Autistic Society.
Haskins, B. G., & Silva, J. A. (2006). Asperger's disorder and criminal behavior: Forensic-psychiatric considerations. *The Journal of the American Academy of Psychiatry, 34*(3), 374–384.
Haw, C., Radley, J., & Cooke, L. (2013). Characteristics of male autistic spectrum patients in low security: Are they different from non-autistic low secure patients? *Journal of Intellectual Disabilities and Offending Behaviour, 4*(1/2), 24–32.
Heeramun, R., Magnusson, C., Gumpert, C. H., Granath, S., Lundberg, M., Dalman, C., & Rai, D. (2017). Autism and convictions for violent crimes: population-based cohort study in Sweden. *Journal of the American Academy of Child & Adolescent Psychiatry, 56*(6), 491–497.
Helverschou, S. B., Bakken, T., & Martinsen, H. (2011). Psychiatric disorders in people with autism spectrum disorders: Phenomenology and recognition. In J. L. Matson & P. Sturmey (Eds.), *International handbook of autism and pervasive developmental disorders* (pp. 53–74). Springer.
Helverschou, S. B., Steindal, K., Nøttestad, J. A., & Howlin, P. (2017). Personal experiences of the Criminal Justice System by individuals with autism spectrum disorders. *Autism,* 1362361316685554.
Hippler, K., Viding, E., Klicpera, C., & Happé, F. (2010). Brief report: No increase in criminal convictions in Hans Asperger's original cohort. *Journal of Autism and Developmental Disorders, 40*(6), 774–780.
Hofvander, B., Delorme, R., Chaste, P., Nydén, A., Wentz, E., Ståhlberg, O., Herbrecht, E., Stopin, A., Anckarsäter, H., Gillberg, C., Leboyer, M., & Råstam, M. (2009). Psychiatric and psychosocial problems in adults with normal-intelligence autism spectrum disorders. *BMC Psychiatry, 9*(1), 35.
Hollander, E., Dolgoff-Kaspar, R., Cartwright, C., Rawitt, R., & Novotny, S. (2001). An open trial of Divalproex Sodium in autism spectrum disorders. *Journal of Clinical Psychiatry, 62,* 530–534.
Howlin, P. (2004). *Autism and Asperger syndrome* (2nd ed.). Routledge.
Im, D. S. (2016a). Template to perpetrate: An update on violence in autism spectrum disorder. *Harvard Review of Psychiatry, 24*(1), 14.
Im, D. S. (2016b). Trauma as a contributor to violence in autism spectrum disorder. *The Journal of the American Academy of Psychiatry and the Law, 44*(2), 184–192.
Junginger, J. (1990). Predicting compliance with command hallucinations. *American Journal of Psychiatry, 147*(2), 245–247.

Junginger, J. (1996). Psychosis and violence: The case for a content analysis of psychotic experience. *Schizophrenia Bulletin, 22*(1), 91–103.
Kawakami, C., Ohnishi, M., Sugiyama, T., Someki, F., Nakamura, K., & Tsujii, M. (2012). The risk factors for criminal behavior in high-functioning autism spectrum disorders (HFASDs): A comparison of childhood adversities between individuals with HFASDs who exhibit criminal behavior and those with HFASD and no criminal histories. *Research in Autism Spectrum Disorders, 6*(2), 949–957.
King, C., & Murphy, G. H. (2014). A systematic review of people with autism spectrum disorder and the criminal justice system. *Journal of Autism and Developmental Disorders, 44*(11), 2717–2733.
Kohn, Y., Fahum, T., Ratzoni, G., & Apter, A. (1998). Aggression and sexual offense in Asperger's syndrome. *The Israel Journal of Psychiatry and Related Sciences, 35*(4), 293–299.
Kumagami, T., & Matsuura, N. (2009). Prevalence of pervasive developmental disorder in juvenile court cases in Japan. *Journal of Forensic Psychiatry and Psychology, 20*(6), 974–987.
Kumar, S., Devendran, Y., Radhakrishna, A., Karanth, V., & Hongally, C. (2017). A case series of five individuals with Asperger syndrome and sexual criminality. *Journal of Mental Health and Human Behaviour, 22*(1), 63.
Långström, N., Grann, M., Ruchkin, V., Sjöstedt, G., & Fazel, S. (2009). Risk factors for violent offending in autism spectrum disorder: A national study of hospitalized individuals. *Journal of Interpersonal Violence, 24*(8), 1358–1370.
Lazaratou, H., Giannopoulou, I., Anomitri, C., & Douzenis, A. (2016). Case report: Matricide by a 17-year old boy with Asperger's syndrome. *Aggression and Violent Behavior, 31,* 61–65.
Lerner, M. D., Haque, O. S., Northrup, E. C., Lawer, L., & Bursztajn, H. J. (2012). Emerging perspectives on adolescents and young adults with high-functioning autism spectrum disorders, violence, and criminal law. *Journal of the American Academy of Psychiatry and the Law Online, 40*(2), 177–190.
Lundström, S., Forsman, M., Larsson, H., Kerekes, N., Serlachius, E., Långström, N., & Lichtenstein, P. (2014). Childhood neurodevelopmental disorders and violent criminality: A sibling control study. *Journal of Autism and Developmental Disorders, 44*(11), 2707–2716.
MacKay, R. (2007). AAPL practice guideline for the forensic evaluation of competence to stand trial: An English legal perspective. *Journal of the American Academy of Psychiatry and Law, 35*(4), 501–504.
Maddox, B. B., & White, S. W. (2015). Comorbid social anxiety disorder in adults with autism spectrum disorder. *Journal of Autism and Developmental Disorders, 45*(12), 3949–3960.
Mandell, D. S., Walrath, C. M., Manteuffel, B., Sgro, G., & Pinto-Martin, J. A. (2005). The prevalence and correlates of abuse among children with autism served in comprehensive community-based mental health settings. *Child Abuse and Neglect, 29*(12), 1359–1372.
Maras, K., Mulcahy, S., & Crane, L. (2015). Is autism linked to criminality? *Autism, 19*(5), 515–516.
Maras, K. L., & Bowler, D. M. (2012). Brief report: Suggestibility, compliance and psychological traits in high-functioning adults with autism spectrum disorder. *Research in Autism Spectrum Disorders, 6*(3), 1168–1175.
Maras, K. L., Crane, L., Mulcahy, S., Hawken, T., Cooper, P., Wurtzel, D., & Memon, A. (2017). Brief report: Autism in the courtroom: Experiences of legal professionals and the autism community. *Journal of Autism and Developmental Disorders, 47*(8), 1–11.
Matson, J. L., & Williams, L. W. (2014). Depression and mood disorders among persons with autism spectrum disorders. *Research in Developmental Disabilities, 35*(9), 2003–2007.
Mawson, D. C., Grounds, A., & Tantam, D. (1985). Violence and Asperger's syndrome: A case study. *The British Journal of Psychiatry, 147,* 566–569.
Mehtar, M., & Mukaddes, N. M. (2011). Posttraumatic stress disorder in individuals with diagnosis of autistic spectrum disorders. *Research in Autism Spectrum Disorders, 5*(1), 539–546.
Melvin, C. L., Langdon, P. E., & Murphy, G. H. (2017). Treatment effectiveness for offenders with autism spectrum conditions: A systematic review. *Psychology, Crime and Law, 23*(8), 1–29.
Milton, J., Duggan, C., Latham, A., Egan, V., & Tantam, D. (2002). Case history of co-morbid Asperger's syndrome and paraphilic behaviour. *Medicine, Science and the Law, 42*(3), 237–244.

Modell, S. J., & Mak, S. (2008). A preliminary assessment of police officers' knowledge and perceptions of persons with disabilities. *Intellectual and Developmental Disabilities, 46*(3), 183–189.

Moss, P., Howlin, P., Savage, S., Bolton, P., & Rutter, M. (2015). Self and informant reports of mental health difficulties among adults with autism findings from a long-term follow-up study. *Autism, 19*(7), 832–841.

Mouridsen, S. E. (2012). Current status of research on autism spectrum disorders and offending. *Research in Autism Spectrum Disorders, 6*(1), 79–86.

Mouridsen, S. E., Rich, B., Isager, T., & Nedergaard, N. J. (2008). Pervasive developmental disorders and criminal behavior: A case control study. *International Journal of Offender Therapy and Comparative Criminology, 52*(2), 196–205.

Mukaddes, N. M., & Topcu, Z. (2006). Case report: Homicide by a 10-year-old girl with autistic disorder. *Journal of Autism and Developmental Disorders, 36*(4), 471–474.

Murphy, D. (2003). Admission and cognitive details of male patients diagnosed with Asperger's Syndrome detained in a Special Hospital: Comparison with a schizophrenia and personality disorder sample. *The Journal of Forensic Psychiatry and Psychology, 14,* 506–524.

Murphy, D. (2010). Extreme violence in a man with an autistic spectrum disorder: Assessment and treatment within high-security psychiatric care. *The Journal of Forensic Psychiatry and Psychology, 21*(3), 462–477.

Murrie, D. C., Warren, J. I., Kristiansson, M., & Dietz, P. E. (2002). Asperger's syndrome in forensic settings. *International Journal of Forensic Mental Health, 1*(1), 59–70.

Newman, S. S., & Ghaziuddin, M. (2008). Violent crime in Asperger syndrome: The role of psychiatric comorbidity. *Journal of Autism and Developmental Disorders, 38*(10), 1848–1852.

Norén Selinus, E., Molero, Y., Lichtenstein, P., Larson, T., Lundström, S., Anckarsäter, H., & Gumpert, C. H. (2015). Childhood symptoms of ADHD overrule comorbidity in relation to psychosocial outcome at age 15: A longitudinal study. *PLoS One, 10*(9), e0137475.

North, A., Russell, A., & Gudjonsson, G. (2008). High functioning autism spectrum disorders: An investigation of psychological vulnerabilities during interrogative interview. *The Journal of Forensic Psychiatry and Psychology, 19*(3), 323–334.

Nylander, L., Lugnegard, T., & Hallerback, M. U. (2008). Autism spectrum disorders and schizophrenia spectrum disorders in adults—Is there a connection? A literature review and some suggestions for future clinical research. *Clinical Neuropsychiatry: Journal of Treatment Evaluation, 5,* 43–54.

Palermo, M. T. (2004). Pervasive developmental disorders, psychiatric comorbidities, and the law. *International Journal of Offender Therapy and Comparative Criminology, 48,* 40–48.

Pelphrey, K. A., Sasson, N. J., Reznick, J. S., Paul, G., Goldman, B. D., & Piven, J. (2002). Visual scanning of faces in autism. *Journal of Autism and Developmental Disorders, 32*(4), 249–261.

Povinelli, D. J., & Preuss, T. M. (1995). Theory of mind: Evolutionary history of a cognitive specialization. *Trends in Neurosciences, 18,* 418–424.

Sandin, S., Lichtenstein, P., Kuja-Halkola, R., Larsson, H., Hultman, C. M., & Reichenberg, A. (2014). The familial risk of autism. *JAMA, 311*(17), 1770–1777.

Santangelo, S. L., & Folstein, S. E. (1999). Autism: A genetic perspective. In H. Tager-Flusberg (Ed.), *Neurodevelopmental disorders* (pp. 431–446). MIT Press.

Satterfield, J. H., Faller, K. J., Crinella, F. M., Schell, A. M., Swanson, J. M., & Homer, L. D. (2007). A 30-year prospective follow-up study of hyperactive boys with conduct problems: Adult criminality. *Journal of the American Academy of Child and Adolescent Psychiatry, 46*(5), 601–610.

Schultz, R. T., Romanski, L. M., & Tsatsanis, K. D. (2000). Neurofunctional models of autistic disorder and Asperger syndrome: Clues from neuroimaging. In A. Klin, F. R. Volkmar, & S. S. Sparrow (Eds.), *Asperger syndrome* (pp. 172–209). Guilford.

Schwartz-Watts, D. M. (2005). Asperger's disorder and murder. *Journal of the American Academy of Psychiatry and the Law Online, 33*(3), 390–393.

Scragg, P., & Shah, A. (1994). Prevalence of Asperger's syndrome in a secure hospital. *The British Journal of Psychiatry, 165*(5), 679–682.

Serra, M., Althaus, M., De Sonneville, L. M. J., Stant, A. D., Jackson, A. E., & Minderaa, R. B. (2003). Face recognition in children with a pervasive developmental disorder not otherwise specified. *Journal of Autism and Developmental Disorders, 33*(3), 303–317.

Sevlever, M., Roth, M. E., & Gillis, J. M. (2013). Sexual abuse and offending in autism spectrum disorders. *Sexuality and Disability, 31*(2), 189–200.

Silva, J. A., Ferrari, M. M., & Leong, G. B. (2002a, February 11–16). What happened to Jeffrey? A neuropsychiatric developmental analysis of serial killing behaviour. In *Proceedings of the American Academy of Forensic Sciences* (Vol. VIII). American Academy of Forensic Sciences.

Silva, J. A., Ferrari, M. M., & Leong, G. B. (2002b, October 24–27). The neuropsychiatric developmental analysis of serial killer behaviour. Annual meeting Program, *American Academy of Psychiatry and the Law*. Newport Beach, CA and Bloomfield, CT.

Silva, J. A., Leong, G. B., & Ferrari, M. M. (2004). A neuropsychiatric developmental model of serial homicidal behavior. *Behavioral Sciences and the Law, 22*(6), 787–799.

Silva, J. A., Ferrari, M. M., & Leong, G. B. (2003a). Asperger's disorder and the origins of the Unabomber. *American Journal of Forensic Psychiatry, 24*(2), 5–44.

Silva, J. A., Smith, R. L., Leong, G. B., Hawes, E., & Ferrari, M. M. (2003b, February 11–16). The genesis of serial killing behavior in the case of Joel Rifkin using the combined BRACE/NDM approach. In *Proceedings of the American Academy of Forensic Sciences* (Vol. IX). Chicago, IL and Colorado Springs, CO: American Academy of Forensic Sciences.

Silva, J. A., Wu, J. C., & Leong, G. B. (2003c, October 16–19). Neuropsychiatric developmental analysis of sexual murder. Annual meeting Program, *American Academy of Psychiatry and the Law*. San Antonio, TX and Bloomfield, CT.

Simblett, G. J., & Wilson, D. N. (1993). Asperger's syndrome: Three cases and a discussion. *Journal of Intellectual Disability Research, 37*(1), 85–94.

Siponmaa, L., Kristiansson, M., Jonson, C., Nydén, A., & Gillberg, C. (2001). Juvenile and young adult mentally disordered offenders: The role of child neuropsychiatric disorders. *Journal of the American Academy of Psychiatry and the Law, 29,* 420–426.

Skokauskas, N., & Gallagher, L. (2010). Psychosis, affective disorders and anxiety in autistic spectrum disorder: Prevalence and nosological considerations. *Psychopathology, 43*(1), 8–16.

Sobsey, D., Wells, D., Lucardie, R., & Mansell, S. (Eds.). (1995). *Violence and disability: An annotated bibliography*. Brookes.

Søndenaa, E., Helverschou, S. B., Steindal, K., Rasmussen, K., Nilson, B., & Nøttestad, J. A. (2014). Violence and sexual offending behavior in people with autism spectrum disorder who have undergone a psychiatric forensic examination. *Psychological Reports, 115*(1), 32–43.

Song, Y., & Hakoda, Y. (2017). Selective impairment of basic emotion recognition in people with autism: Discrimination thresholds for recognition of facial expressions of varying intensities. *Journal of Autism and Developmental Disorders, 48*(6), 1–9.

Tantam, D. (1988a). Lifelong eccentricity and social isolation. I. Psychiatric, social, and forensic aspects. *British Journal of Psychiatry, 153,* 777–782.

Tantam, D. (1988b). Lifelong eccentricity and social isolation. II: Asperger's syndrome or schizoid personality disorder? *British Journal of Psychiatry, 153,* 783–791.

Tantam, D. (1991). Asperger's syndrome in adulthood. In U. Frith (Ed.), *Autism and Asperger syndrome*. Cambridge University Press.

Tantam, D. (2003). The challenge of adolescents and adults with Asperger's syndrome. *Child and Adolescent Psychiatric Clinics of North America, 12,* 143–163.

Taylor, M. J., Charman, T., & Ronald, A. (2015). Where are the strongest associations between autistic traits and traits of ADHD? Evidence from a community-based twin study. *European Child and Adolescent Psychiatry, 24*(9), 1129–1138.

Tick, B., Bolton, P., Happé, F., Rutter, M., & Rijsdijk, F. (2016). Heritability of autism spectrum disorders: A meta-analysis of twin studies. *Journal of Child Psychology and Psychiatry, 57*(5), 585–595.

Tochimoto, S., Kurata, K., & Munesue, T. (2011). Time slip' phenomenon in adolescents and adults with autism spectrum disorders: Case series. *Psychiatry and Clinical Neurosciences, 65*(4), 381–383.
Underwood, L., Forrester, A., Chaplin, E., & Mccarthy, J. (2013). Prisoners with neurodevelopmental disorders. *Journal of Intellectual Disabilities and Offending Behaviour, 4*(1–2), 17–23.
Wachtel, L. E., & Shorter, E. (2013). Autism plus psychosis: A "one-two punch" risk for tragic violence? *Medical Hypotheses, 81*, 404–409.
Wing, L. (1981). Asperger's syndrome: A clinical account. *Psychological Medicine, 11*(1), 115–129.
Woodbury-Smith, M., & Dein, K. (2014). Autism spectrum disorder (ASD) and unlawful behavior: Where do we go from here? *Journal of Autism and Developmental Disorders, 44*(11), 2734–2741.
Woodbury-Smith, M. R., Clare, I. C. H., Holland, A. J., & Kearns, A. (2006). High functioning autistic spectrum disorders, offending and other law-breaking: Findings from a community sample. *The Journal of Forensic Psychiatry and Psychology, 17*(1), 108–120.
Woodbury-Smith, M. R., Clare, I. C., Holland, A. J., Kearns, A., Staufenberg, E., & Watson, P. (2005). A case-control study of offenders with high functioning autistic spectrum disorders. *Journal of Forensic Psychiatry and Psychology, 16*(4), 747–763.
Woodbury-Smith, M., Clare, I., Holland, A. J., Watson, P. C., Bambrick, M., Kearns, A., & Staufenberg, E. (2010). Circumscribed interests and 'offenders' with autism spectrum disorders: A case-control study. *The Journal of Forensic Psychiatry and Psychology, 21*(3), 366–377.

Dr. Clare S. Allely is a Reader in Forensic Psychology at the University of Salford in Manchester, England and is an affiliate member of the Gillberg Neuropsychiatry Centre at Gothenburg University, Sweden. Clare holds a PhD in Psychology from the University of Manchester and has previously graduated with an M.A. (hons.) in Psychology from the University of Glasgow, an MRes in Psychological Research Methods from the University of Strathclyde and an M.Sc. in Forensic Psychology from Glasgow Caledonian University. Clare is also an Honorary Research Fellow in the College of Medical, Veterinary and Life Sciences affiliated to the Institute of Health and Wellbeing at the University of Glasgow. She is also an Associate of the Centre for Youth and Criminal Justice (CYCJ) at the University of Strathclyde. Clare's primary research projects and interests include the pathway to intended violence in mass shooters; serial homicide; investigating how autism symptomology can contribute to different types of offending behaviour and autism in the criminal justice system (police, court, prison and secure psychiatric care). Clare also acts as an expert witness in criminal cases and also contributes to the evidence base used in the courts on psychology and legal issues through her published work.

Chapter 12
Sexual Offending and ASD

Rachel Loftin

This chapter is focused on offending, those situations in which a person with ASD commits unlawful sexual behavior. There is a brief discussion of inappropriate sexual behavior, which may not be illegal but violates social norms and can impact placement and inclusion for people with ASD, as well as sexual behavior that is against the law. A number of factors associated with ASD may increase an individual's risk of unintentionally behaving in sexual ways that are inappropriate and/or illegal, and these are discussed, as are situations in which a behavior appears intentionally and willfully illicit but is, in fact, the result of a person's disability (counterfeit deviance). Chapter 24 of this volume, *Preventing Unlawful Sexual Behavior,* includes a helpful discussion of sexuality education and the reasons that particular aspect of social skills instruction is particularly essential for autistic people.

Intimate and sexual relationships are extremely complex social behaviors. The autism spectrum is defined by difficulty with social interactions. Laws, set up by societies as a means of guiding behavior, are often based on established societal norms. It is not surprising then that sexual relationships, ASD and the law can come into conflict.

The biggest sexual risk to autistic people is most likely victimization. One study, for instance, found that 80% of young autistic adults who were surveyed reported experiencing sexual assault (Brown-Lavoie et al., 2014). Autistic women appear to be at particularly high risk; autistic females are more likely to be victimized than both autistic males and typically developing females (Pecora et al., 2016). (For information on testimony from autistic people, including victims, see Chap. 7, Katie Maras.)

Inclusion of a chapter on sexual offending is not intended to suggest the increased likelihood of a particular autistic individual to offend or to imply that the diagnosis

---

R. Loftin (✉)
Department of Psychiatry and Behavioral Sciences, Northwestern University
Feinberg School of Medicine, Chicago, IL, USA
e-mail: Rachel.loftin@northwestern.edu

F. R. Volkmar et al. (eds.), *Handbook of Autism Spectrum Disorder and the Law*,
https://doi.org/10.1007/978-3-030-70913-6_12

of ASD allows perpetrators to escape responsibility. Rather, it is a reflection of the reality that a small subgroup of people with ASD will be charged with crimes of sexual offending, often as a result of misunderstandings and misperceptions. When criminal charges are brought against an autistic person, professionals can assist the courts and law enforcement officials to understand the role, if any, a person's autism may have played in the situation that lead to the charges.

Problem Sexual Behavior

There is some evidence that as they mature people with ASD may be at an increased risk for displaying a variety of inappropriate sexual behavior that can limit opportunities for placement and inclusion. Adolescents with ASD were found by Stokes and Kaur (2005) to engage in inappropriate sexual behaviors at a higher rate than typically developing adolescents. Problem behaviors cited included touching others without permission, touching their own private areas while in public, masturbating in public, inappropriately disrobing in public, and speaking about sexual activities. This sample included individuals diagnosed with Asperger disorder. This indicates that there were no intellectual disabilities in the sample, yet findings were consistent with older studies that included those with ASD and intellectual disabilities (e.g., Ruble & Dalrymple, 1993). Other investigations have found elevated rates of potential precursors to stalking behavior among adolescents with ASD (see Chap. 14 for a discussion; Stokes et al., 2007) and of sexually aggressive or otherwise inappropriate behavior (Hartmann, et al. 2019). The literature also includes case studies and discussions of the use of medications or hormone suppression to treat severe sexual behavior problems in people with ASD (e.g., Coshway et al., 2016; Coskun et al., 2009). Interestingly, however, other studies have found that autistic people are no more likely to offend than undiagnosed people (Mouridsen, 2012). The discrepancy in findings may be, at least in part, the result of sample selection. Studies employing truly representative samples are needed to better understand whether there are differences in rates of inappropriate sexual behavior among people with ASD.

Criminal Sexual Offending

Sexually inappropriate behaviors and their precursors often first occur within an educational environment. Many inappropriate sexual behaviors that occur in school are addressed and managed through a behavioral support plan created by school personnel, typically without input from law enforcement. However, once a person leaves the education system, the same behaviors that were addressed in school may result in criminal charges. There is rarely a transition or step-down period to help young adults adjust to such a change. For instance, consider the following case example:

> Joe, a 17-year old student, exposed his penis to his teaching assistant in high school. The education team conducted a functional behavior assessment. Results suggested that Joe exposed his penis in order to escape work demands. Thus, Joe's behavior plan dictated that each time he exposed himself, school staff would ignore the behavior and redirect him back to work. With the plan in place, his behavior reduced substantially. However, when Joe started an internship in an employment setting and was faced with new demands, the behavior resurfaced. Joe exposed himself to his supervisor. He lost his job, the supervisor filed a police report, and criminal charges were brought against him.

It is clear that the school team thought they were doing the right thing by providing a function-based behavior plan. However, the plan failed to consider Joe's presentation as an adult in the community.

The available literature on sexual offending in ASD primarily consists of case studies and, of those, a recent systematic review found only 7 (Allely & Creaby-Atwood, 2016). The situations described in the case studies are varied: a marriage, in which the wife experienced sexual abuse because her autistic husband could not understand when she did not want sex (Peixoto et al., 2017); an autistic man forcing himself on a young woman who had rebuffed his first advance (Barry-Walsh & Mullen, 2004); pedophilia (Dowrick & Ward, 1997); other paraphilias (Hellemans, et al., 2007). Likewise, there are few prevalence studies (Allely & Creaby-Attwood found 7 in the 2016 review), and the studies that do exist are fraught with methodological problems or were not designed to estimate prevalence in the larger population.

Sexual Offending Against Children

There are also no studies on the co-occurrence of ASD and paraphilias, which includes pedophilia, although the topic is present in many case studies (e.g., Dorwick & Ward, 1997; Hellemans et al., 2007). Thus, there is no evidence that autistic people are more prone to a pedophilic or hebephiliac sexual attraction than typically developing people. However, there are cases against autistic people, including contact offenses, explicit online communication, and use of sexually explicit media of children.

The concept of "emotional congruence" occurs in numerous models of risk assessment and offending and may provide a helpful tool to increase understanding in some cases of sexual offending against children by autistic people. The term "emotional congruence" was first coined by Finkelhor (1984) to refer to sexual offenders that possessed an exaggerated cognitive and emotional affiliation with children, often defined by others as an overidentification with children. The offender's attachment and dependency needs are more likely to be met by children than adults. Due to the offender's overidentification and emotional congruence with children, they are likely to own children's toys and gaming technology. The hypothesis that emotional congruence is predictive of sexual offendingagainst children was supported in a recent meta-analysis, which found that emotional congruence was a factor in extrafamilial offending (McPhail et al., 2013). Such interests may be independent of one's intellectual abilities but likely congruent with findings of everyday behavior, such as very low scores on the Socialization domain of the Vineland or other adaptive measure.

Whether and how the concept of emotional congruence is applicable to those with ASD is unknown. However, a strong interest in games or activities that are typical of a much younger person is exceedingly common among those with autism. For instance, it is not atypical for an adolescent to enjoy young children's television programs or for an adult to pursue an interest that is more typical of children, such as collecting Pokémon cards. Despite the normalcy of immature interests among autistic adults, the combination of a childish interest with the desire to form friendships and a lack of appreciation of social rules guiding adult contact with children may place both the child and the autistic adult at risk.

Although it has not been specifically established as a risk factor for offending among people with ASD, emotional congruence with children is a common consideration during sexual risk assessments. If an evaluator is not familiar with autism and the tendency for autistic people to pursue interests that typically appeal to a younger age group, they may misperceive an interest in childish topics as a risk factor.

Child Exploitation Material. Charges of possession or distribution of materials that depict child exploitation ("CEM") are sometimes brought against autistic people. As with other cases of sexual offending, a paucity of empirical information about a relationship between ASD and CEM is available. Indeed, little is known about typically developing people with such charges.

Access to the Internet provides relatively new ways for sexual offenders to access children and images of child sexual exploitation (Sheldon & Howitt, 2007). The amount of easily available material and the anonymity with which it can be accessed has increased exponentially as the Internet has skyrocketed in the past 25 years. The number of criminal cases has increased substantially, as prosecutors have devoted more time and resources to investigating and prosecuting creators and collectors of Internet-based images of child maltreatment. Between 1994 and 2006, for instance, federal cases of child pornography in the United States increased from 22 to 69% (Motivans & Kyckelhahn, 2007). The rate of research into online sexual offendingagainst children has increased, but is still not well understood.

The relationship between viewing images of child sexual abuse and committing contact offenses, even without considering the diagnosis of ASD, is still emerging. However, some research has found significant general differences between contact and online offenders (Ly et al., 2018). Consequently, there is an argument that sentences for child pornography possession are too high and disproportionate to the risk posed to society (Hamilton, 2011), and others posit that people who merely view images should not be categorized as contact offenders (Basbaum, 2010).

While there are certainly ASD-associated reasons that a person can become involved with CEM, it is vital to carefully evaluate the risk in each situation. Many people, including a substantial number of prosecutors, assume a link between CEM and pedophilia or hebephilia (Seto et al., 2006). This assumption is consistent with research which finds that CEM is likely to be suggestive of a pedophilic interest or orientation (see Seto et al., 2006; Henshaw et al., 2018). The assumption that people in possession of CEM are likely to commit contact offenses, on the other hand, is not empirically-based or well-supported by current research (see Seto et al., 2011; Seto, 2017).

ASD Characteristics and Risk of Offending

Little is known about the relationship, if any, between sexual offending and ASD and, more specifically, the traits that may distinguish an autistic person at risk for offending. There is heterogeneity in multiple dimensions of ASD, as well as co-occurring conditions that contribute to an individual's presentation which make it extremely difficult to make attributions for behavior.

The intense heterogeneity in presentation across ASD and co-occurring conditions necessitates that the traits, needs, and culpability of each person must be evaluated on a case by case basis to determine if innate vulnerabilities associated with an individual's ASD diagnosis increase the likelihood of the offense (Freckelton, 2011). Evaluations performed in criminal cases, in contrast, are often conducted by forensic specialists with little, if any, specialized ASD training and equipped with tools that, for the most part, have not been normed for this population. Thus, many forensic specialists may be ill-equipped to identify and assess relevant domains that may have been impacted by autism and that could have contributed to unlawful behavior.

Psychiatric Comorbidity

ASD places one at an increased risk for many psychiatric problems, the most common being ADHD, anxiety, and mood disorders (see Kirsch et al., 2020). In the general population, ADHD diagnosis, particularly the features of impulsivity and difficulty regulating emotional responses, has been associated with increased risk of offending (see Young & Thome, 2011). When combined with ASD, it appears that ADHD also increases risk. A Swedish population-based cohort study, for instance, looked at risk and protective factors associated with violent offendingamong people with ASD (Heeramun et al., 2017). While the study focused on a range of violent criminal charges, they included the sexual crimes of rape, sexual coercion, sexual exploitation, indecent exposure, or child molestation. They found increased risk of offending among autistic inmates, overall, but no increased risk of violent offending among autistic people with average or above IQ and *without* ADHD or conduct disorder. Further, the authors found that ADHD, conduct disorder, alcohol and drug abuse, and later-onset psychiatric disorders- all established risk factors for offending in the non-ASD population- were the best predictors of criminal offending in ASD.

There does not appear to be a known increase in psychopathy among people with ASD. There is little research on this topic, but Murphy (2007) did not find a correlation between symptoms of psychopathy and ASD. Even less is known about the co-occurrence of ASD and personality disorders (including antisocial personality disorder [ASPD]) and paraphilias. Given the relatively low incidence of both ASPD and paraphilias in non-autistic samples, the likelihood that a person has both ASD and ASPD or a paraphilia is relatively low. However, there is no reason to assume that both conditions cannot coexist in rare cases. Chapter 13 outlines specific considerations for attorneys tasked with mounting a defense that considers autism-related factors against online offending against children for autistic defendants without comorbid ASPD, psychopathy, pedophilia, or other conditions that may increase offending risk and are related to the offense. Indeed, this is a difficult distinction to make in some cases. Overlapping diagnostic criteria and traits can make it difficult to determine whether ASD is co-occurring with ASPD, psychopathy or pedophilia. For instance, a significant impairment in empathy is one of the core characterological deficits of psychopathy. However, the perceived egocentric traits of a person with ASD may appear similar to other core psychopathic traits of callousness or grandiosity. However, the specific empathy deficits are notably different across the two populations. Both neuroimaging and studies using psychological measures show that autistic traits tend to relate to difficulties with cognitive empathy, while psychopathic traits are associated with problems resonating with others' emotions (e.g., Jones et al., 2010; Lockwood et al., 2013).

More studies on the relationship, if any, between sexual offendingand mood among autistic people are needed in order to understand the role mood may play in risk of sexual offending. One study of adolescent offenders found higher rates of depression among autistic offenders than those without autism (Bleil et al., 2013). Another small study also found higher depression and anxiety symptoms in sexual offenders with ASD, compared with autistic non-offenders (Marshall, 2012). However, neither study was able to measure depression pre-arrest, meaning it was not clear whether depression was present and contributed to offending risk or whether it resulted from the arrest and court case after the offending occurred.

Social-Communication and Social-Cognition

Assessing the culpability of autistic offenders is a complex process. Lack of information about formal and informal social norms may be an be an issue in many instances where an autistic person breaks a law about sexual behavior. While there are certainly cases in which an autistic person knowingly commits an offense, there are also many situations in which the person did not intend to commit a crime or did not realize their actions were illegal because they simply did not understand the social context of the situation. A sample of autistic offenders who were asked about the reasons for their offending reported, among other factors, that misunderstanding of the seriousness of the behaviors were key reasons for offending (Payne et al., 2020). It is easy to see how that may happen. An autistic person who accesses illegal images of child sexual abuse may not have the capacity to understand that something freely accessible on the internet is illegal (Mesibov & Sreckovic, 2017). Or, in cases where the person is aware of laws against contact offending and creation of child pornography, an autistic individual may not know (and were often never taught) that simply viewing images is illegal. Likewise, stalking charges may result when an autistic person does not accept "no" for an answer and, instead, imitates romantic overtures they saw in a romantic comedy. In that instance, the person had no way of understanding that the social norm was different from what was portrayed in a film.

Communication deficits, which are characteristic of ASD, can contribute to confusion about consent. Researchers have suggested that the inability to read and interpret facial expressions, which is established in the ASD population (e.g., Uljarevic & Hamilton, 2013; Woodbury-Smith et al., 2005), may lead to a failure to appreciate when people in images are scared or in pain. And, in turn, a failure to recognize what is "wrong" about viewing such images or continuing to pursue an interaction. The same is likely true of gestures and body language, which someone may try to use to send a message of disinterest but cannot be read by many autistic people.

Restricted Interests and Repetitive Behaviors

Many autistic people have a tendency to become preoccupied with topics and intense interests. Interests may create marked difficulty when circumscribed interests are in a problematic area, such as violent or sexually explicit content (see Woodbury-Smith et al., 2010). Many people with ASD are "completists" who want to possess all of an item within their area of interest. This mentality may extend to accumulating pornography, as well (Mesibov & Sreckovic, 2017). This tendency to collect excessive images can strengthen the charges against them or cause them to appear as more deviant than if fewer images were detected.

Difficulty coping with change and insistence on familiar routines are key diagnostic features of autism. Many people with ASD experience marked distress and anxiety when routines are disrupted.

There have been a handful of studies of the significant life events that can disrupt the normal routines of an autistic person. Payne and colleagues (2020) took the interesting and useful approach of going directly to the source for information. Researchers conducted interviews with convicted autistic sexual offenders who were either incarcerated or on probation in England and Wales and explored reasons the subjects committed the acts that led to their arrest. Analyses of their responses found that themes of social skills challenges, disequilibrium, misunderstandings, poor knowledge or skills with sex and relationships, and inadequate control were key to the offending behaviors. Interestingly, many themes mapped onto models of offending in typical populations, such as the *Integrated Theory of Sexual Offending* (Ward & Beech, 2016).

In addition to the information about characteristics of ASD as they may relate to risk of offending presented here, Chap. 22, contains information that is also relevant to the risk of sexual offending. Specifically, the assessment of features related to ASD and their potential contribution to risk may be helpful in the case of sexual offending as well.

Counterfeit Deviance

In the earlier example of Joe's pattern of sexual behavior, he exposed his penis in order to escape work demands. Through trial and error, Joe learned that exposing his genitals caused a halt in the demands in his environment, which reinforced the exposing behavior. Ordinarily, one would assume that exposing genitals was a sexual activity, undertaken to derive sexual pleasure, and the supervisor who fired Joe made this assumption. Misperception of intention, in which a person's motivations are perceived as sexual when they are not, is known as "counterfeit deviance". The term was first defined by Hingsburger et al. in 1991 to describe people with intellectual disability who appeared to have paraphilia but, in fact, did not. The observed behavior served a function that was unrelated to sexual urges or fantasies. The term has been used in ASD work, although there are no studies of counterfeit deviance using autistic samples. Still, there are anecdotal cases in which an autistic person's behavior is attributed to sexual reasons when, in fact, their behavior services a non-sexual purpose, such as fulfillment of a compulsive routine or pursuit of a sensory interest. It is a complicated issue, however, because behaviors can be multiply-determined. That is, it is possible that Joe used the behavior to escape work demands *and* simultaneously experienced sexual excitement from exposing himself.

Summary

Very little empirical research has been done on unlawful sexual behavior of autistic people, yet there is a need to address the cases that arise. There is, in particular, a need for research which uses inclusive population samples that are representative of the broad spectrum of presentations within ASD (King & Murphy, 2014). Certainly, some of the core features of ASD may play a role in causing unlawful behavior, while it appears that co-occurring conditions, such as ASPD and psychopathy, are much more relevant as risk factors. In the cases in which a person with ASD commits a sexual offense, thorough evaluation is needed to understand an individual's unique profile and the role, if any, ASD features may have played.

References

Allely, C. S., & Creaby-Attwood, A. (2016). Sexual offending and autism spectrum disorders. *Journal of Intellectual Disabilities and Offending Behaviour, 7*(1), 35–51.

Barry-Walsh, J., & Mullen, P. (2004). Forensic aspects of Asperger's syndrome. *The Journal of Forensic Psychiatry & Psychology, 15*(1), 96–107.

Basbaum, J. (2010). Inequitable sentencing for possession of child pornography: A failure to distinguish voyeurs from pederasts. *Hastings Law Journal, 61*(5), 1281–1305.

Bleil Walters, J., Hughes, T. L., Sutton, L. R., Marshall, S. N., Crothers, L. M., Lehman, C., ... & Huang, A. (2013). Maltreatment and depression in adolescent sexual offenders with an autism spectrum disorder. *Journal of Child Sexual Abuse, 22*(1), 72–89.

Brown-Lavoie, S., Viecili, M., & Weiss, A. (2014). Sexual knowledge and victimization in adults with Autism spectrum disorders. *Journal of Autism and Developmental Disorders, 44*(9), 2185–2196.

Coshway, L., Broussard, J., Acharya, K., Fried, K., Msall, M., Lantos, J., & Nahata, L. (2016). Medical therapy for inappropriate sexual behaviors in a teen with Autism spectrum disorder. *Pediatrics, 137*(4), E20154366-e20154366.

Coskun, M., Karakoc, S., Kircelli, F., & Mukaddes, N. (2009). Effectiveness of mirtazapine in the treatment of inappropriate sexual behaviors in individuals with autistic disorder. *Journal of Child and Adolescent Psychopharmacology, 19*(2), 203–206.

Dowrick, P., & Ward, K. (1997). Video feedforward in the support of a man with intellectual disability and inappropriate sexual behavior. *Journal of Intellectual & Developmental Disability, 22*, 147–160.

Freckelton, I. (2011). Autism spectrum disorders and the criminal law. In M. -R Mohammadi (Ed.), *A comprehensive book on autism spectrum disorders* (pp. 249–272). https://doi.org/10.5772/975.

Finkelhor, D. (1984). *Child sexual abuse*. New York, 186f.

Hamilton, M. (2011). The efficacy of severe child pornography sentencing: Empirical validity or political rhetoric? *Stanford Law & Policy Review, 22*(2), 545.

Hartmann, K., Urbano, M., Qualls, L., Williams, T., Clay, W., Kreiser, N., & Deutsch, S. (2019). Sexuality in the Autism spectrum study (SASS): reports from young adults and parents. *Journal of Autism and Developmental Disorders, 49*(9), 3638–3655.

Heeramun, R., Magnusson, C., Gumpert, C. H., Granath, S., Lundberg, M., Dalman, C., & Rai, D. (2017). Autism and convictions for violent crimes: Population-based cohort study in Sweden. *Journal of the American Academy of Child & Adolescent Psychiatry, 56*(6), 491–497.

Hellemans, H., Colson, K., Verbraeken, C., Vermeiren, R., & Deboutte, D. (2007). Sexual behavior in high-functioning male adolescents and young adults with Autism spectrum disorder. *Journal of Autism and Developmental Disorders, 37*(2), 260–269.

Henshaw, M., Ogloff, J., & Clough, J. (2018). Demographic, mental health, and offending characteristics of online child exploitation material offenders: A comparison with contact-only and dual sexual offenders. *Behavioral Sciences & the Law, 36*(2), 198–215.

Hingsburger, D., Griffiths, D., & Quinsey V. (1991). Detecting counterfeit deviance.*Habilitative Mental Healthcare 9*, 51–54.

Jones, A. P., Happé, F. G., Gilbert, F., Burnett, S., & Viding, E. (2010). Feeling, caring, knowing: Different types of empathy deficit in boys with psychopathic tendencies and autism spectrum disorder. *Journal of Child Psychology and Psychiatry, 51*(11), 1188–1197.

King, C., & Murphy, G. H. (2014). A systematic review of people with autism spectrum disorder and the criminal justice system. *Journal of autism and developmental disorders, 44*(11), 2717–2733.

Kirsch, A. C., Huebner, A. R., Mehta, S. Q., Howie, F. R., Weaver, A. L., Myers, S. M., & Katusic, S. K. (2020). Association of comorbid mood and anxiety disorders with Autism spectrum disorder. *JAMA Pediatrics, 174*(1), 63–70.

Lockwood, P. L., Bird, G., Bridge, M., & Viding, E. (2013). Dissecting empathy: High levels of psychopathic and autistic traits are characterized by difficulties in different social information processing domains. *Frontiers in Human Neuroscience, 7*, 760.

Ly, T., Dwyer, R., & Fedoroff, J. (2018). Characteristics and treatment of internet child pornography offenders. *Behavioral Sciences & the Law, 36*(2), 216–234.
Marshall, S. N. (2012). *Self-report anxiety and depression ratings among adolescents with an autism spectrum disorder: A comparison of individuals with and without a history of sexual offending.*
McPhail, I., Hermann, C., & Nunes, K. (2013). Emotional congruence with children and sexual offending against children: A meta-analytic review. *Journal of Consulting and Clinical Psychology, 81*(4), 737–749.
Mesibov, G., & Sreckovic, M. (2017). Child and juvenile pornography and autism spectrum disorder. *Caught in the web of the criminal justice system: Autism, developmental disabilities and sex offences*, 64–94.
Motivans, M., & Kyckelhahn, T. (2007). *Federal prosecution of child sex exploitation offenders, 2006*. US Department of Justice, Office of Justice Programs, Bureau of Justice Statistics.
Mouridsen, S. E. (2012). Current status of research on autism spectrum disorders and offending. *Research in Autism Spectrum Disorders, 6*(1), 79–86.
Murphy, D. (2007). Hare psychopathy checklist revised profiles of male patients with Asperger's syndrome detained in high security psychiatric care. *The Journal of Forensic Psychiatry & Psychology, 18*(1), 120–126.
Murphy, D. (2017). Sense and sensibility: Forensic issues with autism spectrum disorders. In *Autism sectrum disorders in adults* (pp. 247–266). Springer, Cham.
Payne, K.-L., Maras, K., Russell, A. J., & Brosnan, M. J. (2020). Self-reported motivations for offending by autistic sexual offenders. *Autism, 24*(2), 307–320. https://doi-org.turing.library.northwestern.edu/10.1177/1362361319858860.
Pecora, L., Mesibov, G., & Stokes, M. (2016). Sexuality in high-functioning Autism: A systematic review and meta-analysis. *Journal of Autism and Developmental Disorders, 46*(11), 3519–3556.
Peixoto, C., Rondon, D. A., Cardoso, A., & Veras, A. B. (2017). High functioning autism disorder: Marital relationships and sexual offending. *Jornal Brasileiro De Psiquiatria, 66*(2), 116–119.
Ruble, L. A., & Dalrymple, N. J. (1993). Social/sexual awareness of persons with autism: A parental perspective. *Archives of sexual behavior, 22*(3), 229–240.
Seto, M. C. (2017). Research on online sexual offending: what have we learned and where are we going? *Journal of sexual aggression, 23*(1), 104–106.
Seto, M. C., Cantor, J. M., & Blanchard, R. (2006). Child pornography offences are a valid diagnostic indicator of pedophilia. *Journal of Abnormal Psychology, 115*(3), 610–615.
Seto, M. C., Karl Hanson, R., & Babchishin, K. M. (2011). Contact sexual offending by men with online sexual offenses. *Sexual Abuse, 23*(1), 124–145.
Sheldon, K., & Howitt, D. (2007). *Sex offenders and the Internet* (p. 28). Wiley.
Stokes, M. A., & Kaur, A. (2005). High-functioning autism and sexuality: A parental perspective. *Autism, 9*(3), 266–289.
Stokes, M. A., Newton, N., & Kaur, A. (2007). Stalking, and social and romantic functioning among adolescents and adults with autism spectrum disorder. *Journal of Autism and Developmental Disorders, 37,* 1969–1986. https://doi-org.turing.library.northwestern.edu/10.1007/s10803-006-0344-2.
Uljarevic, M., & Hamilton, A. (2013). Recognition of emotions in autism: a formal meta-analysis. *Journal of autism and developmental disorders, 43*(7), 1517–1526.
Ward, T. & Beech, A. R. (2016). The integrated theory of sexual offending—revised. In D. P. Boar (Ed.), *Wiley handbook on the theories, assessment, and treatment of sexual offending* (pp. 123–138). Wiley.
Woodbury-Smith, M. R., Clare, I. C., Holland, A. J., Kearns, A., Staufenberg, E., & Watson, P. (2005). A case-control study of offenders with high functioning autistic spectrum disorders. *Journal of Forensic Psychiatry & Psychology, 16*(4), 747–763.
Woodbury-Smith, M., Clare, I., Holland, A. J., Watson, P. C., Bambrick, M., Kearns, A., & Staufenberg, E. (2010). Circumscribed interests and 'offenders' with autism spectrum disorders: A case-control study. *The Journal of Forensic Psychiatry & Psychology, 21*(3), 366–377.

Young, S., & Thome, J. (2011). ADHD and offenders. *The World Journal of Biological Psychiatry, 12*(sup1), 124–128.

Rachel Loftin is an autism specialist trained in school and clinical psychology. She maintains a private practice that offers diagnosis and assessment, therapy, and consultation on educational and legal cases. She is an Adjunct Faculty in the psychiatry departments of Northwestern and Yale University. She was previously an Associate Professor in the Department of Psychiatry at Rush University Medical Center, where she was the clinical director of the autism program. Dr. Loftin completed fellowship training in developmental disorders at Yale.

Chapter 13
Defending Men with Autism Accused of Online Sexual Offenses

Mark J. Mahoney

General Considerations

There are concerns about autism and criminal justice that can be stated generally, before we get into the particulars of defending cases involving online child exploitation offenses.

A Human Rights Issue

The issue of developmental disabilities, especially for those who are intellectually intact, does not fit neatly into the prevailing criminal law framework. The treatment within the criminal justice system of persons with developmental disabilities must be understood primarily as a matter of human rights. In the United States, we have the Rehabilitation Act, which applies to federal government actors, and the Americans with Disabilities Act, which applies to state governmental actors. Internationally, we have Article 13 of the UN Convention on the Rights of Persons with Disabilities (CRPD), the UK has the Equality Act 2010,[1] and the Canadian Charter of Rights and

[1] The United States has signed but not yet ratified the CRPD. Canada has ratified the CRPD, but it is unclear whether predictions of its usefulness have come true (Canada, 2014; Sala, 2012). At least in the mental health area, it has been observed that "Despite the lack of explicit implementation, the CRPD has helped to facilitate a larger shift in social and cultural paradigms of mental health and disability in Canada" (Hoffman et al., 2016). In the UK, both the CRPD and the Equality Act 2010 have been suggested as sources for an obligation of law enforcement to take autism into account (Holloway, 2018).

M. J. Mahoney (✉)
Harrington & Mahoney, 70 Niagara St 3rd Floor, Buffalo, NY, USA
e-mail: mjm@harringtonmahoney.com

F. R. Volkmar et al. (eds.), *Handbook of Autism Spectrum Disorder and the Law*,
https://doi.org/10.1007/978-3-030-70913-6_13

Freedoms includes an explicit equality rights guarantee for persons with disabilities. [2] The import of these directives is that all governmental officials, with no exception for prosecutors and judges, must meaningfully and substantially take disabilities into account in the exercise of their functions, and follow statutory mandates. There is still no direct precedent for the enforcement of these principles as they relate to prosecutors or judges in their treatment of accused persons with autism. However, that is not going to happen until defense counsel force these principles to be brought to bear on criminal cases.

Extraordinary Goals and Efforts Required

The barriers to an enlightened approach in these cases are substantial. Primarily, prosecutors and judges are overwhelmed by the harm and risks they attribute to child exploitation offenses, and are generally inured to all "excuses" for the behavior. Secondarily, developmental disabilities in general, and ASD in particular, are gravely misunderstood. Autistic "empathy deficits" are confused with antisocial traits, and typical repetitive or compulsive behaviors and rigidity of thinking are mistakenly associated with repeat offending.

With such obstacles, no routine approach by attorneys, clinicians, or advocates will suffice. However, diligent focus by defense counsel on the empirical facts about the characteristics of ASD can undercut moral blameworthiness for such conduct, on the one hand, and counter concerns about risk of future offending, on the other hand, making a difference. In a significant number of cases, prosecutors and judges endorsed dramatic deviations from typical outcomes. This includes diversion, pleas to offenses not involving sex offender registration, or significantly lower sentences and conditions of supervision tailored to the individual needs of those with ASD.

The attainability of such extraordinary and just results lifts the bar for what constitutes effective representation. The prevailing practice at present is to see ASD as merely a mitigating factor, not as something affecting moral culpability. Such an

[2] What about US civil rights laws and the Equal Protection clause of the US Constitution? Treatment of those with developmental disabilities as a suspect class or quasi-suspect class for purposes of the Equal Protection Clause of the 14th Amendment to the US Constitution was foreclosed in *City of Cleburne, Texas v. Cleburne Living Center*, 473 U.S. 432 (1985). The Americans with Disabilities Act was enacted in 1990 in response to *Cleburne,* "to provide a clear and comprehensive national mandate for the elimination of discrimination against individuals with disabilities" (Hoge, 2015). Ironically, later efforts to recognize persons with disabilities as a constitutionally protected class in the US were hindered by the passage of the ADA since that legislation supposedly demonstrated that those with disabilities were not "politically powerless," one of the considerations for determining whether a class of persons might be protected by the Equal Protection clause. See *St. Louis Developmental Disabilities Treatment Ctr. Parents Ass'n v. Mallory*, 591 F. Supp. 1416, 1471 (W.D. Mo. 1984); (Strauss, 2011). While that is an assumption disputed by the four-judge minority in *Cleburne,* and in congressional findings in adopting the ADA, whatever "power" the developmentally disabled community might have has not been exercised in support of the criminally accused with developmental disabilities, especially those charged with a sex offense.

approach may yield appreciable results in the form of reduced charges and sentences, but it does not address the annihilating effects of sex offender registration for disabled persons and their families. While most attorneys have difficulty envisioning even asking for diversion in these cases, it must be the primary objective, putting aside all "local wisdom" about what prosecutors are willing to do to accommodate those with ASD (Allely & Cooper, 2017).

Science not Sympathy

As suggested above, the key to attaining such results is enabling an evidence-based exercise of discretion by prosecutors and judges, and a resulting break from the typical intuitive approach that takes a relatively undifferentiated view of sex offenders. Counsel must bring to bear the mounting data and decades of pertinent research and clinical experience demonstrating persuasively why those with ASD are particularly vulnerable to engaging in objectively offensive behavior without any deviant sexual interest or awareness of wrongdoing; and present no danger, and are very unlikely, with appropriate therapy, to be similarly involved in the future. Prosecutors and judges are in fact capable of coming to a distinctly empirical understanding of what autism experts have known for decades and how this expertise addresses their legitimate concerns for public safety.

A Note About "Wrongfulness"

Throughout this chapter frequent reference is made to the lack of the appreciation of the "wrongfulness" of inappropriate conduct engaged in by the young man with ASD. This always has reference to the *serious* wrongfulness attributed to the conduct by society, to the degree that is thought to warrant the severe criminal and civil sanctions that are authorized and routinely imposed on sex offenders. This is distinct from conduct felt to be embarrassing, and sought to be kept a secret, like masturbation or viewing "adult" pornography, or was known to be proscribed, such as speeding or using marijuana.

Statutory Framework for Online Child Sexual Exploitation Offenses

It will be useful to put this discussion in the larger context of autism and criminal accusations in general and then address the very distinct phenomena that render accusations of online offenses such a "perfect storm" for individuals with ASD.

Brief History of Thinking on Autism and Criminality

We now take it for granted that difficulty appreciating social norms is a core problem in autism and responsible for the most common types of inappropriate public behavior that has been associated with it. When psychologists were first pushed to define the parameters of autism, in 1978, by the parents of children with autism—the National Society for Autistic Children (NSAC)—one of the suggested criteria for the condition was "disturbed quality to relate appropriately to people, events and objects." Eventually, after Asperger's syndrome (AS) was added to the DSM in 1994, it was widely understood as problematic that individuals with ASD see the concrete, do not grasp or "appreciate these unwritten rules of social engagement," and "violate clear social conventions" (Mesibov et al., 2001).

These leading studies noted how Theory of Mind ("ToM") deficits in autism resulted in "[d]eficient social awareness of salient interpersonal and social constraints on behavior" may result in apparently criminal acts (Haskins & Silva, 2006).

Studies demonstrated a lower rate of offending among those with ASD (Woodbury-Smith et al., 2006), and that those with ASD do not have a propensity to offend sexually, or violently (Allely, 2015; Heeramun et al., 2017; Westphal, 2017), or otherwise (King & Murphy, 2014; Mouridsen, 2012). Yet, there is also data suggesting *overrepresentation* of those with intellectual and developmental disabilities in the criminal justice system (Marinos et al., 2020). This seeming paradox is recognized as the product of "innate vulnerabilities which may increase the risk of an individual with ASD being charged with a sexual offence, most notably: impaired ToM, repetitive and stereotyped behavioural patterns and persistent preoccupation" as opposed to sexual deviance (Katz & Zemishlany, 2006). Additionally, these individuals are more likely to falsely confess, or plead guilty to something they did not do, and have less knowledge and support needed to navigate the legal system; they are often seriously misunderstood in the legal system by lawyers, judges, and clinicians, much to their disadvantage (Allen et al., 2008; Allely & Creaby-Attwood, 2016; Marinos et al., 2020). Experienced researchers observed that conviction data, usually never questioned, is not a reliable indicator of criminal propensity when it comes to those with ASD. "Victim empathy deficits and difficulty comprehending the impropriety of viewing, accessing, and/or distributing [child pornograhy] may be secondary to autism spectrum disorder" (Ly et al., 2016).

Acknowledging this underlying dynamic, forensic psychologists and psychiatrists pointed out that "Asperger's syndrome patients come into contact with the legal system due to their social impairments and idiosyncratic interests," and differ from typically developed individuals in that Asperger's may impair one's "capacity to appreciate the wrongfulness of his conduct" (Murrie et al., 2002). These authors suggested that ASD would have an impact on case outcomes if "advances in neurobiology … in the future reveal more precisely the bases of … the autism spectrum disorders" and "demonstrated that the Asperger's syndrome patient has a categorically different experience of subjective reality." Actually, such neurobiological advances had already occurred, and there is no dispute about the "categorically different experience of subjective reality" that those advances illustrated. Nevertheless, this article was forward thinking as to the critical problem: the criminalization of those with developmental disabilities who were unaware of the wrongfulness of their behavior.

Online Child Exploitation Offenses: Overview

There are several categories of child sexual exploitation offenses which are most commonly based on online activity. In trying to master this area clinically or as a legal advocate, we deal with three domains: child exploitation offenses, autism, and the internet. They are equal forces in the powerful "perfect storm" that presents the greatest legal threat to young men with autism.

Child pornography laws need to be discussed first because the environment in which these laws were promulgated continues to dominate the enforcement of all manner of laws designed to protect children from sexual exploitation.

Child Pornography Law Overview

We have to acknowledge the underlying problem: while there are many reasons to question child pornography laws as written and enforced, there is no doubting the pain and harm child pornography victims suffer. The graphic content found in typical child pornography prosecutions, including those of individuals with ASD, does not just consist of sexual photographs of naked teenagers. Prosecutors tend to seek child pornography convictions only where sexually explicit images of prepubertal children are involved.[3] In the average case we see sexually explicit images of children, even infants and toddlers, involved in actual or implied sexual contact with other children or adults, including penetration. In most of these cases, the accused with ASD, though typically having no measurable interest in sexual contact with children, will admit to having masturbated to these images. So, the vigor of those prosecuting these offenses is hardly surprising, and those advocating for the accused cannot be naïve to the shocking content that is involved.

Child pornography laws evolved in a cultivated world of fear and panic.[4] In the United States, the public and legislatures were treated to fabulous accounts of thousands of children being abducted each year to create child pornography. Groundless claims were made in popular magazines, in newspapers, and by Congress members

[3] The primary exception to this is in "sexting" cases where minors, usually over the age of 13, have forwarded a sexual image of themselves to someone who was over 18. Sexting is discussed further below at section "Social Media, Chatting, Sexting, Soliciting, Trolling, and the Internet Context".

[4] Repeatedly, the phrase "moral panic" or "social panic" is referred to in the discussions of the evolution of these laws (see Adler, 2001; Calleja, 2016; Hamilton, 2012; Ost, 2002).

that a child pornography industry existed in the United States with annual revenues as high as $46 billion and involving as many as 2.4 million children (Adler, 2001; Kermani, 1982; Rooney, 1983).[5] In fact, no evidence existed of such a domestic industry, or of such abductions. Yet, fear of the abduction of children by strangers for sexual exploitation of one type or another remains a driving force in legislation and judicial proceedings, despite evidence that it is the rarest of events (Levenson et al., 2016; Meloy et al., 2012; Walker Wilson, 2013).

There can be little quarrel over punishment for those who knowingly create and seek to profit from the sexual exploitation of children. But what about online offenders[6] who generally merely possess or look at child pornography, which is now widely available for free on the internet, unlike when these laws were enacted? The US Supreme Court had long before determined that, while manufacturing and distributing obscene material could be prosecuted, the private possession of obscene material could not, notwithstanding arguments that pornography led to rape, *Stanley v. Georgia*, 394 U.S. 557 (1969). As for those who possess child pornography, though, there is a more legitimate fear that some of these individuals, based on their interests in such images, present an actual danger of hands-on offenses against children.[7]

The legal problem is that fear that a person will commit a crime is generally not enough to imprison that person.[8] Nor is the simple objectionable content of images enough to penalize their private possession, *R. v. Sharpe,* 1 SCR 45 ¶151 (2001). And generally, we do not permit criminalizing mere status, or thoughts, where those thoughts do not result in plans or actions to harm others. It cannot be criminal to be a drug addict, sociopath, or pedophile.[9] Indeed, laws prohibiting the private possession of child pornography were not enacted in England until the Criminal Justice Act of 1988, not upheld by the US Supreme Court until 1990, *Osborne v. Ohio,* 495 U.S. 103 (1990), and not upheld by the Canadian Supreme Court until 2001, in *Sharpe*. How could this be done without expressly criminalizing status or indecent thoughts? The reasons include instrumental arguments that child pornography

[5] See also Statement of Senator DeConcini, 134 Cong. Rec. S645 46 (daily ed. Feb. 4, 1988).

[6] The phrases "online offender" and "offline offender" differentiate those whose activity is only over the internet from those who have had inappropriate sexual contact with children. They are used to refer to actual behavior, not convictions.

[7] Of online offenders with no history of contact offenses, about half have previously engaged in inappropriate sexual contact with a minoro (Seto et al., 2011). This fuels assumptions to the effect that all viewers of child pornography are pedophiles and undetected child molesters. As discussed below, at the section "Advancing the Theory of "Defense,", this is far from the case and even as to those who admit to prior offending behavior, the actual rate of recidivism is very low.

[8] Exceptions include civil commitment of persons who, as a result of mental illness, are a danger to themselves or others, those committed as dangerous sexual predators, and arrestees detained prior to trial on the belief that this is needed to prevent the commission of additional offenses *pendente lite*.

[9] In *Robinson v. California*, 370 US 660 (1962), the US Supreme Court held that it violated the 8th Amendment to the US Constitution, barring "cruel and unusual punishment," to make it a crime to be addicted to narcotics.

possession may contribute to the actual abuse of children,[10] social concerns about sexualizing children, preservation of moral values, or economic propositions.[11]

All of these reasons are directed at morally equating the viewer of child pornography with the person who took the pictures and at prevention of harm to children. Based on the evidence that a significant number of child pornography viewers have committed contact offenses, lawmakers and law enforcers by default treat child pornography enforcement as a vehicle to incapacitate undetected child molesters, no matter what rationales are given to avoid admitting that this is at heart a "status offense" based on one's interests (Hamilton, 2012).

The categories of offenses *as enacted* naturally correlate to positions in the marketplace. Production of child pornography is generally the severest charge, then solicitation, distribution, and possession.

Production of Child Pornography

Production of child pornography envisions the recording of sexual conduct involving children under a certain age. True production cases, as envisioned by legislators, are rare in the USA, Canada, UK, and Western Europe.

Most production cases prosecuted in these countries involve "self-production" by minors of images and videos which are sent using cell phones or web cameras to others. The person asking for or receiving or possessing such images can be prosecuted if an adult or, in some jurisdictions, as a juvenile. Depending on the circumstances and the attitude of the police or prosecutor, production charges might

---

[10] *R. v. Sharpe:* "The evidence establishes several connections between the possession of child pornography and harm to children: (1) child pornography promotes cognitive distortions; (2) it fuels fantasies that incite offenders to offend; (3) it is used for grooming and seducing victims; and (4) children are abused in the production of child pornography involving real children."

[11] It has long been postulated that obtaining child pornography creates a market which encourages more production and therefore more abuse of children. Before the internet, attaining child erotica of all sorts required personal participation in an "underground"—sometimes entered through coded personal ads in swingers club magazines or naturist publications—and some sort of exchange, for money or other erotic images of children. Consequently, there was a kind of marketplace, which was the backdrop for the Supreme Court's holding in *Osborne v. Ohio*, also endorsed in *R. v. Sharpe*, that "If consumption is reduced, presumably production will also be reduced." With the onset of the web and free availability of child pornography to anyone, the idea that the downloading of child pornography creates a marketplace changed fundamentally. The downloading of an image does not decrease the supply and thereby increase the demand. There has been no empirical demonstration, or even anecdotal argument, that producers of child pornography have any knowledge of the number of images that are downloaded off the internet for free or that their behavior is in any way affected by this number. Even the US Sentencing Guidelines Commission now refers to a "growing but *largely non-commercial 'market' for new images,*" in effect conceding the disconnect between today's market and the one that existed before (Sentencing Guidelines Comm'n Report, 2012). The premise that annihilating consumers of child pornography is a means of curbing its production, if it ever had merit, is no longer anything but unmitigated fiction.

be brought against the 18-year-old male who is conceivably complicit in his 16-year-old girlfriend's taking of a sexually explicit photo of herself, a ubiquitous adolescent practice.[12] As the scenario changes—as the difference in age increases, as the familiarity between the correspondents decreases, and perhaps if the accused is perceived as odd or also has been caught with child pornography, it becomes more likely that a prosecutor will actually bring production charges (Leary, 2010). It has greatly bothered Canadian judges, e.g., *R. v. John*, 2018 Ontario Court of Appeal 702, but not judges in the United States, that it would be legal for a young man to have sex with a girl who was 16, but he could face jail—even a mandatory minimum sentences—if she sends him an explicit photograph of herself.

An unintended consequence of extending the charge of production of child pornography to "sexting" is that now criminal justice conviction data will significantly overstate the extent to which there is a real domestic problem of the kind of child pornography production that inspired these laws, enhancing policymakers' and the public's misperception of the problem.

Solicitation

Solicitation for the production of child pornography was modeled on the proposition that commercial producers of child pornography might recruit minor subjects. Most prosecutions arise now in the "sexting" context over cell phones or from internet social medial sites where minors may be asked to self-produce explicit images of themselves. This is a serious problem for young adult men with ASD who get involved in this ubiquitous practice.

Distribution and Transportation of Child Pornography

Charges of distributing and transporting child pornography, like "production," originally envisioned wholesalers financially profiting from marketing child pornography. Such prosecutions are also rare. The most common type of distribution case to be prosecuted is low-level trading of child pornography, persons who have "transported" material on their cell phone or computer, or even "transported" material between devices of their own, and those who have downloaded child pornography using "peer-to-peer file-sharing" programs which, by default upon installation, create a folder for downloaded files that are accessible to other users of this software. Because police are aware of how a charge of distribution can elevate the seriousness of the case and induce an individual to agree to plead to possession to avoid a mandatory minimum

[12] Prevalence of typically developed children and adolescents participating in cell phone and online sexual activity is discussed below at section "Social Media, Chatting, Sexting, Soliciting, Trolling, and the Internet Context".

sentence, they are very focused, at the time of arrest and during interrogations, to elicit anything from the suspect to demonstrate that they were aware of this sharing function.

Receipt of Child Pornography

In the United States, there is an offense of "receipt" of child pornography over the internet. This category of offense does not occur in other countries, for obvious reasons: (1) practically every single case of possession involves the receipt of child pornography over the internet, and (2) it is impossible to articulate how receiving child pornography is more serious than possessing it. This completely irrational criminal category is simply the product of either incompetence or malevolence in fixing a perceived loophole in the original US statute.[13]

Returning to the sexting problem, the 18-year-old male who only receives a sexually explicit photo from his 16-year-old girlfriend by phone or the internet can also be charged under this section, which carries a mandatory 5-year prison sentence.

Possession of Child Pornography

A simple possession offense in the United States carries no mandatory minimum penalty and a maximum term of 10 or 20[14] years of imprisonment at least for the first offense.

Aggravating Factors

Most child pornography laws provide for higher minimum and maximum penalties if the offender has a predicate sex offense conviction.

Under the US Sentencing Guidelines, sentences also can be enhanced significantly based on the number of images or whether the images contain sadistic or masochistic representations, which includes any image involving any sexual contact. There is an

[13] 18 USC § 2252A(a)(2) originally read, "receives *for the purpose of sale or distribution.*" Worrying that some defendant had been acquitted of this charge (though convicted of possession) because they did not intend to "sell" the images but only *trade* them, this original statute was changed by removing the phrase "for sale or distribution for sale." The excuse for this was to make receipt even for *non-commercial* distribution (like trading or making available for others) the equivalent of distribution. But the effect was to remove any purpose to distribute at all from the statute. The consequence, intended or not, was to expand the applicability of the provision to practically every case of mere possession. See *United States v. Malik*, 282 F.Supp.2d 833, 834–835 (N.D. Ill. 2003).

[14] In the case of possession of images of a child younger than 12.

enhancement where persons depicted are under 12 years of age, or for "use of a computer" to commit the offense, or for any video longer than five minutes. Even the US Sentencing Commission has acknowledged the irrationality of the "enhancements," as every one is applicable in almost all cases (US Sentencing Commission 2012). Research has shown that the number and content of images used as aggravating factors for the US Sentencing Guidelines does not relate to culpability or risk of future offending (Seto & Eke, 2015).

Mental Culpability

The vast majority of child pornography laws do not require the accused to be aware of the wrongfulness or illegality of their actions.[15] Except for statutory terms requiring that possession be for the purpose of distribution or the like, they are mainly statutes of general intent and only require that the defendant acted "knowingly." While it is generally assumed that this term merely requires awareness of age or what is depicted in the images, there is an argument, untested in this area, that it carries with it the implication of awareness of wrongdoing. *Liparota v. United States*, 471 U.S. 419, 425, 433 (1985).[16]

One thing is certain: the US Congress, and likely all legislative bodies enacting similar laws in other countries, simply assumes that "everybody knows" the strong social rules and taboos which aim to prevent the sexual exploitation of children. It did not have in mind the problem of the developmentally disabled individual who might not be aware of the social norms and taboos that underlie these statutes. Moreover, although it is certain that a substantial percentage of child pornography offenders have never and will never have sexual contact with a child, and would not even qualify as having paraphilic interests, there is no evident policy for identifying these individuals or sparing them from the harshest criminal penalties and civil disabilities for such offenses. This includes persons who might not even be aware of having engaged in any wrongdoing.

Comparative View of Child Pornography Laws

Internationally, laws related to child pornography differ significantly in the scope of provisions, the severity of available punishment, and the zealousness of enforcement. However, it is difficult to quantify these differences as no single resource exists

---

[15] Canada's statute does allow for a defense that the conduct "(a) has a legitimate purpose related to the administration of justice or to science, medicine, education or art; and (b) does not pose an undue risk of harm to persons under the age of eighteen years." CCC §163.1(6).

[16] "Absent indication of contrary purpose in the language or legislative history of the statute, we believe that 'knowingly' … requires a showing that the defendant knew his conduct to be unauthorized by statute or regulations."

which compares the provisions of different countries and how they are enforced or punished.[17]

United States

The United States is far harsher in its treatment of child pornography offenders than other countries.[18] Over 95% of those charged federally in the United States with child pornography offenses are convicted (Motivans, 2017). For 2019, 99% went to prison, and the average sentence for all "non-production" child pornography offenders is 101 months. For those who were charged with distribution, transportation, advertising, or receipt of child pornography, the average sentence was 133 months. For those convicted of receipt alone, with no prior offense, the average sentence was 87 months. For those charged only with possession, the average was 53 months (US Sentencing Commission, 2020). Most US states achieve comparable results, if not higher.

In the United States, production of child pornography carries a mandatory minimum term of 15 years and a maximum of 40. Even where use of a production statute is objectively outrageous, prosecutors often will charge, or threaten to charge, production as a means of forcing the accused to take a plea, perhaps to an offense which carries a mandatory minimum of a lesser amount. This can be more likely in the case of a person with autism, where the prosecutor fears that otherwise the judge might actually put the person on probation. The ability to charge an offense carrying mandatory minimum, however, arbitrarily, is frequently used by prosecutors to limit the discretion of federal judges in sentencing in the United States.

Soliciting the production of child pornography arises mostly for young men with ASD in the context of social media communications with minors whom they do not know, often more than four years younger than themselves, seeking pictures to be sent. 18 USC 2422(b). This offense carries a mandatory minimum of ten years, with a startling maximum of life in prison.

---

[17] The International Center for Missing and Exploited Children publishes "Child Pornography: Model Legislation & Global Review," a report on the coverage of child pornography laws around the globe (see http://www.icmec.org/wp-content/uploads/2016/02/Child-Pornography-Model-Law-8th-Ed-Final-linked.pdf). The report focuses on several areas, such as whether a particular country criminalizes the possession of child pornography regardless of the intent to distribute; requires internet service providers (ISPs) to report suspected child pornography; or requires ISPs to develop and implement data retention and preservation provisions. But it does not report on specific coverages or sentencing practices. Information like this is hard to obtain and keep current, especially when it comes to actual practice.

[18] For the United States, see 18 U.S.C. §§ 2251, 2252, 2252A, and 2260. See also 18 U.S.C. §§ 1461, *et seq.*, and 1466A(a) and (b). These are obscenity statutes which, when the images are "obscene visual representations of the sexual abuse of children," use the correlative child pornography sentencing schemes.

Transportation, distribution, and reproduction of child pornography, standing between mere possession and production, call for a mandatory minimum sentence of five years and a maximum of 20.

The irrational offense of simple "receipt" of child pornography in the United States allow prosecutors to arbitrarily charge receipt in almost any case for any reason or no reason at all, except that it carries a mandatory minimum sentence of five years and a maximum of 20. There are federal districts where receipt of child pornography is charged in every case possible. As with every offense calling for a mandatory minimum sentence, charging receipt is a ready way to coerce defendants to plead to possession, and also to take sentencing discretion away from judges. This is particularly problematic in cases where the accused has an intellectual or developmental disability on whom prosecutors want to force the judge to impose prison on that accused. There are many young intellectually and developmentally disabled young men suffering in prison solely because of this US statutory anomaly.

There is no exception allowed to a mandatory minimum sentences in the US. A federal judge cannot avoid imposing such a sentence because it would be "cruel and unusual punishment." See, e.g., *United States v. Reingold*, 731 F3d 204 (2013). In Canada, by contrast, a court could make such a finding. *R. v. John*, 2018 Ontario Court of Appeal 702.

Canada

The conviction rate for child pornography in Canada is about 84% (Allen, 2017). Anecdotal information from Canadian defense counsel and autism clinicians indicate that there have been some cases of accommodation for defendants with autism. No actual research confirms the extent of this.

A substantial number of child pornography offenders in Canada also go to prison, but far fewer than in the United States, and for far less time. Mandatory minimum sentences were introduced in 2005 and then enhanced in 2015 (Tougher Penalties for Child Predators Act, S.C. 2015, c. 23, s. 7(2)). As with the U.K., Canada allows prosecutors, for statutory "hybrid offenses," to elect to proceed either by indictment or rather in "summary" proceeding involving lesser penalties. However, as of 2015, the Crown can no longer proceed summarily in production or distribution cases, while possession and accessing remain hybrid offenses. Yet it is widely viewed that Crown counsel is reluctant to proceed summarily in any category of these cases.

Under the 2015 legislation, production or distribution cases each carry a mandatory minimum sentence of one year. For possession and accessing, there was also a one-year mandatory minimum sentence upon an indictment, but six months on summary conviction. The introduction of these mandatory minimums had the effect of increasing sentences for all child pornography offenders (Allen, 2017).[19] Whereas prior to 2005, about half of the makers and distributers of child pornography and more than 70% of possessors and accessors in Canada did not go to jail, after the 2005 and 2015 changes, over 95% of makers and distributers and a little over 90% of those accessing or possessing child pornography went to prison.[20]

The average length of sentences in Canada then approximated the mandatory minimums: it ranges from three to six months for possession and 12–14 months for distribution, depending on the election of the prosecutor to proceed summarily or by indictment.

In a number of provincial decisions (having nothing to do with disabilities) mandatory minimum provisions have been struck down as violative of the "cruel and unusual punishment" clause of §12 of the Charter of Rights and Freedoms, e.g., *R. v. John,* 2018 Ontario Court of Appeal 702. This is of less consequence because many of these courts have indicated that, after most convictions, a sentence at or above the mandatory minimum sentence will be appropriate in any event. Under the 2015 legislation there have been mixed rulings in provincial courts of appeal on the mandatory minimum sentence provision for making and distributing child pornography, and a number striking down these provisions for possession and accessing. However, the Supreme Court of Canada, has deferred ruling on the issue as of this time.

England and Wales

In England and Wales there are no mandatory minimums. A possession conviction by indictment can result in a maximum of five years in custody, whereas on summary it is a maximum of six months (Criminal Justice Act of 1988, §160). Production, distribution, and possession with intent to distribute is punishable by up to 10 years if prosecuted by indictment, and only six months if prosecuted summarily (Protection of Children Act of 1978, §1).

Official UK government data gives us an overall picture (UK Ministry of Justice, 2019). In 2018, England and Wales only "cautions" were given to about one-third of those accused of possessing child pornography and about 8% of those accused of distribution and production.

Only 29% of individuals sentenced for possession of child pornography went to prison, while only 22% of those charged with distribution of production went to prison. The average sentence for 2018 possession convictions was 13.1 months, down

---

[19] See specifically Table 7, entitled "Court outcomes for making or distributing child pornography cases, pre- and post-2012 mandatory minimum penalty (MMP) legislation." It is not known how this has been altered by the direct and ripple effects of the Ontario decision in *R. v. John* (2018).

[20] Note that about 25% of the summary proceeding cases were stayed, withdrawn, dismissed, or discharged, so the reach of the statutes was diminished by these events as well. While 16% of indicted cases were not completed for the same reasons, after the introduction of the mandatory minimum sentences, only 8% of cases were not completed for such reasons.

nine-tenths of a month from 2017, while the average sentence for 2018 distribution or production convictions was 18.7 months, up one month from the previous year.

There does not appear to be any reporting on developmental disabilities being a factor in these data. Anecdotal reports from defense counsel in England support concern that prosecutors there are as resistant to differential treatment of those with developmental disabilities (Allely & Cooper, 2017). There does not appear to be any evidence that the Equality Act of 2010 has been brought to bear (Holloway, 2018).

France

In France, production is punishable by only up to five years' imprisonment and a fine of €75,000. The penalties are increased to seven years' imprisonment and a fine of €100,000 if the internet is used. Possession is punishable only by two years' imprisonment and a fine of €30,000 (about U.S. $41,100).

Australia

Australia punishes child pornography offenses more harshly than other countries, except for the United States. It has a somewhat similar system to the United States, with both national (Commonwealth) and local (state and territorial) legislation and enforcement. Like the United States, results vary widely by region, though sentencing is nominally harsher under Commonwealth rules.

Australia does not have mandatory minimum sentences. Production and nonproduction offenses under the Commonwealth code have a maximum penalty of 15 years, with up to 25 years for "aggravated" offenses (those conducted on three or more occasions and involving two or more people). In contrast, aggravated offenses in states and territories tend to be based on the victim's age and relationship to the assailant, and range from one to 20 years.

Australian government reporting shows "finalised" cases of 1,072 "child pornography offenses" in 2018, but only 568 of them "proven guilty" that year.[21] This possibly suggests that a significant number of cases were diverted in some fashion, begging the question of the extent to which, if any, disabilities were taken into account, a question which seems to be answered persistently in the negative (Allely et al., 2019; Freckelton, 2013).

---

[21] Details—Key Statistics. https://www.abs.gov.au/AUSSTATS/abs@.nsf/DetailsPage/4513.02018-19?OpenDocument.

The Vulnerability of Those with Autism to Sexually Inappropriate Online Behavior

Since child pornography laws do not require the accused to be aware of the wrongfulness or illegality of their actions, see above at section "Mental Culpability," the autism condition of the accused is not likely to provide a substantive defense on the merits. This is hardly the end of the question. The moral foundation of the criminal sanction is blameworthiness (Hart, 1958). Here autism undercuts the moral justification for prosecution and punishment where it has resulted in the lack of understanding of the wrongfulness of the behavior. Prosecutors must exercise discretion as to whether, or how, to prosecute, in every case and "should consider the possibility of a non-criminal ... or other diversionary disposition," "be knowledgeable about ... and ... develop[] alternatives to prosecution or conviction" (ABA, 2017).

Moreover, the enforcement of the criminal law with disproportionately harsh impact on persons with disabilities runs counter to national and international protections for the disabled. See below at sections "The Americans with Disabilities Act and Rehabilitation Act" and "Disability Rights in the Sentencing Context".

Therefore, the first task is to demonstrate how, despite average or even above average intelligence, autism has rendered the accused particularly vulnerable to engaging in objectively offensive sexual behavior online, without substantial awareness of wrongdoing. Further, it is necessary to explore how the client's autism may help demonstrate that the client is very unlikely, with appropriate therapy, to be similarly involved in the future.

So, it is most essential in any case of a person with autism, to make clear above all else that autism is remarkable in that failure of social perception and intuition is the core characteristic among those with autism who come into contact with the criminal justice system (Constantino et al., 2017; DSM-5). This deficit, which goes directly to the question of moral culpability, cannot be brushed aside in a system of law whose validity and integrity rests on the concept of blameworthiness.

It simply is not enough to explain that those with autism are "socially awkward," or "fail to pick up on social cues," or are "naïve" or "childlike" in some variety of ways. These common expressions are superficial and fall far short of capturing the cause, and pervasiveness of autism's effects, or that a particular accused is not morally blameworthy for his conduct.

Chapter 4, "Neuroscience in the Courtroom" discusses the biological causes of autism. It traces the direct instrumental line between the neurological differences in autism and the precise functional deficits that operate prominently in these cases, and undercut assumptions of moral blameworthiness. Common expressions of what is thought to be the problem for those with autism, such as "not picking up on social cues," fall far short of the reality, and give the dangerously false impression that the defendant is at fault for not paying attention to "social cues," from which he would have understood that what he was doing was wrong. In fact, the brains of these individuals stopped seeking social information altogether in early childhood (Constantino et al., 2017), pervasively affecting their lives.

Other Vulnerabilities of Autism

Failure to understand implicit social norms may be the common denominator of most events that can bring those with ASD into contact with the police. However, autism has other typical correlates that can instigate, complicate, or explain these encounters: gullibility, credulity, difficulties in executive functioning, bullying, excessive candor, and inappropriate affect.

Credulity and Gullibility

Mindblindness leads to credulity and gullibility in those with ASD (Attwood, 2007; Greenspan et al., 2001; Sofronoff et al., 2011). While it creates vulnerability to all kinds of victimization, this trait leaves those with ASD extremely susceptible to police "sting" operations, and engaging in behaviors in which they would not ordinarily engage. This is a critical factor in considering entrapment as a defense, and considering the culpability of one with ASD who has been put up to offensive behavior by others.

Executive Functioning

Executive functioning is discussed in Chap. 4. It includes those skills needed to assess one's situation and manage oneself in order to achieve a goal, the ability to envision alternative outcomes from available choices, rationally weigh the risks and advantages of competing choices, the ability to consider alternative goals or means, and mental control and self-regulation. Mindblindness has a catastrophic effect on executive functioning (Ozonoff et al., 1991; Perner & Lang, 2000; Sabbagh et al., 2006). Executive functioning is critical in understanding much offensive behavior and in assessing competence.

Online Addiction

Those with ASD are susceptible to obsessive pursuit of online activities which provide a kind of social involvement and stimulation not easily available in "real life." This is generally understood in terms of circumscribed interests and repetitive behaviors. But those with ASD can easily become addicted to seeking erotica of all sorts, and engaging in sexualized chats with others, without perceiving any boundaries. They can be terribly lonely and the excitement of sexual stimulation online can be the only true stimulation they experience, giving it irresistible attraction.[22]

Bullying

It is rare to encounter a defendant with ASD who was not bullied and otherwise victimized by his peers in school and other social situations. Sometimes they do not interpret this treatment as malicious and frequently mistake any attention at all as being "friendship" (Jawaid et al., 2012). They often do not get how the joke is on them, and tend to be compliant or unresponsive, which can inspire further bullying (Heerey et al., 2005; Sofronoff et al., 2011; Wainscot et al., 2008).

A history of bullying, and the constant state of anxiety and hypervigilance it brings, can affect memory, which may relate to competence, or problems in recollection in interrogation. In jails and prisons, bullying and victimization is the norm for those with ASD, from other inmates and corrections personnel, and they tend to spend inordinate periods of time in solitary confinement for their own protection, or discipline as a result of annoying or inappropriate behavior.

"Not Learning His Lesson"

In cases of a second arrest, for a similar appearing offense, which is rare,[23] a very typical reaction for police and prosecutors is to foreclose discussion of his disabilities, thinking the defendant "should have learned his lesson." Commonly, the two offenses are not actually the same, and the "lesson" learned in the first case, in the mind of the accused, does not seem to cover the new situation.

More important, the learning method for persons with autism is very different. Even parents and therapist might assume that the defendant could not have missed the "message" in the first arrest and prosecution. But without being expressly told, step by step, in the right setting, exactly what was wrong, or why it was wrong, the "rule" evidenced in the first case simply might not "stick" with the accused.

[22] We do not regard seemingly compulsive or obsessive online sexual behavior as a "circumscribed interest" as understood in the diagnosis of ASD. Interest in sex is a common denominator, and those with ASD do not perseverate to others about such interests.

[23] The author's data on cases involving defendants with ASD reveals 0% recidivism for online offenses for those who were diagnosed with ASD and received appropriate therapy at the time of their first conviction.

Inappropriate Affect

Inappropriate facial expressions, including smiling or laughing inappropriately, are diagnostic indicators for ASD (Gillberg & Gillberg, 1989). This is often a serious problem in encounters with police, judges, and juries. Inappropriate facial expressions suggest many negative things *other than* the actual developmental disability that is its cause, such as lack of remorse, sadism, psychopathy, mental illness (Allely & Cooper, 2017; Taylor et al., 2009).

Intelligence Is Not an Antidote to Social Learning Deficits

One of the primary challenges for those with ASD is the difficulty for others to understand how those with ASD who are intelligent enough to graduate from high school, or capable of earning a college, or even graduate degree, might not on their own have perceived the cultural, social, and legal taboos underlying child sexual exploitation offenses and other sex crimes.

As noted above, and discussed in Chap. 1, the deficits in social understanding typical of autism can be severe for those who are also highly intelligent, and this is a fact evidenced by the consensus of the scientific community expressed in the DSM, research, clinical experience, and the personal experience of intelligent persons with autism. Hence, it is appropriate to call "high functioning autism" or "mild autism" a "misnomer" (Alvares et al., 2020; Prizant, 2012; Saulnier & Klin, 2007; Klin et al., 2007; Tillman et al., 2019).

This author conducted an informal online survey, with 350 respondents evenly spread in education level between high school graduates, some college, college degree, graduate degrees, including doctoral level. Of the males with a clinical ASD diagnosis, 10% were not aware of the proscription of child pornography. 25% were not aware of the proscription on receiving sexually explicit photographs from a minor. Among those who claimed to have known these proscriptions, many stated that they learned them by taking the survey. Most others did not learn them until decades after adolescence.

ASD and Sexuality

Sexuality and ASD is discussed in Chap. 24. Specifically in relation to online offenses, where the accused may have spent an inordinate amount of time online looking at pornography, engaging in sexual role play with minors or seeking self-produced images from minors, one still cannot presume typical sexual knowledge. Nor can one accurately deduce from the defendant's behavior exactly what his sexual experience, interests, orientation, or intentions might be. These have to be carefully explored with the defendant. For example, despite all indicators to the contrary, a young man with ASD might have absolutely no interest in real sexual contact with another person.

ASD is not a predictor of pedophilia, or any other paraphilic disorder or sexual offending. Objective testing for sexual interests in these cases rarely evidence any deviant sexual interests.[24] Those with ASD are much more likely to be victims rather than victimizers (Klin et al., 2005). Their social deficits render most men with ASD unable to strike up conversations with strangers, even children. What gets young adults with ASD into legal trouble is not abnormal sexual desires, but their tendency to express or pursue normal interests in a manner outside social conventions.

Advancing the Theory of "Defense"

As noted above at section "The Vulnerability of Those with Autism to Sexually Inappropriate Online Behavior", the approach advanced here does not aim at a trial on the merits. The approach is to persuade prosecutors and judges to accommodate the developmentally disabled accused with the favorable exercise of discretion. As it happens, in a significant number of cases, appreciation of the empirical facts about the nature of ASD, and how it undercuts moral blameworthiness for such conduct, on the one hand, and counters concerns about risk of future offending, on the other hand, has led prosecutors, and judges, to support dramatic deviations from the typical results in the ordinary child pornography case and other cases. This includes diversion, pleas to offenses not involving sex offender registration, no imprisonment, or significantly lower sentences, and conditions of supervision tailored to the individual needs of those with ASD.

The task is not an easy one. Here are some specific practice considerations.

Developmentally Disabled Offenders Are Likely the Least Dangerous

Before it can be accepted that the accused with ASD differs from the "typical" offender, the prosecutor, probation officer, and judge need to be reminded of the reality that viewers of child pornography are not homogeneous. Viewers of child pornography include "recreational users" and "at-risk users" who would never have looked at child pornography but for the Internet; but only "sexual compulsives" were

[24] Deviant sexual interests can be ruled out with the Abel Assessment for Sexual Interest (AASI-3) or the Abel-Blasingame Assessment System, for individuals with an intellectual disability (ABID), and a polygraph ruling out prior "hands-on" offenses can often practically obviate the need for any separate "risk assessment" or full psychosexual evaluation.The AASI does not appear to be validated for women.

identified as "hav[ing] a specific interest in children as sexual objects" (Wortley & Smallbone, 2012). The US Sentencing Commission observed that "not all child pornography offenders are pedophiles, and not all child pornography offenders engage in other sex offending" (US Sentencing Commission, 2012). Even the discredited "Butner Report" noted that it "is indisputable that certain factors (e.g., psychiatric disorders, developmental and psychological vulnerabilities)" may be at work in some cases' and that a "small minority" of child pornography offenders "are motivated by non-sexually deviant interests" (Bourke & Hernandez, 2009).

This "minority" may be as much as 45% (Seto et al., 2011). But the best research available (Babchishin et al., 2015), differentiates "child pornography only" (CPO) offenders from exclusively "sex offenders against children" (SOC) and "mixed" offenders, indicating that CPO offenders are least likely to present a future problem. Both as to CPO's and those who solicit images from minors on the internet, these researchers, and others (Briggs et al., 2011) further differentiate between "fantasy driven" and "contact-driven" offenders. Further meta-analysis of this data could likely to identify the least risky, most "fantasy driven" group as developmentally disabled.[25]

Despite knowledge that there are online offenders who are not the "child predators" at whom these criminal laws and sex offender registration are aimed, there is generally no legal or policy structure aimed at diverting those who present no danger, and perhaps have no knowledge of wrongdoing, from the harshest consequences.

Also, prosecutors and judges often have the bias of thinking that the diagnosis of autism is subjective, or trivial ("everybody is a little autistic"), or that "mild" or "high functioning" autism does not have severe consequences, and that thus ASD cannot be an "excuse." They are always suspicious of diagnoses attained after the arrest.

The task in confronting this has to be a scientifically based explanation as to why young men might be looking at child pornography or communicating sexually with minors without being motivated by deviant sexual interests, or presenting cognizable risk of hands-on offending, and without appreciating the socially and culturally inculcated boundaries underlying these laws.

[25] The study identifies a number of protective "meta-variables" in the source studies that point away from risk of further offending that correlate with autism: youth, loneliness, emotional empathy with actual children, greater internet use, sexual preoccupation, higher intelligence, lack of antisocial traits and prior criminal history, adherence to rules, absence of sexual deviance, dissociation between sexual fantasy and action, less severe mental illness, never lived with a partner, underassertiveness, loneliness. Other "meta-variables" related to higher risk point away from autism: cognitive distortions, lack of emotional empathy, antisociality, hostility, problems with supervision, impression management. However, these data have not been analyzed with a view to correlation of ID/DD to CPOs or within category differences. Surprisingly, suggestions for clarifying different typologies of CPOs still do not expressly consider the possibility of the non-deviant, developmentally disabled viewer as a distinct category of CPO, e.g. Henshaw et al. (2017).

While Autism Can Make Young Men Vulnerable to Unwittingly Transgressing Social Norms, It Often Renders Them "Rule Bound" and Assiduous at Following the Social Rules About Which They Are Expressly Told

The pervasive effects of the inability to develop socially intuitive thinking leaves most of those with ASD desperate to figure out the important social rules they cannot intuit and which no one has expressly shared with them. DSM-5 observes that being rule-bound is a trait under both domains of diagnostic criteria. This is a trait which all clinicians, teachers, and others who work with those on the autism spectrum know well.

Being rigidly rule-bound can be a problem for children with ASD. But being rule-bound is an asset in persuading prosecutors and judges that, despite rendering most seriously affected individuals vulnerable to committing online offenses, autism may, especially when well-evidenced in the developmental history, minimize the risk of reoffending or worse.[26] Some research bears this out (Cheely et al., 2012).

Educating the Prosecutor and the Judge

The goal is to help prosecutors and judges educate themselves about autism. This begins with a comprehensive autism-centric evaluation which addresses all of the problematic behaviors in the case from the viewpoint of autism. See below at section "Clinical Evaluations in Cases of Online Offending" and Chap. 4.

However, it is never sufficient or wise to simply hand over a clinician's reports and test results and hope the prosecutor draws the correct conclusions. The report has to be supplemented with other information explaining the research and experience outlined in this volume, and policy statements from autism organizations and researchers that will help in the prosecutor's and judge's education process. Community support from autism organizations should be sought, and brought to bear. Anything which can be done, such as videos of the client, to assist the prosecutor, and possibly the court, to understand the mind of the accused, and his disability from the perspective of the parents and clinicians and teachers, must be considered.

---

[26] While there can be a significant occurrence of Oppositional Defiant Disorder or Conduct Disorder, or their symptoms, in conjunction with ASD, is not clear the extent to which these conditions actually militate against rigid adherence to social rules considered to be morally important, once learned.

Meeting the Prosecution

At the initial stage of a case get a commitment from the prosecutor to sit down with defense counsel and the clinician after all this material has been provided. The point of this is not to negotiate, but to complete the education process. It is important not to just duplicate what has been provided to the prosecutor previously. Most important is to anticipate and listen to the concerns of prosecutors and law enforcement and address those concerns with empirical evidence related to the defendant's autism condition.

Let us turn to specific issues in encountered in cases of online offending by persons with ASD.

Child Pornography Issues

Viewing and possessing child pornography seems to be the most common online criminal trap for the unwary young man with ASD. It is also the kind of online offending which has most often has resulted extraordinary accommodations by prosecutors and judges, perhaps because this is the easiest to explain in terms of autism.

The Path to Viewing Child Pornography

Many of the risk factors described in Chap. 22 also apply here. An interest in illegal pornography is not an anticipated characteristic of people with ASD (Attwood, 2014). Nevertheless, there are clear ways a young man with ASD is vulnerable to viewing child pornography, and without appreciating the serious wrongfulness of the behavior. Experience with many of these cases shows that for those with ASD, the path to child pornography does not begin with pursuit of sexual images of children on the internet, unless they started seeking naked pictures of other children when they were children themselves.

In many cases, the developmentally disabled child has been lured by an older person with these curious images that may seem fascinating rather than revolting. Or these images might be posted in chat rooms about computer games or topics attractive to those with ASD, such as Japanese style animations (anime, hentai, manga) or "furries" or "My Little Pony," etc.

Most often it seems that it is the exploration of the online world of pornography that has resulted in exposure to child pornography. The typically developed young man can also start down the same path. However, because of his socialization experience, when he comes across sexual images of young teens, not on "legitimate" porn sites, he is going to see a "yellow flag." He may hesitate, because he knows that he is nearing a boundary. If he sees images of young teens engaged in sexual activity, or prepubescent children, a "red flag" will go up in his mind.

In contrast, the young man with ASD, socially isolated and sexually naïve, is intensely curious about sex and romance and turns to the Internet for his education. He may be oblivious to the taboos implicated here and does not see these boundaries when he approaches them. No yellow or red flags go up. He may be completely unaware of any moral or legal boundaries when it comes to looking at sexual images of young adolescents or children. "The lack of sociosexual knowledge is always the major issue" (Henault, 2014).

What Are They Looking at?

Most frequently, when questioned about what actually interests them in such images, young men with ASD will simply say that it is the sexual body parts they're looking at. They do not, it seems, as a pedophile might, see the child in these images as a child.

This should not be surprising in light of what we now know about how differently those with ASD actually "see" the world as discussed in Chap. 4. With such a huge difference in the way persons with autism see the world, why would we even suspect that a young man with autism "sees" the same thing in an erotic image that a typically developed persons sees?

By the same token, put aside any illusion that because young men with ASD are so naïve sexually that they are not looking at "hard core" images, or are not aroused by much of what they look at. Moreover, while they may through accident or curiosity come across underage images, often they will actively seek out such images specifically, though rarely exclusively. The point is that what we often see here is a relatively undifferentiated interested in sexual stimulation from viewing sexual body parts in action—oblivious therefore to the social attributes of this behavior, or the behavior they are observing.

The Problem of Interpreting Social Scenes

Not "seeing" the social world, as discussed in Chap. 4, takes us an important step further. Failure to intuit the social taboos related to viewing child pornography explains why a "red flag" would not go up when encountering this material to begin with. But when typically developed persons actually see child pornography feelings of disgust and revulsion are the rule. One who appears to be seeking out this material appears pathologically callous to the abuse, pain, and harm it depicts.

Those with ASD are simply not seeing the social attributes and implications of the entire scenes presented in these images (Baez et al., 2012). Time after time in these cases the answer is the same: until asked about it after arrest, these young men likely never gave a thought to how these images came about or why they were made or how the children in them might feel about this or be hurt by it. When it is all explained to them, they are generally horrified at what they have done, even though they do not naturally display this.

Here a very important point must be made. The disgust and revulsion experienced by the typically developed person looking at these images is not innate. It is the product of a lifetime of seeking social information, and the resulting internalization of social norms, something those with ASD have missed.

Social Media, Chatting, Sexting, Soliciting, Trolling, and the Internet Context

Cases involving sexualized online communications and exchanging photographs with minors are increasingly common and more challenging than simple cases of possession of child pornography. However common "sexting" may be among minors, for example, when it involves an adult encouraging a minor to send photographs it is considered predatory and a precursor to "hands on" offending, even though in the case of those with ASD it may be fantasy rather than contact-seeking. If the children seeking sexual experience on the internet have underlying emotional, social, and psychological problems, things these defendants may not intuit or understand, their behavior can be seen as even more egregious.

Defending such cases requires thorough understanding of the Internet environment in which this occurs and the effect of that environment on the youth who spend so much time there, both typically developed and developmentally disabled. It is necessary to objectively evaluate not only the behavior of the accused but also the behavior of his minor counterparts. While any discussion of the behavior of the latter evokes reflexive accusations of "victim blaming," justice requires looking at this milieu as the young man with ASD sees it. The ultimate point is that both the defendant and those minors with whom he is engaging are the victims of the Internet environment.

At alarmingly young ages, many children are seeking sexually charged experiences on the Internet (Strassberg et al., 2013). Those who had sent or received explicit sexual messages described sexual messaging, sexual role play, cybersex experiments, and discussions related to sex among peers as fun and pleasurable (Nielsen et al., 2015). Emotionally identifying with these younger individuals, and unable to socially connect to their peers, young men with ASD seek to participate in this online environment, generally oblivious to how seriously this is viewed and the potential harm to these children. While their older age exposes them to criminal prosecution, they are usually significantly less socially mature and sexually knowledgeable than the children and teenagers they communicate with.

The challenge here is to help prosecutors and judges to consider the matter from the viewpoint of the accused, which perceives these children as equal, willing participants in widespread activity that is most akin, in their minds, to online computer games. Blind to the social implications of these encounters, and to the complete difference their age makes, they are often astonished at how seriously wrong their behavior is viewed.

Counsel first has to take the conduct involved—chatting, sexual role play, sexting, soliciting, trolling—and demonstrate how "normal" that behavior is among typically-developing children. As the above research shows, typically developed people, including children and adolescents, say and do things on the internet that they would not ordinarily say or do in person. The explanation for this is what is called the "Online Disinhibition Effect" (Suler, 2004). Essentially, the Internet creates the sense of an anonymous environment where "anything goes," everyone is equal, and if trouble does arise, it is easy to escape. This is especially true for adolescents whose underdeveloped brain does not fully grasp the impact their online sexual behaviors.

Those with ASD do not have culturally fostered "inhibitions" needing to be dulled. They are not *escaping* the rules of the social world, they do not "get" these rules to begin with. But they see this behavior by their peers as a model and therefore remain oblivious to how seriously inappropriate this behavior, or their participation in it, would be viewed. Like their typically developed peers, they also see no limitations on the internet, and feel that "everyone is equal." And they are more likely to talk about sex and send naked pictures or movies of themselves or of others and engage in Cybersex (Dewinter et al., 2015). However, they are far less equipped than their neurotypical peers to understand the opprobrium for this behavior or the potential consequences.

It is not enough to speak to generalities, however. Each different kind of internet conduct, and each specific path to that conduct in the internet experience of the accused, has to be explored in detail. Then all that experience has to be examined in its relation to the accused's autism and related deficits, and compared with the often very different understanding and motivation that may be involved in that type of behavior by typically developed persons. So, this is partly a sociological inquiry into each kind of behavior and its prevalence among typically developed children, and then how that appears to those with autism who are drawn to it, and the accused in particular.

Autism expertise is needed to recognize how autism figures into online activity. For example, young men with autism encounter minors, sometimes very young, who appear to them as willing and equal participants in explicit sexual "role play." Here players adopt scripted roles such as "Submissive/Dominant," and "Master/Slave" or "Daddy/Baby." This may involve playing games such as "Truth or Dare." These are all vehicles for explicit sexual fantasy sometimes about meeting personally, which rarely happens, and the exchange of explicit photographs.

The primary problem for young men with autism in this kind of role play is that they do not see how inappropriate it is for them to be involved with minors who seem too willing to engage in this fashion. Additionally, the language they use can appear clever, manipulative, and coercive and, for prosecutors and judges not familiar with these games, confirm the assumption that the accused is an antisocial predator. Rather this is generally an example of very common adaptive skills adopted by those with autism to overcome their lack of intuitive social understanding. Those with ASD learn is to mimic the expressions of neurotypical individuals. They are very quick to pick up on the wording and expressions and gestures of others that seem to work in the environment. This is related to what is generally called "social scripting," which Tony Attwood, describes as "borrowed phrases" (Attwood, 2007, pp. 39–40). Calculated mimicry of these successful representations of what is considered socially acceptable in a particular milieu helps mask their social confusion (Ormond et al., 2018).

Thus, the young man with ASD will come off as far cleverer and more manipulative than he really is, because he is scripting and mimicking others. Additionally, such encounters and efforts to connect on social media can be pursued obsessively with very little capability to assess the utility or appropriateness of the behavior. While this persistence can appear pathological, it needs to be interpreted in light of autistic traits of obsessiveness and lack of executive function.

Childhood Sexual Experimentation

In a small percentage of cases, young men with ASD admit to or are accused of having sexual contact with children, sometimes when they were children themselves but sometimes, more problematically, when they are four or five years older. This almost exclusively involves relatives, cousins or siblings, or very familiar neighborhood children. For police and prosecutors this supports an intuition that the young man is a child predator. Therefore, it is essential that such conduct, whether charged as part of the offense or not, be addressed and considered in the contexts of both normal childhood development and ASD. This provides a rational basis to differentiate, for those with ASD, between what is essentially "normal" child sexual experimentation, and something more concerning.

Child sexual experimentation, beginning as early as toddler-age, is a normal part of sexual development (Finkelhor, 1980; Haugaard, 1996; Lamb & Coakley, 1993). Over 80% of children have engaged childhood sexual play (Kellogg, 2010; Larsson & Svedin, 2007; Lamb & Coakley, 1993). Counterintuitively, the type of sexual acts, like kissing, exposing or fondling genitalia, oral sex, or intercourse, is not associated with how positively or negatively the behavior was thought of in adulthood (Haugaard & Tilly, 1988; Lamb, 2002). It is usually a friend, cousin, or sibling with whom the child has their first sexual experimentation (Finkelhor, 1980). Thus, where a report of child sexual behaviors involves contacts with such close relations, normal child sexual experimentation should be first be explored as a differential explanation from "molesting."

The big problem is that young people with ASD are typically delayed five years or more in their social and sexual development and can often engage in behavior seen as age inappropriate, including touching younger children who are seen as peers by the individual with ASD (Ashley, 2007).

These encounters are categorized as "age discordant sexual play" (Bruce et al., 2012; Lee et al., 2003; O'Sullivan & Thompson, 2014),[27,28] and not "molestation," because when this experience ends there is no more experience with younger minors, or, very often, anyone else thereafter. In other words, this behavior does not represent the beginning of a pattern of seeking out sexual or romantic experiences with minors.

Therefore, when it comes to reports or allegations of a young man with ASD involved in sexual contact with minors that might, but for the age differential, fall into the category of "child sexual experimentation," it is essential to determine whether this might more accurately be considered to be a case of age discordant sex play, rather than molesting behavior.

Competency Issues

Problems with receptive language, rigid thin Leslie abstract thinking, memory, working memory, intellectual or reasoning impairments, emotional regulation, sensory processing problems, and especially executive function, all may give rise to serious concerns about the ability of a person with ASD to "understand the nature and consequences of the proceedings against him or to assist properly in his defense." 18 USC 4241(a).[29] These may impair understanding the attorney, providing useful narrative of events, being able to be attentive or follow court proceedings, and understanding the import of testimony or what the lawyers say in court. Difficulties in working memory and executive function especially impact on the necessary ability to make autonomous decisions that the accused needs to make. ToM deficits and working memory and literal and concrete thinking may impact on the ability to give a narrative as a witness or follow questions or see traps being laid by a cross-examiner, or avoid being led into inconsistent or damaging answers that are not correct.

The difficulty here is that forensic psychologists or psychiatrists rarely have significant experience diagnosing and treating adults with ASD. This is why it is so important, before having a forensic evaluation, to already have a thorough autism evaluation pertinent to the charges that also highlights all the relevant deficits and illustrating how they might impair function in the areas that are important to competence.

---

[27] See also the Declaration of Nancy Thaler in *Markelle Seth v. District of Columbia, et al.*, 18-cv-01034-BAH, Document 29-3, 10/26/18 ("In some cases, individuals with IDD engage in sexual activity with individuals who are not of an appropriate age, which is sometimes called "age discordant sex play").

[28] "5 Facts Attorneys Need to Know When Representing or Working with Citizens with Intellectual and Developmental Disabilities (I/DD)" https://thearc.org/wp-content/uploads/forchapters/NCCJDTipSheet_Attorney_CopyrightBJA.pdf.

[29] "An inability to make any meaningful contribution to his defense marks a defendant as incompetent to stand trial." *United States v. Gigante*, 982 F. Supp. 140, 166 (E.D.N.Y. 1997). The issue is "whether the defendant has sufficient competence to take part in a criminal proceeding and make the decisions throughout the course." *Godinez v. Moran*, 509 U.S. 389, 403 (1993; Kennedy, J. concurring).

There are compelling reasons to delay actually raising the issue of competence. Making a motion for a competency determination sets the case on an automatic roller coaster of litigation. This will divert attention from educating prosecutors. Rather, concerns about competency may serve best as a backdrop for discussions about the suitability of the defendant with ASD for being prosecuted criminally, or some other favorable outcome.[30]

Lack of Criminal Responsibility

The arguments on behalf of the ASD defendant in an online offending case closely parallel the argument that the person lacks criminal responsibility. The argument is that as a result of his disability he was unaware of the nature (in its cultural context), or wrongfulness, of his conduct.

However, the person with ASD, who is not also intellectually disabled, was *capable* of understanding the nature of his conduct or its extreme wrongfulness had it been explained to him at that time. Rather, because of his ASD he may have been sufficiently impaired in intuiting on his own the social norms and taboos that pertain to the conduct. Thus, absent having received explicit instruction on these rules, he was incapable of knowing them on his own. Whether this semantically distinguishable, but functionally equivalent formulation of lack of criminal responsibility would meet the standard for lack of criminal responsibility does not appear to have been discussed in any cases.

The main argument for caution in raising lack of criminal responsibility is that one found not responsible by reason of a mental disease or defect for a sex offense will still have to register as a sex offender, once discharged, in many jurisdictions (Weiss & Watson, 2008). That may be less of a concern where the alternative is a lengthy prison sentence.

The Role of Treatment in Advocacy

Knowing options for appropriate treatment for clients with ASD is essential to effective advocacy in these cases. Identifying accessible and effective treatment reassures prosecutors and judges that the defendant will not re-offend. Explaining the differences between appropriate therapy and typical sex offender treatment programs can

[30] One can imagine a sort of ethical conundrum where counsel, seeing obvious deficits which call into question certain aspects of competency, fears that it is inappropriate to proceed without a determination of competency by the court. First, a premature determination of the question is unlikely to succeed. Second, since the primary aim of the representation is diversion of the case, very little "competence" is required for that. Diversion also being better in many respects than the uncertain "roller coaster" of competency litigation. So, it is clearly in the client's best interest to hold off the question of competency until it is ripe and necessary.

help ensure that conditions for pretrial diversion, probation, or post-release supervision are actually appropriate and effective, while at the same time enhancing the quality of supervision.

Most important, the consensus of clinicians in this area is that what individuals with ASD who have sexually offended actually need roughly boils down to giving them sociosexual information and social communication skills. This supports the understanding that the condition being addressed is not one rooted in deviance or sociopathy. The cure is telling us something about the condition. These methods of treatment are successful because they give these individuals an ability to make up for what they missed due to their neurologically based social learning deficits.

For a discussion of offender treatment and sex education, see Chaps. 24 and 26.

Counterfeit Deviance

An extremely useful way to conceive of the problem presented in some cases where an individual with ASD faces online sex offense charges is in the term "counterfeit deviance," first used by Hingsburger, Griffiths, and Quinsey in 1991 (Hingsburger et al., 1991). Counterfeit deviance occurs when an individual engages in behavior that "topographically look[s] like a Paraphilia but lack[s] the recurrence of and the pathological use of sexual fantasies, urges, or behavior" (Griffiths et al., 2007). The fourth edition of the DSM acknowledges that in certain individuals "there may be a decrease in judgment, social skills, or impulse control that, in rare instances, leads to unusual sexual behavior" that is distinguishable from Paraphilia and considered a differential diagnosis.

Under the Diagnostic Manual-Intellectual Disability (DM-ID-2), "counterfeit deviance" is a differential diagnosis for Paraphilia. There is significant overlap between those with ID and ASD, including "lack of sociosexual skills and knowledge, decreased opportunities for sociosexual behavior, sexual victimization, difficulties projecting consequences, and difficulties recognizing and expressing emotions" (Griffiths et al., 2007). This overlap makes the concept of counterfeit deviance equally applicable to both ID and AS because the person's IQ has no real bearing on this adaptive deficit (Griffiths & Fedoroff, 2009; Kellaher, 2015).

Clinical Evaluations in Cases of Online Offending

Chapters 2, 21, and 22 include information about evaluation of people with ASD in criminal cases in general. In the case of an individual with ASD charged with online sexual offending, beyond a compelling autism diagnosis, a high degree of empirical input is needed to overcome the assumptions and heuristics that dominate the current law enforcement approach to these cases.

The clinician can help make the case, discussed above at section "Developmentally Disabled Offenders Are Likely the Least Dangerous," that these are individuals with a neurological difference, the most salient consequence of which is the lack of the social intuition necessary to discern, on their own, the implicit social mores and taboos that may have been being violated by their conduct.

The report must directly address the appropriateness of possible prosecutorial decisions. If the person who knows the most about autism and its effects on the accused is not making it compelling and clear that diversion from the criminal process is appropriate, the prosecutors will never come to this conclusion on their own.

The clinician needs to explain how the accused was impaired in appreciating the wrongfulness of all aspects of his conduct—not just the actual charges, but other things that investigators or prosecutors or judges might view negatively. Often what seems like a very bad thing is simply an innocuous symptom (Allely & Cooper, 2017). One defendant who was "smirking" during police interrogation was taken to be sociopathic, which is "inappropriate affect," discussed at section "Inappropriate Affect". Police thought that all the Disney videos in another defendant's bedroom were devices to lure children, when interest in such things is nearly ubiquitous among adults with ASD.

In addressing the severity of social learning deficits, adaptive testing is essential, preferably the comprehensive Vineland Adaptive Behavior Scales using the caregiver interview form.

Familiarity with the contents of images and videos is required, not because it is of particular significance (see Seto and Eke (2015) and section "Aggravating Factors" above) but so the examiner does not later appear naïve as to exactly what the defendant had done, or in suggesting that he might not process the social implications of what he has looked at or solicited.

In cases where there are "chats" with minors, the prosecutor need only focus on a handful of worst things said by the defendant to make the point. This evidence can only be addressed objectively and effectively in the context of the chats *overall*, which are always instructive. Any of the vulnerabilities described above at sections "The Vulnerability of Those with Autism to Sexually Inappropriate Online Behavior" and "Other Vulnerabilities of Autism" need to be addressed.

It is essential to investigate in a structured way exactly what the defendant was thinking at the time of the relevant events. After the arrest it can be a challenge for him to remember what he was thinking before his arrest. Careful probing is needed to test the degree to which, and how, his actual appreciation of the wrongfulness of the conduct was impaired. Note that the significant question is not whether or not the defendant was aware that there might be something *illegal* about the conduct, although that is most often the case also.

Statements during interrogations need to be evaluated by the clinician for signs of impairment and suggestiveness and acquiescence. Research on the vulnerabilities of those with autism in the interrogation setting must be reviewed.

In the case of a second arrest, the first arrest also has to be contextualized in the framework of autism. The failure of the defendant to have "learned his lesson" from that prosecution heavily affects the attitude of the prosecutor and the judge, and thus needs to be addressed. See above at the section "Not Learning His Lesson". This almost certainly will trace back to not having had a correct diagnosis at the time, or the failure to have received appropriate therapy, or the failure of the accused to see the two incidents as involving the same sociosexual rule.

Reference should be made to resources from the autism community helping to reinforce the points made, including appropriate policy statements by experts and organizations (Klin et al., 2008; The Arc, 2014, 2015, 2017).

Neuroimaging research or actual imaging, discussed in Chap. 4, may be considered to assist in confirming the diagnosis or ruling out other conditions, for example, antisocial personality traits. E.g. Wallace et al. (2012), or simply illustrating that the defendant is indeed neurologically different in a manner expected for those with ASD.

The Americans with Disabilities Act and Rehabilitation Act

At the outset of this chapter, it was observed that the issue of the treatment of persons with developmental disabilities in criminal courts is in fact a human rights issue. Reference was made to conventions and treaties and domestic statutes. The Americans with Disabilities Act and its similarly interpreted antecedent, the Rehabilitation Act are discussed generally in Chap. 20. In connection with gaining prosecutor's favorable discretion in the resolution of these cases, these principles need to be brought to bear.

Disability laws apply to those enforcing the criminal law (Dinerstein & Wakschlag 2019). These laws impose a duty upon prosecutors and judges to meaningfully and substantially take developmental disabilities into account in exercising their discretion in relation to the developmentally disabled accused person. Discrimination, under these statutes, generally includes: (1) intentional discrimination; (2) discriminatory impact of decisions and policies; and (3) a refusal to make a reasonable accommodation to the disabled. *Alexander v. Choate*, 469 U.S. 287, 295–296 (1985). Thus, when treating the autistic accused "like anyone else," the results, even if unintended, may establish discrimination because of the disproportionate effect such a "neutral" approach is having and will have on him because of his disability. See Dinerstein and Wakschlag (2019).

Authoritative pronouncements from the Department of Justice, the agency tasked with enforcing the ADA and Rehabilitation Act, expressly call on prosecutors and judges to take the defendant's disability into account, both as a consequence of these laws, and as a moral proposition (Gupta, 2016; Rubin & McCampbell, 1995; US Department of Justice, 2006, 2016, 2017a, 2017b).

The Department of Justice has stated the goal of nondiscrimination requirements is to "avoid [ ] unnecessary criminal justice involvement for people with disabilities" emphasizing the importance of "assessing individuals for diversion programs" on the basis of developmental disabilities. This guidance goes further to insist that "governments must prevent unnecessary institutionalization of people with disabilities" (US Department of Justice, 2017b).

Sentencing

If the defense has taken advantage of earlier opportunities to inform the judge about the defendant's autism condition and its consequences, the judge will have a better chance of learning what he or she needs to know about ASD, and how it is presented in this individual.

In the sentencing presentation, there will be more emphasis on prison, and how tortuousness, harmful, and counterproductive it is for those with autism spectrum disorder. As the alternative, focus must be on the success of community treatment actually suited to the young man with ASD, and so much more effective for him and the safety of the community than if delayed by years of gratuitous incarceration devoid of habilitation. The issue of blameworthiness remains the same: to what extent was the accused, because of his neurological difference, unaware of the wrongdoing and potential harm involved in his behavior? This, and the "rule bound" tendency of those with ASD to follow important social rules, once they understand them, are critical factors in imposing sentence.

A Human Rights Issue

Sentencing, where the judge does have the choice not to imprison, squarely involves a choice about treatment of persons with disabilities, and the human rights concern addressed at the outset of this chapter.

Judges everywhere are required to take individual characteristics into account, especially factors that would affect blameworthiness of the individual or the degree to which incarceration is needed to protect society. There is every reason to believe that they will understand the need to take developmental disabilities into account, out of simple fairness (Allely & Cooper, 2017; Berryessa, 2014a, 2014b, 2016; Berryessa et al., 2015).

This author has attempted to identify and track state and federal criminal cases in the United States involving defendants with ASD, and especially where a significant effort was made to educate the judge about the role of ASD in the offense and its significance for estimating the risk of reoffending. Most of the cases involve online sexual offenses. Of those cases, excluding the dismissals, and pretrial diversion, but including cases involving reduced charges not implicating sex offender registration, there are 33 cases.[31]

Of the federal cases, on average, judges departed 84% downward from the bottom end of the federal Sentencing Guideline range. And for those defendants not subject to a mandatory minimum, 54% of the defendants were not sent to prison. For those defendants not subject to a mandatory minimum who were sent to prison, the average sentence was 32 months, significantly below the average.

In the 17 state cases, where there was no diversion or dismissal, none of the defendants were sent to prison.

[31] Of these 33 cases, 16 were not placed on the registry. Contact author for current data.

These results, despite the limited number of cases, reflect extraordinarily different results than would be expected in similar cases involving typically developed defendants. This is not to say that there are not plenty of cases where horrific results have occurred. But it is evident that many judges in the United States will respond positively to efforts to edify them concerning autism and its effects.

Disability Rights in the Sentencing Context

The anti-discrimination provisions in United States disability statutes have a provision particularly applicable to the imposition of sentence. This is called the "community integration mandate." Section 504 of the Rehabilitation Act requires agencies to conduct their programs and activities in "the most integrated setting" appropriate for the individual with a disability. 29 U.S.C. § 794(a). The "community integration mandate" applies broadly to judges at all stages (US Department of Justice, 2017b). The integration mandate applies to the choice of imposing incarceration, stopping the "school-to-prison-pipeline" for those with intellectual and developmental disabilities, and avoiding unjustified imprisonment. Judges having discretion to do so, and no compelling reason not to do so, should be bound to impose community treatment rather than prison (Dinerstein & Wakschlag, 2019).

Conclusion

Representing persons with ASD in online sex offenses presents an extraordinary challenge for the advocate. We must mediate between two worlds: a world overcome with fear for the sexual exploitation of children, and which tends to demonize those who exhibit any potential sexual interest in children; and another world that struggles on a daily basis to assist those with ASD to adapt to a social world they do not naturally understand. A big part of success for the defense of these cases is having the faith that prosecutors and judges will respond appropriately to the consensus of the scientists, researchers, and organizations about the realities of ASD and the evidence of how directly that relates to the blameworthiness of the accused.

References

Adler, A. (2001). The perverse law of child pornography. *Columbia Law Review, 101,* 209.

Allely, C. S. (2015). Experiences of prison inmates with autism spectrum disorders and the knowledge and understanding of the spectrum amongst prison staff: A review. *Journal of Intellectual Disabilities and Offending Behaviour, 6*(2), 55–67.

Allely, C. S., & Cooper, P. (2017). Jurors' and judges' evaluation of defendants with autism and the impact on sentencing: A systematic Preferred Reporting Items for Systematic Reviews and

Meta-analyses (PRISMA) review of autism spectrum disorder in the courtroom. *Journal of law and medicine, 25*(1), 105–123.
Allen, D., Evans, C., Hider, A., Hawkins, S., Peckett, H., & Morgan, H. (2008). Offending behaviour in adults with Asperger syndrome. *Journal of Autism and Developmental Disorders, 38*, 748–758. https://doi.org/10.1007/s10803-007-0442-9.
Allely, C. S., & Creaby-Attwood, A. (2016). Sexual offending and autism spectrum disorders. *Journal of Intellectual Disabilities and Offending Behaviour, 7*(1), 35–51.
Allely, C., Kennedy, S., & Warren, I. (2019). A legal analysis of Australian criminal cases involving defendants with autism spectrum disorder charged with online sexual offending. *International Journal of Law and Psychiatry, 66,* 101016.
Allen, M. (2017). Mandatory minimum penalties: An analysis of criminal justice system outcomes for selected offences. *Juristat.* Available via Statistics Canada Catalogue no. 85-002-X: https://www150.statcan.gc.ca/n1/pub/85-002-x/2017001/article/54844-eng.htm. Accessed Apr 2020.
Alvares, G. A., Bebbington, K., Cleary, D., et al. (2020). The misnomer of 'high functioning autism': Intelligence is an imprecise predictor of functional abilities at diagnosis. *Autism, 24*(1), 221–232.
Ashley, S. (2007). *The Asperger's answer book: The top 300 questions parents ask.* Sourcebooks.
Attwood, T. (2007). *The complete guide to Asperger's syndrome.* Jessica Kinglsey.
Attwood, T. (2014). The pathway to accessing child pornography. In T. Attwood, I. Henault, & N. Dubin (Eds.), *The autism spectrum, sexuality, and the law: What every parent and professional needs to know.* Jessica Kingsley.
Attwood, T., Henault, I., & Dubin, N. (2014). *The autism spectrum, sexuality, and the law: What every parent and professional needs to know.* Jessica Kingsley.
Babchishin, K., Hanson, R., & VanZuylen, H. (2015). Online child pornography offenders are different: A meta-analysis of the characteristics of online and offline sex offenders against children. *Archives of Sexual Behavior, 44,* 45–66.
Baez, S., Rattazzi, A., Gonzalez-Gadea, M. L., Torralva, T., Vigliecca, N. S., Decety, J., Manes, F., & Ibanez, A. (2012). Integrating intention and context: Assessing social cognition in adults with Asperger syndrome. *Frontiers in Human Neuroscience, 8*(6), 302.
Berryessa, C. M. (2014a). Judiciary views on criminal behaviour and intention of offenders with high-functioning autism. *Journal of Intellectual Disabilities and Offending Behaviour, 5*(2), 97–106.
Berryessa, C. M. (2014b). Judicial perceptions of media portrayals of offenders with high functioning autistic spectrum disorders. *International Journal of Criminology and Sociology, 3,* 45–60.
Berryessa, C. M. (2016). Brief report: Judicial attitudes regarding sentencing of offenders with high functioning autism. *Journal of Autism and Developmental Disorders, 46*(8), 2770–2773.
Berryessa, C. M., Milner, L. C., Garrison, N. A., & Cho, M. K. (2015). Impact of psychiatric information on potential jurors in evaluating high functioning autism spectrum disorder (hfASD). *Journal of Mental Health Research in Intellectual Disabilities, 8*(3–4), 140–167.
Bourke, M. L., & Hernandez, A. E. (2009). The "Butner Study Redux": A report of the incidence of hands-on child victimization by child pornography offenders. *Journal of Family Violence, 24,* 183–191.
Bruce, D., Harper, G. W., Fernández, M. I., & Jamil, O. B. (2012). Age-concordant and age-discordant sexual behavior among gay and bisexual male adolescents. *Archives of Sexual Behavior, 41,* 441–448.
Canada. (2014). *Convention on the rights of persons with disabilities: First report of Canada.* ISBN 978-1-100-21419-1.
Constantino, J. N., Kennon-McGill, S., Weichselbaum, C., Marrus, N., Haider, A., Glowinski, A. L., Gillespie, S., Klaiman, C., Klin, A., & Jones, W. (2017). Infant viewing of social scenes is under genetic control and is atypical in autism. *Nature, 547*(7663), 340–344.
Dinerstein, R. and Wakschlag, S. (2019). Using the ADA's 'Integration Mandate' to Disrupt Mass Incarceration. 96 Denver Law Review 917. http://dx.doi.org/10.2139/ssrn.3424085.

Finkelhor, D. (1980). Sex among siblings: A survey on prevalence, variety, and effects. *Archives of Sexual Behavior, 9,* 171–194.

Freckelton, I. (2013). Forensic issues in autism spectrum disorder: Learning from court decisions, Ch. 8. In M. Fitzgerald (Ed.), *Recent advances in autism spectrum disorders—Volume II*. IntechOpen.

Gillberg, C., & Gillberg, C. (1989). Asperger syndrome—Some epidemiological considerations: A research note. *Journal of Child Psychology and Psychiatry, 30*(631), 631–638.

Greenspan, S., Loughlin, G., & Black, R. S. (2001). Credulity and gullibility in people with developmental disorders: A framework for future research. *International review of research in mental retardation, 24,* 101–135.

Griffiths, D., et al. (2007). Sexual and gender identity disorders, in diagnostic manual-intellectual disability: A textbook of diagnosis of mental disorders in persons with intellectual disability.

Griffiths, D., & Fedoroff, J. P. (2009). Persons with intellectual disabilities who sexually offend, Ch 25. In F. M. Saleh, A. J. Grudzinskas, J. M. Bradford, & D. J. Brodsky (Eds.), *Sex offenders: Identification, risk, assessment, treatment, and legal issues* (pp. 352–374). Oxford University Press.

Gupta, V. (2016). *Head of the civil rights division Vanita Gupta delivers remarks at the national disability rights network's annual conference.* Retrieved from https://www.justice.gov/opa/speech/head-civil-rights-division-vanita-gupta-delivers-remarks-national-disability-rights.

Hamilton, M. (2012). The child pornography crusade and its net widening effect. *Cardozo Law Review, 33,* 1.

Hart, H.M., Jr. (1958, Summer). The aims of the criminal law. *Law and Contemporary Problems, 23,* 401–441.

Haskins, B., & Silva, J. A. (2006). Asperger's disorder and criminal behavior: Forensic-psychiatric considerations. *Journal of the American Academy of Psychiatry and the Law, 34,* 374.

Haugaard, J. (1996). Sexual behaviors between children: Professionals opinions and undergraduates recollections. *Families in Society: The Journal of Contemporary Social Services, 77,* 81–89.

Haugaard, J., & Tilly, C. (1988). Characteristics predict-ing children's responses to sexual encounters with other children. *Child Abuse and Neglect, 12,* 209–218.

Heeramun, R., Magnusson, C., Gumpert, C. H., et al. (2017). Autism and convictions for violent crimes: Population-based cohort study in Sweden. *Journal of the American Academy of Child and Adolescent Psychiatry, 56,* 491–497.

Heerey, E. A., Capps, L. M., Keltner, D., & Kring, A. M. (2005). Understanding teasing: Lessons from children with autism. *Journal of Abnormal Child Psychology, 33*(1), 55–68.

Henault, I. (2014). Sex education and intervention. In T. Attwood, I. Henault, & N. Dubin (Eds.), *The autism spectrum, sexuality, and the law: What every parent and professional needs to know.* Jessica Kingsley.

Henshaw, M., Ogloff, J. R. P., & Clough, J. A. (2017). Looking beyond the screen: A critical review of the literature on the online child pornography offender. *Sexual Abuse, 29*(5), 416–445.

Hingsburger, D., Griffiths, D., & Quinsey, V. (1991). Detecting counterfeit deviance: Differentiating sexual deviance from sexual inappropriateness. *The Habilitative Mental Healthcare Newsletter, 10,* 51–54.

Hoffman, S. J., Sritharan, L., & Tejpar, A. (2016). Is the UN convention on the rights of persons with disabilities impacting mental health laws and policies in high-income countries? A case study of implementation in Canada. *BMC International Health and Human Rights, 16*(1), 28. https://doi.org/10.1186/s12914-016-0103-1.

Hoge, S. (2015). Cleburne and the pursuit of equal protection for individuals with mental disorders. *Journal of the American Academy of Psychiatry and the Law, 43,* 416–422.

Holloway, C. (2018). *Facilitating access to justice: Exploring the experiences of autistic individuals arrested and detained in police custody.* https://www.researchgate.net/publication/328172042_Facilitating_Access_to_Justice_Exploring_the_Experiences_of_Autistic_Individuals_Arrested_and_Detained_in_Police_Custody. Accessed Apr 2020.

Jawaid, A., et al. (2012). 'Too withdrawn' or 'too friendly': Considering social vulnerability in two neuro-developmental disorders. *Journal of Intellectual Disability Research, 56,* 335–350.

Katz, N., & Zemishlany, Z. (2006). Criminal responsibility in Asperger's syndrome. *Israel Journal of Psychiatry and Related Sciences, 43*(3), 166–173, 171.

Kellaher, D. (2015). Sexual behavior and autism spectrum disorders: An update and discussion. *Current Psychiatry Reports, 17,* 25.
Kellogg, N. D. (2010). Sexual behaviors in children: Evaluation and management. *American Family Physician, 82*(10), 1233–1238.
Kermani, K. (1982, April 25). Kid porn: A billion dollar scandal. *Albany Times Union.*
King, C., & Murphy, G. H. (2014). A systematic review of people with autism spectrum disorder and the criminal justice system. *Journal of Autism and Developmental Disorders, 44*(11), 2717–2733.
Klin, A., et al. (2008). Principles for prosecutors considering child pornography charges against people with Asperger profiles. From AANE. Available online at https://www.aane.org/principles-for-prosecutors/. Accessed May 2020.
Klin, A., McPartland, J., & Volkmar, F. (2005). Asperger syndrome. In F. Volkmar, et al. (Eds.), *Handbook of autism and pervasive developmental disorders* (pp. 88–125). Wiley.
Klin, A., Saulnier, C. A., Sparrow, S. S., Cicchetti, D. V., Volkmar, F. R., & Lord, C. (2007). Social and communication abilities and disabilities in higher functioning individuals with autism spectrum disorders: The Vineland and the ADOS. *Journal of Autism and Developmental Disorders, 37*(4), 748–759.
Lamb, S. (2002). *The secret lives of girls: What good girlsreally do-sex play, aggression, and their guilt.* Free Press.
Lamb, S., & Coakley, M. (1993). 'Normal' childhood sexual play and games: Differentiating play from abuse. *Child Abuse and Neglect, 17,* 515–526.
Larsson, I., & Svedin, C.-G. (2007). Sexual behaviour in Swedish preschool children, as observed by their parents. *Acta Paediatrica, 90,* 436–444.
Leary, M. G. (2010). Sexting or self-produced child pornography? The dialog continues—Structured prosecutorial discretion within a multidisciplinary response. *Virginia Journal of Social Policy and the Law, 17*(3), 488.
Lee, J. K., Jennings, J. M., & Ellen, J. M. (2003). Discordant sexual partnering: A study of high-risk adolescents in San Francisco. *Sexually Transmitted Diseases, 30,* 234–240.
Levenson, J., Grady, M., & Leibowitz, G. (2016). Grand challenges: Social justice and the need for evidence-based sex offender registry reform. *Journal of Sociology & Social Welfare, 43,* 3.
Ly, T., Murphy, L., & Fedoroff, P. (2016). Understanding online child sexual exploitation offenses. *Current Psychiatry Reports, 18,* 74.
Marinos, V., Griffiths, D., Stromski, S., & Whittingham, J. (2020). Complexities and gaps in understanding persons with intellectual and developmental disabilities and the criminal justice system, Ch. 1. In V. Marinos, D. Griffiths, S. Stromski, & J. Whittingham (Eds.), *Intellectual and developmental disabilities & the criminal justice system.* NADD Press.
Meloy, M., Curtis, K., & Boatwright, J. (2012). The sponsors of sex offender bills speak up: Policy makers' perceptions of sex offender, sex crimes, and sex offender legislation. *Criminal Justice and Behavior, 40,* 438–452.
Mesibov, G., Shea, V., & Adams, L. (2001). Understanding Asperger syndrome and high-functioning autism. In G. Mesibov (Ed.), *The autism spectrum disorders library* (Vol. 1, p. 10). Springer.
Mouridsen, S. E. (2012). Current status of research on autism spectrum disorders and offending. *Research in Autism Spectrum Disorders, 6*(1), 79–86.
Murrie, D. C., Warren, J., Kristiansson, M., & Dietz, P. E. (2002). Asperger's syndrome in forensic settings. *International Journal of Forensic Mental Health, 1*(1), 59–70.
Nielsen, S., Paasonen, S., & Spisak, S. (2015). 'Pervy role-play and such': Girls' experiences of sexual messaging online. *Sex Education, 15*(5), 472–485.
Ormond, S., Brownlow, C., Garnett, M. S., Rynkiewicz, A., & Attwood, T. (2018). February). Profiling autism symptomatology: An exploration of the Q-ASC parental report scale in capturing sex differences in autism. *Journal of Autism and Developmental Disorders, 48,* 389–406.
Ozonoff, S., Pennington, B. F., & Rogers, S. J. (1991). Executive function deficits in high-functioning autistic individuals: Relation to theory of mind. *Journal of Child Psychology and Psychiatry, 32*(7), 1081–1105.
Perner, J., & Lang, B. (2000). Theory of mind and executive function: Is there a developmental relationship? In S. Baron-Cohen, H. Tager-Flusberg, & D. Cohen (Eds.), *Understanding other*

minds: Perspectives from autism and developmental cognitive neuroscience (2nd ed., pp. 150–181). Oxford University Press.
Prizant, B. (2012). High- and low-functioning autism: A false (harmful?) dichotomy? *Autism Spectrum Quarterly,* 31–33.
Sabbagh, M. A., Xu, F., Carlson, S. M., Moses, L. J., & Lee, K. (2006). The development of executive functioning and theory of mind: A comparison of Chinese and U.S. preschoolers. *Psychological Science, 17*(1), 74–81.
Sala, J. (2012). *How the UN convention on the rights of persons with disabilities (CRPD) Might be used in Canadian litigation.* CCD.
Saulnier, C., & Klin, A. (2007). Brief report: Social and communication abilities and disabilities in higher functioning individuals with autism and Asperger syndrome. *Journal of Autism and Developmental Disorders, 37,* 788–793.
Seto, M. C., & Eke, A. W. (2015). Predicting recidivism among adult male child pornography offenders: Development of the Child Pornography Offender Risk Tool (CPORT). *Law and Human Behavior, 39*(4), 416–429.
Seto, M. C., Hanson, R. K., & Babchishin, K. M. (2011). Contact sexual offending by men with online sexual offenses. *Sexual Abuse, 23,* 124–145.
Sofronoff, K., Dark, E., & Stone, V. (2011). Social vulnerability and bullying in children with Asperger syndrome. *Autism, 15*(3), 355–372.
Strassberg, D., McKinnon, R., Sustalia, M., & Rullo, J. (2013). Sexting by high school students: An exploratory and descriptive study. *Archives of Sexual Behavior, 42*(1), 15, 18.
Strauss, M. (2011). Reevaluating suspect classifications. *Seattle University Law Review, 35,* 135.
Suler, J. (2004). The online disinhibition effect. *Cyberpsychology & Behavior, 7,* 321–326.
Taylor, K., Mesibov, G., & Debbaudt, D. (2009). *Asperger syndrome in the criminal justice system.* Available via AANE: http://www.aane.org/asperger-syndrome-criminal-justice-system/. Accessed Apr 2020.
The Arc. (2014). *Position statement criminal justice system.* Retrieved from http://www.thearc.org/document.doc?id=3636.
The Arc. (2015). *Sex offenders with intellectual/developmental disabilities: A call to action for the criminal justice community.* Retrieved April 30, 2020, from http://thearc.org/wp-content/uploads/2019/07/NCCJD-White-Paper-2_Sex-Offenders-FINAL.pdf.
The Arc. (2017). *Competency of individuals with intellectual and developmental disabilities in the criminal justice system: A call to action for the criminal justice community.* Retrieved April 30, 2020, from http://thearc.org/wp-content/uploads/2019/07/16-089-NCCJD-Competency-White-Paper-v5.pdf.
The International Center for Missing and Exploited Children. (2016). *Child pornography: Model legislation & global review.* Available via ICMEC: http://www.icmec.org/wp-content/uploads/2016/02/Child-Pornography-Model-Law-8th-Ed-Final-linked.pdf. Accessed Apr 2020.
UK Ministry of Justice. (2019). Criminal justice system statistics quarterly (2018): December 2018, outcomes by offence data tool. https://www.gov.uk/government/statistics/criminal-justice-system-statistics-quarterly-december-2018.
U.S. Department of Justice. (1993). Americans with disabilities act: Title II technical assistance manual 1994 supplement § II- 7.1000(B), illustration 3. Retrieved from http://www.ada.gov/taman2up.html.
U.S. Department of Justice. (2006). Commonly asked questions about the Americans with disabilities act and law enforcement, section I, question 2. Retrieved from https://www.ada.gov/q&a_law.htm.
U.S. Department of Justice. (2016). Deputy Assistant attorney general eve hill of the civil rights division delivers remarks at the White House Forum on criminal justice reform and people with disabilities. Retrieved from https://www.justice.gov/opa/speech/deputy-assistant-attorney-general-eve-hill-civil-rights-division-delivers-remarks-white.

U.S. Department of Justice. (2017a). Ensuring equality in the criminal justice system for people with disabilities. In *Information and technical assistance on the Americans with disabilities act*. Retrieved from https://www.ada.gov/criminaljustice/.

U.S. Department of Justice. (2017b). *Examples and resources to support criminal justice entities in compliance with title II of the Americans with disabilities act*. Retrieved from https://www.ada.gov/cjta.html.

U.S. Sentencing Commission (USSC). (2012). *Report to the congress: Federal child pornography offenses*. Available online at: https://www.ussc.gov/research/congressional-reports/2012-report-congress-federal-child-pornography-offenses. Accessed Apr 2020.

U.S. Sentencing Commission (USSC). (2020). *Quick facts on child pornography offenders*. https://www.ussc.gov/sites/default/files/pdf/research-and-publications/quick-facts/Child_Pornography_FY19.pdf.

Wainscot, J. J., Naylor, P., Sutcliffe, P., Tantam, D., & Williams, J. V. (2008). Relationships with peers and use of the school environment of mainstream secondary school pupils with Asperger syndrome (high-functioning autism): A case-control study. *International Journal of Psychology and Psychological Therapy, 8*(1), 25–38.

Walker Wilson, M. (2013). The expansion of criminal registries and the illusion of control. *Louisiana Law Review, 73*(509), 519–522.

Wallace, G. L., Lee, N. R., Clasen, L. S., et al. (2012). Distinct cortical correlates of autistic versus antisocial traits in a longitudinal sample of typically developing youth. *The Journal of Neuroscience, 32*(14), 4856–4860.

Weiss, K., & Watson, C. (2008). NGRI and Megan's law: No exit? *Journal of the American Academy of Psychiatry and the Law Online, 36*(1), 117–122.

Westphal, A. (2017). Public perception, autism, and the importance of violence subtypes. *Journal of American Academy of Child & Adolescent Psychiatry, 56*(6), 462.

Woodbury-Smith, M. R., Clare, I. C. H., Holland, A. J., & Kearns, A. (2006). High functioning autistic spectrum disorders, offending and other law-breaking: findings from a community sample. *The Journal of Forensic Psychiatry & Psychology, 17*(1), 108–120. https://doi.org/10.1080/14789940600589464.

Wortley, R., Smallbone, S. (2012). Child pornography on the Internet. Problem-Oriented Guides for Police Problem-Specific Guides Series No. 41. ISBN 1-932582-65-7. https://popcenter.asu.edu/content/child-pornography-internet-0. Available online at: www.cops.usdoj.gov. Accessed Apr 2020.

Mark J. Mahoney exclusively defends people with social learning differences on criminal accusations in the United States. He is currently a Partner at Harrington & Mahoney, Buffalo, NY. Previously: Lecturer, University of Buffalo Law School; Founder, President, New York State Association of Criminal Defense Lawyers; Board of Directors, National Association of Criminal Defense Lawyers (USA).

Chapter 14
Stalking, Autism, and the Law

Laurie A. Sperry, Mark A. Stokes, Melanie E. Gavisk, and David C. Gavisk

Defining Stalking

From a behavioral perspective, stalking is not marked by a singular instance; rather, the behaviors must occur over time and be unwanted, at that time, by the target. They must also result in the target experiencing fear or distress to qualify as stalking (Dell'Osso et al., 2015). In the U.S., the National Institute of Justice (NIJ, 2007) more broadly defines stalking to include physical or visual proximity to the victim, unwanted communications, and threats that are made in writing, verbally, or implied. These threats may be directed toward damaging the victim's property or character by maligning them in public or via the internet. Stalking may also include waiting for the person at places they frequent, such as school, work, or place of worship. Giving unwanted presents or leaving items for the person can also be considered stalking. Stalking laws vary by state, and depending on the facts of the case, additional charges may be levied against the perpetrator, such as breaking and entering, trespassing, and intimidating a witness (Stalking Resource Center, 2017).

L. A. Sperry (✉)
Autism Services And Programs, Wheat Ridge, CO, USA
e-mail: drsperry@asapsperry.com

M. A. Stokes
School of Psychology, Faculty of Health, Deakin University, Melbourne, VIC, Australia
e-mail: mark.stokes@deakin.edu.au

M. E. Gavisk
Assistant Federal Public Defender, District of Wyoming, Cheyenne, WY, USA
e-mail: melanie.gavisk@fd.org

D. C. Gavisk
College of Contemporary Liberal Studies, Regis University, Denver, CO, USA
e-mail: dgavisk@regis.edu

F. R. Volkmar et al. (eds.), *Handbook of Autism Spectrum Disorder and the Law*,
https://doi.org/10.1007/978-3-030-70913-6_14

On a more granular level, typologies of stalking include hyper-intimacy, mediated contact (cyber-stalking), interactional contacts (efforts to see the person), surveillance, invasion (of home or work), harassment, intimidation, coercion, and aggression (Spitzberg & Cupach, 2007). People on the spectrum may be more prone to engaging in some of these behaviors while less prone to engage in others. For example, a rush to intimacy may occur as the result of a person on the spectrum not recognizing that intimacy develops over time. If their primary source of information is the media, where stalking and over-the-top expressions of love are celebrated and win over romantic targets, those on the spectrum may be at risk for misunderstanding and engaging in exaggerated or inappropriate expressions of their interest. Cyber stalking may result from the inordinate amount of time people with ASD spend on the computer. People on the spectrum spend more time online than pursuing any other leisure pursuits (Engelhardt et al., 2013; Engelhardt & Mazurek, 2014; Must et al., 2015; Jones et al., 2017). Excessive time online combined with resultant anonymity and the falsely perceived safety of online relationships may make people on the spectrum more likely to engage in cyber stalking than other stalking behaviors (Benford & Standen, 2009).

Extinction bursts are sharp increases in a particular behavior despite the lack of any reward for the behavior. When a person on the spectrum is denied access to the target of their affections, they may engage in increasingly persistent and invasive interactional contact behavior that intensifies before it resolves. If this burst of intensified behavior is successful, meaning it results in contact with the victim, the behavior has been inadvertently strengthened (Domjan, 2015). Difficulty seeing how others or their romantic target may perceive their behavior could lead to surveilling the victim and failing to think through the legal consequences of their actions, which may lead some people on the spectrum to go so far as to invade a person's home or work place. While ASD may increase the likelihood of the aforementioned behaviors, it may decrease the likelihood that a person would deliberately manipulate others through intimidation, coercion, and threat, which require an understanding of power dynamics and perspective taking from the viewpoint of the victim.

Risk Factors

Those diagnosed with autism, having both impoverished social communication skills and a tendency toward restricted interests (American Psychiatric Association, 2013), would appear predisposed to become fixated with another person and unaware of the impact of their unwanted attention on the focus of their social/romantic interest (Howlin, 2004). There is some evidence of this in the research literature. For instance, Stokes et al. (2007), using a sample of 25 adolescents with ASD compared to a group of 38 typically developing (TD) peers, found that those with ASD were more likely to persist in unwelcome advances (including threats of violence) than TD peers, despite requests to cease.

A person perceived of as stalking, as described above, must both persist inappropriately and either not understand the impact of this behavior or not care. Successful courting behavior in humans usually requires some persistence in order to succeed, and knowing when to persist and when to desist is a skill reliant upon sound social communication (Gersick & Kurzban, 2014). These skills are among the most affected by a diagnosis of ASD. Persistence with an incorrect strategy, or perseveration, is a hallmark of ASD (Mullins & Rincover, 1985; Frith, 1996; Konstantareas & Lunsky, 1997; Keenan et al., 2017). It is as if those with ASD are unable to find another solution to their problem while involved in the situation. Broadbent and Stokes (2013) wondered if this could be because the social demands of these interactions might be blocking those with ASD from stopping and reconsidering the problem. Using the Wisconsin Card Sort Task (WCST), used to evaluate perseveration, and having modified it by removing socially mediated negative feedback in one condition (an instructor saying "no" when the response was wrong), those with ASD ($n = 50$) were expected do as well as typically developing (TD) respondents ($n = 50$). To their surprise, Broadbent and Stokes found that those with ASD actually performed better than TD respondents in the adjusted condition. Thus, it was possible to reduce inappropriate perseveration in those with ASD in this nonsocial context. Landry and Al-Taie (2016) undertook a meta-analysis of WCST results from 31 studies, and their results supported this finding. Therefore, it is likely that the social expectations of a situation may itself be contributing to stalking behavior.

Stokes et al. also found that those with ASD were more likely to have used inappropriate courting techniques such as making threats, using inappropriate gestures, or touching others improperly, and these individuals displayed a profound lack of understanding of the impact of their behavior upon others and the consequences thereof. Although it has not yet been explored, it would be interesting to know if the use of poor strategies and inappropriate perseveration result from executive function deficits noted in ASD (South et al., 2007) and thought to underlie perseveration (Frith, 1996). Together, the perseveration, the poor choice of courting strategies, and the lack of insight into how this effects the other leads those with ASD into situations where they fall afoul of any number of laws in many jurisdictions.

Psychologically, there appears to be a compounded relationship between social naïveté, poor sexual education, inappropriate reliance upon the media as an educational source, and a lack of a functional peer group. This relationship, in turn, appears to lead to sexual behavioral problems. Social naïveté associated with ASD may lead to those with ASD becoming victims of sexual aggression and violence (Brown-Lavoie et al., 2014; Hancock et al., 2017). The difficulty those with ASD have in understanding social intentions (Happé et al., 2001) may lead to confusion and false beliefs about appropriate sexuality, and it may result in missing or misunderstanding important opportunities for intimacy and healthy sexual engagement (Hénault, 2006). Such inaccurate beliefs have been identified by Stokes et al. (2007) and Brown-Lavoie et al. (2014), among others.

Another element in this system failure is the lack of suitable education around sex and intimacy for those with ASD. This has been widely recognized, and many have called for this urgent need to be remedied (e.g.: Byers et al., 2012; Dewinter et al.,

2017; Dewinter et al., 2013; Ginevra et al., 2016; Hancock et al., 2017; Hellemans et al., 2007; Nichols & Blakeley-Smith, 2009; Pecora et al., 2016; Visser et al., 2017a, 2017b). Among others, Brown-Lavoie et al. (2014) as well as Visser et al. (2017a, 2017b) have demonstrated the impact of a lack of education in this group. Mistaken beliefs around sexuality abound in males with ASD, which in turn have consequences for their choices of behavior and may result in lifelong outcomes that limit, reduce, and penalize them.

The lack of suitable sources of learning leaves individuals with ASD open to inappropriate sources of information. Mehzabin and Stokes (2011) and Stokes et al., (2007) noted that among 24 respondents with ASD, the nominated sources of learning about sex were the media and "by making mistakes." The media in this context was explicit sexual material and pornography conveyed by print, film, and television, but in the time since Mehzabin and Stokes's work, consumption of internet pornography has increased dramatically (Hald & Štulhofer, 2016; Baltieri et al., 2016). With a lack of useful, healthy knowledge about sex, is it hardly surprising that many young individuals with ASD are attracted to and misinterpret the offerings of pornography (Brown-Lavoie et al., 2014).

Peer group pressure can serve as a strong behavioral correction system (Cialdini & Goldstein, 2004). Where behavior becomes aberrant, peers can act to correct this. In the case of stalking, social influence from peers would serve to help shape accurate perceptions and respond appropriately which in turn serves to maintain social relationships and protect one's image within a social group. However, many individuals with ASD do not have a functional peer group (Head et al., 2014; Kasari et al., 2011) and do not often consult with peers if they do have them, particularly about sexuality (Stokes et al., 2007; Mehzabin & Stokes, 2011). Consequently, the behavioral correction that arises from peer group feedback (Park & Shin, 2017) is largely absent for those with ASD. Note that in addition to peers having a correcting influence on appropriate sexual behavior, they can also serve as a guide for appropriate attempts to contact and communicate with an object of affection. Without peer correction, people with ASD can often inadvertently progress toward behavior that may meet the definition of stalking.

When social naïveté, poor sexual education, consumption of media not designed to educate but to titillate, and a lack of peer control and feedback are combined, it is unsurprising that those with ASD may not understand how to appropriately court and initiate romantic or intimate interactions. In turn, such distorted information sources increase the propensity for false and erroneous beliefs about appropriate behavior. This may even lead to dire and concerning thoughts and behaviors as identified by Palermo and Bogaerts (2015), who found obsessional consumption of violent, aggressive, and misogynistic pornography in a small sample of five high functioning males with ASD. Moreover, juvenile sexual offenders with autistic traits show increased consumption of pornography and increased likelihood of having been sexually victimized in the past (Baarsma et al., 2016). Consequently, it would appear very likely that social naïveté combined with poor education, a reliance upon misleading sources of information, and a lack of a suitable peer group may be major risk factors. It seems unlikely, though, that the problematic issues of media as a source of learning and poor formal sexual education would exert as much influence if the social naïveté of ASD were absent.

Restrictive and repetitive interests, a diagnostic feature, can result in the stalking victim becoming the circumscribed interest of the person with ASD. Stalkers without ASD tend to pursue their victims for an average duration of 16 months with most episodes lasting approximately 1 month (Mohandie et al., 2006). By comparison, a study of a non-forensic population by Stokes et al. (2007) found that adolescents with ASD tend to pursue their romantic target for up to 11 days longer than adolescents who were not on the spectrum, even when faced with threats to their person to leave the target alone.

Challenges interpreting non-verbal language can present additional risks for the person with ASD. Information is communicated through both words and non-verbal means including body language, facial expression, tone, and volume. According to Mehrabian (1972) when a disconnect exists between the spoken word and the accompanying non-verbals, body language should reign supreme in accurately determining the intent of the message. People on the spectrum frequently struggle to interpret non-verbals that add meaning to words. In their case study, Dell'Osso and colleagues (2015) found that case study subject G.C. had considerable difficulty distinguishing between the literal meaning of a communication versus its actual intent. Therefore, it is reasonable that this difficulty with mentalizing may play a role in the failure of people with ASD to accurately interpret the rebuffs from their romantic targets. The body language of ignoring, turning of the back, failure to pause during an ongoing conversation to acknowledge the presence of another, and dismayed or disgusted facial expressions may be signals of disinterest given off by the romantic target that are misinterpreted by the person on the spectrum resulting in a new, more intrusive strategy to secure the attentions and affections of their intended partner.

Challenges understanding the nature and trajectory of intimacy may also present a risk factor. When presented with illustrations of sexual situations, adolescents with ASD are able to judge severely inappropriate hypothetical situations as accurately as their typically developing peers (Visser et al., 2017b). However, adolescents with ASD tend to struggle with identifying acceptable situations and those that are only mildly inappropriate. This suggests that while the obvious, acutely inappropriate sexual situations are clear to them, those requiring nuanced judgment are less clear. Moreover, they are likely to err on the side of caution when presented with an appropriate situation and deem it as inappropriate (Visser et al., 2017b). When unsure of what constitutes typical adolescent sexualized behavior, such as flirting, crushes, and contacting each other through social media, adolescents with ASD may avoid it altogether either because they have been taught that these behaviors are off limits or because they have not been taught how to engage in these nascent sexual behaviors. Therefore, inappropriate sexual behaviors such as obsessive interest in a romantic target, missing the rebuff and signs of rejection when they are adults may be reflective of the social errors their neurotypical peers engaged in during adolescence.

Risk Assessment

The four factors outlined above—social naïveté, poor sexual education, inappropriate reliance upon the media as an educational source, and a lack of a functional peer group—have outward assessable traits. Tests such as Constantino and Gruber's (2012) Social Responsiveness Scale (version 2; SRS-2) evaluate social awareness, social cognition, social communication, social motivation, and restrictive interests and repetitive behavior. Other tests are available that assess for social naïveté and social understanding, such as the Test of Problem Solving (Version 3; TOPS-3; Bowers et al., 2005; Manjiviona, 2003).

Nonetheless, evaluating an individual's social naïveté alone does not provide sufficient information to conclude they may be at risk for stalking. Many who are socially incompetent do not engage in this behavior. As detailed above, several other factors appear to be involved. One factor that may be strongly protective is the presence of a functional peer group in an individual's life (Park & Shin, 2017). Assessment of this is not as straightforward as it might be hoped. Simple questions about the number and quality of friends may result in individuals counting raw numbers of pseudo-friends, such as those they have "friended" on Facebook or online role-playing video games and who bear little relationship to actual friendship networks (Reich et al., 2012). Consequently, a careful assessment of this should be undertaken in ecologically valid situations by professionals trained to make these observations. For instance, parents or teachers often report that a child or adolescent may have a social network, yet when this is explored by establishing the details and depth of contact beyond the school setting, this social network is absent (Mazurek & Kanne, 2010; Head et al., 2014). Children with ASD are more commonly on the fringes of their social circles (Kasari et al., 2011). Baron-Cohen and Wheelwright's (2003) Friendship Questionnaire (FQ) is one test used to establish the quality and depth of a group of friends. However, clinical assessment of friendships and social connection by a qualified psychologist would be the best practice for determining the strength and quality of these relationships.

The remaining two factors addressed above, appropriate education and reliance upon inappropriate information sources, are also best addressed by clinical assessments. There has been a number of attempts to develop such tests, starting with the Acquisition of Sexual Information Test (Monge et al., 1977) and the Sexual Knowledge and Attitudes Test (Miller & Lief, 1979). Other more modern tests have been developed (*cf.* Weinstein et al., 2007), but thus far none have been widely adopted. For instance, sexual understanding and knowledge was evaluated by Visser et al. (2017a, 2017b) for their well-regarded psychosexual training program, yet they were obliged to develop their own test of sexual knowledge. Consequently, clinical interview is the most suitable means to evaluate these matters. These may be facilitated by the use of these instruments and by other tests containing sexual knowledge subscales that have been recently developed, such as the Sexual Behavior Scale—III (*cf*. Hancock, 2017; Hancock et al., 2017). In summary, the risks of these behaviors may be evaluated for, but are most suitably undertaken by clinical interview.

Stalking Typologies: Intimacy Seeking and Incompetent Suitor

When the law, the mental health field, and disability providers look at stalking through their own lens, each professional may understandably come to a different conclusion about the genesis and motivation of the behavior. Thus, standard typologies, often mutable, frequently fail to consider the characteristics of ASD that may be implicated in the commission of a stalking offense. Dell'Osso and colleagues (2015) propose that in addition to typologies that consider the relationship with the victim, motivation, and context of the behavior, increased emphasis should be ascribed to psychiatric diagnoses as an additional criterion for classification purposes. The incompetent suitor classification may most aptly describe the type of stalking usually perpetrated by people on the spectrum. These individuals are often socially awkward and bereft of friendships or intimate relationships (Racine & Billick, 2014). Impairment in relational functioning can manifest as maladaptive patterns of behavior (Perkins, 2010) and result in severe difficulties in establishing intimate relationships.

Mohandie et al. (2006) completed a review of stalking cases ($N = 2300$) derived from prosecutors, police agencies, security departments, and their own case files for the purpose of providing a comparison to people on the spectrum. Males stalk at a slightly higher than 4:1 ratio to females. Nearly half of the sample (46%) demonstrated a DSM IV-TR diagnosis and 24% had a potential psychiatric diagnosis. The majority of males who stalk (63%) are without an intimate partner, being either single, separated or divorced, and only a minority (22%) were fully employed. There are a number of similarities when compared to the population of people with ASD: A 4:1 ratio of males to females (American Psychiatric Association, 2013), more than 66% unemployment rate, and of those who were employed, 80% were employed part-time (Haber et al., 2016). Though many people with ASD report wanting an intimate relationship, many are unsuccessful in obtaining or maintaining a relationship (Sperry & Mesibov, 2005). These social deficits and lack of intimate relationships may make people on the spectrum more likely to be reported for stalking as studies have demonstrated that a previous intimate relationship moderates how victims perceive their experience, thus making it less likely for them to report the behavior of former intimate partners to the authorities (Dennison & Thomson, 2005). In short, a desire for intimacy, coupled with time on one's hands due to unemployment and social isolation sets the stage for intimacy-seeking behaviors that could reach the level of criminality.

G.C.: An Incompetent Suitor Case Study

Dell'Osso and colleagues (2015) provide a case study of a 25-year-old man (G.C.) initially diagnosed with delusional disorder, erotomanic type was assessed using the Ritvo Autism and Asperger Diagnostic Scale-Revised (RAADS-14) following his hospitalization for suicide attempts and stalking behaviors related to a break-up with his girlfriend. The dissolution of the relationship had occurred six years prior to his hospitalization. The relationship with the young woman took on an order of magnitude that was not warranted by the duration of the romance given that it lasted only a few weeks before she ended it. While many people with ASD desire an intimate relationship, only a small minority report having one (Mehzabin & Stokes, 2011), and this may have been the young man's first and subsequently only intimate relationship. G.C. described himself as socially inept, and he labeled socially nuanced dating behaviors as "tricks" that he lacked. The authors have had clients who described seeing people flirt as "like watching aliens interact." While they understand the purpose, which is to attract an intimate partner, they seem to lack the social wherewithal to engage in the behaviors in a fluid manner. In the case of G.C., he self-reported a history of behaviors that could be considered stalking. He sent repeated and invasive messages to young women and ignored their multiple rebuffs. He maintained a persistent, mistaken belief that there was mutual interest on the part of these young women. This may lend additional support to the idea that the first and possibly only intimate relationship, albeit brief, took on an order of magnitude because it initially was reciprocal on some level.

A parallel could be drawn here to the difficulties people on the spectrum have with maintaining social conversation (Gantman et al., 2012). They can become adept at initiating a conversation but may struggle with the social fluidity and perspective taking required to maintain a conversation. It is possible that in the case of G.C. and other individuals who stalk following the break-up of a relationship that they had the basic skills required to start a relationship but lacked the requisite skills to maintain it. Specifically, difficulties with social-emotional reciprocity and perspective taking could make maintaining a relationship particularly difficult for the suitor with ASD. In the absence of a circle of friends or sufficient outside activities toward which to direct their time and attention post break-up, their former partner becomes the target of obsessional thoughts and behaviors.

Overview of Basic Elements of Stalking Laws

In contrast to crimes like murder, assault, and battery, the crime of stalking is a new crime. California was the first U.S. state to pass an anti-stalking law, and now stalking is a criminal offense in all 50 states and interstate stalking is a federal offense. Within the EU, all member states with the exception of Denmark are signatories to the Council of Europe Convention on Preventing and Combating Violence against Women and Domestic Violence, which obligates signatories to criminalize stalking. The most common thread among stalking laws is that they require repeated conduct directed toward another person. But the elements of a stalking offense vary considerably across jurisdictions, particularly regarding what precise conduct constitutes stalking, what mental state or states the defendant must have *(mens rea)*, and whether the victim must subjectively experience fear.

Conduct

In terms of the conduct required to constitute stalking, jurisdictions vary in some important ways. Some allow a prior stalking conviction, in addition to one additional contact, to satisfy the repeated-course-of-conduct element. For example, in an Iowa case, a man was convicted of stalking because he parked his car in an area where he could look directly into the victim's office, and he had previously been convicted of stalking her. *State v. Lindell*, 828 N.W.2d 1, 3 (Iowa 2013). Other jurisdictions, however, require an entirely separate transaction. In Colorado, for example, for a defendant to be "convicted of a second stalking offense, he would have had to so act, in a separate transaction that is factually distinct from the first, on at least two more occasions." *People v. Herron*, 251 P.3d 1190, 1194 (Colo. App. 2010); *see also State v. Stewart*, 234 P.3d 707 (Idaho 2010). In the U.S., most states do not specify a time frame when the repeated acts or conduct must take place, but a few do. For instance, Arkansas requires the acts to be "separated by at least thirty-six (36) hours, but occurring within one (1) year." Ark. Code Ann. § 5-71-229.

Some U.S. states do not require "unequivocally hostile conduct" for a stalking conviction. The Georgia appellate court explained that under its law, "[e]ven behavior that is not overtly threatening can provide the requisite degree of intimidation and harassment if is it ongoing, repetitious, and engaged in despite the communicated wishes of the victim." *Placanica v. State*, 693 S.E.2d 571, 574 (2010).

Mens Rea

Just as jurisdictions vary in terms of the conduct required for stalking conviction, they vary in terms of what mental state (called *mens* rea) is required. Most, but not all, stalking statutes require a particular mental state for *both* the underlying conduct *and* the result of the conduct.

Consider, for example, a stalking statute that requires a perpetrator "*knowingly* repeatedly followed, approached, contacted, placed under surveillance, or made any communication with another person" and also that he "*knew or should have known*" that his conduct would cause a reasonable person to suffer serious emotional distress. In this exemplar statute, the perpetrator must have knowingly engaged in repeated stalking-type conduct and either actually knew or should have known that conduct would cause a reasonable person to suffer serious emotional distress.

In terms of the mental state required for the conduct itself, it's important to make the distinction between intent and a mental state like "knowingly." The defendant must *know* he was following, contacting, surveilling, or communicating with the victim. However, under a statutory scheme like the one outlined above, the prosecution need not prove "that the stalker actually intended to cause fear in the victim, but rather that the stalker consciously engaged in conduct." *State v. Neuzil*, 589 N.W.2d 708, 711 (Iowa 1999). If a defendant repeatedly but accidentally called the victim, or they just happened to be traveling the same route several times, the "knowingly" mental state would not be met. But if he intentionally repeatedly followed the victim, but never intended to cause any upset or harm, the *mens rea* element would still be met. *See New Jersey v. Gandhi*, 989 A.2d 256, 271 (N.J. 2010). In many U.S. states, the perpetrator must "intentionally" or "purposefully" engage in the conduct, but this mental state is distinct from the one required for the harm caused.

In terms of the mental state required for the harm caused, some jurisdictions—unlike the exemplar statute above—require that the defendant *intend* to put the victim in fear or mental distress. E.g., Cal. Penal Code § 646.9; Ga. Code Ann. § 16-5-90; Mass. Gen. Laws Ann. ch. 265, § 43; Mo. Ann. Stat. § 565.225; N. M. Stat. Ann. § 30-3A-3; S.C.C. Ann. § 16-3-1700.

But many other jurisdictions—as in the exemplar statute above—require only that the perpetrator either actually knew or "should have known" that his conduct would cause fear. E.g., Minn. Stat. Ann. § 609.749; Va. Code Ann. § 18.2-60.3; Wash. Rev. Code Ann. § 9A.46.110. The "should have known" standard is an objective one based on what a reasonable person should have known. Under this standard, a defendant can be convicted so long as a "reasonable person" would have known his conduct would cause fear, even if the defendant did not actually know that his conduct would cause fear or mental distress.

Not all stalking statutes require any mental state regarding the harm caused by the stalking. In Colorado, for example, the Supreme Court explained that "the legislature recognized that the stalker in pursuing the victim may be oblivious to objective reality; he or she may not be aware that the repeated acts engaged in would cause a reasonable person to suffer serious emotional distress" and therefore, the statute did not require the perpetrator to be "aware that his or her acts would cause a reasonable person to suffer serious emotional distress." *People v. Cross*, 127 P.3d 71, 77 (Colo. 2006).

For someone with autism, the ramifications of a statutory scheme that does not require any mental state for the harm caused by the conduct or uses the "knew or should have known" standard are apparent. People with autism often persist at failing strategies. (Mullins & Rincover, 1985; Frith, 1996; Konstantareas & Lunsky, 1997; Keenan et al., 2017). Unable to adjust when attempts for romance or friendship floundered, someone on the spectrum may doggedly pursue someone without understanding that their attempts are scary or threatening, and they may never intend any harm. As the New Jersey Supreme Court put it, the "statutory offense reaches and punishes one who engages in a course of stalking conduct even if that person is operating under the motivation of an obsessed and disturbed love that purportedly obscures appreciation of the terror that his or her conduct would reasonably cause to the victimized person." *New Jersey v. Gandhi*, 989 A.2d 256, 271 (N.J. 2010). The Iowa Supreme Court similarly explained that allowing a defendant to excuse conduct based on his affection for the victim "would effectively negate the purpose of the anti-stalking statute—to enable law enforcement to get involved in a harassing situation before physical confrontation results" *People v. Neuzil*, 589 N.W.2d 708, 712 (Iowa 1999).

Victim's Subjective Fear

Some states in the U.S., for example Utah, do not require the victim to actually experience fear or emotional distress. *See State v. Bingham*, 348 P.3d 730, 736 (Utah App. 2015). In Utah, the criminal stalking statute requires that a person "intentionally or knowingly engages in a course of conduct directed at a specific person and knows or should know that the course of conduct would cause a reasonable person: (a) to fear for the person's own safety or the safety of a third person; or (b) to suffer emotional distress." Utah Code Ann. § 76–5–106.5. The use of a "reasonable person" standard rather than the subjective standard is consistent with a more modern approach to stalking laws. *See Bott v. Osburn*, 257 P.3d 1022, 1025 (Utah App. 2011). However, the majority of states still require the victim to actually experience fear or mental distress and require that the fear or mental distress was reasonable. Stalking, 2 Subst. Crim. L. § 16.4(d) (3d ed.).

Considerations Regarding Defendant Testimony

Most criminal defense attorneys usually counsel their clients to not testify at trial. The prosecution has the burden of proving guilt beyond a reasonable doubt, meaning the defense need not say or do anything at trial—it can simply argue that the prosecution failed to meet its burden. In practice, defense attorneys do more than that, but many practitioners believe that putting on defense witnesses—including the defendant himself—tends to shift the burden of proof away from the prosecution. Instead of asking whether the prosecution proved its case, attorneys worry that jurors will weigh the relative evidence and come out in favor of the prosecution if the defendant is not believable, irrespective of the weight of the evidence against him.

The potential challenges related to a defendant's testimony are further complicated when a defendant has ASD. First, someone on the spectrum may have a hard time understanding the risks of testifying and may be less likely to heed his attorney's advice. Second, juries may respond negatively to the atypical behaviors sometimes associated with autism. They may mistake flat affect with evasiveness or a lack of remorse or awkwardness with a guilty conscience. Third, people with ASD may be especially vulnerable to the unpredictability of cross-examination and may respond inappropriately or in ways that undermine their defense (Chaplin et al., 2017). Finally, anxiety and stress compromise verbal comprehension (Twachtman-Cullen, 2006) and further reduce the ability to understand the legal jargon of a trial.

Sentencing

Someone with ASD also faces challenges at the sentencing phase of a stalking case. The receptive and expressive communication challenges for many people on the spectrum create vulnerabilities, particularly because judges often want to hear from and speak to defendants at sentencing. This stress may result in semantic errors, difficulty establishing timelines, and the use of echolalia. Failure to read communicative intent of the prosecutor and the tendency to be literal increases the potential that people on the spectrum may inadvertently self-incriminate through excessive candor. Affective control theory suggests, in part, that criminals who are perceived negatively by the individuals in charge of sentencing are given harsher sentences (prison vs. probation) and longer sentences than those who are perceived positively (Tsoudis, 2000). These perceptions are impacted by neutral, negative, or ambiguous displays of affect and could place the person with ASD at a disadvantage during the sentencing phase of a trial.

One recent case is worth examining to see how some behaviors could play out at sentencing. In *State v. Jason*, a defendant with Asperger's syndrome was convicted of three counts of stalking and sentenced to the maximum sentence, an indeterminate sentence of up to 45 years. *State v. Jason*, 872 N.W.2d 409 (Iowa Ct. App. 2015). Even though the underlying conduct for these convictions was not particularly egregious (he sent 19 emails and left two voicemails), the court determined the long sentence was appropriate. The court concluded that the defendant "showed no lack of remorse for his actions" and had previously stalked the same victim. The defendant also exhibited bizarre behavior in court and throughout the proceedings that likely impacted the sentence. He filed a disciplinary complaint against his attorney, threatened to "file judicial qualification complaints" about the judge to a disciplinary board, and told the judge to "get the hell off this case." He sent a letter to the chief judge of the court to complain about the judge assigned to his case, calling him a pedophile and accusing him of drawing "sexually inappropriate" artwork. At one point, he told the judge he planned to sexually abuse the judge's granddaughter. When the defendant challenged the sentence as excessive based on his diagnosis, the appellate court rejected his argument. Despite recognizing that the defendant had "a long history of difficulties with social skills, obsessional thinking, and intermittent depressive symptoms," the court concluded that the defendant's "actions previous to and during this case appear to have been tactics intended to manipulate the judicial system to get what he wanted, and whenever something did not go his way, he blamed his Asperger's Syndrome diagnosis."

Parole

Depending on the jurisdiction of conviction, a defendant sentenced for a stalking conviction may eventually be eligible for parole. Parole is an administrative action taken after a defendant has served some portion of his prison sentence that allows him to serve the rest of his sentence outside of prison but still under government supervision. *See* Law of Probation & Parole § 2:1 (2nd Ed.). If granted parole, parolees must abide by often stringent requirements or they end up back in prison to serve the remainder of their term. People with autism face unique challenges when it comes to first getting parole and then successfully completing a parole term.

Parole boards have discretion concerning whether to grant or deny parole. *E.g., Terrell v. United States*, 564 F.3d 442 (6th Cir. 2009). While the specific criteria vary by jurisdiction, parole boards are essentially tasked with determining whether, considering an inmate's crime(s) and his conduct while his prison, he should be reintegrated into society. In most states, the parole board (whose members are appointed by the governor) reviews the inmate's history and holds a hearing to decide whether the inmate should be granted parole. Law of Probation & Parole § 4:1 (2d). Often, board members are not required to have any particular experience or education. Law of Probation & Parole § 4:2 (2d).

There are few empirical studies examining the rate at which people with ASD are granted parole compared to the general population. According to the National Autism Indicators Report: Transition into Young Adulthood (Roux et al., 2015), only 0.5% of the study population ($N = 11{,}270$) reported having been on probation or parole during a two-year period. People with ASD may be at a disadvantage during a parole hearing when compared to the general population for a number of reasons. First, parole boards may consider an inmate's expressions of remorse when deciding whether to grant parole, and people with ASD often have difficulty expressing emotions or understanding how their actions affected others. Second, parole boards often consider an inmate's institutional adjustment, including their participation in available rehabilitative programs and educational classes, and people with ASD may not adjust well to prison or succeed in these types of programs and classes. Third, parole boards may consider an inmate's support structure. People with ASD tend to be more isolated than the general population.

If someone with ASD is granted parole, they are not simply released into society. Rather, they must comply with whatever conditions of release are imposed by statute, regulation, and/or the parole board. These conditions run from seemingly mild (for example, a requirement that the parolee does not break any criminal laws) to more demanding (for example, regularly reporting to a parole officer for in-person meetings). Typical parole conditions also include payment of fines or restitution, refraining from using drugs and alcohol, refraining from associating with certain people or going to certain places, requiring someone to be employed or volunteering, participation in educational or counseling programs, submitting to searches, and getting permission before moving, traveling, or changing jobs. Complying with these conditions can be challenging for anyone, but they present special challenges for people with ASD.

Participation in educational and counseling programs can also be a challenge, particularly because states may not have programs equipped to address the special circumstances presented by someone with autism. Worse, some of the required programs may be incompatible with programs specifically geared to people with autism, meaning that someone who is paroled could be forced to participate in a one-size-fits-all program instead of one more appropriate for people with ASD.

Probation and Parole Violations

If someone with autism is on parole or probation and fails to comply with a condition, they may go back to prison (in the case of a parole violation) or be sentenced to prison instead of probation (in the case of a probation violation). It is important to note that parole and probation officers generally have discretion about what happens in the case of a violation, including whether to report it to the court. People with ASD may be able to avoid being sent to prison (at least for minor or isolated violations) if someone works on their behalf to make sure their parole or probation officer understands ASD. And they may be able to work with the court at sentencing to fashion conditions that are tailored toward ASD and perhaps even include participation in ASD-specific programs or accessing state-level disability services.

Please see Chaps. 24 and 26 for information about treatment and rehabilitation.

Conclusion

Important legal considerations surround ASD and stalking. If a person with ASD is charged with stalking, that person is normally subject to the same legal framework used for neurotypical perpetrators. The core deficits associated with ASD can create problems in areas such as determining intent and a victim's perspective. If convicted, the person's ability to represent themsevles in a fashion deemed sufficiently remorseful at sentencing and parole hearings can also be compromised, and adhering to parole guidelines can often be difficult.

The risk of first or future stalking offenses cannot simply be reduced by further isolating people who are already at risk of isolation due to their social challenges. Proactive intimacy education, social opportunities, and teaching the skills necessary to attain the individual's definition of a "Good Life" are all critical elements in reducing the risk and reoccurrence of stalking behaviors. Effective education and therapy combined with a thorough understanding of how the complexities of ASD might create difficulty in a legal context can go a long way toward preventing stalking from occurring and ensuring fair and just outcomes when stalking does occur.

References

American Psychiatric Association. (2013). *Diagnostic and statistical manual of mental disorders* (5th ed.). Author.
Baarsma, M. E., Boonmann, C., 't Hart-Kerkhoffs, L. A., de Graaf, H., Doreleijers, T. A., Vermeiren, R. R., & Jansen, L. M. (2016). Sexuality and autistic-like symptoms in juvenile sex offenders: A follow-up after 8 years. *Journal of Autism & Developmental Disorders, 46*(8), 2679–2691. https://doi.org/10.1007/s10803-016-2805-6.
Baltieri, D. A., de Souza, L., Gatti, A., Henrique de Oliveira, V., Junqueira Aguiar, A. S., & Almeida de Souza Aranha e Silva, R. (2016). A validation study of the Brazilian version of the pornography consumption inventory (PCI) in a sample of female university students. *Journal of Forensic and Legal Medicine, 38,* 81–86. https://doi.org/10.1016/j.jflm.2015.11.004.
Baron-Cohen, S., & Wheelwright, S. (2003). The friendship questionnaire: An investigation of adults with Asperger syndrome or high-functioning autism, and normal sex differences. *Journal of Autism and Developmental Disorders, 33,* 509–517.
Benford, P., & Standen, P. (2009). The internet: A comfortable communication medium for people with Asperger syndrome (AS) and high functioning autism (HFA)? *Journal of Assistive Technologies, 3*(2), 44–53.
Björklund, K., Häkkänen-Nyholm, H., Sheridan, L., & Roberts, K. (2010). The prevalence of stalking among finnish university students. *Journal of Interpersonal Violence, 25*(4), 684–698. https://doi.org/10.1177/0886260509334405.
Bowers, L., Huisingh, R., & LoGiudice, C. (2005). *TOPS 3 elementary*. Linguisystems.
Broadbent, J., & Stokes, M. (2013). Removal of negative feedback enhances WCST performance for individuals with Asperger's syndrome. *Research in Autism Spectrum Disorders, 7*(6), 785–792.
Brown-Lavoie, S. M., Viecili, M., & Weiss, J. (2014). Sexual knowledge and victimization in adults with autism spectrum disorders. *Journal of Autism and Developmental Disorders, 44,* 2185–2196.
Byers, E. S., Nichols, S., Voyer, S. D., & Reilly, G. (2012). Sexual well-being of a community sample of high-functioning adults on the autism spectrum who have been in a romantic relationship. *Autism, 17*(4), 418–433. https://doi.org/10.1177/1362361311431950.
Chaplin, E., McCarthy, J., & Forrester, A. (2017). Defendants with autism spectrum disorders: What is the role of the court liaison and diversion? *Advances in Autism, 3*(4), 220–228.
Cialdini, R., & Goldstein, N. (2004). Social influence: Compliance and conformity. *Annual Review of Psychology, 55,* 591–621.
Constantino, J., & Gruber, C. P. (2012). *Social responsiveness scale—Second edition (SRS-2)*. Western Psychological Services.
Dell'Osso, L., Luche, R. D., Cerliani, C., Bertelloni, C. A., Gesi, C., & Carmassi, C. (2015). Unexpected subthreshold autism spectrum in a 25-year-old male stalker hospitalized for delusional disorder: A case report. *Comprehensive Psychiatry, 61,* 10–14.
Dennison, S. M., & Thomson, D. M. (2005). Criticisms or plaudits for stalking laws? What psychological research tells us about proscribing stalking. *Psychology, Public Policy and Law, 11,* 384–406.
Dewinter, J., De Graaf, H., & Begeer, S. (2017, June 9). Sexual orientation, gender identity, and romantic relationships in adolescents and adults with autism spectrum disorder. *Journal of Autism & Developmental Disorders*. https://doi.org/10.1007/s10803-017-3199-9.
Dewinter, J., Vermeiren, R., Vanwesenbeeck, I., & Nieuwenhuizen, C. (2013). Autism and normative sexual development: A narrative review. *Journal of Clinical Nursing, 22,* 3467–3483.
Domjan, M. (2015). *The principles of leaning and behavior* (7th ed.). Cenage Learning.
Engelhardt, C. R., & Mazurek, M. O. (2014). Video game access, parental rules, and problem behavior: A study of boys with autism spectrum disorder. *Autism, 18*(5), 529–537. https://doi.org/10.1177/1362361313482053.
Engelhardt, C. R., Mazurek, M. O., & Sohl, K. (2013). Media use and sleep among boys with autism spectrum disorder, ADHD, or typical development. *Pediatrics, 132*(6), 1081–1089. https://doi.org/10.1542/peds.2013-2066.

Frith, U. (1996). Cognitive explanations of autism. *Acta Paediatrica Supplement, 416,* 63–68.

Gantman, A., Kapp, S. K., Orenski, K., et al. (2012). *Journal of Autism and Developmental Disorders, 42,* 1094. https://doi.org/10.1007/s10803-011-1350-6.

Gersick, A., & Kurzban, R. (2014). Covert sexual signaling: Human flirtation and implications for other social species. *Evolutionary Psychology, 12*(3), 549–569.

Ginevra, M. C., Nota, L., & Stokes, M. A. (2016). The differential effects of autism and down's syndrome upon sexual behavior. *Autism Research, 9*(1), 131–140. https://doi.org/10.1002/aur.1504.

Haber, M. G., Mazzotti, V. L., & Mustian, A. L. et al. (2016). What works, when, for whom, and with whom: A meta-analytic review of predictors of postsecondary success for students With disabilities. *Review of Educational Research, 86*(1), 123–162. https://doi.org/10.3102/0034654315583135.

Hald, G. M., & Štulhofer, A. (2016). What types of pornography do people use and do they cluster? Assessing types and categories of pornography consumption in a large-scale online sample. *Journal of Sex Research, 53*(7), 849–859. https://doi.org/10.1080/00224499.2015.1065953.

Hancock, G. I. (2017). *Socio-sexual functioning in autism spectrum disorders.* Unpublished Doctoral thesis, Deakin University.

Hancock, G. I., Stokes, M. A., & Mesibov, G. B. (2017). Socio-sexual functioning in autism spectrum disorder: A systematic review and meta-analyses of existing literature. *Autism Research, 10*(11), 1823–1833. https://doi.org/10.1002/aur.1831.

Happé, F., Briskman, J., & Frith, U. (2001). Exploring the cognitive phenotype of autism: Weak "central coherence" in parents and siblings of children with autism: I. Experimental tests. *Journal of Child Psychology and Psychiatry, 42*(3), 299–307. https://doi.org/10.1111/1469-7610.00723.

Head, A., McGillivray, J., & Stokes, M. (2014). Gender differences in emotionality and sociability in children with ASD. *Molecular Autism, 5,* 1–9. https://doi.org/10.1186/2040-2392-5-19.

Hellemans, H., Colson, K., Verbraeken, C., Vermeiren, R., & Deboutte, D. (2007). Sexual behavior in high-functioning male adolescents and young adults with autism spectrum disorder. *Journal of Autism and Developmental Disorders, 37,* 260–269.

Hénault, I. (2006). *Asperger's syndrome and sexuality: From adolescence through adulthood.* Jessica Kingsley.

Howlin, P. (2004). Legal issues. In P. Howlin (Ed.), *Autism and Asperger syndrome: Preparing for adulthood* (Vol. 2, pp. 300–312). Routledge.

Jones, R. A., Downing, K., Rinehart, N. J., Barnett, L. M., May, T., McGillivray, J. A., Papadopoulos, N. V., Skouteris, H., Timperio, A., & Hinkley, T. (2017). Physical activity, sedentary behavior and their correlates in children with autism spectrum disorder: A systematic review. *PLoS One, 12*(2), e0172482. https://doi.org/10.1371/journal.pone.0172482.

Kasari, C., Locke, J., Gulsrud, A., & Rotheram-Fuller, E. (2011). Social networks and friendships at school: Comparing children with and without ASD. *Journal of Autism and Developmental Disorders, 41,* 533–544.

Keenan, E. G., Gotham, K., & Lerner, M. D. (2017, July 1). Hooked on a feeling: Repetitive cognition and internalizing symptomatology in relation to autism spectrum symptomatology. *Autism, 22*(7), 814–824, 1362361317709603. https://doi.org/10.1177/1362361317709603.

Konstantareas, M. M., & Lunsky, Y. J. (1997). Sociosexual knowledge, experience, attitudes, and interests of individuals with autistic disorder and developmental delay. *Journal of Autism and Developmental Disorders, 27*(4), 397–413.

Landry, O., & Al-Taie, S. (2016). A meta-analysis of the Wisconsin card sort task in autism. *Journal of Autism and Developmental Disorders, 46*(4), 1220–1235. https://doi.org/10.1007/s10803-015-2659-3.

Manjiviona, J. (2003). Specific learning difficulties. In M. Prior (Ed.), *Learning and behavior problems in Asperger syndrome.* The Guilford Press.

Mazurek, M. O., & Kanne, S. M. (2010). Friendship and internalizing symptoms among children and adolescents with ASD. *Journal of Autism and Developmental Disorders, 40,* 1512–1520.

Mehrabian, A. (1972). *Nonverbal communication.* Aldine Transaction.

Mehzabin, P., & Stokes, M. A. (2011). Self-assessed sexuality in young adults with high functioning autism. *Research in Autism Spectrum Disorders, 5*, 614–621.
Miller, W. R., & Lief, H. I. (1979). The sex knowledge and attitude test (SKAT). *Journal of Sex and Marital Therapy, 5*(3), 282–287.
Mohandie, K., Meloy, J. R., McGowan, M. G., & Williams, J. (2006). The RECON typology of stalking: Reliability and validity based upon a large sample of North American stalkers. *Journal of Forensic Sciences, 51*(1), 147–155.
Monge, R. H., Dusek, J. B., & Lawless, J. (1977). An evaluation of the acquisition of sexual information through a sex education class. *The Journal of Sex Research, 13*(3), 170–184.
Mullins, M., & Rincover, A. (1985). Comparing autistic and normal children along the dimensions of reinforcement maximization, stimulus sampling, and responsiveness to extinction. *Journal of Experimental Child Psychology, 40*(2), 350–374.
Must, A., Phillips, S., Curtin, C., & Bandini, L. G. (2015). Barriers to physical activity in children with autism spectrum disorders: Relationship to physical activity and screen time. *Journal of Physical Activity & Health, 12*(4), 529–534. https://doi.org/10.1123/jpah.2013-0271.
National Institute of Justice, Office of Justice Programs. (2007). *Stalking*. Retrieved from https://www.nij.gov/topics/crime/stalking/Pages/welcome.aspx.
Nichols, S., & Blakeley-Smith, A. (2009). "I'm not sure we're ready for this…": Working with families toward facilitating healthy sexuality for individuals with autism spectrum disorders. *Social Work in Mental Health, 8*, 72–91.
Palermo, M. T., & Bogaerts, S. (2015). Violent fantasies in young men with autism spectrum disorders: Dangerous or miserable misfits? Duty to protect whom? *International Journal of Offender Therapy & Comparative Criminology, 61*, 1–16.
Park, S., & Shin, J. (2017). The influence of anonymous peers on prosocial behavior. *PLoS One, 12*(10), https://doi.org/10.1371/journal.pone.0185521.
Pecora, L., Mesibov, G., & Stokes, M. A. (2016). Sexuality in high functioning autism: A systematic review and meta-analysis. *Journal of Autism and Developmental Disorders, 46*(11), 3519–3556. https://doi.org/10.1007/s10803-016-2892-4.
Perkins, D. (2010). Mentally disordered offenders. In J. Brown & E. Campbell (Eds.), *The Cambridge handbook of forensic psychology* (pp. 221–229). Cambridge handbooks in psychology. Cambridge University Press. https://doi.org/10.1017/cbo9780511730290.028.
Racine, C., & Billick, S. (2014). Classification systems for stalking behavior. *Journal of Forensic Science, 59*(1), 250–254.
Reich, S. M., Subrahmanyam, K., & Espinoza, G. (2012). Friending, IMing, and hanging out face-to-face: Overlap in adolescents' online and offline social networks. *Developmental Psychology, 48*(2), 356–368. https://doi.org/10.1037/a0026980.
Roux, A. M., Shattuck, P. T., Rast, J. E., Rava, J. A., & Anderson, K. A. (2015). *National autism indicators report: Transition into young adulthood*. Life Course Outcomes Research Program, A.J. Drexel Autism Institute, Drexel University.
South, M., Ozonoff, S., & McMahon, W. M. (2007). The relationship between executive functioning, central coherence, and repetitive behaviors in the high-functioning autism spectrum. *Autism, 11*(5), 437–451.
Sperry, L. A., & Mesibov, G. B. (2005). Perceptions of social challenges of adults with autism spectrum disorder. *Autism, 9*(4), 362–376. https://doi.org/10.1177/1362361305056077.
Sperry, L. A, & Stokes, M. A. (2017). Stalking. In *Encyclopedia of autism spectrum disorders*. A Springer major reference work. http://refworks.springer.com/autism.
Spitzberg, B. H., & Cupach, W. R. (2007). Cyberstalking as (mis)matchmaking. In M. T. Whitty, A. J. Baker, & J. A. Inman (Eds.), *Online matchmaking* (pp. 127–146). Palgrave Macmillan.
Stalking Resource Center, Criminal Stalking Laws. (2017). Retrieved from http://victimsofcrime.org/our-programs/stalking-resource-center/stalking-laws/criminal-stalking-laws-by-state.
Stokes, M., Newton, N., & Kaur, A. (2007). Stalking, and social and romantic functioning among of adolescents and adults with autistic spectrum disorder. *Journal of Autism and Developmental Disorders, 37*(10), 1969–1986.

Tsoudis, O. (2000). Relation of affect control theory to the sentencing of criminals. *Journal of Social Psychology, 4,* 473–485.
Twachtman-Cullen, D. (2006). Communication and stress in students with autism spectrum disorders. In M. G. Baron, J. Groden, G. Groden, & L. P. Lipsitt (Eds.), *Stress and coping in autism.* Oxford University Press.
Visser, K., Greaves-Lord, K., Tick, N. T., Verhulst, F. C., Maras, A., & van der Vegt, E. J. M. (2017a). An exploration of the judgement of sexual situations by adolescents with autism spectrum disorders versus typically developing adolescents. *Research in Autism Spectrum Disorders, 36,* 35–43.
Visser, K., Greaves-Lord, K., Tick, N. T., Verhulst, F. C., Maras, A., & van der Vegt, E. J. M. (2017b). A randomized controlled trial to examine the effects of the tackling teenage psychosexual training program for adolescents with autism spectrum disorder. *Journal of Child Psychology and Psychiatry and Allied Disciplines, 58,* 840–850. https://doi.org/10.1111/jcpp.12709.
Weinstein, R. B., Walsh, J. L., & Ward, L. M. (2007). Testing a new measure of sexual health knowledge and its connections to students' sex education, communication, confidence, and condom use. *International Journal of Sexual Health, 20*(3), 212–221.

Laurie A. Sperry is a Board Certified Behavior Analyst-Doctoral and the Director of Autism Services And Programs in Wheat Ridge, Colorado. She has worked as a developer of the Neurodiverse Student Support Program at Stanford University, School of Medicine, Department of Psychiatry. Prior to joining Stanford, she was an Assistant Clinical Faculty at Yale University, Department of Psychiatry.

In 2006 she was added to the Fulbright Scholarship's Senior Specialist Roster for Autism. She moved to Australia in 2010 and worked at Griffith University in the Department of Arts, Education and Law. Her research focuses on people with ASD who come in contact with the criminal justice system to ensure their humane and just treatment. She has served as a Special Interest Group Chairwoman at the International Meeting for Autism Research (IMFAR) providing mentoring and leadership in the field of criminality and ASD. She has provided training to secure forensic psychiatric facility staff in England and presented at the International Conference for Offenders with Disabilities. She has published numerous articles and book chapters and was an expert panelist at the American Academy of Psychiatry and Law conference where she spoke on Risk Assessment, Management, and ASD. She has completed ADOS evaluations in prisons, has testified as an expert witness in sentencing hearings, has written *amicus curiae* briefs and has participated in cases that have been considered before state supreme courts.

Mark A. Stokes is a registered psychologist, and has been involved in Autism research since 1992; he obtained his PhD from La Trobe University in 1996 in circadian rhythms and sleep control. Following this, Mark has had appointments at La Trobe, Monash University, and Vanderbilt University. In 1999 Mark returned to Monash University as Director of the Victorian Injury Surveillance Unit at Monash University's Accident Research Centre. In 2002 Mark was appointed to Deakin University where he established a research group—the Healthy Autistic Life Lab (HALL). HALL collaborates with many researchers globally and covers research programs into autism addressing sexuality; relationship development; the female profile of autism; mirror neurons in autism; and the transition to adulthood in autism. HALL seeks to understand how to support autistic adolescents and adults through the major transitions to adulthood, such as finding employment, finding a life partner, developing intimacy, to assist people to obtain a life that supports outcomes of mental health and positive well-being. Mark has published over 150 peer-reviewed publications, book chapters, and reports to government as well as more than 140 conference presentations. Mark has supervised over 30 doctoral and PhD completions. Mark actively supports research into autism through his role as former President of the Australasian Society for Autism Research and as National Lead for Australia to INSAR. Mark has also been involved in Child Injury Prevention and Intervention for 25 years. Mark has been a board member of Kidsafe since 2000 and is a life member and former President of Kidsafe Victoria and Kidsafe Australia.

Mark is currently Vice President of Kidsafe Victoria. https://www.deakin.edu.au/about-deakin/people/mark-stokes.

Melanie E. Gavisk is an Assistant Federal Public Defender based in Cheyenne, Wyoming. She represents criminal defendants charged with federal crimes in the District of Wyoming. In addition to her law degree, Ms. Gavisk has a master's degree in psychology.

She previously worked with the Federal Public Defender in Las Vegas, Nevada, representing criminal defendants, including those sentenced to death, in post-conviction proceedings, and at a large international law firm as a civil litigator, where she worked on a wide variety of civil cases and on white collar criminal defense. Ms. Gavisk was also a law clerk to the Honorable Lewis Babcock at the United States District Court for the District of Colorado.

David C. Gavisk received his Ph.D. in Educational Psychology from the University of Georgia. Dave also has an M.A. in Educational Psychology from the University of Colorado, Denver. Since 2014, he has been an Affiliate Faculty member at Regis University in Denver.

Chapter 15
The Right to Special Education

Stacey Therese Cherry

Introduction

In response to concerns that the majority of children with disabilities were not receiving an appropriate education and over a million children were completely excluded from school, the United States' Congress passed the Education for All Handicapped Children Act of 1975 ("EHA") (P.L. 94–142) (20 U.S.C. § 1400(b)(4)(1998)). The goal of the EHA and its successor legislation is to ensure that all children with disabilities receive a free and appropriate public education ("FAPE") in the least restrictive environment ("LRE"); and that they are educated, to the maximum extent appropriate, with their non-disabled peers (20 U.S.C. § 1400(d)(1)). The primary mechanism for meeting this goal is the student's Individualized Education Program ("IEP"), which provides for "special education and related services designed to meet the child's unique needs and prepare them for further education, employment, and independent living" (20 U.S.C. §§ 1400(d)(1), 1414(d); 34 C.F.R. § 300.1(a)). To ensure that the purpose is met, parents and students are also afforded specific procedural safeguards that protect their rights (20 U.S.C. §§ 1400(d)(2), 1415; 34 C.F.R. § 300.1(b)). The EHA was amended in 1983 (P.L. 98–199) and 1990 (P.L. 101–476), when the name was changed to the Individuals with Disabilities Education Act ("IDEA"). Subsequent revisions were enacted in 1997 (P.L. 105–17) and 2004 (P.L. 108–446), when the IDEA was renamed the Individuals with Disabilities Education Improvement Act, although it is still commonly called the IDEA.

S. T. Cherry (✉)
Fogarty & Hara, 21-00 Route 208 South, Fair Lawn, NJ 07410, USA
e-mail: scherry@fogartyandhara.com

F. R. Volkmar et al. (eds.), *Handbook of Autism Spectrum Disorder and the Law*,
https://doi.org/10.1007/978-3-030-70913-6_15

Among those recognized as eligible for special education and related services, children with autism qualify—if they meet the IDEA's eligibility requirements—since first being recognized as a separate eligibility category in the 1990 amendments (P.L. 101–476). In 1991–1992, the school year that autism was first added to the IDEA, the United States Department of Education ("US DOE"), which reports to Congress annually regarding the implementation of the IDEA, reported that there were 5,415 school-aged (ages 6–21) students classified with autism (24th Annual Report, 2002: II–20). By 2000–2001, school-aged students classified with autism had increased to 78,749 (24th Annual Report, 2002: II–20) and by 2004, there were 165,552 school-aged students and an additional 25,664 preschool (ages 3–5) students classified with autism (28th Annual Report, 2006: 10, 13). In 2018, the most recent year for which data is provided by the US DOE, there were 663,098 school-aged students receiving services under the category of autism (10.5 percent of all classified school-aged children) and autism represented the fourth most prevalent disability category (following specific learning disability at 37.7 percent, speech or language impairment at 16.4 percent, and other health impairment at 16.2 percent) (42nd Annual Report, 2020: 41–42). There were also 92,911 preschool students identified under the category of autism (11.4 percent of preschool-aged children with disabilities), which represented the third largest category for preschool-aged children (following speech and language impairment at 41.4 percent and developmental delay at 37.7 percent) (42nd Annual Report, 2020: 29–30). The increase in students with autism served under the IDEA is consistent with the increase in children estimated by the United States Center for Disease Control and Prevention ("CDC") identified with Autism Spectrum Disorder ("ASD"), which estimates that in 2018 approximately 1 in 54 children has been identified with an ASD; an increase from 1 in 150 in 2000.[1] Given the number of children diagnosed with ASD and the increase in students eligible for special education and related services under the category of autism, it is important to understand a local education agency's ("school district") obligation to meet these students' needs.

Fundamentally, the IDEA is a Spending Clause statute (U.S. Const. Art. 1, § 8, cl. 1). That is, to receive funding available under the IDEA, a State must agree to implement the IDEA's requirements. The States implement the IDEA by adopting their own statues and regulations, which must offer at least as much protection as required by the IDEA but can offer more. This Chapter discusses the dual requirements imposed by the IDEA: (1) the procedural safeguards, including the steps that a school district must follow, and the protections afforded students and parents, and (2) the substantive provision of a FAPE. Practitioners are urged to review their State's statues and regulations for information specific to implementation in their State.

---

[1] https://www.cdc.gov/ncbddd/autism/data.html (accessed on May 13, 2021). The data is based on estimates from the CDC's Autism and Developmental Disabilities Monitoring Network of children at eight years of age. Diagnosis, however, is not equivalent to eligibility for special education and related services.

Child Find and Referral for Special Education

The right to a FAPE begins with the school district's obligation to identify, locate, and evaluate children who are in need of special education and related services (20 U.S.C. § 1412(a)(3)(A); 34 C.F.R. § 300.111). This obligation extends to children who are homeless, wards of the state, or attending private schools (20 U.S.C. § 1412(a)(3)(A); 34 C.F.R. § 300.111). Accordingly, the school district must take affirmative action to find students who may be eligible for special education and related services, to conduct a nondiscriminatory evaluation, and to provide them with the services they need at no cost.

If a child receives services through a State's early intervention ("EI") system,[2] a direct referral is made to the school district so that an IEP is in place by the time the child turns three (20 U.S.C. § 1412(a)(9); 34 C.F.R. § 300.323(b)). If the child is not receiving EI or is between the ages of three and twenty-one when the need for special education is suspected, the parent or the school district can refer the child for an evaluation[3] (20 U.S.C. § 1414(a)(1)(B), 34 C.F.R. § 300.301(b)).

Consent

Before conducting an initial evaluation, the school district must obtain informed consent from the parent (20 U.S.C. § 1414(a)(1)(D), 34 C.F.R. § 300.300(a), 300.301(a)). Consent is only valid when the parent is provided all of the information relevant to the school district's proposal—the evaluation—in the parent's native language or another mode of communication, and the parent understands and voluntarily agrees in writing to the school district's proposed action (34 C.F.R. § 300.9(a)&(b)). The parent must also know that consent can be revoked, but that revocation is not retroactive (34 C.F.R. § 300.9(c)(1)&(2)).

The written notification of the initial evaluation must include the following content:

1. A description of the proposed action;
2. An explanation of why the school district proposes the action;
3. A description of each evaluation, procedure, assessment record, or report the school district used to determine the proposed action;
4. A statement that the parents have procedural safeguards[4];
5. Sources the parent can contact to obtain assistance understanding their rights and the provision of special education;
6. A description of other options that were considered and why they were rejected;

---

[2] Children between birth and age three can receive services under 20 U.S.C. § 1431 *et seq.*

[3] The referral can also be made by the State educational agency or another State agency.

[4] For an initial evaluation, parents must be provided a copy of their procedural safeguards (20 U.S.C. § 1415(d)(A)(i)).

7. A description of any other factors relevant to the decision (34 C.F.R. § 300.503(b)).

Once the parent provides informed consent, the school district has sixty days, or the timeframe established by the State, to complete the initial evaluation unless the parent fails or refuses to produce the child for the evaluation or the child enrolls in a new school district (34 C.F.R. § 300.301(c)(1)&(d)). If the parent refuses to provide consent, the school district can seek to compel the evaluation through a due process hearing[5] (20 U.S.C. § 1414(a)(D)(ii)(I); 34 C.F.R. § 300.507(a)(1)).

Evaluation

The purpose of an evaluation is to determine if the student has a disability and, if the child is eligible, the content of the IEP (20 U.S.C. § 1414(b)(2), 34 C.F.R. § 300.304(b)(1)). Therefore, the evaluation must assess the student in all areas of suspected disability, which includes gathering information on the student's functional, developmental, and academic needs, and the contribution of any cognitive, behavioral, developmental, or physical factors (20 U.S.C. § 1414(b)(2)(A), (b)(2)(C) and (b)(3)(B)). In conducting the evaluation, the school district cannot use a single measure or assessment to determine a student's eligibility or a student's IEP, and it must administer the assessment in the child's native language, unless that is clearly not feasible (20 U.S.C. § 1414(b)(2)(B), (b)(3)(A)(ii), 34 C.F.R. § 300.304(b)(2)&(3), (c)(1)). The assessment used must be technically sound, non-discriminatory, and valid, and reliable (20 U.S.C. § 1414(b)(2)(C), (b)(3)(A)(i)&(iii); 34 C.F.R. § 300.304(c)(1)(i)&(iii)). Finally, the person administering the assessment has to be trained, knowledgeable, and follow the instructions of the producer of the assessment (20 U.S.C. § 1414(b)(3)(A)(iv)&(v), 34 C.F.R. § 300.304(c)(1)(iv)&(v)).

A comprehensive assessment for a student suspected to have autism often includes: an assessment of cognitive abilities, an assessment of academic skills, a speech and language assessment including social pragmatics, a medical assessment such as one conducted by a neurodevelopmental pediatrician, a developmental history, and observations of the student. Depending on the student's suspected needs, the evaluation could also include an occupational therapy assessment, including a sensory profile, a physical therapy assessment, an augmentative communication assessment, an assistive technology assessment, or a functional behavioral assessment. If there are other areas of suspected need, those must also be addressed through the evaluation (see, e.g., New Jersey Department of Education, 2004; North Dakota Department of Public Instruction, 2014; Oregon Department of Education, 2010).

Once the evaluation is complete, the parent must be given a copy of the evaluation (20 U.S.C. § 1414(b)(4)(B), 34 C.F.R. § 300.306(a)(2)). If the parent disagrees with an evaluation, the parent has the right to request an evaluation by someone not

[5] A due process hearing is an administrative procedure by which a party can ask a hearing officer for certain relief, including compelling an evaluation.

employed by the school district—an independent educational evaluation ("IEE")—at the school district's expense (34 C.F.R. § 300.502(a)). Upon receipt of a request for an IEE, the school district must, without unnecessary delay, either file a due process request to show that its evaluation was appropriate or pay for the evaluation (34 C.F.R. § 300.502(b)(2)). The results of an IEE or a private evaluation submitted by the parent must be considered by the school district (34 C.F.R. § 300.502(c)).

Reevaluation

A reevaluation shall not be conducted more than once a year, but must be conducted at least every three years, unless the parent and district agree that no additional information is needed to determine that the student is eligible and to determine the student's needs (20 U.S.C. § 1414(b)(2); 34 C.F.R. § 300.303(b)). A reevaluation must also be conducted before determining that a student is no longer a child with a disability; when needed to plan for the student's education, including because of improved performance; and upon the request of the parent or teacher (20 U.S.C. § 1414(b)(2); 34 C.F.R. § 300.303(a)).

Eligibility

After the evaluation is complete, the school district and parent determine if the student is a child with a disability (34 C.F.R. § 300.306(a)(1)). To qualify as a child with a disability, the student must meet the eligibility criteria for one of the thirteen eligibility categories[6] and, because of the disability, need special education and related services (34 C.F.R. § 300.306(b)(2), 300.8(a)). If a student's needs are a result of a lack of appropriate instruction in reading, a lack of instruction in math, or a lack of English proficiency, the student shall not be determined to be a child with a disability (20 U.S.C. § 1414(b)(5), 34 C.F.R. § 300.306(b)(1); 34 C.F.R. § 300.306(b)(1)(i)).

For purposes of this chapter, the eligibility category of autism is most relevant; however, it is important to note that a student with autism could be considered under other eligibility categories.[7] Autism is defined as:

---

[6] The eligibility categories are: intellectual disability, hearing impairment, speech or language impairment, visual impairment, serious emotional disturbance, orthopedic impairment, autism, traumatic brain injury, other health impairment, specific learning disability, deaf-blindness, or multiple disabilities (34 C.F.R. § 300.8(a)(1)). A child between the ages of three to nine (or a subset of that range) may qualify if they have a developmental delay as defined by the State and need special education and related services (34 C.F.R. § 300.8(b)).

[7] For example, a student with autism could also have an intellectual disability, a specific learning disability, or an other health impairment. If these are the primary disability, the student could be found eligible under these categories. Where the student has multiple disabilities that result in

> a developmental disability significantly affecting verbal and nonverbal communication and social interaction, generally evident before age three, that adversely affects a child's educational performance. Other characteristics often associated with autism are engagement in repetitive activities and stereotyped movements, resistance to environmental change or change in daily routines, and unusual response to sensory experiences. (34 C.F.R. § 300.8(c)(1)(i))

A student does not meet the criteria for autism if the primary impact is due to an emotional disturbance (34 C.F.R. § 300.8(c)(1)(ii)).

Just because a student has a medical diagnosis of ASD does not mean they qualify as a student with a disability. A student must also need special education and related services. Special education means "specially designed instruction . . . to meet the unique needs of a child with a disability" and can be provided in a school, home, hospital, or other settings, and instruction in physical education (34 C.F.R. § 300.39(a)(1)). Specially designed instruction is further defined as "adapting, as appropriate to the needs of [the student], the content, methodology, or delivery of instruction" to meet the student's needs that result from their disability and to ensure access to the general education curriculum (34 C.F.R. § 300.39(b)(3)). Related services are "transportation and such developmental, corrective, or other supportive services as required to assist a child with a disability to benefit from special education" (34 C.F.R. § 300.34(a)). Notably, if a student only needs related services then the student is not a child with a disability, unless the State considers the related service special education under State standards (34 C.F.R. § 300.8(a)(2)).

The Individualized Education Program

When a student is determined to be a child with a disability, the school district, through the IEP Team, must develop an IEP (34 C.F.R. § 300.306(c)(2)). The IEP Team is the group of individuals who collectively determine the content of the IEP. At a minimum the IEP Team must include the following: (1) the parents; (2) a general education teacher if the child is or may be participating in the general education environment; (3) a special education teacher, or where appropriate, a special education provider of the child; (4) a representative of the school district who is qualified to provide or supervise special education services and is knowledgeable about the curriculum and the school district's resources; (5) an individual who can interpret the instructional implication of evaluation results; (6) individuals invited by the parent or district; and (7) the child, if appropriate (20 U.S.C. § 1414(d)(1)(B); 34 C.F.R. § 300.321(a)).

The IEP is a document that, at its most basic, sets forth the student's needs and services. It also serves to guide the teacher and allows the school district and parent to monitor the student's progress. IEPs include the following components:

---

severe needs such that the student's needs cannot be met in a program that is designed solely for one impairment, the student is considered multiple disabled (34 C.F.R. § 300.8(c)(7)).

1. The present levels of academic achievement and functional performance ("PLAAFP"), including how the student's disability affects their progress and involvement in the general education curriculum.
2. Measurable annual goals, including academic and functional goals that meet the student's needs that result from their disability and enable the student to be involved in and progress in the general education curriculum. The goals should be challenging based on the child's profile. *Endrew F. v. Douglas County School Dist.*, 137 S.Ct. 988, 1000 (2017).
3. A description of how the student's progress on the goals and objectives will be monitored and when the parent will be informed regarding the student's progress.
4. A statement of the special education and related services, and supplementary aids and services based on peer-reviewed research to the extent practicable that will be provided to the student.
5. A statement of the program modifications or supports for school personnel.
6. A statement explaining the extent to which the student will not participate with general education peers.
7. The accommodations the student requires on any State or districtwide assessments.
8. The commencement, frequency, location, and duration of services provided in the IEP.
9. Transition planning beginning with the IEP developed for the year the child turns 16, and updated annually thereafter, including:

   (a) Appropriate, measurable postsecondary goals based on a transition assessment;
   (b) The transition services needed to reach the transition goals;
   (c) Beginning not later than one year before the student reaches the age of majority, notification that the rights of the IDEA will transfer to the student at the age of majority (20 U.S.C. § 1414(d)(1)(A)(i); 34 C.F.R. § 300.320).

When developing the IEP, the IEP Team must consider the student's strengths, the concerns of the parent, the results of the initial or most recent evaluation, and the academic, developmental, and functional needs of the child (20 U.S.C. § 1414(d)(3)(A); 34 C.F.R. § 300.324(a)(1)). If the student has behaviors that impact their learning or the learning of others, the IEP has to consider including positive behavioral interventions, which may include a behavior intervention plan ("BIP"), or other strategies (20 U.S.C. § 1414(d)(3)(B); 34 C.F.R. § 300.324(a)(2)(i)). The IEP Team must also consider the child's communication needs, the language needs of children with limited English proficiency, the Braille needs of children who are blind or visually impaired, the communication needs of the student, the communication and language needs of children who are deaf or hard of hearing, and whether the child needs assistive technology devices or services (20 U.S.C. § 1414(d)(3)(B); 34 C.F.R. § 300.324(a)(2)(ii)–(iv)).

Related Services

Related services must be provided by the school district to the extent that they are needed for the student to benefit from their education (20 U.S.C. § 1401(26)(A); 34 C.F.R. § 300.34(a)). Examples of related services are speech and language services, audiology services, interpreting services, psychological services, physical and occupational therapy, recreation, counseling, orientation and mobility services, and medical services for diagnostic and evaluation purposes (34 C.F.R. § 300.34(c)). Medical devices that are surgically implanted, the optimization of that device's functioning (e.g., mapping), maintenance of that device, or the replacement of that device are not considered related services (34 C.F.R. § 300.34(b)(1)). Related services also do not include medical services that are performed by a physician, except for the purpose of evaluation and diagnosis (34 C.F.R. § 300.34(c)(5)).

The Supreme Court has twice addressed the extent to which a school district must provide related services to a student with disabilities, and in particular services that the school district considered medical. In *Irving Independent School Dist. v. Tatro*, the Court determined that clean intermittent catheterization ("CIC")[8] is a related service that must be provided by the school district when it is necessary for a student to benefit from special education. 468 U.S. 883 (1984). In reaching its determination, the Court found that: (1) CIC is a supportive service without which the student could not stay in school, and (2) CIC is not a medical service, which a school district need only provide for purposes of diagnosis or evaluation. 468 U.S. at 890–91. CIC was considered a supportive service, which is under the category of related services, and not a medical service because it can be performed by a school nurse and because the student needed the procedure every three to four hours in order to remain in school. 468 U.S. at 885, 894. More specifically, the Court found that excludable medical services are only those that require a physician (except for diagnostic and evaluation), not a nurse. 468 U.S. at 892.

Almost fifteen years later, the Court again addressed the extent to which a school district must provide nursing services to a student when Garrett F., a student dependent on a ventilator, required continuous nursing services to attend school. *Cedar Rapids Community School Dist., v. Garrett F.*, 526 U.S. 66 (1999). Following its reasoning in *Tatro*, the Court found that, even though there were legitimate financial concerns, the school district had to provide Garrett F. with nursing services so that he could access his education. 526 U.S. at 78–79. In reaching its decision, the Court held that school districts must pay for related services, such as nursing, in order to help guarantee the inclusion of students with disabilities in the public schools. 526 U.S. at 79. Central to the Court's decision is the purpose of the IDEA, "to assure that all children with disabilities have available to them . . . a free appropriate public education which emphasizes special education and related services designed to meet their unique needs" 526 U.S. at 68, *citing*, 20 U.S.C. § 1400(c).

---

[8] CIC is a procedure that involves inserting a catheter into the urethra to drain the bladder. It is a relatively simple procedure that can be performed by a lay person with less than an hour of training. 468 U.S. at 885.

Least Restrictive Environment/Continuum of Placements

One of the central tenets of the IDEA is that students with disabilities must be included in the general education environment with nondisabled peers to the maximum extent appropriate (20 U.S.C. § 1412(a)(5); 34 C.F.R. § 300.311(a)(2)). To that end, students with disabilities cannot be denied access to the general education setting unless the nature and severity of their disability is so severe that they cannot receive their education in a general education class even with supplemental supports and aids (20 U.S.C. § 1412(a)(5), 34 C.F.R. § 300.114(a)(2)(ii)). The IEP Team determines a student's placement; however, the IDEA emphasizes that any decision regarding a student's placement must include the parents (20 U.S.C. § 1414(e), 34 C.F.R. § 300.327). While students with disabilities must be included to the maximum extent appropriate, the IDEA recognizes that a general education setting is not appropriate for all students. Therefore, school districts must have a continuum of placements available (34 C.F.R. § 300.315(a)). The continuum of placements includes regular classes, special classes, special schools, home instruction, and instruction in hospitals and institutions (34 C.F.R. § 300.315(b)(1)). School districts must also provide for supplementary services such as resource room or itinerant instruction provided in conjunction with a general education program (34 C.F.R. § 300.315(b)(2)). In addition, if a residential placement is necessary to provide the student with special education and related services, a school district has to fund the non-medical care and room and board (34 C.F.R. § 300.104).

With regard to students eligible under the category of autism, as of 2018, the US DOE reports that less than half of school-aged students spend 80 percent or more of their day in a general education setting. More specifically, 39.7 percent spend 80 percent or more of their day in general education, 18.4 percent spend between 40 percent and 79 percent of their day in general education, 33.4 percent spend less than 40 percent of their day in general education, and 8.5 percent are in other environments (42nd Annual Report, 2020: 56). Given the distribution of students with autism in more restrictive settings, the IEP Team must consider if the student is included in the LRE to the maximum extent appropriate.

A consensus standard has not emerged from the Circuit Courts or the Supreme Court with regard to implementation of the LRE standard[9]; however, the most often articulated standard is set forth in *Oberti v. Board of Educ.*, 995 F.2d 914 (3d. Cir., 1993). *Oberti* sets forth a three-factor test:

1. Whether the school district has made reasonable efforts to accommodate the child in a general education classroom.
2. The educational benefits available to the child in a general education class, with appropriate supplementary aids and services, as compared to the benefits provided in a special class.

[9] See, e.g., *P. v. Newington Board. of Educ.*, 546 F.3d 111 (2nd Cir., 2008); *Daniel R.R. v. State Board. of Educ.*, 874 F.2d 1036 (5th Cir., 1989); *Roncker v. Walter,* 700 F.2d 1058 (6th Cir., 1983).

3. The possible negative effects of the inclusion of the child on the education of the other students in the class.
   Oberti, 995 F.2d at 1217–18.

This test is consistent with provisions in the 2006 IDEA regulations, such as considering any harmful effects of the placement on the student and the quality of services the student will receive (34 C.F.R. § 300.116(d)) and including positive behavioral interventions and supports if a student's behavior impeded the learning of the student or others (34 C.F.R. § 300.324(a)(2)(i)).

Annual Review

The IEP must be reviewed at least annually to determine if the student's goals are being achieved and to revise the IEP to address any lack of progress toward the goals and in the general education curriculum, any information about the child provided to or by the parents, the child's anticipated needs, and other matters (20 U.S.C. § 1414(d)(4)(A); 34 C.F.R. § 300.324(b)(1)(i)). After the annual IEP is developed, it can be amended without an IEP meeting if the parents and school district agree in writing to amend the IEP (20 U.S.C. § 1414(d)(3)(D)&(F); 34 C.F.R. § 300.324(a)(4)).

A Free and Appropriate Public Education

When crafted correctly the IEP meets both the procedural requirements and substantive requirements of the IDEA and, therefore, affords the student a FAPE. Twice the Supreme Court has addressed the question of what constitutes a FAPE. First, in *Board of Educ. of Hendrick Hudson Central School Dist. v. Rowley*, 458 U.S. 176 (1982) and then again in *Endrew F. v. Douglas County School Dist.*, 580 U.S. ___, 137 S.Ct. 988 (2017).

In *Rowley*, the parents of a student with minimal residual hearing sought a sign language interpreter in all of her academic classes, but the school district did not agree. 458 U.S. at 184. Following an administrative hearing, the hearing officer found that a sign language interpreter was not needed because the student "was achieving educationally, academically, and socially" without the assistance. 458 U.S. at 185. The New York Commissioner of Education reviewed the decision and affirmed the hearing officer's determination. 458 U.S. at 185. On appeal, even though the student was performing better than the average peer and she was advancing from grade to grade, the District Court found in favor of the parents because she was not performing as well as she would have if she were not handicapped. 458 U.S. at 185–86. The Second Circuit affirmed. 458 U.S. at 186. The Supreme Court reversed. 458 U.S. at 209–10.

In reaching its decision, the Supreme Court found that the IDEA did not require that States maximize the potential of students with disabilities. 458 U.S. at 189. Rather, the IDEA provides access to an education that confers "some educational benefit" upon the student with a disability. 458 U.S. at 200. More specifically, it consists of access to specialized instruction and related services that are individually tailored to meet the needs of the child. 458 U.S. at 201. The Court also found that the IDEA's procedural requirements were as important as the substantive offering of the IEP. 458 U.S. at 205–6. Considering these tenets, the Supreme Court set forth a two part test to determine if a student received a FAPE: (1) Has the school district complied with the procedures set forth in the IDEA, and (2) Is the IEP reasonably calculated to enable the child to receive educational benefits? 458 U.S. at 206–7. Based on this standard, the Court found that the student was receiving an adequate education since she performed better than the average student and she was advancing from grade to grade. 458 U.S. at 209–10.

Rowley explained that students with disabilities have a substantive right to a FAPE and set forth that a student in general education classes who was advancing from grade to grade was receiving a sufficient educational benefit to meet the requirements of the IDEA. However, when the Court considered *Rowley*, it did not endorse any one standard and did not address the level of benefit necessary for a student not in general education classes. Therefore, thirty-five years later, the Court was presented with the question of what constituted a FAPE for a student with autism who was not in general education classes. *Endrew F.*, 137 S.Ct. 988, 993–94.

The student at the center of *Endrew F.* was diagnosed with autism. 137 S.Ct. at 996. Endrew attended public school until fourth grade; however, by that point his parents were concerned that his progress had stalled. 137 S.Ct. at 996. While he had many strengths, he also had significant behaviors including screaming, climbing on furniture, and running away from school, and he had severe fears of commonplace things. 137 S.Ct. at 996. These difficulties inhibited his ability to learn. Ultimately, his parents placed him in a private school where he did much better and, after meeting with the school district to consider a new IEP which the parents determined also did not address his needs, they sought reimbursement for the private placement. 137 S.Ct. at 996–97.

At the administrative hearing, the administrative law judge ("ALJ") disagreed with the parents and denied their request for relief. 137 S.Ct. at 997. They appealed to the District Court, which affirmed the decision. 137 S.Ct. at 997. In reaching its decision, the District court noted that the changes to Endrew's IEP showed "at the least, minimal progress." 137 S.Ct. at 997. On appeal to the Tenth Circuit, the school district again prevailed, with the Tenth Circuit citing *Rowley* for the proposition that Endrew had received "some educational benefit" and that an IEP is appropriate so long as it is calculated to provide a benefit that is "merely . . . more than *de minimus*." 137 S.Ct. at 997, *citing* 798 F.3d at 1338.

The Supreme Court granted *certiorari*, vacated the Tenth Circuit decision, and remanded the case. 137 S.Ct. at 1002. In reaching its decision, the Court re-affirmed the holding in *Rowley* that the IDEA imposes a substantive standard for the provision of FAPE. 137 S.Ct. at 998. The Court then set forth the standard for FAPE as applied to students who are not in general education progressing from grade to grade: "To meet its substantive obligations under the IDEA, a school must offer an IEP reasonably calculated to enable a child to make progress appropriate in light of the child's circumstances." 137 S.Ct. at 998–99. Further elucidating this standard, the Court stated that the IEP must be "reasonable," not "ideal." 137 S.Ct. at 999. In addition, the IEP must be calculated so that the student makes progress, with a focus on meeting the student's unique needs through specially designed instruction. 137 S.Ct. at 999. The Court recognized that the determination of progress varies depending on each child's needs, but the IEP should be "appropriately ambitious in light of the child's circumstances" and provide "challenging objectives" for the student to meet. 137 S.Ct. at 999–1001. For a student in general education, advancement from grade to grade is appropriately ambitious; "merely more than *de minimis*" for students with more significant needs is not sufficient. 137 S.Ct. at 1001.

Procedural Safeguards

Imbedded in the IDEA are procedural safeguards designed to ensure that students receive the education to which they are entitled. The IDEA requires school districts to inform parents of their procedural safeguards on an annual basis, upon initial referral, upon filing a complaint, and if requested by the parents (20 U.S.C. § 1415[d][1][A]; 34 C.F.R. § 300.504(a)). The procedural rights have to be in the parent's native language, if feasible, and understandable (20 U.S.C. § 1415(b)(4)&(d)(2)).

Among the parental rights, is the right to prior written notice whenever the school district proposes to or refuses to make a change related to the identification, evaluation, or educational placement of a student or the provision of FAPE (20 U.S.C. § 1415(b)(3); 34 C.F.R. § 300.503(a)). The parent also has the right to review records and the right to obtain an IEE under certain circumstances (20 U.S.C. § 1415(b); 34 C.F.R. § 300.501&300.502). In addition, if there is a dispute, either party may file a complaint or utilize the mediation and due process procedures to resolve the issues (20 U.S.C. §1415(b)(5)–(7); 34 C.F.R. § 300.506, 300.507). A complaint or due process request must be filed within two years of the date the party knew or should have known about the alleged action that formed the basis for the complaint, unless the State has a specific timeline for requesting a hearing (20 U.S.C. § 1415(b)(6)(B), 1415(f)(3)(C); 300.507(a)(2)). Finally, during the pendency of mediation or due process, the student remains in the then-current educational placement unless the parents and school district agree to change the placement-commonly referred to as "stay-put" (20 U.S.C. § 1415(j); 34 C.F.R. § 300.518(a)).

When a party files a due process request, it must include the name of the student, the address, the school the child attends, a description of the problem including the facts related to the problem, and a proposed resolution (20 U.S.C. §1415(b)(7); 34 C.F.R. § 300.508(b)). The State has to provide a form for the parent to utilize to assist the parent in filing a complaint or request for due process (20 U.S.C. §1415[b][8]). After receiving a due process request, a school district has to respond to the parent within 10 days, unless the school district already gave prior written notice on the issue in the due process request (20 U.S.C. § 1415(c)(2)(B)(i)(I); 34 C.F.R. § 300.509). The school district's response has to explain why the school district took the action it took, describe the other options the IEP Team considered and why the IEP Team rejected those options, describe the evaluations, assessments, records, or other information the IEP Team considered in making the decision, and describe any other factors that were relevant to the decision (20 U.S.C. § 1415(c)(2)(B)(i)(I)(aa)–(dd); 34 C.F.R. § 300.508(e)). If the school district filed the due process request, the parent has 10 days to submit a response that addressed the issues raised in the complaint (20 U.S.C. U.S.C. § 1415(c)(2)(B)(i)&(ii); 34 C.F.R. § 300.508(f)).

Mediation

Each State is required to facilitate mediation with an impartial mediator; however, participation is voluntary and mediation cannot delay a parent's right to a due process hearing (20 U.S.C. § 1415(e); 34 C.F.R. § 300.506(b)(1)). The State has to absorb the cost of mediation and maintain a list of mediators (20 U.S.C. § 1415(e)(2)(C)&(D); 34 C.F.R. § 300.506(b)(3)&(4)). If the parties reach an agreement, it is documented in a written agreement, signed by both parties, and is enforceable in any State court of competent jurisdiction or United States District Court (20 U.S.C. § 1415(e)(2)(F); 34 C.F.R. § 300.506(b)(6)). To encourage frank discussions, mediation is confidential and any discussion in mediation cannot be used in a subsequent due process hearing (20 U.S.C. § 1415(e)(2)(G); 34 C.F.R. § 300.506(b)(8)).

Resolution Session

Before a due process hearing, the school district must offer the parent a resolution session within 15 days of receipt of the complaint, unless the parties agree in writing to waive the resolution session or the parties agree to use mediation in lieu of a resolution session (20 U.S.C. § 1415(f)(1)(B)(i); 34 C.F.R. § 300.510(a)(1)). The resolution session has to include a representative from the school district with decision-making authority (20 U.S.C. § 1415(f)(1)(B)(i)(II); 34 C.F.R. § 300.510(a)(1)(i)). An attorney for the school district cannot participate unless an attorney representing the parent attends (20 U.S.C. § 1415(f)(1)(B)(i)(III); 34 C.F.R. § 300.510(a)(1)(ii)). If an agreement is reached, it has to be recorded in writing and signed by representatives for both parties (34 C.F.R. § 300.510(d)). Either party can void the agreement within three days, after which it is enforceable in any State court of competent jurisdiction or United States District Court (20 U.S.C. § 1415(f)(1)(B)(iii)&(iv); 34 C.F.R. § 300.510(d)(2)&(e)).

Due Process

Due process is a formal procedure overseen by a hearing officer (in some jurisdictions referred to as ALJ) (20 U.S.C. § 1415(f)(3)(A); 34 C.F.R. § 300.511(b)&(c)). At a hearing, the parties have the right to be advised by counsel, although the parent can appear *pro se*,[10] and individuals with special knowledge or training regarding students with disabilities; the right to present evidence, confront, cross-examine, and compel the attendance of witnesses; the right to a record of the hearing; and the right to a written decision (20 U.S.C. § 1415(h); 34 C.F.R. § 300.512(a)). Parties must also abide by certain procedures. For example, a least five business days prior to a due process hearing, the parties have to disclose all evaluations and recommendations based on those evaluations that will be used in the hearing (20 U.S.C. § 1415(f)(2)(A); 34 C.F.R. § 300.512(b)(1)). If they are not disclosed, they may be barred from admission in the hearing (20 U.S.C. § 1415(f)(2)(B); 34 C.F.R. § 300.512(b)(2)).

In reaching a decision, the hearing officer considers both procedural and substantive violations of the IDEA; however, the decision must be made on substantive grounds based on whether the student received a FAPE (20 U.S.C. § 1415(f)(3)(E)(i); 34 C.F.R. § 300.513(a)(2)). In considering procedural violations, the hearing officer can only find that a student did not receive a FAPE if the procedural violations impeded the student's right to a FAPE, significantly impeded the parent's opportunity to participate in the decision-making regarding the provision of FAPE to the student, or caused a deprivation of educational benefits (20 U.S.C. § 1415(f)(3)(E)(ii); 34 C.F.R. § 300.513(a)(2)). Even if the hearing officer cannot find that the procedural violations caused a substantive deprivation of FAPE, the hearing officer can order the school district to meet the procedural requirements of the IDEA (20 U.S.C. § 1415(f)(3)(E)(iii); 34 C.F.R. § 300.513(c)).

Burden of Proof

The IDEA is silent regarding which party bears the burden of proof, which encompasses the burden or persuasion—which party wins or loses if the evidence is closely balanced—and the burden of production—which party has to present evidence first at different time during a hearing—in a due process hearing; however, the Supreme Court addressed the burden of persuasion in *Schaffer v. Weast*, 546 U.S. 49 (2006). In *Schaffer*, the parents sought services from the public school district when the student was in middle school. 546 U.S. at 55. After determining that the IEP offered was not appropriate, the parents unilaterally placed the student and sought reimbursement. 546 U.S. at 54–55. The proceedings traversed through appeals and remands as it

[10] In *Winkelman v. Parma*, the Supreme Court found that parents have rights under the IDEA and, therefore, they can prosecute IDEA claims on their own behalf in the District Court. 550 U.S. 516 (2007).

progressed to the Supreme Court with the evidence in equipoise, thus turning on the burden of persuasion. 546 U.S. at 55. The Supreme Court granted certiorari and held that "the burden of persuasion in an administrative hearing challenging an IEP is properly placed on the party seeking relief." 546 U.S. at 62. The Court left open whether a State law or regulation[11] placing the burden of persuasion on the school district was valid. 546 U.S. at 61–62.

Appeal and Appropriate Relief

The decision of the hearing officer is final; however, either party may appeal the decision (20 U.S.C. § 1415(g); 34 C.F.R. § 300.514(a)). The appeal must be filed within 90 days from the date of the hearing officer's decision unless the State has a specific timeline (20 U.S.C. § 1415[g][2][B]). The court hearing the appeal receives the records of the administrative decision, can hear additional evidence at the request of the parties, bases its decision on a preponderance of the evidence, and has the power to grant "appropriate relief" (20 U.S.C. § 1415(g)(2)(C); 34 C.F.R. § 300.514(b)(2)). While the reviewing court can hear additional evidence, it must give due weight to the administrative proceedings and leave questions of methodology to the States. *Rowley*, 458 U.S. at 208.

Appropriate relief can include changes in placement, new or additional services, and reimbursement for expenses, including attorneys' fees. The Supreme Court specifically addressed the scope of relief available to parents who unilaterally place their children when they disagree with the IEP; first at a State-approved school and later at an accredited, but not approved school.

In *Burlington*, after disagreeing with the IEP, the parents placed their son, Michael, at a State-approved school to address his learning needs without the consent of the school district. *School Committee of the Town of Burlington, Mass. v. Dept. of Education of the Commonwealth of Mass*, 471 U.S. 359, 362–63 (1985). They filed for due process to obtain reimbursement for their expenses. 471 U.S. at 362. After the administrative hearing and a series of appeals, the Supreme Court granted certiorari to address two issues: (1) whether the potential relief available under the IDEA includes reimbursement to parents for the costs of a private school, and (2) whether there is a bar to reimbursement if the school district does not agree to the placement. 471 U.S. at 367.

The Court found that the IDEA directs courts to "grant such relief as [it] determines is appropriate . . . in light of the purposes of the [IDEA]" and that the IDEA grants "broad discretion" to the Court in granting relief. 471 U.S. at 369–70. As such, reimbursement for a private school placement that is proper when the school district's IEP was not appropriate is permitted. 471 U.S. at 370. In reaching this decision, the

[11] Some states have adopted statutes or regulations placing the burden of proof on school districts. See e.g., Del.Code.Ann., Tit. 14, § 3140 (adopted before *Schaffer*) and N.J.S.A. 18A:46–1.1 (adopted after *Schaffer*).

Court noted that the time it takes to complete an administrative and judicial review is protracted and that it would be an "empty victory" if parents prevailed but could not be reimbursed. 471 U.S. at 370.

The Court also found that the parents did not waive their right to reimbursement by placing Michael without consent of the school district, which the school district considered a violation of the "stay-put" provision of the IDEA. 471 U.S. at 370–71. Preliminarily, the Court noted that once the ALJ found in favor of the parents, the parents had consent for the placement because the decision was equivalent to agreement from the State. 471 U.S. at 372. However, the Court also found that parents can obtain reimbursement for the period before the Court issues a decision because interpreting the IDEA to require a school district's agreement would force parents to leave their child in an inappropriate placement or give up their right to a free education. 471 U.S. at 372.

The Supreme Court extended the reasoning in *Burlington* when it decided *Florence County School District Four v. Carter*, 510 U.S. 7 (1993). Like in *Burlington*, the parents in *Carter* unilaterally placed their daughter, Shannon, in a private school when they disagreed with the school district's IEP. 510 U.S. at 10. However, the school the parents' chose was not approved by the State and it did not meet all of the procedural requirements of the IDEA; it did provide an "excellent education in substantial compliance with all of the substantive requirements" of the IDEA. 510 U.S. at 10–11. Upon review, the Supreme Court found that the private school's failure to meet the requirements of the IDEA did not bar the parents' request for reimbursement. 510 U.S. at 13–15. The Court did recognize, however, that in determining the relief available to the parents, the Court can consider all relevant factors, including if the cost of the parents' choice of school is reasonable. 510 U.S. at 16.

Attorneys' Fees

In addition to relief related to the services or placement, the IDEA is a fee shifting statute that provides parents who are the prevailing party reasonable attorneys' fees (20 U.S.C. § 1415(i)(3)(B)(i); 34 C.F.R. § 300.517(a)). The fee awarded is determined based on the prevailing rate in the community for the kind and quality of service provided (20 U.S.C. § 1415(i)(3)(C); 34 C.F.R. § 300.517(c)(1)). Unless the State or school district unreasonably protracted the litigation, parents' attorneys' fees reimbursement can be reduced if (1) the parent, or their attorney, unreasonably protracted the litigation; (2) the hourly rate unreasonably exceeds the rate for attorneys with similar skills, reputations, and experience; (3) the time spent by the attorney was excessive; or (4) the attorney for the parent did not provide the information required—name, address, school, nature of the problem, and proposed resolution—in the notice of the complaint (20 U.S.C. § 1415(i)(3)(F)&(G); 34 C.F.R. § 300.517(c)(4)). In addition, if the school district makes a written offer of settlement at least 10 days before the hearing and the parent is not substantially justified in rejecting the settlement offer,[12] the offer is not accepted within ten days, and the court finds that the relief the parents obtain through the hearing is not more favorable to the parents then the offer, then the parents are not entitled to fees for any services performed after the offer (20 U.S.C. § 1415(i)(3)(D)(i), 20 U.S.C. § 1415(j)(3)(E); 34 C.F.R. § 300.517(c)(2)&(3)).

A school district can also obtain attorneys' fees in limited circumstances. The attorney for the parent may be liable for attorneys' fees, if the attorney files a complaint that is "frivolous, unreasonable, or without foundation," or if the attorney continues the proceedings when it clearly becomes "frivolous, unreasonable, or without foundation" (20 U.S.C. § 1415(i)(3)(B)(i)(II); 34 C.F.R. § 300.517(a)(1)(ii)). A school district can also obtain attorneys' fees from the attorney for the parent or the parent, if the complaint was brought for "an improper purpose, such as to harass, to cause unnecessary delay, or to needlessly increase the cost of litigation" (20 U.S.C. § 1415(i)(3)(i)(II); 34 C.F.R. § 300.517(a)(1)(iii)).

While parents are entitled to attorneys' fees if they are the prevailing party, they are not entitled the cost of experts. *Arlington Central School Dist. Board. of Educ. v. Murphy*, 548 U.S. 291 (2006). In *Arlington*, the parents sought reimbursement for the costs of an educational consultant that assisted them prior to and during the hearing. 548 U.S. at 294. The District Court rejected the request for any fees provided prior to the filing of the request and found that only fees related to consultation, not legal representation were reimbursable; but found that all of the remaining fees could be characterized as consultation. 548 U.S. at 294. The Second Circuit affirmed. 402 F.3d 332 (2005). The Supreme Court subsequently reversed, holding that because the IDEA is a statute enacted pursuant to the Spending Clause—that is, States accept funds in exchange for implementing the IDEA—the IDEA must "unambiguously" set forth the conditions for receipt of the funds so that the State's acceptance is "knowing and voluntary." 548 U.S. at 295–96. As expert costs were not clearly identified as a condition for a State's receipt of funding, they are not recoverable by parents. 548 U.S. at 300, 304.

Student Discipline

Students with disabilities have additional protections related to discipline that are intended to balance the need for order in the school with the student's right to a FAPE. In disciplining a student with a disability, the following considerations are set forth in the IDEA:

1. The school district may consider any unique circumstances in determining if a change of placement is appropriate for a child with a disability (20 U.S.C. § 1415(k)(1)(A); 34 C.F.R. § 300.530(a));

[12] If the mater is before the Federal Court, the offer must be made in accordance with Rule 68 of the Federal Rules of Civil Procedure (20 U.S.C. § 1415(i)(3)(D)(i)(I)).

2. A school district may remove—suspend—a child with a disability for not more than 10 school days (to the extent that removal is also applied to students without disabilities) (20 U.S.C. § 415(k)(1)(B); 34 C.F.R. § 300.530(b));
3. If the behavior that gave rise to the discipline is not a manifestation of the student's disability, the school district may impose the same disciplinary procedures as applied to students without disabilities (20 U.S.C. § 1415(k)(1)(B); 34 C.F.R. § 300.530(c));
4. If a student's placement is changed because the behavior is not a manifestation of the student's disability or because special circumstances apply, the student shall continue to receive educational services so that they can continue to participate in the general education curriculum and make progress toward the goals in their IEP and, as appropriate, receive a functional behavioral assessment ("FBA"), behavior intervention services and modifications (20 U.S.C. § 1415(k)(1)(B); 34 C.F.R. § 300.530(d)); and
5. No later than the day the decision is made to take disciplinary action, notify the parents of the decision and their procedural safeguards for disciplinary matters (20 U.S.C. § 1415(k)(1)(H); 34 C.F.R. § 300.530(h)).

When a student's placement will be changed for more than ten school days (e.g., for a suspension of more than ten school days), the school district must hold a manifestation determination within ten school days of the decision to change the student's placement (20 U.S.C. § 1415(k)(1)(E); 34 C.F.R. § 300.530(e)). At the manifestation determination, which includes parent and relevant members of the IEP Team, they must review the current IEP, teacher observations, and any relevant information provided by the parent to determine if the student's conduct "was caused by, or had a direct and substantial relationship to, the child's disability" or if the conduct was the "direct result of the [school district's] failure to implement the IEP (20 U.S.C. § 1415(k)(1)(E)(i); 34 C.F.R. § 300.530(e)(1)). If either inquiry is applicable, then the student's conduct is deemed a manifestation of the student's disability and the IEP Team must:

1. conduct a Functional Behavioral Assessment ("FBA") and implement a BIP, unless the school district already conducted an FBA;
2. if there is already a BIP, review the BIP and modify it as necessary;
3. return the child to the placement unless the school district and parent agree to a change in placement as part of the modification to the BIP (20 U.S.C. § 1415(k)(1)(F); 34 C.F.R. § 300.530(f)).

Even if a student's behavior is a manifestation of their disability, a school district can move the student to an interim alternative setting[13] for up to 45 school days[14] if the student

---

[13] The interim alternative educational setting is determined by the IEP Team (20 U.S.C. § 1415(k)(2); 34 C.F.R. § 300.533).

[14] The time that a school district can remove a student to an interim alternative setting under the special circumstances provision can be reduced by State law. For example, in New Jersey, the maximum amount of time is 45 calendar days (N.J.A.C. 6A:14–2.8(d)).

1. carries a weapon to or possesses a weapon at school, on school grounds, or at a school sponsored function;
2. knowingly possesses or uses illegal drugs, or sells or solicits the sale of a controlled substance while at school, on school grounds, or at a school sponsored function;
3. inflicts serious bodily injury on another person while at school, on school grounds or at a school sponsored function (20 U.S.C. § 1415(k)(1)(G); 34 C.F.R. § 300.530(g)).

A parent that disagrees with the decision regarding placement or the manifestation determination or a school district that believes that maintaining the current placement will likely result in injury to the child or others can request a hearing (20 U.S.C. § 1415(k)(3)(A); 34 C.F.R. § 300.532(a)). The hearing officer can order a change of placement that returns the child to their original setting or to an interim alternative educational setting for up to 45 school days when the hearing officer determines that staying in the current placement is "substantially likely to result in injury to the child or others" (20 U.S.C. § 1415(k)(3)(B)(ii); 34 C.F.R. § 300.532(b)). During the appeal, the child remains in the interim alternative setting until the hearing officer's decision or the time period—45 school days—expires, unless the parent and school district agree otherwise (20 U.S.C. § 1415(k)(4)). However, the hearing is expedited and has to be held within twenty school days of the date it is requested and decision rendered within ten school days after the hearing (20 U.S.C. § 1415(k)(4)(B); 34 C.F.R. § 300.532(c)).

A student who has not been determined eligible for special education has the same protections as a student who is eligible if the school district had knowledge that the child was a child with a disability before the behavior occurred (20 U.S.C. § 1415(k)(5)(A); 34 C.F.R. § 300.534(a)). The school district is deemed to have knowledge if (1) the parent expressed concern that the student was in need of special education and related services in writing to supervisory or administrative personnel or the child's teacher; (2) the parent requested an evaluation of the child to determine if the child is eligible for special education and related services; or (3) the teacher or other school district staff expressed specific concerns about a pattern of behavior directly to the director of special education or other supervisory personnel in the school district (20 U.S.C. § 1415(k)(5)(B); 34 C.F.R. § 300.534(b)). However, if a parent did not allow an evaluation of the child, then the school district is not deemed to have knowledge (20 U.S.C. § 1415(k)(5)(C); 34 C.F.R. § 300.534(c)). Should a student be referred for an evaluation during the discipline period, the evaluation must be conducted in an expedited manner and, if the student is eligible for special education and related services, the student must be provided special education and related services (20 U.S.C. § 1415(k)(5)(D); 34 C.F.R. § 300.534)(d)(2)(i). While the evaluation is pending, the student remains in the educational setting determined by the school district (20 U.S.C. § 1415(k)(5)(D)(ii); 34 C.F.R. § 300.534(d)(2)(ii)).

While there are limitations regarding the discipline imposed on a student with a disability, the IDEA clearly authorizes a school district to report a crime committed by a child with a disability to local law enforcement (20 U.S.C. § 1415(k)(6)(A); 34

C.F.R. § 300.535(a)). In addition, the school district must share copies of the special education and disciplinary records with the agency to which the crime was reported (20 U.S.C. § 1415(k)(6)(B); 34 C.F.R. § 300.535(b)).

Conclusion

The increasing identification of children with autism, both as a diagnosis and as eligible for special education and related services, requires consideration of their rights in school. Under the IDEA, students with disabilities and their parents have clearly defined rights and protections. While the procedures are unambiguous, disputes regarding implementation of those rights and whether the student is receiving an appropriate education are common. For students with autism, issues arise at all stages of the special education process. Among them: Was the evaluation sufficiently comprehensive? Is the student eligible for special education and related services? Were the student's behaviors a manifestation of the student's disability? Does the IEP provide FAPE? A comprehensive understanding the IDEA and the State's implementation of the statue and regulations will allow you to answer these questions for your clients.

References

20 U.S.C. § 1400 et seq.

34 C.F.R. § 300.01 et seq.

Arlington Central School Dist. Board. of Educ. V. Murphy, 548 U.S. 291 (2006).

Board of Educ. of Hendrick Hudson Central School Dist. v. Rowley, 458 U.S. 176 (1982).

Cedar Rapids Community School Dist., v. Garrett F., 526 U.S. 66 (1999).

Daniel R.R. v. State Board. of Educ., 874 F.2d 1036 (5th Cir. 1989).

Endrew F. v. Douglas County School Dist., 580 U.S. ___, 137 S.Ct. 988 (2017).

Florence County School District Four v. Carter, 510 U.S. 7 (1993).

Irving Independent School Dist. v. Tatro, 468 U.S. 883 (1984).

Newington Board. of Educ., 546 F.3d 111 (2nd Cir. 2008).

New Jersey Department of Education. (2004). *Autism program quality indicators*, 9–10 https://www.nj.gov/education/specialed/info/autism.pdf. Last Accessed 12 Jan 2019.

North Dakota Department of Public Instruction. (2014). *Guidelines for serving students with autism spectrum disorders in educational settings*, 11–12. https://www.nd.gov/dpi/uploads/60/NDGuidelinesforServingStudentswithASDFINAL914.pdf. Last Accessed 12 Jan 2019.

Oberti v. Board of Educ., 995 F.2d 914 (3d. Cir. 1993).

Office of Special Education and Rehabilitative Services, U.S. Department of Education. (2006). *28th Annual Report to Congress on the Implementation of the Individuals with Disabilities Act* (Vol. 2, pp. 10, 13). https://www2.ed.gov/about/reports/annual/osep/2006/parts-b-c/28th-vol-2.pdf. Last Accessed 12 Jan 2019.

Office of Special Education and Rehabilitative Services, U.S. Department of Education. (2020). 42nd Annual Report to Congress on the Implementation of the Individuals with Disabilities Act, pp. 29-30, 41-42, 56. https://www2.ed.gov/about/reports/annual/osep/2020/parts-b-c/42nd-arc-for-idea.pdf. Last Accessed 13 May 2021.

Oregon Department of Education. (2010). *Autism spectrum disorder: Evaluation, eligibility, and goal development (Birth-21) Technical Assistance Paper*, 11–18. https://www.ode.state.or.us/groups/supportstaff/specializedservices/autism/autismtap.pdf. Last Accessed 12 Jan 2019.
Roncker v. Walter, 700 F.2d 1058 (6th Cir. 1983).
Schaffer v. Weast, 546 U.S. 49 (2006).
School Committee of the Town of Burlington, Mass. v. Dept. of Education of the Commonwealth of Mass, 471 U.S. 359 (1985).
U.S. Department of Education. (2002). *24th Annual Report to Congress on the Implementation of the Individuals with Disabilities Act*, II–20. https://www.govinfo.gov/content/pkg/ERIC-ED479983/pdf/ERIC-ED479983.pdf. Last Accessed 12 Jan 2019.
U.S. Department of Health and Human Services, Centers for Disease Control and Prevention, Autism Spectrum Disorders, Data and Statistics. https://www.cdc.gov/ncbddd/autism/data.html. Last Accessed on 5 July 2020.
Winkelman v. Parma, 550 U.S. 516 (2007).

Stacey Therese Cherry is a partner with Fogarty & Hara. Mrs. Cherry graduated magna cum laude from Pepperdine University School of Law in 2004. She graduated magna cum laude from Hope College with a Bachelor of Arts degree in Learning Disabilities in 1999. After obtaining her B.A., Mrs. Cherry taught inclusion and self-contained special education classes and is a New Jersey certified Teacher of the Handicapped and Elementary School Teacher.

Mrs. Cherry represents boards of education in all areas, including labor and employment, student discipline, and harassment, intimidation and bullying, and has particular expertise in special education law. She is admitted to practice in New Jersey and New York, the United States District Court for the District of New Jersey, and the United States Court of Appeals for the Third Circuit. Mrs. Cherry was named to New Jersey's Super Lawyers: Rising Stars list, which was published in the 2017 issue of New Jersey Super Lawyers magazine.

In addition, Mrs. Cherry has volunteered for over 15 years with the New Jersey Branch of The International Dyslexia Association, where she has been a Director, the Vice President for Community Affairs, the Fall Conference Chair, and a member of the Nominating Committee. She also serves as an invited speaker for boards of education and parents as well as for organizations including the New Jersey Association of Pupil Services Administrators, the New Jersey Association of Learning Consultants, the Somerset County Association of Directors of Special Services, and Fairleigh Dickinson University.

Chapter 16
Navigating the Transition to Adulthood—Preparing for Life Under the U.S. Legislative Model

Gary S. Mayerson

For students with autism and other special needs living in the U.S., the transition to adulthood marks a process that, over time, ends at least in one sense when a classified student with an Individualized Education Plan (IEP) ages out of *entitlement-based* programming mandated under the federal Individuals with Disabilities Education Act (IDEA) (20 U.S.C. Sec. 1415 *et seq.*) and transitions into *eligibility-based services* and programming that may or may not be available or funded at the state level.

At least "on paper," transition services in the U.S. under the federal IDEA statute represent Congress' ambitious and optimistic blueprint to prepare classified[1] students for adulthood by grooming them to become included, to the extent of each student's potential and capabilities, as independent and contributing members of society. "Transition services" constitute the mechanism designed by Congress to effectuate this process and its hoped-for inclusive outcome: 20 U.S.C. §§ 1401(34), 1414(d)(l)(A)(i)(VIII). Just as autism is a spectrum disorder, there exists a broad spectrum of ultimate transition goals and options, including but not limited to college and vocational experiences (Lazer, 2018; Lei et al., 2018; Rast et al., 2019).

Some countries, especially those receiving significant aid from other nations, may not be in a position to fund transition services and its necessary components. Other nations who might appear to have the economic resources to "invest" in transition services may nevertheless lack the optimism and high *expectations* needed to believe that with education, training, and support, individuals with autism and other special needs can ever become included as independent and contributing members of society.

[1] Students with autism and other special needs who have been declared as eligible for special education services.

G. S. Mayerson (✉)
Mayerson and Associates, New York City, NY, USA
e-mail: info@mayerslaw.com

F. R. Volkmar et al. (eds.), *Handbook of Autism Spectrum Disorder and the Law*,
https://doi.org/10.1007/978-3-030-70913-6_16

The U.S., the U.K., Sweden,Norway, and Israel are among those nations that offer some of the more robust transition supports and opportunities for social inclusion (Baric et al., 2017). Israel, for example, offers individuals who are on the autism spectrum training for suitable positions within its National Service and IDF (Israel's defense forces).

Having high expectations for the autism population normally goes hand in hand with the growing acceptance of "neurodiversity." However, just as certain nations may be thinking of neurodiversity when they think of autism, other nations (e.g., Brazil) may still be viewing autism as representing generic "mental suffering" for which there is little hope.

Accordingly, just as a professional sports franchise must first *believe* that it can "win" to be truly competitive, in order for a nation to make the policy decision to invest substantial funds and personnel in transition infrastructure, I would urge that it is essential for that country to be genuinely optimistic about the efficacy of vocational training and other transition services. Having high expectations is pretty much a prerequisite for any nation thinking about providing transition supports and services.

For the autism community in the U.S., the metrics and related challenges associated with the transition to adulthood are compelling. Each year, more than 50,000 Americans with autism will transition to adulthood and lose all of their IEP-mandated, IDEA-based services and programming. At that same juncture, approximately 85% of that group (approximately 42,000) will "graduate" to a state of perpetual unemployment with most living at home, typically with a parent or other relative (Remnick, 2019).

This precarious time frame is often referred to as "going off the services cliff." Normally, when we hear of some poor soul going off a cliff, we are envisioning a terrible accident attributable to mechanical failure or human error. Here, however, the cliff at issue is no accident. It is the recognized, designed-by-Congress terminus of the IDEA statute and its many protections. Inasmuch as going off the IDEA cliff is part of Congress's blueprint for the transition to adulthood, how, if at all, can school districts, families, and caregivers located in the U.S. arrange for smoother landings?

Going off the IDEA services cliff is not the only threat. At the time this chapter is being completed, the COVID-19 pandemic is far from over. The immediate damage resulting from what remains an active pandemic has so far included tens of millions of Americans losing their jobs and livelihoods, more than 100,000 deaths in the U.S. alone, unemployment rates that have not been seen since the Great Depression, the closure of U.S. schools and countless businesses, and the substitution of remote "telehealth" teaching for in-person instruction.

Recently, as a direct result of the COVID-19 pandemic and crisis, parents in the U.S. have faced some serious threats to transition and other entitlements mandated under the federal IDEA statute. At least one of those threats was a political effort to water down the IDEA statute itself. Buried within the CARES stimulus package enacted by Congress on March 27, 2020 was a provision requiring the U.S. Secretary of Education, Betsy DeVos, to identify portions of the federal IDEA statute that, in the opinion of the Secretary, are provisions that Congress should "waive."

On April 27, 2020, the special needs community in the U.S. breathed a collective sigh of relief when Secretary DeVos delivered a letter to ranking members of Congress in which she made clear that she is not requesting waiver authority for any of IDEA's "core tenets." Thankfully, the few waivers being sought by Secretary DeVos will not have any impact on transition services and other IDEA-based entitlements.

Accordingly, to the extent that there remains a great deal of legitimate concern and uncertainty as to the financial and other consequences of the pandemic for the autism community, it is absolutely critical that parents living in the U.S. timely secure and enforce their children's IDEA-based transition entitlements in the years *before* the services "cliff" looms ahead.

There is another significant reason why preserving IDEA's entitlements in the face of the pandemic and its resulting economic and other consequences is absolutely essential. In 2017, in the *Endrew F.* case,[2] a unanimous Supreme Court clarified the statutory right to a "free and appropriate public education" (FAPE) as being "markedly" more robust than a number of federal circuit courts had ruled during the prior 35 years. IEP goals must now be challenging and sufficiently ambitious. For the first time, the Supreme Court has identified a child's "potential" as something the school system needs to consider. Transition planning has a great deal to do with building on a student's interests and potential (Browning & Pease, 2018).

Protected by this more robust and clarified national standard of care from the highest court in the U.S., a window of opportunity had opened to empower the next generations. Had U.S. Secretary of Education DeVos gone further with her IDEA waiver recommendations, Congress could easily have materially diluted or even nullified the Supreme Court's clarified FAPE standard—something that could have adversely impacted transition entitlements throughout the U.S.

It is just a matter of time before science catches up to and neutralizes the threat and impact of the COVID-19 virus. The uncertainty is "when?" Whatever the future may bring, parents in the U.S. can never take for granted the IDEA statute's essential statutory protections and entitlements. Parents should be sure to take full advantage of the IDEA statute's transition mandates. No parent or school district should defer transition services and supports, thinking that there is plenty of time remaining to implement those supports.

The federal IDEA statute requires that school districts in the U.S. take steps to start the transition process long before a student is getting ready to exit from the public educational system. To the extent of each student's potential and capabilities, school districts are required to prepare classified students for adulthood by grooming them to become independent and contributing members of society: 20 U.S.C. §§ 1401(34), 1414(d)(l)(A)(i)(VIII) (Schall et al., 2014; Van Schalkwyk & Volkmar, 2017).

For students with autism and other special needs, "transition services" under the federal IDEA statute are supposed to be an integrated and well "coordinated" bundle of procedural and substantive rights that include: (a) assessments of the student's

---

[2] 137 S. Ct. 29 (2017).

needs, capabilities, and interests (such as vocational evaluations); (b) planning by educators and families to create appropriate post-secondary goals for the student; (c) notices to parents and students to facilitate their participation in determining the student's interests and creating the student's goals; and (d) the development of programs and services to develop skills (whether academic skills, vocational skills, employment skills, and/or life skills) that are designed and reasonably calculated to reach those goals: 20 U.S.C. §§ 1401(34); 1414(d)(1)(A)(i)(VIII), 1415(b)(3), 1415(c)(1); 34 C.F.R. §§ 300.320(b), 300.321(b).

Some school systems will offer vocational assessments, transition planning and the like but may do so without *coordinating* and reconciling their availability or import. Let it suffice to say that parents should not have to become detectives to find out where basic entitlements are buried. *Note to School Districts*: It is the school district's obligation to inform parents of the existence of these resources even if parents do not ask (Hatfield et al., 2018; Hewitt &Weiss, 2015).

When Is Transition Planning Required to Start in the U.S.?

It is a well-accepted rule that while individual states in the U.S. are mandated and under a duty to meet the standards set forth under federal law (i.e., the federal IDEA statute), any individual state can always decide to offer a *greater* level of protection than the federal statute requires. Nationally, the IDEA statute requires transition planning to be underway during the school year when the student turns 16. New York State, on the other hand, provides for transition support to start somewhat earlier, when the student turns 15. While New York is to be congratulated for recognizing how important the transition process is, the State of Connecticut deserves even higher honors for triggering the start of transition during the school year when the student is turning 14.

Pioneer states like Connecticut are on to something. The fact that some state legislatures are willing to go out on a financial limb to *advance* the start of transition services in the absence of any legal obligation to do so tells us something. The message is that the earlier that effective services can start, the greater are the chances that there will be a good outcome by the time that the student is about to exit the educational system. Accordingly, for parents and school systems alike, it is important to view transition-related services and supports in the same manner as they may look at early intervention i.e., the earlier the better.

There is a section in every IEP document that pertains to the transition process and the development of "post secondary goals." Year after year, a parent attending their child's IEP meeting may notice that the IEP team skips over this section of the IEP and leaves it blank. Finally, the school year arrives when someone on the IEP team remarks "Hey, don't we have to address transition this year?" That year will be the first year that the transition section of the IEP is filled out. It is essential that the school district, the student, and the child's parents properly and timely develop this "foundation." Otherwise, the parties will lose valuable time kicking the transition can down the road.

While a child with special needs is still receiving services from the local school district, it is essential that the IEP visibly promote increasing levels of independence and self-sufficiency with goals that are genuinely ambitious and challenging and take the student's potential into account. Making sure that a student gets what he or she is entitled to during the school experience is part of supporting the transition process.

It is important to bear in mind that the extent of a student's independence and self-sufficiency at the time that student ages out of the public education system often will turn on the extent to which the student and his or her parents were successful in "mining" the transition-related supports and services under IDEA while such supports and services were still available. It is not at all effective to wait until graduation to teach basic daily living skills such as personal hygiene, food preparation, dressing and undressing, having a functional system of communication, and doing the laundry or dishes. Early acquisition of those skills may mean the difference between the student who resides and works as an adult in their community and one who may require a more restrictive and supported setting (Depeolu et al., 2015).

Unfortunately, while transition planning is supposed to start in earnest years *before* a student ages out of the public educational system (normally at age 21), it is my sense that all too many school systems and parents are content to begin addressing transition right about the time that the school system is thinking of scheduling the student's exit interview. For the student who is about to lose all of his or her IDEA entitlements and "go off the services cliff," this represents a missed opportunity that the student really cannot afford to miss. The school system may think that it just saved a great deal of time and money. The school system may, in fact, have saved some money, but in actuality, it just kicked the student's needs and entitlements to the curb.

To access services that a particular state may have available for individuals who are exiting the educational system, a student must be registered and must meet that state's eligibility requirements. If, for example, a student and his or her parents happen to live in New York State, they should not wait until graduation day to register with state agencies such as the OPWDD (the Office for People With Developmental Disabilities) or ACCES—VR (Adult Career and Continuing Education Services—Vocational Rehabilitation). The earlier that a student is registered, the better.

In New York State, OPWDD is the state agency that provides programs and oversees the funding of agencies that deliver services to people with autism and other developmental disabilities. OPWDD provides a wide variety of support and service options that can be tailored to address an individual's needs. New Yorkers can log onto OPWDD's user-friendly website (www.opwdd.ny.gov) that describes "person-centered planning" with supports and services that may include:

- Help for living in a home in the local community.
- Support to live in their family home with supports.
- Help for people who want to work in the community, and
- Help for those who need intensive residential and day services.

Most OPWDD services are funded through Medicaid by way of a "Medicaid Waiver." It's considered a waiver system because eligibility does not turn on the consideration of parental income. Assuming that a child meets eligibility, requirements and has a qualifying diagnosis that affects the independent living, services can also include counseling, respite, recreation, sibling support groups, training, adaptive devices, behavioral services, supported employment opportunities, job coaching, social skills training, equipment, and more.

Before receiving any Medicaid-funded services through OPWDD, an applicant must arrange for a review of records showing evidence of a qualifying disability that arose before age 22 and is serious enough to affect that child's ability to live independently. The documents OPWDD will be looking for and reviewing include:

- OPWDD's eligibility form (available online).
- A psychological assessment less than three years old that includes adaptive behavior scales and a written summary by the person who did the testing.
- A social or psychosocial history.
- A medical report less than one year old.
- Other documents specifically requested by OPWDD, such as an IEP.

Assuming that a child is declared to be eligible for the Medicaid waiver, at age 18, the Medicaid waiver magically converts into standard Medicaid for that child without having to go through a separate application process. If, however, a parent does not have the Medicaid waiver in hand when a child turns 18, a separate application will need to be filed. That is because once children age out of educational programs, Medicaid benefits are needed for their acceptance into adult programs. For this reason, parents have every incentive to explore eligibility under the Medicaid waiver program early on.

Currently, Medicaid waiver funding can cover a wide range of services through OPWDD including but not limited to summer and other special needs recreational programs, music and arts programs, parent training and consultation, behavioral services, support groups for parents and siblings, physical therapy, nurses, occupational therapy, medical and dental services, equipment and devices, transportation, respite services, and community programs.

The Medicaid waiver emphasizes "person-centered" planning—planning in which the child's family members and service providers focus on the child's desires and interests for their future. The waiver also is the mechanism and key for the child to unlock and receive federal and state funds to pay for necessary services that are designed to empower the child so they might live at home, reside in the local community, and have a meaningful and fulfilling life.

One of the most important eligibility factors that OPWDD looks at is a child's level of independence. It is important for a parent to answer any interview questions truthfully and be mindful not to allow ego to inadvertently overstate the child's level of independence. Independence for eligibility purposes means that the child can reliably perform the task at issue on their own without any support or additional prompting. If a parent were to brag about how independent their child is, eligibility might be denied on that basis.

Assuming that a child qualifies for the Medicaid Waiver, a parent may want to consider moving into a program called "self-direction." Some years ago, New York

State had 35,000 adults living in group homes. This was one-sixth of the total group home residents for the whole country! In addition to what New York was spending on operating and sustaining its group homes, there were some other serious problems, including instances of sexual abuse and other assaults. All of the above precipitated a move by New York to close down and otherwise move away from its group home[3] model in favor of a "self-direction" or consumer-oriented model that would allow a family or agency to construct a customized program and budget around the needs of the individual. Some families prefer having the control that self-direction offers. Other families feel more comfortable continuing with a professional care coordinator.

Once a family's self-direction budget is approved, the family can purchase services directly from a provider agency (at the agency's rates) or may choose to hire and train their own providers. Services that are available to be supported in the context of self-direction programs include but are not limited to supported employment, respite, and having a live-in caregiver. The budget, subject to limitations, can also cover individual services such as laundry, transportation, camp, health club memberships, parent training, and even massages.

How Telehealth Communication Technology Can Support Transition

When schools and offices in the U.S. went into lockdown mode after the COVID-19 pandemic arrived, the nation quickly adapted to working and learning from home using Zoom and other forms of telehealth technology. The technology works, is easy if not fun to use, and costs next to nothing. Telehealth technology is here to stay.

Whether used on the "entitlement" or "eligibility" sides of the transition process, telehealth technology is a natural support that we are likely to see much more of going into the future. The technology is easily adaptable for numerous applications including:

- Vocational assessments.
- Vocation sampling.
- Parent training.
- Job training.
- Check-ins for individuals living on their own or with roommates.
- Supervision.
- Counseling.
- Probing for generalization and independence.
- Staff meetings.
- Eligibility interviews.
- Behavioral and other consultation.
- Development of goals and objectives.

[3] Group homes are also sometimes referred to as IRAs (individual residential alternatives).

- Convening IEP and other meetings.

While we may be living in an era of relative uncertainty, what is certain is that each year, more than 50,000 Americans with autism will be transitioning to adulthood, needing a variety of services and supports. The U.S. Congress, in enacting the IDEA statute's transition-related mandates, did so while communicating the importance of having high expectations. At least on paper, the U.S. legislative model of services and supports available to effectuate the transition to adulthood represents today's "gold standard" capable of helping people with autism to become more independent, self-sufficient, contributing and included members of society.

The overarching objective of providing transition services and supports, of course, is not simply to have an individual with autism simply "graduate" from school-age services, but rather for the individual to graduate *to* something that is fulfilling, worthwhile, and sustainable for them. As perceptions and attitudes toward autism, inclusion, and neurodiversity change over time, we can expect more nations to enact and implement statutory entitlements that meaningfully support the transition process.

References

Baric, V. B., Hemmingsson, H., Hellberg, K., & Kjellberg, A. (2017). The occupational transition process to upper secondary school, further education and/or work in Sweden: As described by young adults with Asperger syndrome and attention deficit hyperactivity disorder. *Journal of Autism and Developmental Disorders, 47*(3), 667–679.

Browning, S., & Pease, L. (2018). Higher education transitions and autism. In *Autism spectrum disorders: Breakthroughs in research and practice* (pp. 281–290). Information Science Reference/IGI Global.

Depeolu, A. O., Storlie, C., & Johnson, C. (2015). College students with high functioning Autism Spectrum Disorder: Best practices for successful transition to the world of work. *Journal of College Counseling, 18*(2), 175–190.

Hatfield, M., Ciccarelli, M., Falkmer, T., & Falkmer, M. (2018). Factors related to successful transition planning for adolescents on the autism spectrum. *Journal of Research in Special Educational Needs, 18*(1), 3–14.

Hewitt, L. E., & Weiss, A. L. (2015). Issue editor foreword: Transition to college for students with language disorders on and off the autism spectrum. *Topics in Language Disorders, 35*(4), 297–299.

Lazer, D. J. (2018). Transition from high school to college for students with high functioning Autism Spectrum Disorder: A qualitative study. *Dissertation Abstracts International Section A: Humanities and Social Sciences, 79*(10-A(E)).

Lei, J., Calley, S., Brosnan, M., Ashwin, C., & Russell A. (2018). Evaluation of a transition to university programme for students with Autism Spectrum Disorder. *Journal of Autism and Developmental Disorders, 50,* 2397–2411.

Rast, J. E., Roux, A. M., & Shattuck, P. T. (2019). Use of vocational rehabilitation supports for postsecondary education among transition-age youth on the autism spectrum. *Journal of Autism and Developmental Disorders, 50,* 2164–2173.

Remnick, N. (2019). The coming care crisis as kids with autism grow up. *The Atlantic.*

Schall, C., Wehman, P., & Carr, S. (2014). Transition from high school to adulthood for adolescents and young adults with autism spectrum disorders. In *Adolescents and adults with autism spectrum disorders* (pp. 41–60). Springer Science + Business Media.

Van Schalkwyk, G. I., & Volkmar, F. R. (2017). Autism spectrum disorders: Challenges and opportunities for transition to adulthood. *Child and Adolescent Psychiatric Clinics of North America, 26*(2), 329–339.

Gary S. Mayerson is a graduate of the Georgetown University Law Center and the S.I. Newhouse School of Public Communications at Syracuse University. In 2000, Gary founded Mayerson & Associates as the first civil rights law firm in the nation dedicated to representing individuals with autism and related developmental disorders.

Chapter 17
Legal Issues and Academic Accommodations in Higher Education

Jane Thierfeld Brown and Lorre Wolf

Portions of this chapter were originally printed in Disability Compliance in Higher Education, January 2018, "Students with Autism: Challenges with Conduct and Title IX" and are reprinted here with permission.

Colleges and universities are quite familiar with the academic and other needs of students with disabilities and most do an excellent job working with this population of students. However, students with autism differ from students with other disabilities in that their pervasive struggles present throughout all aspects of the higher education experience including cognitive, social, and regulatory domains.

For most college personnel (faculty, administrators, and staff) the challenges lie in understanding that students with autism need to make a great effort to manage their social, executive, and self-regulatory functioning. College is a period of independence for all students but those who have difficulty establishing meaningful social interactions may especially be at risk. For example, making friends in the residence halls and sharing space with a roommate can be quite challenging—for both parties. Thus, residential life staff may not know how to approach roommate conflicts when one partner may not understand interpersonal negotiations. Outside of residential life, the same relational issues which can impact a young adult with autism—e.g., altered eye contact or lack of understanding of unwritten social codes—can also be a challenge in the classroom. Again, the professor with this student in his or her class may not know how to hold productive 1:1 meetings with someone who does not meet their gaze. These factors make the college student with autism unfamiliar and often unique for university personnel to understand. This chapter reviews some of the basic legal underpinnings of disability service in higher education and aims to better prepare colleges to improve service provision to students with autism.

J. T. Brown
Yale Child Study, College Autism Spectrum, 41 Crossroads Plaza #221, West Hartford, CT, USA
e-mail: jane.brown@yale.edu

L. Wolf (✉)
Disability Services, Boston University, Boston, MA, USA
e-mail: lwolf@bu.edu

F. R. Volkmar et al. (eds.), *Handbook of Autism Spectrum Disorder and the Law*,
https://doi.org/10.1007/978-3-030-70913-6_17

Accommodating Students with Autism

Accommodations are defined as adjustments to an academic program or environment intended to mitigate the impact of the functional limitations of a disability on participation in that environment. Extended time for exams, use of assistive technology, relocating classrooms to enable physical access and alternate-format textbooks (digital audio rather than print) are all examples of accommodations commonly provided on college campuses. Intended to "level the playing field" accommodations render the academic environment manageable without fundamentally altering the curriculum.

The ADA states that "Institutions must make *modifications* to academic requirements as necessary to ensure that such requirements do not discriminate against students with disabilities, or have the effect of excluding students solely on the basis of disability. An institution may not impose rules or restrictions that have the effect of limiting participation of students with disabilities in educational programs or activities" (ADA.gov). This means that students with disabilities have the right to receive accommodations, which mitigate the impact of their disability on their academic performance and which allow them to compete equitably with their peers without disabilities. In simple terms, providing extended exam time to a student who reads slowly would mean that the student would be assessed based on their ability not their reading speed.

Reasonable Accommodations: Reasonable accommodations mitigate the impact of impairment and level the playing field for students who need them. For students with disabilities, extended time, a notetaker, or some other reasonable accommodation puts them on an equal basis for being evaluated with other students. This is the same as an accessible entrance or ramp for someone in a wheelchair. For students with autism, accommodations allow them to better learn and demonstrate proficiencies in an educational environment, preventing them from drowning in an atmosphere far too social for most students on the spectrum to survive.

Determining reasonable accommodations for students with autism requires careful planning, dialogue and understanding of the spectrum. Many accommodations are straightforward and flow directly from the student's functional limitations and the provider's understanding of the essentials of autism. For example, it would be reasonable for a student on the spectrum to take an exam in a separate room to control for anxiety. Other reasonable accommodations for a student on the spectrum might be extra time on an exam, changing a classroom or moving a class to reduce sensory issues (e.g., dim lights, away from sources of noise) or a single room in the residence hall. All accommodations must follow the crucial part of the law; the students must engage in an interactive process with the designated college or university agent, usually in Disability or Access Services office in requesting and monitoring their accommodations.

Are there Typical Accommodations for students with autism? Every student with autism is different; therefore, it is impossible to offer a laundry list of reasonable and unreasonable accommodations. Further, accommodations must be individualized for the student and not prescribed per any particular diagnosis. One does not "accommodate autism," but rather accommodates a *student* with an autism spectrum diagnosis that affects them in a uniquely individual manner. Successful accommodations stem from understanding the diagnosis, the way it affects an individual student, and the fundamental requirements of a course or program.

Many academic difficulties in autism are related to difficulties in integration of sensory, information processing, executive functioning, and self-regulation. Examples could include challenges in planning and organizing, synthesizing large amounts of reading with lecture information, and managing criticism and feedback. Understanding these factors can lead to the best route to accommodating the students. While we are reluctant to offer a list of recommended accommodations for the reasons outlined above, the table below provides some of the more common adjustments with which college personnel and faculty are most familiar.

Some Common Academic Accommodations

Exams:

- Extra time
- Low distraction (or solo) environment
- Computer for essay exams
- Clarification of questions or answers (written or oral)
- Space apart major exams
- Breaks as needed
- Drinks or food
- Oral supplement to essay exams
- No "scantron forms" (bubble sheets)
- Extra scrap paper
- Paper in lieu of digital exams

Presentations:

- Webcast or video recorded presentation
- Present to smaller group (or professor only)
- Notes during presentation
- Breaks during presentation (if feasible)
- Alternate assignment (unless presentation is a fundamental requirement)

Classroom:

- Avoid cold-calling in class (call on student and return later)
- Permission to bring sensory objects
- Permission to bring drinks or food
- Breaks as needed
- Notetaker/audio record/digital "smart pen" in class
- Laptop or tablet for note taking

We also encourage personnel to consider requests that may be somewhat unfamiliar but might make sense in the context of the struggles of a student with autism. For example, a student who struggles with understanding the personal motivations of a character in a Shakespeare play might well struggle in an English class, which requires an essay analyzing such motivations and ask to be excused from these assignments. This student should not be offered a waiver of the University English requirement but rather, may be permitted to substitute a paper on the historical or sociological factors operating in Elizabethan England. In another example, the student who requests to be exempted from in-class presentations due to social anxiety might rather be permitted to deliver their presentation via webcam from their residence hall or to present to the professor alone in their office. These examples illustrate how unreasonable requests might be changed into reasonable accommodations with understanding and creativity.

Unreasonable Accommodations

We have provided some examples of reasonable accommodation for students with autism. The compelling issues of many neurodiverse students can tempt college personnel to go to great lengths to find the right type of assistance. However, this should be tempered by legal parameters. For example, accommodations must not provide students with autism an unfair advantage over other students. ADA Title II defines an accommodation as a "modification of the institute's rules, policies, or practices; environmental adjustments, such as the removal of architectural or communicative barriers; or auxiliary aids and services" (ADA.gov). In meeting the need for accommodations, what is reasonable for universities and colleges to do? Accommodations maybe either reasonable or unreasonable. Reasonable accommodations are guaranteed under the law to level the playing field for a person with a disability. On the other hand, unreasonable accommodations are adjustments, which would (1) confer an unfair advantage of the recipient, (2) compromise the fundamental requirements, technical standards, or essential functions of a course program or position, (3) pose an undue burden to the provider, or (4) be inappropriate per the diagnosed condition and its functional limitations.

Unreasonable accommodations would be those which alter the curriculum, confer an unfair advantage, or create an undue burden. For example, an unreasonable accommodation may be a tutor to accompany the student to all exams and classes and to clarify all of the student's answers to their professor.

Other examples of unreasonable academic accommodations include waiving required courses that are deemed fundamental to the course of study (such as the English requirements for the student who struggles with composition), permitting papers in lieu of exams for the student with test anxiety, assigning a tutor to attend class and prepare individualized study guides, permitting independent or directed studies for courses with attendance requirements, assigning fewer readings or less homework, waiving lab attendance, unlimited time for exams, and unlimited extensions for homework, papers, or out-of-class assignments.

Students who qualify for accommodations must be able to attend classes and complete the required work—academic standards don't change. For example, students with autism are expected to complete the same assignments and are evaluated using the same academic standards as students without disabilities. Students are not excused from reading the same books, writing the same term papers, and attending the same classes simply by virtue of their classification as a student with a disability. However, certain modifications maybe necessary, which will be discussed at greater length, such as extended time or a lighter course load.

To reiterate, a request becomes unreasonable when it would confer an unfair advantage—such as allowing unlimited time to complete an assignment, having professionally prepared study guides that are not available to students without disabilities, or having a personal tutor attend classes with the student. Unreasonable requests may also not pose an undue burden to the grantor of the accommodation. An example of this might be a student whose sensory sensitivities overwhelm them in the dining hall and request the university build an apartment for them on campus with a kitchen (presuming no such apartments exist on campus).

Finally, accommodations must not fundamentally alter the nature of a course, examination, or program of study, such as never writing a paper in college. It is also unreasonable if it compromises the academic integrity, standards, or fundamental requirements for the course or program.

Conduct and Behavior

All colleges and universities have written enforceable academic and community standards and conduct codes that apply to all students, with or without disabilities. Campuses differ considerably in how they handle and adjudicate violations (student conduct board, dean, conduct office, etc.). Regardless of the process, however, students with disabilities must maintain appropriate behavioral standards with no exceptions for students with autism. For example, a student who has an outburst in class and argues with a professor, intimidating the class and the instructor, maybe subject to conduct code charges. The fact that the student has autism might become relevant in the process and could be part of determining any sanctions. However, the presence of any disability does not excuse the student's behavior or eliminate the prohibition on disruption of the educational environment.

Title IX

Most students with autism will have few (if any) conduct issues, however, for others, challenging behaviors can emerge on campus and in class. This is often due to inherent difficulty with communication, including processing verbal and nonverbal cues, understanding and anticipating social situations ("reading between the lines"), and identifying and extrapolating information/directions that are both implicit and explicit in nature. In class, students with autism may ask many questions, hold rigid or inflexible opinions, correct the professor, and/or monopolize the discussion. Elsewhere on campus interpersonal challenges and violation of behavioral and conduct codes can arise from lack of awareness of social norms, poor social skills, and social anxiety (3).

Disability Laws

Students on the autism spectrum who have spent their K-12 school career under the protective cloak of special education can encounter marked challenges as they transition to college, partly due to the change in applicable laws (from the Individuals with Disabilities Education Act to the Americans with Disabilities Act). Behavioral issues often create the most challenging scenarios for families who are accustomed to special education where consequences for infractions may be excused under a loophole called "manifestation determination" which does not exist in college. The chart 1 below illustrates the differences in premise, responsibility, services, and focus that underlay these important changes (1).

	IDEA	ADA
Type of Law	Education, Entitlement	Civil rights statute, Eligibility
Responsibility	Parent and school	Student
Ensures	Success	Equal Access
Services	Evaluation, remediation, special accommodations	Reasonable accommodations
Focus	Diagnostic label	Level of functional impairment
Disability	One of 13 categories	**Impairment in major life activity**

Chart 1 College Autism Spectrum 2021

Title IX

A part of the Education Amendments Act of 1972, Title IX is a civil law that prohibits discrimination based upon sex in any federally funded program or activity (3). The application of the law includes the prohibition of unequal treatment based on sex, unequal power dynamics based on sex, harassment based on sex, and sexual violence. Colleges and Universities receiving federal funding must have processes and procedures to ensure equal treatment and processes for complainants to be supported in the college environment. This includes mandated training for faculty, staff, and students. Title IX has become the largest mechanism college campuses use to prevent unwanted sexual advances, stalking, and other sexually based acts of misconduct (see Chap. 14). This is a hot-button topic, as the guidance for what does and does not constitute sexual misconduct is ephemeral. Neurotypical students as well as college personnel struggle to grasp these subtleties.

Title IX and the Student with Autism

The developmental impact of autism on social information processing thus poses particular challenges in understanding the requirements for Title IX compliance both as a potential respondent or victim. For example, student trainings often focus on standards of consent. However, the student with autism who lacks nuance around social norms and dating behaviors can unknowingly violate the statutes because they may not perceive physical signs, facial expressions, or verbal cues that indicate an advance is unwelcome. Indeed, research has demonstrated that students on the spectrum maybe more likely to be accused of stalking. Conversely, students with autism maybe at risk for becoming the victims of sexual abuse and misconduct as lack of social exposure may make students vulnerable to offensive practical jokes, over trusting others, and an inability to discriminate atypical social behaviors. Thus, through possible deficits in social information processing, poor understanding of social norms, and a lack of awareness of the interpretations of their behaviors, students with autism may not recognize the nexus between their behavior as it might impact Title IX.

Per federal mandate, to comply with Title IX campuses must be proactive in training all students However, trainings and education can take many forms. Some campuses utilize popular videos such as "Tea and Consent" which portrays standards of consent in humorous cartoon format. Other schools use online and video-based tutorials that are mandatory for incoming students prior to registration, residence hall meetings, and/or public student trainings with deans or judicial officers. Students on politically active campuses may stage and organize rallies such as "Take Back the Night" to raise awareness of sexual assault resources.

Regardless of the methodology, students with autism require additional support to benefit from Title IX training. To best support students on the spectrum in those trainings, and in conduct training overall, campus administrators must rethink the way trainings are offered to students, and when necessary, partner with the disability service providers to ensure the trainings are effective. Best practices for trainings that impart information about nuanced social behavior should involve an opportunity for one-to-one teaching, repetition, and role playing. Students should be encouraged to confidentially request individualized training with a professional who both understands autism and Title IX. The curriculum should optimally include (but not be limited to) dating, consent, stalking, good and bad touch, rules for texting and online dating, recognizing signs of assault, and reporting of misconduct and abuse. Students with autism may be rule bound, therefore explicit guidelines and templates can be utilized (e.g. "how many times can you text a student before its considered stalking," how to write a neutral email, etc.).

Code of Conduct and Investigations

On most campuses, Title IX augments robust codes of conduct that govern acceptable behavior in the curricular and noncurricular domains. Few campus officials (other than individuals directly involved in judicial proceedings) and fewer students and their parents have actually read these codes but in most cases, they are prohibitive rather than prescriptive. In other words, they do a good job outlining prohibited behaviors but do not provide any information about what constitutes acceptable standards of behavior. We tell students what not to do but we do not tell them how they should act. Students with autism greatly benefit from the latter forms of instruction, therefore a sensitive code of conduct would provide explicit guidance about how to behave (rather than how not to). Conduct officers and disability services can work together to create informal guides as well as bulleted lists of how to behave on campus in addition to what is not allowed.

All conduct code statements, whether inverted or traditional, should be presented according to the principles of Universally Designed Instruction. In other words, multiple forms of presentation (written, video, etc.), with alternate means for assessing student's comprehension. Underlying all of these must be the clear message that disability does not excuse behavior. If an infraction has occurred and is being investigated, it is crucial to make sure the student and their family understand the seriousness of the process, the potential impact on the student, and the protocol of the investigation. In addition, the process of investigating a violation of any conduct code for a student on the spectrum should be accommodated (permission to bring a parent or other nonparticipating advocate, behavior coach, materials in writing in advance, repetition of questions or instructions, permission to ask questions, etc.). In short, standards are not compromised, however, the process is accommodated and sanctions may be creative.

College students are treated as adults and those expectations are enforced. Students with disabilities in college are included in the adult expectations. No disability excuses behavior. For students with autism, behaviors must be under control in order to remain on a college campus. For those with challenging behaviors (a very small number of college students with autism), the standards do not change, however, the process is accommodated.

Disclosure and Confidentiality

Questions often arise as to when and whether autism should be disclosed to roommates, professors, and others on campus. Students and families may assume that relevant personnel will automatically be informed as they were in high school. This is not, however, the case in higher education.

College students are legal adults who have full access to their academic records (including disability files) with full protection of confidentiality. However, campuses differ in how they regard disclosure of disability. For example, some institutions maintain a strict interpretation of FERPA (Federal Education Rights and Privacy Act; www.ferpa.gov) which prohibits sharing information with anyone without the student's written permission, while other campuses share certain information such as grade reports, judicial sanctions, and health information. Schools should consider what information students on the spectrum are comfortable sharing and with whom. Additional questions arise determining what information can be shared with parents, particularly when there are judicial or mental health issues. For example, it can be useful for students and their parents to work with the school to identify resources for students when stressed, however, it is up to the student to determine what and how much information may be disclosed.

The Legal Transition from High School

As students move forward to higher education, the legal focus shifts from entitlement and remediation to protection from discrimination and equal access. Increasingly, the student must be able to self-identify as a person with a disability and demonstrate that they are qualified as a member of a protected group. Adult students must take charge of their own education and their disability. This comes as a shock to many highly (sometimes overly) involved families who find their function limited by the policies of the university. Families discover that documentation guidelines and the review processes for eligibility are more stringent, as the diagnosis alone is no longer the only criterion for services. Students may for the first time face a rejection for accommodations and services. Even when approved, families discover that services and accommodations are usually more limited than what they enjoyed in high school.

Section 504 of the Rehabilitation Act and the Americans with Disabilities Act prohibit discrimination solely on the basis of disability in employment, education, and physical plant (see below), and thus protect individuals with disabilities from discrimination. There are many key differences between the special education laws and the disability statutes that protect college students with disabilities. These will be summarized below.

Section 504 of the Rehabilitation Act of 1973 (http://www.hhs.gov/ocr/504.pdf)

This is a civil rights law that prohibits discrimination on the basis of disability in programs and activities, public and private, which receive federal financial assistance. This is the law that mandates accommodations in higher education, for the most part. No funding to the student or the campus is associated with this law.

Section 504 states that

> No otherwise qualified individual with a disability in the United States, as defined in section 7(20), shall, solely by reason of her or his disability, be excluded from the participation in, be denied the benefits of, or be subjected to discrimination under any program or activity receiving Federal financial assistance or under any program or activity conducted by any Executive agency or by the United States Postal Service. (Sec 504, a)

The Americans with Disabilities Act (ADA) www.ada.gov

The ADA was enacted in 1990 as a federal civil rights law that extends Section 504 to protect against discrimination for reasons related to disabilities in employment, education, and accommodations. It applies to public and private entities that receive federal funds, and thus covers access in most places of employment, colleges, and universities. Titles II and III of the ADA prohibit discrimination on the basis of disability in employment, government, public accommodations, commercial facilities, transportation, and telecommunications. It includes building and facilities access, employment practices, self-evaluation of the services provided, and grievances.

University Rights and Responsibilities

Under 504/ADA, a college or university must provide the qualified student with a disability equal access to all educational programs, services, facilities, and activities. The university must also provide reasonable accommodations, academic adjustments, and/or auxiliary aids and services to eligible persons with disabilities. The university or college is also responsible for maintaining student confidentiality as far as their disability is concerned, and must establish and maintain written policies and procedures (including procedures for filing grievances).

In addition to the university's responsibilities, the educational institutions hold certain rights. Universities have the right to maintain academic standards, integrity, and freedom, and to determine the fundamental requirements of their individual courses and programs. Fundamental requirements are essential aspects of a course or program that do not need to be altered or modified for a student with a disability. One example might be a math or foreign language requirement in a liberal arts course of study. Just because a student is an Engineering major who never intends to read a non-technical book or travel abroad, he or she is expected to meet the same foreign language or general education requirements as other students if it has been determined that these are essential to the Engineering education.

Once a fundamental requirement has been established (following the legal guidelines for such determination, *Wynne v. Tufts Univ. School of Medicine*, 932 F.2d 19, 26, 1st Cir. 1991; also see Macurdy & Geetter, 2008), the college or university does not need to waive or modify the requirement as an accommodation for a student with a disability even if the student had demonstrated that she would benefit from such an adjustment. As mentioned, universities also have the right to maintain and enforce conduct codes without regard to a student's disability as a mitigating factor (unlike public K-12 schools, which often cannot discipline unless disability is considered).

With regard to accommodations, the university may determine what is reasonable and appropriate and select among effective alternatives. This means that despite the student's request for a notetaker, for example, the university may determine that another alternative would be reasonable and appropriate (such as audio taping lectures). Finally, the university may deny unreasonable or inappropriate accommodation requests. An accommodation request is considered unreasonable when the accommodation would confer an unfair advantage on the student receiving the adjustment, pose an undue burden on the agency being asked to provide the accommodations, compromise the academic integrity of academic standards of a course, degree, or program, or fundamentally alter the nature of a course, examination, or program of study (See *Southeastern Community College v. Davis*, 442 U.S. 397, 423 [1979], where the Supreme Court determined that colleges and universities are not required to make changes to program standards that can be demonstrated to be fundamental or essential to the program of study; also see Macurdy & Geetter, 2008).

Student Rights and Responsibilities

Under the law, students with disabilities have the right to equal access to all university programs and activities. Other rights that the universities must recognize include the right to receive effective, appropriate, and reasonable accommodations. This is often the first point of intersection between the student with AS and the university, as the student and/or his family contact the university to arrange accommodations for tests or in residence halls. Unlike high school, students must engage in an interactive process with the disability services office in requesting and monitoring their accommodations.

Along with student rights come the student's responsibilities. Students are ultimately responsible for self-disclosing their disability to the designated entity on campus. Failure to do so means that the university is not obligated to recognize the student as having a disability or offer the legal protection appropriate disclosure affords. Self-disclosure also includes providing documentation of disability in compliance with campus policy. The student is responsible for requesting their own accommodations and monitoring their effectiveness. Finally, the student must follow established policies and procedures with regard to disabilities accommodations and must meet required academic and behavioral standards (e.g., be otherwise qualified).

Conclusion

The laws change from high school to postsecondary education and students and their families must be informed before making transition decisions. Accommodations also change substantially and only through research and questioning will a student feel prepared to make the leap to the college campus. Secondary schools need to prepare students academically for the next step and teach as much independence as possible. Families need to educate themselves about the changes and applicable laws in transitioning from high school to college.

Accommodations for students with autism flow from understanding the individual student, the characteristics of the condition as it affects the individual's academic and nonacademic domains of higher education. Also to be considered are established policies and practices at different institutions and the fundamental requirements of the student's course or program. Balancing these factors permits the determination of reasonable accommodations while avoiding unreasonable recommendations. Alterations to established University conduct codes are most often unreasonable.

College and University campuses need to understand students with autism and the challenges they may face on campus along with the richness and diversity they bring. Training and acceptance of difference will go far in integrating people with autism into the campus community.

Resources

1. Americans with Disabilities Act of 1990 and Revised ADA Regulations, ADA.gov.
2. Brown, Jane Thierfeld; Wolf, Lorre; Sullivan, Linda. Students with Autism: Challenges with Conduct and Title IX, In Disability Compliance in Higher Education, January 2018, Wiley and Co.
3. Brown, Sarah. "What Colleges Need to Know About the New Title IX Rules," Chronicle of Higher Education, May 6, 2020.
4. FERPA. https://www2.ed.gov/policy/gen/guid/fpco/ferpa/index.html.

5. Individuals with Disabilities Education Act, 2004. https://sites.ed.gov/idea/.
6. Office for Civil Rights, Title IX and Sex Discrimination, revised April, 2015. https://www2.ed.gov/about/offices/list/ocr/docs/tix_dis.html.
7. *Section 504 of the Rehabilitation Act of 1973*. http://www.hhs.gov/ocr/504.
8. *Southeastern Community College v. Davis*, 442 U.S. 397, 423 [1979].
9. Universal Design for Learning. https://udlguidelines.cast.org/.
10. *Wynne v. Tufts Univ. School of Medicine*, 932 F.2d 19, 26, 1st Cir. 1991; also see Macurdy, A. H, Geetter, E. (2008). Legal Issues for Adults with Learning Disabilities in Higher Education and Employment. In C. Weinstein, L. E. Wolf, H. Schreiber, J.Wasserstein (Eds.), *Adult learning disorders: Contemporary issues*.

Jane Thierfeld Brown is Director of College Autism Spectrum, Assistant Clinical Professor at Yale Child Study, Yale Medical School, and former Director of student Services at the University of Connecticut School of Law. She has worked in Disability Services for 42 years. She holds an Ed.D from Columbia University, Teachers College and received an honorary Doctorate of Letters from Muhlenberg College in 2020. Dr. Brown consults with many families, students, school districts, and institutions of higher education. Dr. Brown has appeared on Good Morning America, CBS News, and NPR. She has co-authored "Students with Asperger's: A Guide for College Professionals," (2009) published in Japanese in 2017, "The Parent's Guide to College for Students on the Autism Spectrum," (2012) and "Behavior Management and Self-Regulation," (2012) along with many textbook chapters and articles. She received the Ron Blosser Dedicated Service Award from AHEAD in 2019. Dr. Brown is married and has three children, the youngest being a 29-year-old son with Autism.

Dr. Lorre Wolf is the Director of Disability Services at Boston University. She holds a doctorate in clinical neuropsychology from the City University of New York and has over 30 years of experience working with children, adolescents, and adults with neurodevelopmental disorders. She has taught experimental psychology, assessment, and neuropsychology at the undergraduate and graduate levels. Dr. Wolf has published and presented nationally and internationally on issues for students with attention and learning disorders, psychiatric disabilities, and autism spectrum disorders. She holds faculty appointments in psychiatry and in rehabilitation sciences at Boston University. She was a co-editor of Adult Attention Deficit Disorders: Brain Mechanisms and Life Outcomes (2001, New York Academy of Sciences), is the senior co-editor of Learning Disorders in Adults: Contemporary Issues (Psychology Press, 2008), and is the co-author of Students with Asperger Syndrome: A Guide for College Personnel (Autism Asperger Publishing Company, 2009) and Students on the Spectrum: A College Guide for Parents (AAPC, 2011). Dr. Wolf's interests include the neuropsychology of attention disorders, and developing effective services for students with autism spectrum and other psychiatric disabilities in higher education. Along with her co-presenter Jane Thierfeld Brown, she developed a model of service delivery for college students entitled "Strategic Education for Students with Autism Spectrum Disorders." She is the parent of twins, one of whom is on the spectrum, which gives her a unique insight into these courageous young people.

Chapter 18
Autism Spectrum Disorder and the Workplace

Michael Selmi

Introduction

Employment, for disabled and non-disabled individuals, can provide a crucial link to economic security and independence, as well as alleviating social isolation. Unlike the education setting where there has been considerable focus on Autism Spectrum Disorder ("ASD"), integrating autistic individuals into the workplace has received far less attention. According to a recent study conducted by the A.J. Drexel Autism Institute, young adults with autism had the lowest employment rate (57%) compared to individuals with similar disabilities (AJ. Drexel Autism Institute, 2015). The study also found that employees with ASD tended to hold low-wage part-time jobs. There have also been relatively few cases to arise under the primary federal statute that prohibits discrimination among those defined as disabled, the Americans With Disabilities Act ("ADA"), and in those cases, it has often proved difficult for individuals to establish a claim of discrimination.

Fortunately, the news regarding the employment of individuals with ASD is not all gloomy. In recent years, a number of major companies such as Microsoft and Walgreens have begun specific initiatives designed to hire individuals who are on the Autism spectrum, and those efforts, discussed later in this chapter, may help guide courts and other employers toward fuller integration of individuals with ASD into the workplace by demonstrating what works best to enable individuals to perform their jobs. A key aspect of the ADA is that employers are required to provide reasonable accommodations to those with disabilities, and the recent private initiatives should provide guidance regarding the kinds of accommodations that may be most helpful.

This chapter will begin by discussing some common workplace issues that arise with individuals with ASD that may make some workplaces challenging. Next, the

M. Selmi (✉)
Arizona State College of Law, Phoenix, AZ, USA
e-mail: Michael.Selmi@asu.edu

F. R. Volkmar et al. (eds.), *Handbook of Autism Spectrum Disorder and the Law*,
https://doi.org/10.1007/978-3-030-70913-6_18

Americans with Disabilities Act will be discussed, including the requirement that employers make a good faith effort to accommodate individuals with disabilities. The third section will explore recent company initiatives targeting individuals on the autism spectrum for employment, and how those initiatives may illustrate ways employers can best integrate autistic workers into their workplaces.

Individuals with ASPD in the Workplace

One of the key insights regarding employment opportunities is that individuals with ASD differ substantially in their workplace abilities. Many or perhaps most such individuals will encounter no greater problems than non-disabled workers in the workplace and no particular accommodation will be necessary. And for others with more severe conditions, obtaining meaningful employment may prove difficult, which is generally true for individuals with severe disabilities regardless of the nature of the disability. As a result, the group of individuals most likely to require some workplace accommodation is those who fall somewhere in between, those with behavioral issues that many employers and co-employees may view as problematic.

For example, individuals with ASD often lack social skills that can prove important to workplace success, including difficulty in reading social cues or communicating directly with others. These conditions might manifest themselves in what might be described as a difficulty getting along with others, as will be discussed more fully below given that most of the legal cases that have arisen involving individuals with ASD implicate getting along with others in one form or another. Additionally, many individuals with ASD may require detailed instructions for their job tasks and may perform best in positions that offer routine and repetition rather than requiring frequent modifications or new tasks (Hendricks, 2010). Relatedly, individuals with ASD may be most successful in jobs where they can fulfill one task at a time rather than juggling multiple assignments.

As such, there is no one-size-fits-all blueprint or accommodation for individuals with ASD but rather the specifics of both the workplace and the individual will dictate successful integration strategies. As we will see, virtually all of the legal cases that have arisen involve individuals who are employed and encounter difficulties in their workplace, whereas likely a more important issue is getting into the workplace. This is again not an issue unique to ASD individuals but runs across disabilities and discrimination claims involving hiring cases are far less common than termination cases. But with respect to ASD, many individuals may be faced with the question of whether they should disclose their condition at the time of an interview or even at the application stage. There is no definitive answer to this question. Under existing law, there is no requirement that individuals disclose a disability, and in fact, employers are prohibited from asking about disabilities. Employers can, however, list a task and ask applicants if they can perform that task, at which point the applicant has a duty to respond truthfully. So, for example, if an employer noted that working with others, or handling multiple tasks simultaneously, was a required job duty, an individual might be required to indicate any difficulty she might have in fulfilling those duties.

There is a related advantage to disclosing one's disability—for some, though certainly not all employers, obtaining information regarding a disability may make them more cautious and careful in their decision so as to avoid the possibility of a lawsuit. Some employers may even react favorably, particularly if they are interested in increasing diversity within their workforce. And, as discussed in the next section, it would be impermissible for an employer to fail to hire someone because of the disclosed disability, although hiring lawsuits are notoriously difficult to prove because the evidence necessary to establish such a claim is often lacking. Moreover, many applicants who are turned down for a job will fail to even explore why they were rejected. But disclosing a disability may also trigger stereotypic responses so that someone who mentions in an interview that they are on the autism spectrum may then be associated with the kind of odd behavior portrayed in the popular media, such as in Rain Man or the more recent television show The Good Doctor, that may have little to do with the applicant's actual behavior. Depending on the employer, these stereotypic assumptions might lead an employer to decline to hire an individual with ASD for fear that the person may be too difficult to manage. While that decision would likely be legally impermissible, it again might be difficult to prove. Accordingly, whether someone should disclose a condition will likely depend on the particular situation, the relevance of the condition to the job, and some educated guess of how the employer might respond.

The Americans with Disabilities Act

The landmark Americans With Disabilities Act ("ADA") prohibits discrimination against those who the statute defines as disabled. Originally passed in 1991, the statute was subsequently interpreted very narrowly by the Supreme Court in a way that restricted the reach and force of the statute (Selmi, 2008). In turn, Congress amended the statute in 2008 in the awkwardly named Americans with Disabilities Act Amendments Act of 2008 ("ADAAAA") so as to restore the statute to its original purpose. The Amendments have had a particular effect on individuals with ASD and the amended Act rather than the original Act will be the focus of the rest of this chapter.[1]

The ADA prohibits employers with more than 15 employees from discriminating against those who are defined as disabled. Unlike something like age discrimination, there is no consensual definition of who is disabled for purposes of statutory protection and the statute offers a specific definition that requires proof of four different

[1] Under the original Act, individuals with autism were frequently defined as not disabled because the court concluded that the individuals were not substantially limited in a major life function, a condition for protection both under the original and amended statute. However, the amended statute broadened the scope and individuals with autism are not routinely defined as disabled.

elements. The statute prohibits discrimination against the disabled who are qualified to perform the essential functions of the job, either with or without a reasonable accommodation. Each of these terms—disabled, qualified, essential functions and reasonable accommodations—requires definition, and all of the terms are susceptible to varying interpretations.

Defining Disability

The statute defines "disabled" as someone who is substantially limited in a major life function. This is a term that the 2008 Amendments sought to clarify, as prior to the passage of those Amendments, there were many cases seeking to interpret what constituted a major life function, a term that generally encompasses things like walking, talking, eating, and other daily functions. Before the Amendments were passed, in some cases, individuals with Asperger's were deemed not sufficiently limited in their daily life functions and therefore were not considered disabled under the terms of the statute, and in a large number of nonautism related cases, courts struggled to determine whether certain daily tasks like brushing one's teeth constituted a major life activity. In the context of those with Asperger's, in response to an employer's claim that the employee was not substantially limited in a major life function, the individual employee often responded that she was substantially limited in the major life function of getting along with others. Most courts accepted this position but some courts were reluctant to see getting along with others as a major life function, and indeed, the ability to get along with others continues to serve as a hurdle to obtaining protection under the ADA.

One issue that has arisen in several of the cases is that an individual with Asperger's, by far the most common ASD condition present in the court cases, is also identified as having ADHD, which has long been a controversial diagnosis. Although courts appear to readily accept Asperger's diagnoses, their general skepticism over ADHD may influence their analysis, particularly when it comes to determining whether the individual is qualified to perform the job. In any event, the key point here is that prior to the 2008 Amendments, many cases, including those focusing on ASD individuals, turned on whether the individual was defined as disabled under the terms of the statute.

For the most part, the statutory changes have caused that debate to recede, and today, individuals with Asperger's or other related conditions are generally defined as disabled without meaningful inquiry or discussion, a conclusion that is consistent both with the statutory language and the interpreting regulations promulgated by the EEOC. In its interpretive regulations, the EEOC has made it clear that those with ASD should be defined as disabled in that it substantially limits brain functions.[2] Indeed, consistent with the regulations, the statutory Amendments have largely been interpreted to define disability broadly and to avoid lengthy disputes about whether

[2] 29 C.F.R. § 1630(h)(3)(iii) (2016).

someone falls within the scope of the statute. But, as a practical matter, what that means is that the focus of inquiry has shifted from whether the individual is disabled to whether the person is qualified to perform the essential functions of the job, and that inquiry often results in finding the person is unqualified. Again, this has been true not just for individuals with ASD but across the board on disability claims, which remain extremely difficult to win.

Qualified to Perform the Essential Functions of the Job

Cases involving ASD, most commonly Asperger's, turn on some common facts but it is also important to note that the ADA requires an individualized inquiry in all circumstances. Assuming the individual has been defined as disabled, the inquiry then turns to whether the person can perform the essential functions of the job, and there is a separate question of whether there are reasonable accommodations that would enable the person to perform those essential functions. As a result, a court will carefully analyze the particular situation both to identify the essential functions of a job, and to determine whether the individual is able to perform those functions, with, or without, a reasonable accommodation. Both the focus on essential functions and reasonable accommodations are unique to the operation of the ADA, and require judicial interpretation.

Under the statute, disabled individuals are only required to perform the essential functions of the job—any job requirement that is not deemed essential can effectively be disregarded in determining whether someone is qualified for the position. In cases involving those with Asperger's, the employee was often disciplined or terminated because of a difficulty getting along with others, or in some instances the difficulty interacting with customers. In those cases, the initial question becomes whether getting along with others or interacting positively with customers is an essential function of the job. There is no definitive test to determine what constitutes an essential function; the statute defines essential function as "fundamental," but courts often defer to employers in defining the specific requirements of the job. Other courts have sought to provide a quantitative measure, seeking to assess how much of a particular job requires interacting with customers, for example, or getting along with others. One court explained:

> An "essential function" is a fundamental job duty of the position at issue … [it] does not include the marginal functions of the position. Whether a job function is "essential" is determined by looking at numerous factors, including: the employer's judgment as to which functions are essential; written job descriptions of the job prepared before considering applicants; the amount of time spent on the job performing the function; the consequences of not requiring the incumbent to perform the function; and the work experience of past and current incumbents of the job. In the absence of evidence of discriminatory animus, [courts] generally give[s] substantial weight to the employer's view of job requirements.[3]

[3] Kinghorn v. General Hosp. Corp., 2014 WL 3058291, *6 (D. Mass. 2014).

Once the essential functions of the job are defined, the next and typically most important question is whether the individual is qualified to perform those functions with or without a reasonable accommodation. These two questions—performing the job and reasonable accommodations—should be analyzed together, but courts typically split them and focus primarily on whether the person is qualified without regard to available accommodations. This is not an analysis unique to individuals with ASD but instead reflects how courts analyze disabilities more generally, and it has led to many cases being lost because the court determines the individual is not qualified for the position without ever assessing whether a reasonable accommodation is available. For example, in one well-known case involving a police officer who had interpersonal problems with his subordinates, which the plaintiff alleged resulted from his ADHD, the court simply concluded that his behavior meant he was not qualified to perform his duties.[4] The court never considered whether there was any reasonable accommodation that might have allowed him to perform his job satisfactorily but simply concluded that his personality made him unsuited for the supervisory position he held.

The same has occurred in several cases involving individuals with Asperger's. In one case involving a Bioinformatics Specialist at a Hospital, the employee, Brian Kinghorn, got into an argument with his supervisor after only two days on the job, which was quickly followed by other negative interactions with co-workers. After the employee informed his employer that he had Asperger's, the employer provided him with a detailed agenda and sought to provide a more structured day for him. He was nevertheless fired after less than a month on the job, which the court found did not violate the ADA. The court concluded that the employee was unqualified to perform his job because he was unable to "follow instructions and work collaboratively with others," two essential functions of his work. The court added, "The record is replete with examples of Plaintiff failing to follow directions even after a structured daily training plan was reduced to writing for him."[5] In a similar case involving a medical resident, the court concluded that the plaintiff's Asperger's interfered with his ability to communicate with colleagues and patients and that he had failed to demonstrate that there was any way to accommodate his disability. As an accommodation, the plaintiff sought to have his colleagues undergo training to provide "knowledge and understanding" of Asperger's, something the court noted would not affect his interaction with patients, and thus rejected the suggestion as a permissible reasonable accommodation.[6]

Both of these cases touch on what has been a divisive issue within courts and which has particular application to those with ASD—how should courts analyze a situation of workplace misconduct when that misconduct is directly attributable to one's disability. Two approaches have arisen. In one, which is currently the majority approach among courts, it does not matter if the misconduct is attributable to the disability—workplace misconduct is a legitimate reason for discipline or termination

[4] Weaving v. City of Hillsboro, 763 F.3d 1106 (9th Cir. 2014).

[5] Kinghorn v. General Hospital Corp., 2014 WL 3058291 (D. Mass. 2014).

[6] Jakubowski v. Christ Hospital, 627 F.3d 195 (6th Cir. 2010).

regardless of its source. As the Second Circuit Court of Appeals explained in a recent case: " The fact that such aberrant behavior may be a result of [the employee's] Asperger's is immaterial, inasmuch as workplace misconduct is a legitimate and nondiscriminatory reason for terminating employment, even when such misconduct is related to a disability."[7] This principle has been applied to all manner of disability cases and when applied, it invariably means that the employer's actions will be upheld. In these cases, courts rarely seek to determine whether the employer might have been able to accommodate an individual's disability, perhaps by hiring a job coach, an issue that will be discussed shortly, and likewise fail to ask whether the misconduct justified termination.

The other approach, which has been adopted by the Ninth Circuit Court of Appeals, is far more protective of employee rights, and more consistent with the statute's intent of providing protections to the disabled. Within the Ninth Circuit, an employer may be held liable if the plaintiff can demonstrate a causal link between what the court labels "disability-produced conduct" and an employee's termination. In other words, if the employee can show that she was terminated for conduct that was directly traceable to her disability, she may be able to prevail in her disability claim. In a case involving a T-Mobile retail store manager with Asperger's, the trial court explained that "conduct that results from a disability is part of the disability and not a separate basis for termination."[8] This does not mean that the employee will always prevail on her claim but it shifts the focus to determining whether a reasonable accommodation might be available, or in some instances to determining whether the employer might have been motivated by fear or animus regarding one's disability.

One such case involved an individual with Asperger's who worked as a bagger at a grocery store. The employee, Gary Taylor, often spoke loudly on the job, was overly talkative and occasionally made inappropriate comments to customers. When a customer complained, the employee was fired, and the employee later sued claiming his termination was in violation of the ADA. The employer did not contest that Taylor was disabled under the terms of the statute, nor did the employer contest that Taylor's behavior was a manifestation of his Asperger's but instead the employer claimed that Taylor could not do his job without offending customers. But upon reviewing the entire record, the Court of Appeals concluded that Taylor had received only a couple of complaints from customers or co-workers and more importantly, he did not receive any more complaints than other non-disabled employees.[9] This latter point is important and goes to what it means to discriminate based on stereotypes because it will often be the case that an employer will effectively exaggerate the behavior of those who are different so that a mishap by a disabled employee might be noticed while a mishap by a non-disabled employee will be ignored. This was one of the central objectives the ADA was designed to eradicate—allowing employers to operate on stereotypes or assumptions regarding the abilities of those with disabilities.

---

[7] Krasmer v. City of New York, 580 Fed. Appx. 1 (2nd Cir. 2014).

[8] Bacon v. T-Mobile USA, Inc., 2010 WL 340517 (W.D. Wash. 2010).

[9] Taylor v. Food World, Inc., 133 F.3d 1419 (11th Cir. 1998).

Defining Reasonable Accommodations

This leads to the last, and what Congress intended to be the most important inquiry, namely whether there is a reasonable accommodation that would allow the employee to perform the essential functions of her job. The reasonable accommodation requirement is a core and distinctive feature of the ADA, and at the time the statute was passed, it was seen as critical to integrating the disabled into the workplace. Under the provision, employers have an affirmative obligation to provide a reasonable accommodation and to explore along with the employee what kind of accommodation may be helpful. Yet, in the way the statute has unfolded, there has been surprisingly little development regarding what constitutes a reasonable accommodation. At the same time, the reasonable accommodation provision is crucial to ensuring successful workplace protections and integration.

The basic principles regarding the duty to accommodate are well established: an employer must only provide a reasonable accommodation, not the accommodation an employee prefers. What constitutes a "reasonable" accommodation will depend on the nature of the job, the employee's requirements, and also the nature of the employer. The statute specifically acknowledges that costs are relevant and what might be reasonable for a large employer may prove unreasonable for a smaller employer, or for a large employer in a precarious financial situation. An employer is also obligated to engage in an interactive process with the employee to determine whether a reasonable accommodation exists, and it is not necessary for the employee to request an accommodation. Rather, once an employer has notice of an employee's disability, whether by disclosure or observation, the employer's obligation to consider an accommodation arises.

The issue of the essential functions of the job also plays a role in the accommodation inquiry. If a part of a job is deemed not to be essential, say customer interaction is not essential to the position, then that part of the job can be eliminated, whereas it is not considered reasonable to eliminate an essential function of a job, or to require another employee to perform essential functions. Essential functions must be accommodated, if at all, in a way that allows the disabled employee to perform them.

To date, there have been very few cases assessing what might constitute a reasonable accommodation in the context of individuals with ASD. As mentioned previously, in one case, a medical professional requested that his colleagues be provided with educational training regarding ASD but the court held that such an accommodation would not have addressed the difficulty the individual had communicating with patients. Nevertheless, workplace education of co-workers could constitute a reasonable accommodation in appropriate circumstances so long as the education could ameliorate the workplace conflict. While education should make co-workers more knowledgeable and sensitive to behavioral issues associated with ASD, it may not alleviate workplace performance issues attributable to ASD, although it may make employers and colleagues more tolerant of any such behavior. Another possible accommodation could be a job coach, and a number of employers have voluntarily provided job coaches as part of their initiatives to hire individuals with ASD. Job coaches may be effective in helping employees with ASD navigate complex workplace social interactions. Obviously, the cost of a job coach might prove prohibitive for smaller employers but could likely be reasonable for larger employers, particularly if several employees share the coach. Job coaches may also be available through community organizations and outside the workplace to help train individuals with ASD in the social mores of the workplace.

One of the issues that may arise with a job coach or some other instruction as a possible reasonable accommodation is whether such coaching will help change what the employer considers disruptive behavior. If it does not, then a court is likely to view such an accommodation as ineffective and therefore unreasonable, and it may be necessary at the time the accommodation is requested to demonstrate the potential efficacy of coaching. A number of studies have shown that an individual with ASD can successfully modify her behavior through coaching or instruction (Chen, 2015), though it is also likely the case that it may not always work and may likewise be difficult to establish that coaching will lead to improvement before it is implemented. Coaching may work for some but not others and whether it will prove to be a reasonable accommodation will turn not just on the cost but whether its effectiveness can be demonstrated in the particular situation. With that in mind, coaching or job mentoring is more likely to be voluntarily adopted by employers upon request rather than mandated by a court as a required accommodation.

Individuals with ASD are often sensitive to light and noise, and depending on the workplace, some modest accommodations may be helpful. Changing out harsh fluorescent lights for softer LED lights would rarely pose a financial hardship for employers and may go a significant way toward alleviating some workplace stress for employees on the spectrum; similarly, allowing individuals to wear noise cancelling headphones may enable workers to be more productive and, in the words of the statute, perform the essential functions of the job. There are, indeed, a large number of small shifts in workplace culture that can enable autistic individuals (and others) to perform their job, ranging from providing written instructions to advance notice regarding any changes in workplace routine. Again, these kinds of accommodations are unlikely to impose a financial burden even on smaller employers and may significantly enhance the workplace productivity of employees.

Two frequently requested accommodations have proved more controversial. For many individuals, including those with ASD, working at home would alleviate some of the difficulties they encounter in the workplace, and this applies to those with social deficits, sensitivity to light, noise, or smells, and individuals for whom getting to work can prove difficult. Courts, however, have been particularly hostile to requests for working at home, and as a result most (though not all) such requests have been deemed unreasonable.[10] The primary reason courts deny such requests is that they conclude that showing up to work, or being at work, is an essential function of the job, and therefore cannot be accommodated by eliminating that requirement. This does not mean that requests for a flexible schedule or even to work exclusively at

[10] EEOC v. Ford Motor Co., 782 F.3d 753 (6th Cir. 2015) (en banc).

home will always be rejected as unreasonable, and courts may reconsider some of their earlier decisions in light of the sharp increase in remote work resulting from the coronavirus pandemic. Whether a request will be granted will likely depend on whether the job lends itself to being done outside of the office, and also whether the request is for limited flexibility or a broader request to always work at home. It should also be noted that there is a potential downside to such requests, as the employee can become quite isolated working away from the office and may also limit his or her potential advancement within the company.

Another common accommodation request is to be transferred to a different job one that fits the individual's skills better. In all circumstances, such a request will be reasonable only if a job is open, as it will generally be per se unreasonable to try to bump a person out of a job. However, the statute and courts have determined that transferring an individual with a disability to an open job can constitute a reasonable accommodation.[11] The issue becomes more complicated when there might be another candidate who is more qualified for the open position, or when a union contract determines how the position should be filled, in which case the union contract will typically govern.[12]

Courts have divided over whether companies should be required to allow a transfer as a reasonable accommodation regardless of the qualifications of other applicants or whether companies are only required to allow disabled individuals to compete for a position, which turns out to be not much of an accommodation since qualified individuals would presumably be permitted to apply and compete for any open position (Hensel, 2017: 93). One thing is clear, transferring to another job is only available to the extent that the individual is not capable of performing the essential functions of the current position taking into account the possibility of a reasonable accommodation. In other words, it is not available when an individual would prefer a different job, only when the transfer is necessary to allow the individual to continue working.

Hiring Tests

One emerging area in the employment setting that could pose difficulties for individuals with ASD involves the use of games as part of the interview process. These games, typically played on a tablet or other device, are often used in lieu of more traditional tests and are designed to provide employers with information regarding the likelihood of success in a particular workplace or for a particular job. Many of these games would pose no problems for individuals with ASD but some seek to test for the kind of soft workplace skills that individuals with ASD may have trouble with, such as reading social cues and even the facial expressions of characters portrayed in a game (Morgan, 2013).

[11] Aka v. Washington Hospital Center, 124 F.3d 1302 (D.C. Cir. 1997).

[12] U.S. Airways v. Barnett, 535 U.S. 391 (2002).

These games are relatively new and there have yet to be any legal challenges to them but to the extent they disadvantage disabled applicants, including those with ASD, the ADA strictly regulates their use. In order to use a test during the application process, an employer would be required to demonstrate that the test was job related in that it provided information that was deemed essential to success in the workplace (Carle, 2017). It is not necessary to establish that the employer chose the test so that it would exclude individuals with ASD only that the test does so, and the employer's burden to establish the test is job related can be a hefty one.

Recent Employer Initiatives

As should be obvious from the above, the law offers only limited protections for individuals with ASD (and those with disabilities more generally) and has to date focused almost exclusively on individuals with jobs rather than helping individuals obtain jobs. This latter issue is likely to be of greater significance since many ASD individuals may have difficulty navigating the demands of a traditional interview process, and thus will never make it into the workplace.

Recently, a number of employers have voluntarily begun initiatives designed to hire individuals on the autism spectrum, and these initiatives offer insights into best practices for employers who want to reach out to individuals with ASD. A number of the initiatives were started by company executives who have ASD children but just as many are designed to target individuals because of their underemployed but valuable skills.

Microsoft, for example, has started a small-scale initiative that is notable for its restructured interview process. Realizing that the interview process can pose problems for individuals with ASD often by adding anxiety to the process, the company has created a lengthy introductory process, one that initially lasted up to four weeks, that essentially enables the worker to try out for the position. Several other companies, often working with the Danish company Specialisterne, have adopted similar programs to provide an interview process that will likely lead to less anxiety among those with ASD and will also demonstrate to employers the valuable skills individuals with ASD can bring to the workplace. Walgreens has even constructed a mock store in a Chicago suburb as a way of allowing applicants or new employees gradually to adjust to the workplace setting. Many companies have also provided training to employees regarding autism and have likewise found that buy-in from other employees and managers can provide an important link to long-term employment for those with ASD.[13]

These initiatives have filled a wide range of jobs. For example, the large software company SAP has successfully placed individuals with ASD in software positions,

[13] The various initiatives have been widely chronicled in the popular media. For one such example see J. Che, "Why More Companies Are Eager to Hire People with Autism," Huffpost, Mar. 29, 2016.

IT, graphic design, finance, and marketing, in other words, many of the most common jobs at the firm (and many of which could be performed remotely). Other companies have sought to place ASD individuals in jobs that may best fit their skills. Bank of America has a group of disabled employees, including a number of high-functioning autistic individuals, who process written checks, a task that involves repetition while rewarding careful attention to detail, two tasks that many individuals with ASD can thrive at. And at the Rising Tide Car Wash chain based in Florida—known for its expert attention to detail—all of the employees are on the autism spectrum.

These programs are a variation of what is known as "supported" employment, which provides various supports to allow disabled individuals to work in an integrated competitive workplace. The supports can vary from on-site job coaches to off-site community support in the form of general job training, interview practice, or learning the specific requirements of a job (Wehman et al., 2012). A key feature of supported employment is that the coach, or a designated individual, will initially work to find a job that matches the individual's skills, a step that has proved crucial to maintaining long-term employment. Supported employment is often funded by state or federal vocational offices, although the programs discussed earlier are typically funded by the companies without governmental support, and supported employment has been associated with improving cognitive functioning outside of the workplace as well as leading to more stable employment (Garcia-Villamisar & Hughes, 2007).

An alternative but the more controversial approach is known as "sheltered employment," where disabled individuals often including those with ASD will work in a separate environment often at sub-minimum wages (Pendo, 2016). These programs are authorized under the federal Fair Labor Standards Act, and are controversial in large part because the employees are paid poorly while the employers receive federal grant funds. Some of the programs are designed as transitional employment that would allow individuals to move into competitive integrated workplaces whereas others are intended as long-term employment. In contrast to supported employment, there is little evidence to suggest that sheltered employment has improved the quality of life for individuals with ASD and the programs are now in decline with several states moving to ban them altogether.

These private initiatives mentioned above remain relatively new and have typically been implemented on a small scale, though several employers have stated their desire to increase their scale. To date, the programs have been successful in their goals and as they expand and gain greater publicity, other employers may adopt similar programs, or perhaps will be more willing to hire an applicant with ASD. Stereotypes die hard but, particularly in tight job markets, employers should be willing to reach out to a potentially broad and talented pool of applicants that have encountered too many barriers to entering the workplace.

Conclusion

Despite the current low levels of employment, individuals with ASD can be productive employees often with no necessary accommodation at all, and when accommodations are necessary they will often prove of minimal cost. The recent private initiatives by companies to reach out to individuals with ASD should help change the perception of the abilities of such individuals, leading, one would hope, to greater employment opportunities in meaningful work.

References

AJ. Drexel Autism Institute. (2015). *National autism indicators report: Transition into young adulthood*.

Carle, S. D. (2017). Analyzing social impairments under title I of the Americans with disabilities act. *University of California Davis Law Review, 50,* 1109–1164.

Chen, J. L. (2015). Trends in employment for individuals with autism spectrum disorder: A review of the literature. *Review Journal of Autism Developmental Disorders, 2,* 115–127.

Garcia-Villamisar, D., & Hughes, C. (2007). Supported employment improves cognitive performance in adults with autism. *Journal of Intellectual Disability Research, 51,* 142–150.

Hendricks, D. (2010). Employment and adults with autism spectrum disorders: challenges and strategies for success. *Journal of Vocational Rehabilitation, 32,* 125–134.

Hensel, W. F. (2017). People with autism spectrum disorder in the workplace: An expanding legal frontier. *Harvard Civil Rights–Civil Liberties Law Review, 57,* 74.

Morgan, J. (2013, December 17). Want to work here? Play this game first. *Forbes*.

Pendo, E. (2016). *Hidden from view: Disability, segregation, and work, in invisible labor* (W. Poster, M. Crain, & M. Cherry, Eds.). University of California Press.

Selmi, M. (2008). Interpreting the Americans with disabilities act: Why the Supreme Court rewrote the statute and why congress did not care. *George Washington University Law Review, 76,* 101.

Wehman, P., et al. (2012). Supported employment for young adults with autism spectrum disorder: Preliminary data. *Research and Practice for Persons with Severe Disabilities, 37,* 160–169.

Michael Selmi is Foundation Professor of Law at Arizona State College of Law where he teaches courses on employment discrimination, employment law, and law and social change. Prior to entering academia, he was an attorney with the Civil Rights Division of the Department of Justice and the Lawyers' Committee for Civil Rights.

Chapter 19
Laws Affecting the Health, Security, Autonomy, and Well-Being of People with ASD

Alison Morantz and Lorri Unumb

Introduction

Individuals with Autism Spectrum Disorder (ASD) confront numerous challenges in the educational and employment arenas, which several preeminent federal laws in the United States (such as the Individuals with Disabilities Education Act and the Americans with Disabilities Act of 1990) are designed to address. Yet the welfare of people with ASD and their families is also influenced by myriad other civil laws, regulations, and entitlement programs across the life cycle. Some of these, such as Supplemental Security Income (SSI) and Medicaid, affect people with a wide range of disabilities. Others, such as state insurance mandates that require private insurers to provide in-home Applied Behavior Analysis (ABA) therapy to children diagnosed with autism, are ASD-specific. For some individuals, especially those who require significant support after attaining the age of legal majority, navigating these laws and programs successfully can make the difference between living in highly restrictive settings and leading full and meaningful lives in the community.

This chapter provides a brief overview of these heterogeneous laws and entitlement programs in the United States, highlighting the ways in which they can improve the health, security, autonomy, and well-being of individuals with ASD and their families. We survey six domains: Health Care; Public Benefits, Services and Supports; Custody and Child Support; Economic Security and Financial Planning; Legal Decision-Making Capacity; and Workforce Readiness and the Transition to Adulthood. The list of statutes and benefits discussed is not exhaustive, nor do we

A. Morantz (✉)
Stanford University, Stanford, CA, USA
e-mail: amorantz@law.stanford.edu

L. Unumb
The Council of Autism Service Providers, Lexington, SC, USA
e-mail: lunumb@casproviders.org

F. R. Volkmar et al. (eds.), *Handbook of Autism Spectrum Disorder and the Law*,
https://doi.org/10.1007/978-3-030-70913-6_19

describe any provisions in great detail or catalogue which ones apply in which jurisdictions. Rather, our goal is to introduce the diverse array of laws and programs that currently exist under state and federal law, and provide a few illustrative examples.

Health Care

Meeting the health care needs of individuals with ASD can pose daunting challenges. Parents of young children who exhibit developmental delays may struggle to obtain an initial ASD screening and evaluation, and to pay for therapies that a clinician recommends following an ASD diagnosis. Adults on the autism spectrum with little income or assets likewise may find it difficult to secure adequate health insurance. In this section, we summarize a variety of laws and programs that affect the capacity of individuals with ASD to meet their medical and behavioral health care needs.

Medicaid

Passed as part of the Social Security Act of 1965 (Centers for Medicare & Medicaid Services [CMS], 2015), Medicaid is a joint federal-state program that provides publicly funded health care to specified categories of children and adults. Medicaid is the largest single provider of health insurance in the United States (Godbolt, 2017), and as such, is an important conduit for medical and behavioral health care services for many individuals with ASD.

Although a detailed description of the numerous pathways to Medicaid eligibility is beyond the scope of this chapter, a few general observations can be made. First, broadly speaking, there are two types of eligibility criteria: means-tested criteria that depend on indicators of economic status such as income and assets; and categorical/demographic criteria that depend on each individual's personal attributes or life circumstances. For many types of Medicaid applicants—such as children, pregnant women, parents, and adults—the family's modified adjusted gross income (MAGI) is the predominant criterion for determining eligibility for a large cluster of means-tested programs (CMS, n.d.-a). The Patient Protection and Affordable Care Act (ACA), passed into law in 2010, significantly relaxed the MAGI-based eligibility criteria and expanded the rate at which the federal government subsidizes program benefits, although the uptake of these provisions has varied by state (Medicaid and CHIP Payment and Access Commission [MACPAC], 2019).

Some individuals with ASD, however, may not be subject to MAGI-based eligibility requirements. For example, the eligibility of those who meet the definition of "disabled" adopted by the Social Security Administration (SSA), are blind, or are over the age of 65[1] is generally determined using the SSA's other income—and resource-based criteria, discussed below. Additionally, adults with ASD who meet the SSA's definition of disability may, in some states, qualify for Medicaid through other channels as long as they do not exceed certain, less restrictive, income- or asset-based thresholds.[2] Finally, some state Medicaid programs cover severely disabled children, including those with ASD, even if their families are relatively well off.[3]

Importantly, even if individuals with ASD are initially deemed ineligible for Medicaid because they exceed the relevant income and/or asset requirements, they sometimes can exploit special legal provisions that reduce their income or assets for purposes of Medicaid eligibility without lowering their standard of living. For example, if a state agency deems an applicant's support needs to be sufficiently profound and extensive that they meet the level of care (LOC) typically provided in an institutional setting,[4] means-tested criteria sometimes can be relaxed, enabling them to enroll in Medicaid regardless of whether their parents (or spouse) earn significant income or hold significant assets (CMS, n.d.-b). Individuals with ASD who do not meet an institutional LOC may still be able to utilize other provisions discussed later in this chapter—Special Needs Trusts, ABLE Accounts, and "Cafeteria Plans"—to achieve a similar result.[5]

Secondly, Medicaid eligibility criteria vary widely across the United States because states are allowed considerable discretion to opt in (or out) of many programs, and to adjust each program's requirements. For example, although every state deems children of age 18 years or younger with family income up to 133% of the federal poverty level eligible for Medicaid, some states extend eligibility to children whose family incomes exceed this threshold (KFF, 2020). Another source of cross-state variation involves the connection between Supplemental Security Income (SSI), discussed in more detail below, and Medicaid. Although in most states, individuals who receive SSI qualify automatically for Medicaid, a minority of states—collectively known as the 209(b) states—use additional criteria to determine the Medicaid

[1] For these elderly "dual eligible" individuals, Medicare generally pays for covered medical services, as Medicaid is the payer of last resort. Medicaid may cover medical costs that Medicare does not cover or only partially covers (such as nursing home care, personal care, and home and community-based services) (CMS, 2020).

[2] For example, in California, there are three Medicaid eligibility pathways for individuals with disabilities who would not otherwise qualify for Medicaid benefits: the Aged and Disabled Federal Poverty Level Medi-Cal program; the Aged, Blind, and Disabled Medically-Needy Medi-Cal program; and the 250% Working Disabled Program (Disability Benefits 101, 2020).

[3] For example, certain states offer the Katie Beckett or TEFRA option, originally enacted in 1982. This option allows states to provide Medicaid coverage to children with disabilities—who require an institutional level of care—who would otherwise be ineligible due to their parents' income or resources (O'Keeffe et al., 2010).

[4] Since the Supreme Court's decision in *Olmstead v. L.C.* (1999), there has been an increasing effort to serve these individuals in non-institutional settings through the use of home and community-based services, discussed in detail below.

[5] For further discussion of these provisions, see *infra* section "Economic Security and Financial Planning".

eligibility of SSI recipients (CMS, n.d.-c; U.S. Social Security Administration [SSA], 2017).

Finally, Medicaid eligibility criteria often differ between children and adults. For example, some individuals with ASD who do not qualify for SSI (and by extension, Medicaid) as children because their parents' income and assets do not meet the relevant criteria may become eligible after age 18, when parental income is no longer considered.[6] In addition, a number of Medicaid eligibility pathways are explicitly limited to children,[7] whereas others are confined to adults.[8]

The scope of benefits available to Medicaid beneficiaries is likewise complex and highly variable. Part of this complexity stems from the fact that the Centers for Medicare and Medicaid Services (CMS) do not require all states to provide the same array of benefits to all recipients. Rather, federal law sets a "floor" of mandatory benefits that every state must provide, and lets each state choose whether to raise this floor by offering additional services. States can raise the federal floor either by amending their Medicaid plans to make additional services available to *all* eligible individuals, or by making targeted Waiver programs available to specific groups of consumers. Importantly, the federal government permits states to ration Waiver services by capping enrollment at pre-specified levels. As a consequence, the provision of Waiver services in some states is characterized by long waiting lists (Foster et al., 2019).

Another contributing factor to the complexity of Medicaid benefits is the fact that the federal floor has shifted over time, and varies considerably by age. For example, the Early and Periodic Screening, Diagnostic and Treatment (EPSDT) program, first enacted in 1967 (U.S. Health Resources & Services Administration [HRSA], 2018), sets the benefits floor at a relatively high level for children, requiring states to provide "access to any Medicaid-coverable service in any amount that is medically necessary, regardless of whether the service is covered in the state plan" (MACPAC, n.d.-b). The EPSDT program covers screening and diagnostic services to identify any physical or mental impairments in recipients under age 21, along with the medical treatments and other services necessary to correct or ameliorate them (HRSA, 2018).

Prior to 2014, many states did not treat Applied Behavior Analysis (ABA), the leading behavioral treatment for children with ASD, as medically necessary, and thus only covered it through a Medicaid Waiver if they covered it at all. As a result,

---

[6] This age-based distinction does not apply to all Medicaid eligibility pathways. For example, MAGI-based pathways take parental and spousal income into account regardless of age, as long as the claimant is treated as a member of the same household in tax filings (CMS, n.d.-a). Moreover, even though many Medicaid eligibility pathways do not consider parental income when evaluating the eligibility of adult claimants, if a claimant is married, spousal income is typically considered (SSA, 2020a).

[7] For example, 48 states have implemented the Children's Health Insurance Program (CHIP), at least partly, as an expansion of the Medicaid Program (MACPAC, n.d.-a).

[8] Many of the 1915(c) Home and Community-Based Services (HCBS) Waiver programs, discussed below, are specifically targeted toward adults with disabilities. For example, the Colorado Supported Living Services Waiver program specifically targets individuals with developmental disabilities who are 18 years of age or older (Colorado Department of Health Care Policy and Financing, 2019).

many children diagnosed with ASD could not access ABA therapy through their Medicaid plans. In July 2014, however, CMS issued a memorandum to all state Medicaid agencies specifying that "medically necessary" care included the screening, diagnosis, and treatment of ASD (Autism Speaks, 2018; Mann, 2014). Following this policy directive, most states began to cover ABA for children diagnosed with ASD through their EPSDT programs (Autism Speaks, 2018).

Generally speaking, the scope of Medicaid benefits is far more limited for adults than it is for children. Although adults are still entitled to a sizable array of mandatory benefits—such as in-patient hospital care, nursing and home health services, and physician services—they may not receive many of the additional (optional) benefits that EPSDT mandates for minors (MACPAC, n.d.-c). Yet here again, the scope of benefits available can vary markedly across state lines. For example, although the guarantee of ABA services through the EPSDT program applies only to children under age 21, in 2019, New Mexico enacted legislation requiring mandatory (i.e., non-Waiver) Medicaid coverage of ABA and other therapeutic care (such as occupational therapy, speech therapy, and physical therapy) to *all* Medicaid recipients with ASD who require these services, regardless of age (H.B. 322, 2019).

Affordable Care Act

As noted above, the Affordable Care Act, passed in 2010, significantly expanded the number of individuals who qualify for Medicaid. Some of the ACA's other provisions have also, at least indirectly, helped individuals with ASD access health care benefits. For example, the ACA prohibits insurers from denying coverage on the basis of pre-existing conditions whose onset pre-dated the issuance of the insurance policy (U.S. Department of Health & Human Services [HHS], 2017). This prohibition can be vitally important for people with ASD who change insurance plans following a job change or other significant life event. Before the ACA's passage, people with ASD who sought to change insurance carriers could be denied coverage on the ground that their ASD diagnosis was a pre-existing condition. The ACA expressly prohibited this practice.

Moreover, before the passage of the ACA, children of covered adults generally could only obtain coverage through their parents' private insurance plans until they turned 19 (or graduated from college if they were full-time students) (Andrews, 2013; Goldman, 2013). Although private insurance policies occasionally covered the disabled children of beneficiaries beyond age 18, such policies often relied upon highly restrictive definitions of disability that excluded some individuals with ASD. The passage of the ACA did not affect this variability in insurance companies' coverage of policy holders' disabled adult children. Yet some young adults (aged 18–26) with ASD benefitted from a provision in the ACA allowing *all* individuals (regardless of disability status) to claim benefits through their parents' insurance policies through age 26 (U.S. Department of Labor, n.d.-a).

A separate provision of the ACA that conceivably could affect the provision of medical services to individuals with ASD, known as the "nondiscrimination provision," prohibits discrimination on the basis of race, color, national origin, sex, age, or disability in the provision and administration of most health insurance plans (HHS, 2021). Federal regulations passed in 2016 interpreted this clause to prohibit insurers from denying, canceling, limiting, or renewing a health insurance policy; denying or limiting coverage of a claim; or designing benefits in a way that discriminates on the basis of disability. This provision could be used to ensure that health insurance plans do not construe or administer plan provisions in ways that disproportionately burden or disadvantage individuals with ASD. In 2020, however, the U.S. Department of Health and Human Services (HHS) reversed course by removing the 2016 interpretation and making numerous other changes to the provision's governing regulations, including some that narrow the range of businesses to which the law applies, and potentially reduce the accessibility of health care information to individuals with disabilities (Musumeci et al., 2020a). The regulations were widely opposed by disability rights organizations (Autistic Self Advocacy Network, 2019; Disability Rights California, 2019), but as of this writing, the Biden Administration has not yet proposed new ones pertaining to disability discrimination (HHS, 2021).

State Insurance Mandates for Treatment of ASD

As recently as the turn of the millennium, very few private health insurance plans provided adequate treatment to individuals with ASD. Some insurance companies classified ASD as "uninsurable," effectively depriving those who carried the diagnosis of many medical services (Indiana Resource Center for Autism, 2016). Even if individuals with ASD were deemed eligible for insurance coverage, the benefits they received were often inadequate or nonexistent. For example, an individual with ASD whose doctor recommended Applied Behavior Analysis (ABA) might find that the family's insurance policy specifically excluded ABA, or that other plan provisions could be used to effectively deny coverage. If other forms of therapy—such as speech therapy, occupational therapy, and physical therapy—were covered at all, they often conferred little therapeutic benefit because of low caps on the number of sessions covered.

Frustrated by the lack of adequate insurance coverage, families of individuals with ASD and nonprofit organizations began to lobby elected officials, urging them to require health insurance providers to meet the health care needs of individuals with ASD. Since private health insurers are regulated by state law, these campaigns were generally organized at the state level, and by the first decade of the twenty-first century they began to bear fruit. As of this writing, all fifty states mandate that state-regulated health insurance plans cover ASD treatments (Autism Speaks, 2019), albeit with different caps on ABA expenditures (National Conference of State Legislatures, 2018). Importantly, state insurance mandates apply only to conventional health insurance policies, not to health benefit plans offered by large employers that self-insure (i.e., manage the risks associated with the provision of health care benefits internally, rather than transferring them to a third party). Yet despite being excluded from the scope of these state law reforms, many self-insured employers have opted to provide ABA and other behavioral therapies to individuals with ASD (Autism Law Hub, 2019).

Employment Retirement Income Security Act of 1974 (ERISA)

The Employee Retirement Income Security Act of 1974 (ERISA) is a federal law that sets minimum standards for a variety of employee benefits, including voluntarily established health benefit plans offered by large companies that opt to self-insure (U.S. Department of Labor, n.d.-b). As noted above, large companies that offer self-funded health benefit plans are not covered by state insurance mandates. Although many self-insured companies still choose to offer ASD and ABA coverage, individuals covered by such plans must look to ERISA, not state law, to challenge the scope of coverage or contest claim denials.

ERISA imposes "fiduciary" responsibilities on the individuals involved in controlling the company plan's assets, management or administration, which means that they must act prudently, diversify the plan's investments, adhere to the terms of the plan documents, and "run the plan solely in the interest of participants and beneficiaries and for the exclusive purpose of providing benefits and paying plan expenses" (U.S. Department of Labor, n.d.-c). In a highly publicized class action lawsuit, *Wit v. United Behavioral Health* [UBH] (2019), the U.S. District Court for the Northern District of California found that "financial self-interest was a critical consideration [in UBH's decision] regarding what criteria would be used to make coverage decisions and when Guidelines would be revised," which constituted a breach of UBH's fiduciary duty. Among the facts that the court cited in reaching this conclusion was UBH's decision in 2016 not to amend its guidelines on the provision of ABA services to individuals with ASD—despite the company's Utilization Management Committee's recommendation that the coverage be expanded—because of the CEO's desire to cut costs.

As of this writing, it is unclear how much practical recourse ERISA will provide to individuals with ASD and their families seeking to challenge adverse benefit determinations or claim denials by self-insured health care plans. Yet *Wit v. UBH* suggests, at the very least, that self-insured employers may not allow financial self-interest to taint the process of developing or revising coverage guidelines for the treatment of ASD, especially if those guidelines purportedly adhere to generally accepted behavioral standards of care.

Mental Health Parity and Addiction Equity Act of 2008 (MHPAEA)

In many health insurance plans, the devil is in the details when it comes to accessing benefits. Fine-print exclusions and limitations can make the difference between covered treatments that are robust and readily accessible, and those that are difficult to obtain or so negligible in quantity that they confer little therapeutic benefit. Albeit with some exceptions, the ACA requires health plans to cover ten Essential Health Benefits including, for example, emergency services and mental health treatment (CMS, n.d.-d, n.d.-e; Fernandez et al., 2018; Keith, 2018). Importantly, federal law also prohibits insurers from covering mental health treatments in a more restrictive manner than they cover other forms of treatment. Under the Paul Wellstone and Pete Domenici Mental Health Parity and Addiction Equity Act of 2008 (MHPAEA), limitations or financial requirements imposed on mental health benefits can be no more restrictive than those imposed on medical and surgical benefits.

Unlike state health insurance mandates, the MHPAEA applies to most group health plans—including both conventional health insurance and self-funded health benefit plans offered by large employers (U.S. Department of Labor, 2010)—as well as Medicaid Managed Care Plans, the Federal Employees Health Benefits Program, State Children's Health Insurance Programs (S-CHIP), health plans purchased through the Health Insurance Marketplaces, and most individual health plans purchased outside the Health Insurance Marketplaces (National Alliance on Mental Illness, n.d.). Although from a neurodiversity standpoint it is inaccurate (and arguably offensive) to describe ASD as a "mental health disorder," it is generally treated as such in insurance contexts because it is included in the Diagnostic and Statistical Manual of Mental Disorders (DSM). As a consequence, ASD-related treatments are included in the scope of protection that the MHPAEA provides (Graham, 2017).

In effect, the MHPAEA may help individuals with ASD ensure that their covered therapies are provided at the same level, and subjected to the same limitations, that apply to other forms of treatment. For example, the financial requirements that apply to speech therapy for an individual with ASD—such as deductibles, copayments, coinsurance, and out-of-pocket expenses—cannot be more restrictive than the financial requirements that apply to substantially all of the medical/surgical benefits covered by the policy. The same parity requirement applies to restrictive treatment limitations, such as the frequency or geographic location of treatments; the number of visits; and the duration of coverage. MHPAEA also establishes parity requirements for other limitations relating to:

- Medical management standards limiting or excluding benefits based on medical necessity or medical appropriateness, or based on whether the treatment is experimental or investigative;
- Formulary design for prescription drugs;
- For plans with multiple network tiers (such as preferred providers and participating providers), network tier design;

- Standards for provider admission to participate in a network, including reimbursement rates;
- Plan methods for determining usual, customary, and reasonable charges;
- Refusal to pay for higher-cost therapies until it can be shown that a lower-cost therapy is not effective (also known as fail-first policies or step therapy protocols);
- Exclusions based on failure to complete a course of treatment; and
- Restrictions based on geographic location, facility type, provider specialty, and other criteria that limit the scope or duration of benefits for services provided under the plan or coverage (26 C.F.R. § 54.9812–1(c)(4)(ii)).

Again, it is important to note that federal law does not ban any of these cost-containment practices; it requires only that they be applied in an evenhanded manner to mental health, medical, and surgical benefits alike. Before the passage of the ACA, the mental health parity protections described above were not available to people insured through individual or small group plans; the ACA extended the MHPAEA's protections to the latter groups (Beronio et al., 2013).

Finally, it is worth noting that some states have passed their own mental health parity laws whose provisions may complement, and in some cases augment, the protections of the MHPAEA (Douglas et al., 2018).

Health Insurance Coverage Provided to Active-Duty Military, Veterans, and Their Families

Many individuals in the armed forces and their dependents receive treatment and services through TRICARE, a set of healthcare plans offered by the Department of Defense to active duty and retired military personnel and their families through the Defense Health Agency (DHA) (U.S. Defense Health Agency [DHA], 2019a). Benefits are also available temporarily to veterans transitioning out of the military (DHA, 2019b). Although speech and language therapy is considered a basic TRICARE benefit and as such is available to all beneficiaries, ABA is considered "experimental in nature" and thus outside the scope of basic coverage. The DHA originally offered ABA benefits to discrete groups of TRICARE beneficiaries through a patchwork of programs with varying eligibility requirements, but in 2014, all of these programs were consolidated into the Comprehensive Autism Care Demonstration Project (Autism Care Demo), which covers ABA for all eligible TRICARE beneficiaries with ASD (DHA, 2020a; U.S. Department of Defense [DOD], 2014). Originally scheduled to sunset in 2018, the Autism Care Demo has been renewed until 2023 (DHA, 2020a; DOD, 2014). Yet since the DHA currently *only* covers ABA through the temporary Autism Care Demo, it is unclear whether coverage will be provided after the program sunsets (DHA, 2020b).

Due to a recent policy change, individuals with ASD can also receive ABA benefits through the Civilian Health and Medical Program of the Department of Veterans Affairs (CHAMPVA), a separate health benefit plan available to the family members of veterans who do not qualify for TRICARE and are either deceased or permanently and totally disabled as the result of service-related conditions (U.S. Department of Veterans Affairs, 2020a, 2020b).

Public Benefits, Services, and Supports

Although laws that improve access to health care can significantly improve quality of life, some individuals with ASD may require non-medical services and supports, including income support, to achieve long-term stability and pursue their life goals. Several federal programs, including Medicaid, can help individuals with ASD cover non-medical costs.

Medicaid Long-Term Services and Supports Delivered in Institutional Settings

In addition to the health care benefits discussed above, Medicaid provides a variety of non-medical services and supports to consumers with disabilities. For example, consumers who require extensive around-the-clock care may receive long-term services and supports (LTSS), including a mix of medical and non-medical services, in institutional environments. The provision of LTSS in institutional settings, such as Skilled Nursing Facilities, is a mandatory component of each state's Medicaid program (Sowers et al., 2016) and accounts for about a third of all Medicaid expenditures (Thach & Wiener, 2018). At such facilities, Medicaid consumers receive extensive support with activities of daily living (such as eating, bathing, and dressing), as well as longer-term tasks such as housekeeping, transportation, and budget management (Thach & Wiener, 2018).

Home and Community-Based Services

In recent decades, a growing proportion of individuals with disabilities, including ASD, have begun to receive Medicaid services and supports, including LTSS, in their own homes or in community-based settings. The federal government provides states with three major conduits for accessing these resources, which are collectively referred to as Home and Community-Based Services (HCBS).

About 13% of Medicaid consumers receiving HCBS do so through federally mandated Home Health State Benefit Plan Policies (Watts et al., 2020), which provide basic HCBS benefits to all Medicaid recipients, such as medical supplies and equipment, nursing care, and home health aide services (Musumeci et al., 2020b).

Another 52.5% of HCBS recipients participate in the Medicaid Waiver programs described in Section I (Watts et al., 2020), which are generally referred to by their respective statutory sections. Recall that the Waiver programs are implemented at each state's discretion, and expand HCBS provision to designated populations. Importantly, states can cap enrollment in Waiver programs, and only individuals who meet an institutional level of care are eligible to participate. The Waiver program that serves the largest number of individuals with ASD, the Section 1915(c) Waiver, allows states to tailor services to meet the needs of a particular target group (CMS, n.d.-b). Notably, states can only require 1915(c) Waiver participants to enroll in capitated managed care plans if they obtain that authority through a separate Medicaid provision.[9] Thirteen states have chosen to make 1915(c) Waiver programs available to individuals with ASD (CMS, n.d.-f).[10] Another important HCBS Waiver, the Section 1115 Waiver, permits states to target several populations at once and "can be used to authorize both HCBS and mandatory managed care enrollment" without the need to obtain that authority through a separate Medicaid provision (Musumeci et al., 2020b). The Section 1915(c) Waiver served 1.81 million enrollees in FY 2018, compared to 698,500 served through the Section 1115 Waiver, including some diagnosed with ASD (Watts et al., 2020).

The remaining 34.5% of Medicaid HCBS consumers benefit from "State Plan Options" (Watts et al., 2020), also known as "State Plan Amendments," through which states can elect to provide certain services to *all* Medicaid consumers who meet pertinent eligibility requirements (Watts et al., 2020). For example, thirty-four states offer personal care services as an additional benefit in their State Plans. Nearly all of these states cover assistance with household activities, such as meal preparation and housekeeping, and a significant portion also cover additional services, such as transportation (Musumeci et al., 2020b). Another eight states have taken advantage of the ACA's Community First Choice (CFC) State Plan Option. The CFC Plan Option provides states with extra federal funds[11] in exchange for offering HCBS benefits to all individuals who would otherwise qualify for an institutional level of care (Musumeci et al., 2020b). Finally, thirteen states offer HCBS to targeted groups of consumers—which in four states includes consumers with intellectual and developmental disabilities (I/DD)—through the 1915(i) State Plan Option (Musumeci et al.,2020b), which permits states to provide HCBS benefits to certain Medicaid consumers who do not require an institutional level of care.[12]

[9] These other provisions include the Section 1932 State Plan Option, and the respective Waivers contained in Sections 1915(a) and 1915(b) (Musumeci et al., 2020b).

[10] This figure does not include Waiver programs that target the population of individuals with ASD as part of a broader program for those with I/DD.

[11] Service expenditures related to the CFC plan option are reimbursed by CMS at a rate that is six percentage points higher than the standard rate they receive for most Medicaid expenditures (CMS, n.d.-g; Mitchell, 2018).

[12] In most states that provide HCBS through Section 1915(i), beneficiaries must already be eligible for Medicaid through a different pathway (Musumeci et al., 2020b). In three states (Ohio, Indiana, and Idaho), however, 1915(i) can be used as an independent pathway to Medicaid eligibility.

Social Security Benefits: SSI and SSDI

For many individuals with ASD living in the community, the cash assistance available through the Social Security Administration (SSA) is critical to secure basic necessities, such as food and housing, that cannot be obtained through the HCBS programs discussed above.

SSA distributes cash benefits through two programs: the Social Security Disability Insurance (SSDI) program and the Supplemental Security Income (SSI) program. Both programs provide monthly cash payments and (in most states) entitle recipients to publicly-funded health insurance;[13] both also require recipients claiming that they are disabled to meet SSA's definition of disability.[14] To qualify as disabled, a child under age 18 must have a medically determinable physical or mental impairment (including emotional or learning problems) that results in marked, severe, and functional limitations, and is expected to last longer than a year or else result in death (SSA, 2020b). Meanwhile, an adult recipient must have a completely disabling condition that will last longer than a year or result in death (SSA, 2020b). A key difference between the two programs is that SSDI requires recipients themselves (or in certain situations, their parents or spouses) to have amassed long enough work histories to qualify for benefits, whereas the SSI program contains no such requirement. Therefore, SSI is more relevant to individuals with ASD who lack significant work experience and cannot claim SSDI benefits through family members.

In order to qualify for SSI benefits, an individual's assets and "countable" income may not exceed specified thresholds (SSA, 2020a, 2020c). Broadly speaking, countable income includes earned income (wages and net self-employment earnings); unearned income (including Social Security and unemployment benefits, pensions, state disability payments, interest, cash, and dividends); and in-kind income (such as food and shelter obtained for free or purchased at below-market rates). Importantly, however, countable income *does not* include the value of Supplemental Nutrition Assistance Program (SNAP) benefits; need-based food or shelter provided by nonprofit entities; or wages used to pay for items or services that help the individual work (SSA, 2020a). The amount of countable income determines the level of benefits to which an SSI recipient is entitled, and the benefit level declines as income rises.

It is also important to note that in calculating SSI eligibility, the SSA may take into account parental and/or spousal assets and income. This provision is especially important for children under the age of 18 living with their families, since a portion

[13] As noted above, nine "209(b)" states impose additional eligibility restrictions beyond SSI enrollment for Medicaid eligibility. However, all individuals receiving SSDI qualify for Medicare after a 24-month waiting period (SSA, 2017, n.d.-a).

[14] SSI also has pathways for individuals who are blind, or age 65 or older.

of parental income and resources are included in eligibility determinations.[15] After a child turns 18, parental resources no longer factor into these calculations.[16]

Protection & Advocacy Services

As part of the Developmentally Disabled Assistance and Bill of Rights Act of 1975 (DD Act), Congress mandated the creation of state-level Protection and Advocacy Systems (P&As) for the purpose of protecting, and advocating for, the rights of individuals with disabilities (U.S. Administration for Community Living [ACL], 2017a, 2019). Every state and U.S. territory has a P&A authorized to "pursue legal, administrative, and other appropriate remedies or approaches to ensure the protection of, and advocacy for, the rights of such individuals [with disabilities] within the State" (42 U.S.C. § 15043). P&As have been active in ensuring the implementation of the U.S. Supreme Court's decision in *Olmstead v. L.C.* (1999), which bars the unnecessary segregation of individuals with disabilities and helps ensure that they receive services in the least restrictive environment. P&As typically help individuals engage in self-advocacy, and in some cases also conduct investigations, monitor compliance with laws affecting individuals with I/DD, and provide direct legal representation (ACL, 2017b, 2019).

P&As may also coordinate their activities with other state-level entities authorized by the DD Act, such as State Councils on Developmental Disabilities and University Centers for Excellence in Developmental Disabilities Education, Research, and Services (UCEDDs) (ACL, 2019).

Custody, Visitation, and Child Support

Although published family law cases involving children with ASD are relatively scant, two general patterns seem to apply in most jurisdictions. First, parents' duty to support a child with ASD does not necessarily terminate when the child reaches adulthood. In the majority of states, the duty of parental support may continue for as long as a child's disability prevents him/her from earning a living and performing adequate self-care. Consequently, parents may have a duty to provide ongoing support to their adult children with ASD—or in the wake of divorce, non-custodial parents may be required to pay child support to custodial parents—even after children reach the age of legal majority. States differ, however, on whether the level of support is

[15] Certain resources and sources of parental income, such as Temporary Assistance for Needy Families (TANF) and Veterans Affairs pension benefits; foster care payments; and court-ordered child support payments, are not included in these calculations (SSA, 2020d).

[16] If the adult child marries, however, his or her spouse's income and resources could be considered in SSI eligibility calculations (SSA, 2020a, 2020c).

fixed by child support guidelines, or adjusted to a level that balances the parents' economic circumstances with the needs of the disabled child (National Council of State Legislatures, 2020).

Secondly, in situations where parents seek to acquire or retain custody or visitation rights, published opinions reflect a commitment to several goals: ensuring that the parent or guardian of a child with ASD can address the child's unique needs; providing the child with a consistent routine; and attaining continuity in the provision of services and supports (Dicker & Marion, 2012). Before determining which arrangement is in the child's best interest, courts frequently appoint a *guardian ad litem* (GAL). Although the formal training of GALs may vary and their precise duties vary across jurisdictions, they generally are expected to advocate on the child's behalf for the duration of a legal action. In so doing, GALs may carry out investigatory functions such as reviewing records; interviewing family members; and consulting with clinicians, school personnel, and other individuals with relevant knowledge (Boumil et al., 2011).

The question of whether the parent fully understands the child's disability and can provide appropriate support often looms large in decisions regarding custody and visitation. For example, in *Martocchio v. Savoir* (2008) a father, who had not known that he was a parent for more than two years, petitioned for custody of his child, a four-year-old boy with severe ASD. Not only did the court grant the father sole custody on the ground that he had "immersed himself, almost to a fault, in the study of autism and proper treatment of his son," but the court also ordered the child's mother and maternal grandparents to "endeavor to learn all they can regarding autistic children." The issue of parental capacity has also arisen in child protection cases in which an agency is considering whether to remove a child with ASD from the family home. For example, in *In re Juan R.* (2007), the court affirmed that the Connecticut Department of Children and Families had made sufficient efforts to prevent the removal of an autistic child, opining that the "mother had been unable to significantly benefit" from the services provided from the Department, and could not ensure the health and safety of her son.

Courts also have emphasized the need to maintain consistency in a child's schedule and routine. For example, in *Suleman v. Egenti* (2016) the Maryland Court of Special of Appeals upheld the visitation schedule set by a prior court, noting that an "abrupt return to overnight visitation" by the father "could be disruptive to [the child with ASD] and cause him to regress." Similarly, in *LaGuardia v. LaGuardia* (2005), the Court of Appeals of Tennessee affirmed the visitation schedule determined by the trial court, citing expert testimony that children with ASD require "sameness and consistency."

In addition to maintaining the consistency of schedules and routines, courts have often emphasized the need to maintain continuity in the mix of services provided. For example, in *Ermini v. Vittori* (2013), the U.S. Court of Appeals for the Second Circuit denied a father's petition to relocate his son from New York, where he had been receiving treatment for ASD, to Italy on the ground that such a move posed a "grave risk of harm" to the child by risking "a significant regression in his skills." The court expressed concern that "without such an intensive, structured program, [the child would] not develop ... cognitive, language, social, emotional and independent living skills." Moves across state lines can raise similar risks by disrupting relationships with therapists and networks of community support that can take months or years to rebuild; altering the mix of services that school-age children with ASD receive from public schools; and forcing individuals who receive Medicaid Waiver services to forfeit their spot upon their departure and join the Medicaid Waiver waitlist in a new state.

Economic Security and Financial Planning

If individuals with ASD earn significant income from paid employment or hold a sufficient amount of assets in their name, they may be disqualified from some of the means-tested entitlement programs described in prior sections. However, three special legal mechanisms can enable some of these individuals to overcome eligibility barriers without reducing their standard of living: ABLE Accounts, Special Needs Trusts, and Cafeteria Plans.

ABLE Accounts

The Achieving a Better Life Experience Act (ABLE Act), passed in 2014, was designed to mitigate the deterrent effects of means-tested eligibility criteria on disabled individuals' incentives to accumulate savings. In addition to "encourage[ing] and assist[ing] individuals and families in saving private funds for … health, independence, and quality of life," the ABLE Act aims to "provide secure funding for disability-related expenses of beneficiaries that will *supplement, but not supplant*, benefits provided through private insurance" and "[the SSI and Medicaid sections] of the Social Security Act" (ABLE Act, 2014).

Under the ABLE Act, people with ASD and/or other disabilities and their families can establish ABLE Accounts, tax-advantaged savings accounts for qualified disability expenses (QDEs). QDEs can include expenses related to education, housing, transportation, employment training, and other costs generally related to the person's disability (SSA, 2020e). With rare exception, savings accrued in an ABLE Account do not affect eligibility for means-tested public benefits, including SSI and Medicaid. (The two primary exceptions are the fact that ABLE Accounts *are* included in the means tests for SSI distributions for housing expenses, and that SSI benefits are suspended if the amount held in an ABLE Account surpasses $100,000) (Disability Benefits 101, 2020).

To qualify for the ABLE program, an individual with a disability must be able to prove that his/her disability onset before the age of 26 (ABLE National Resource Center [ABLENRC], n.d.-a). Yet the program places few additional restrictions on qualifying applicants. For example, an ABLE Account can be opened at any stage of the life cycle, and sometimes can be opened in a state other than the consumer's state of legal residence (ABLENRC, n.d.-b, n.d.-c).

Contributions to an ABLE Account are capped at $15,000 per year, and starting in 2018, employed account beneficiaries can additionally contribute a portion of their income (Internal Revenue Service [IRS], 2018). The maximum allowable *total* savings in an ABLE Account, however, varies by state. For example, while the limit on allowable savings is $520,000 in New York as of this writing, the limit is only $370,000 in Nevada (ABLENRC, n.d.-d, n.d.-e). While federal tax treatment of ABLE Accounts is complex and evolving (American Bar Association, 2017; IRS, 2018, 2019), some aspects of their tax treatment also vary by state (ABLENRC, n.d.-f).

Special Needs Trusts

Like ABLE Accounts, Special Needs Trusts (SNTs) can help individuals with disabilities accumulate assets while preserving their eligibility for public benefit programs such as SSI and Medicaid (Neale, 2017; SSA, 2020f).

There are two main types of SNTs: First Party SNTs and Third Party SNTs. First Party SNTs are funded directly by the assets of the beneficiary, including, for example, money acquired from personal injury settlements or inheritances (Special Needs Alliance [SNA], 2013). Sometimes, multiple beneficiaries can pool their assets in a so-called Pooled Special Needs Trust, which allows them to maintain individual accounts while investing their assets together (California Department of Health Care Services, 2019). In contrast, Third Party SNTs cannot be funded by the beneficiary's assets, and usually contain direct inheritances or life insurance policy proceeds from family members (SNA, 2013).

Although both ABLE Accounts and SNTs are intended to preserve a beneficiary's eligibility for public benefits, there are important differences between the two. With regard to eligibility, only ABLE Accounts require the beneficiary to document that his/her disability onset before age 26. While ABLE Accounts may be created at any age, SNTs must be established before the intended beneficiary turns 65 (SSA, 2018). The two programs also include different sets of restrictions, with corresponding trade-offs. For example, while ABLE Accounts have monthly contribution limits, SNTs do not; SNT contributions are subject to gift tax restrictions, while ABLE Accounts are not (SNA, 2020; Special Needs Answers, 2020). Whereas ABLE Account assets can only be spent on QDEs, as mentioned above, SNT assets can be used for *anything* that directly benefits the beneficiary (SNA, 2020). Finally, ABLE Accounts can be directly managed by the beneficiary him/herself, whereas SNT assets must be controlled by a trustee.

Cafeteria Plans

A Cafeteria Plan is an employee benefit plan that permits a participating company's employees, regardless of their disability status, to select at least one item from a menu of "qualified benefits" in exchange for a reduction in pre-tax earnings (SSA, 2012). Qualified benefits can include, but are not limited to, health plans, life insurance coverage, and childcare expenses (IRS, 2020a, 2020b). Unlike ABLE Accounts and SNTs, Cafeteria Plans cannot help individuals with ASD shelter their savings, but may render them eligible for federal entitlement programs by helping them or their family members reduce their earned income (and, in turn, their modified adjusted gross income). Although employers are not required to offer Cafeteria Plans to their workers, many large companies choose to do so, and some smaller employers offer "Simple Cafeteria Plans" with slightly different eligibility criteria (IRS, 2020b). In short, by helping to reduce the earned income of disabled workers or their family members, Cafeteria Plans can help some individuals with ASD qualify for means-tested public benefit programs.

Legal Decision-Making Capacity

When a person with ASD turns 18, the question sometimes arises of whether he or she is capable of making important life decisions on his/her own behalf. Parents who believe that their child's ASD, which may be combined with other impairments, significantly impairs his/her decision-making capacity sometimes consider special legal arrangements whereby decision-making authority can be transferred to parents or other individuals after the individual reaches the age of legal majority.

Guardianship/Conservatorship

Legal provisions that grant parents, family members, or other individuals the authority to make decisions on behalf of adults with developmental disabilities, including ASD, are generally known as "guardianship" arrangements. Some states, such as California and Massachusetts, instead use the term "conservatorship" to refer to the entirety (or a subset) of these arrangements (California Courts, n.d.; Government of Massachusetts, n.d.). For simplicity's sake, we use the term "guardianship" throughout this section.

Broadly speaking, if a court concludes that an individual is unable to make important life decisions on his or her own behalf, the court may appoint a guardian whose authority encompasses one or both of two domains: guardianship of the person, and guardianship of the estate (Barton et al., 2014). Guardianship of the person includes decisions pertaining to the person's daily activities, health and welfare, such as "choosing a residence, consenting to medical treatment, and making end-of-life decisions" (Barton et al., 2014: 27). Meanwhile, guardianship of the estate empowers the guardian to assert control over the individual's assets and personal finances.

Because (essentially by definition) traditional guardianship arrangements strip individuals with disabilities of the authority to make decisions about their daily lives and/or their personal finances, they have become increasingly disfavored. For example, the Uniform Guardianship, Conservatorship And Other Protective Arrangements Act of 2017, a model law designed to harmonize different states' approaches toward guardianship issues, emphasizes that "guardianship and conservatorship should be options of last resort," and "recognizes the role of, and encourages the use of, less restrictive alternatives" (National Conference of Commissioners on Uniform State Laws [NCCUSL], 2018: 1–2).

One alternative to full guardianship is a *limited* guardianship, which, as the name implies, limits the scope of the guardian's authority to specific domains, allowing the individual with a disability to retain decision-making power in others (e.g., Cal. Prob. Code § 1801(d); Mo. Rev. Stat. § 475.080; North Carolina Judicial Branch, n.d.). However, the availability, scope, and procedural aspects of limited guardianships vary by state. In New York, for example, the duties of a limited guardian are left entirely to the judge's discretion, whereas in California, a limited guardian (called a conservator) is precluded by statute from choosing a residence or making financial decisions on the disabled person's behalf without express judicial authorization (Barton et al., 2014; Cal. Prob. Code § 2351.5).

Power of Attorney and Supported Decision-Making

Drawing on the United Nations' Convention on the Rights of Persons with Disabilities, which recognizes the right to legal capacity regardless of disability, and the Americans with Disabilities Act's mandate to provide services in the least restrictive environment, Supported Decision-Making (SDM) is emerging as an increasingly popular alternative to guardianship (Bach & Kerzner, 2010; Salzman, 2010; Thinking Person's Guide to Autism, 2017). SDM is a process whereby "people with disabilities use friends, family members, and professionals to help them understand the situations and choices they face, so they make their own decisions" (Francisco & Martinis, 2017: 2). In the SDM framework, the individual with ASD assembles a team of supporters, including friends, family, and various professionals, to assist with important decisions (Francisco & Martinis, 2017). Some states, including Texas and Rhode Island, have statutorily recognized the use of SDM as an alternative to guardianship and created standardized SDM agreement forms that enable supporters to assist in the individual's decision-making and communication (National Resource Center for Supported Decision-Making, n.d.-a, n.d.-b). In other contexts, the SDM team may utilize informal agreements to establish the SDM relationship and outline the duties of the team (Francisco & Martinis, 2017).

A different legal device that does not require judicial approval, and sometimes can be used in combination with SDM, is the "power of attorney," a written authorization whereby an adult (called the "grantor") can grant another person the authority to make decisions on his/her behalf under circumstances specified in the authorization (American Bar Association, n.d.). "Limited" or "special" powers of attorney are limited by their terms to specific domains (such as health care or personal finances); "durable" powers of attorney are designed to endure (unless they are revoked) until the grantor's death, even if the grantor becomes incapacitated (American Bar Association, n.d.). Some individuals with ASD may use powers of attorney to cede to others the authority to make decisions in specified areas, without the need for court involvement. Yet it is important to note that legally, an individual who grants a power of attorney must do so voluntarily and possess the requisite level of legal capacity. Therefore, a power of attorney bearing the signature of an individual with ASD whom the court deems to be incapacitated, or who did not assent knowingly and voluntarily to the arrangement, may not be enforced if its validity is challenged.

The Social Security Administration's Representative Payee Program

Some individuals with ASD who receive benefits from the Social Security Administration (SSI and SSDI) may not be well equipped to handle the various financial transactions required to meet their ongoing needs, such as food and housing, or to manage their own budgets. In such situations, it may be helpful to designate another individual or agency, known as a "representative payee," to receive and manage these funds for the "current needs of the beneficiary and in their best interests" (SSA, n.d.-b). The SSA makes its own determination regarding whether a recipient can manage his or her own benefits, or whether the appointment of a representative payee is warranted (Wynn, 2016). If the benefit recipient expresses preferences regarding which individuals should (or should not) be appointed to serve as representative payees, the SSA generally takes those preferences into account in making its determination (Disability Rights California, 2018). Most individuals for whom representative payees are appointed do not have court-appointed guardians (Belbase & Sanzenbacher, 2017). If guardianship arrangements are in place, guardians are not required to serve as representative payees, but do so in the majority of cases (Special Needs Alliance, 2015).

Workforce Readiness and Transition to Adulthood

Securing paid employment poses significant challenges for many adults with ASD. In 2017, for example, only 29% of surveyed adults with ASD were employed, and about half of those who did earn wage income did so in segregated "sheltered workshop[s]" (Roux et al., 2017: 50). In contrast, the nationwide employment rate[17] was about 60% in the same year (Bureau of Labor Statistics [BLS], 2018). Particularly for the estimated 50,000 individuals with ASD who turn 18 each year (Shattuck et al., 2012), accessing programs and resources designed to help individuals with disabilities secure paid employment can be critical to facilitate the transition to adulthood.

Vocational Rehabilitation Agencies

The Rehabilitation Act of 1973 requires state vocational rehabilitation (VR) agencies to provide an array of employment services to people with ASD and other disabilities (34 C.F.R. § 361.48). In accordance with federal law, every U.S. state operates a VR agency that uses a mixture of state and federal funding to provide employment services and resources to people with disabilities (Employer Assistance and Resource Network, n.d.; U.S. Department of Education, 2017). Although the number of people with ASD applying for VR services has increased dramatically in the past decade, an ASD diagnosis alone is not sufficient to qualify for VR services (Roux et al., 2016). The applicant must also demonstrate that his/her impairment "substantially interferes with the ability to get a job" and consequently that he/she "require[s] VR services to prepare for, secure, or regain employment" (Roux et al., 2016: 18).

If an applicant with ASD qualifies for VR services, the VR agency must complete vocational assessment(s) and, ultimately, an Individual Plan for Employment (IPE). The IPE specifies the VR services to which the applicant is entitled, which may include training, counseling, job placement, assistive technology, and supported employment (Autism Speaks, 2013). The average time required for the agency to complete an IPE can vary widely by state. For example, while over 80% of transition-age youth with ASD in California whose VR cases were closed between fiscal years 2014 and 2016 obtained their IPEs within 90 days of their eligibility determination, the comparable figure for Iowa was just 23% (Roux et al., 2020).

Workforce Innovation and Opportunity Act

The Workforce Innovation and Opportunity Act (WIOA), passed in 2014, was intended to address the unique needs of workers with disabilities. Among WIOA's key reforms were provisions requiring VR agencies to provide additional resources

[17] In calculating the "employment-population ratio" (i.e., the employment rate), the Bureau of Labor Statistics only considers "persons 16 years of age and older residing in the 50 states and the District of Columbia, who are not inmates of institutions (e.g., penal and mental facilities, homes for the aged), and who are not on active duty in the Armed Forces" (BLS, 2018; Federal Reserve Bank of St. Louis, 2020).

to disabled workers in subminimum wage employment (34 C.F.R. § 397.40), and to allocate at least 15% of their federal funding to pre-employment transition services for students transitioning from high school to college or the workforce (U.S. Rehabilitation Services Administration, 2015). The resources funded through WIOA include job exploration counseling, workplace readiness training, instruction in self-advocacy, and other related services (U.S. Department of Education, 2016).

State Laws Designed to Ease Transition to Adulthood

In part because the breadth of federally funded VR services varies widely across states (Roux et al., 2020), some states have passed other laws to help people with ASD and their families better navigate the transition into adulthood. Some of these laws require public schools to take specific steps to prepare students with disabilities for the labor market. In Connecticut, for example, school districts must provide a "Transition Bill of Rights" to parents and guardians of children receiving special education services in middle school and high school, explaining the full range of resources available to students who graduate from (or leave) the public education system (Connecticut State Department of Education, 2016). Some states have also expanded post-secondary education for people with disabilities. In 2013, for example, California appropriated special funds to the community college system to expand the range of educational offerings available to students with disabilities (California Adult Education, n.d.).

Conclusion

Civil rights laws designed to protect the rights of disabled individuals in the workforce and in public education are familiar to many disability rights advocates and stakeholders. Yet numerous other civil statutes, regulations, and entitlement programs, some of which are available to disabled and non-disabled individuals alike, may be just as consequential for individuals with ASD and their families. Many of these diverse laws—such as those that broaden access to affordable health care, provide cash benefits, encourage savings, or fund individualized services and supports—can improve health, stability, and well-being throughout the life span. Others—such as those that pertain to custody and child support, the transition to adulthood, or legal decision-making capacity—only rise to prominence during important life transitions. Overall, our survey of this varied legal landscape suggests that although the rights of individuals with ASD have evolved rapidly in recent decades, there are many areas in which the law is inconsistent or under-developed, leaving plenty of room for continued reform and innovation.

References

26 C.F.R. § 54.9812–1(c)(4)(ii). (2020). https://www.ecfr.gov/cgi-bin/text-idx?SID=dd11b5b2933ccf1ec79422247f6399a4&mc=true&node=se26.19.54_19812_61&rgn=div8. Accessed 7 July 2020.

34 C.F.R. § 361.4. (2020). https://www.ecfr.gov/cgi-bin/text-idx?SID=303c42f31788292ae4edd19db63bd959&mc=true&node=se34.2.361_14&rgn=div8. Accessed 7 July 2020.

34 C.F.R. § 397.40. (2020). https://www.ecfr.gov/cgi-bin/text-idx?SID=dd11b5b2933ccf1ec79422247f6399a4&mc=true&node=se34.2.397_140&rgn=div8. Accessed 7 July 2020.

42 U.S.C. § 15043. (2021). https://www.govinfo.gov/app/details/USCODE-2010-title42/USCODE-2010-title42-chap144-subchapI-partC-sec15043. Accessed 18 May 2021.

ABLE Act of 2014. H.R. 647. 113th Cong., 2nd sess. (2014). https://www.congress.gov/bill/113th-congress/house-bill/647. Accessed 23 June 2020.

ABLE National Resource Center. (n.d.-a). *About ABLE Accounts.* https://www.ablenrc.org/what-is-able/what-are-able-acounts/. Accessed 7 July 2020.

ABLE National Resource Center. (n.d.-b). *Colorado.* https://www.ablenrc.org/state-review/colorado/. Accessed 7 July 2020.

ABLE National Resource Center. (n.d.-c). *Missouri.* https://www.ablenrc.org/state-review/missouri/. Accessed 7 July 2020.

ABLE National Resource Center. (n.d.-d). *New York.* https://www.ablenrc.org/state-review/new-york/. Accessed 7 July 2020.

ABLE National Resource Center. (n.d.-e). *Nevada.* https://www.ablenrc.org/state-review/nevada/. Accessed 7 July 2020.

ABLE National Resource Center. (n.d.-f). *Iowa.* https://www.ablenrc.org/state-review/iowa/. Accessed 7 July 2020.

American Bar Association. (2017). *ABLE Accounts: What trusts and estates lawyers need to know.* https://www.americanbar.org/groups/real_property_trust_estate/publications/probate-property-magazine/2017/may_june_2017/2017_aba_rpte_pp_v31_3_article_krooks_rubin_able_accounts/. Accessed 7 July 2020.

American Bar Association. (n.d.). *Power of attorney.* https://www.americanbar.org/groups/real_property_trust_estate/resources/estate_planning/power_of_attorney/. Accessed 7 July 2020.

Andrews, M. (2013). Young adult insurance quandary: Stay with parents, or go it alone? *NBC News.* https://www.nbcnews.com/healthmain/young-adult-insurance-quandary-stay-parents-or-go-it-alone-8C11300070. Accessed 7 July 2020.

Autism Law Hub. (2019). *Self-funded companies with ABA benefits.* https://www.autismlawhub.com/self-funded-companies-with-aba-benefits. Accessed 7 July 2020.

Autism Speaks. (2013). *Employment tool kit.* https://www.autismspeaks.org/sites/default/files/2018-08/Employment%20Tool%20Kit.pdf. Accessed 23 June 2020.

Autism Speaks. (2018). *Medicaid EPSDT.* https://www.autismspeaks.org/medicaid-epsdt. Accessed 7 July 2020.

Autism Speaks. (2019). *Autism Speaks commends Tennessee as it becomes 50th state requiring that insurance plans cover autism.* https://www.autismspeaks.org/press-release/autism-speaks-commends-tennessee-it-becomes-50th-state-requiring-insurance-plans. Accessed 7 July 2020.

Autistic Self Advocacy Network. (2019). *ASAN opposes proposed changes to Section 1557.* https://autisticadvocacy.org/2019/08/asan-opposes-proposed-changes-to-section-1557/. Accessed 7 July 2020.

Bach, M., & Kerzner, L. (2010). *A new paradigm for protecting autonomy and the right to legal capacity.* Law Commission of Ontario. https://www.lco-cdo.org/wp-content/uploads/2010/11/disabilities-commissioned-paper-bach-kerzner.pdf. Accessed 7 July 2020.

Barton, R., Lau, S., & Lockett, L. L. (2014). *The use of conservatorships and adult guardianships and other options in the care of the mentally ill in the United States.* World Guardianship Congress. https://www.guardianship.org/IRL/Resources/Handouts/Family%20Members%20as%20Guardians_Handout.pdf. Accessed 7 July 2020.

Belbase, A., & Sanzenbacher, G. T. (2017). *Guardianship and the representative payee program.* Center for Retirement Research at Boston College. https://crr.bc.edu/wp-content/uploads/2017/08/wp_2017-8.pdf. Accessed 7 July 2020.
Beronio, K., Po, R., Skopec, L., & Glied, S. (2013). *Affordable Care Act expands mental health and substance use disorder benefits and federal parity protections for 62 million Americans.* U.S. Department of Health and Human Services. https://aspe.hhs.gov/report/affordable-care-act-expands-mental-health-and-substance-use-disorder-benefits-and-federal-parity-protections-62-million-americans. Accessed 7 July 2020.
Boumil, M. M., Freitas, C. F., & Freitas, D. F. (2011). Legal and ethical issues confronting guardian ad litem practice. *Journal of Law and Family Studies, 13*(1), 43–80. https://epubs.utah.edu/index.php/jlfs/article/view/491/358. Accessed 7 July 2020.
Cal. Prob. Code § 1801(d). (2019). https://leginfo.legislature.ca.gov/faces/codes_displaySection.xhtml?lawCode=PROB§ionNum=1801. Accessed 7 July 2020.
Cal. Prob. Code § 2351.5. (2019). https://leginfo.legislature.ca.gov/faces/codes_displaySection.xhtml?lawCode=PROB§ionNum=2351.5. Accessed 7 July 2020.
California Adult Education. (n.d.). *About AEBG.* https://caladulted.org/ContentSystem/Home/AB86. Accessed 7 July 2020.
California Courts. (n.d.). Conservatorship. https://www.courts.ca.gov/selfhelp-conservatorship.htm?rdeLocaleAttr=en. Accessed 7 July 2020.
California Department of Health Care Services. (2019). *Special Needs Trust.* https://www.dhcs.ca.gov/services/Pages/Special-Needs-Trust.aspx. Accessed 7 July 2020.
Centers for Medicare & Medicaid Services. (2015). *Program history.* Medicaid.gov. https://www.medicaid.gov/about-us/program-history/index.html. Accessed 7 July 2020.
Centers for Medicare & Medicaid Services. (2020). *Dually eligible beneficiaries under Medicare and Medicaid.* https://www.cms.gov/Outreach-and-Education/Medicare-Learning-Network-MLN/MLNProducts/downloads/Medicare_Beneficiaries_Dual_Eligibles_At_a_Glance.pdf. Accessed 7 July 2020.
Centers for Medicare & Medicaid Services. (n.d.-a). *Eligibility.* https://www.medicaid.gov/medicaid/eligibility/index.html. Accessed 7 July 2020.
Centers for Medicare & Medicaid Services. (n.d.-b). *Home & Community-Based Services 1915(c).* https://www.medicaid.gov/medicaid/home-community-based-services/home-community-based-services-authorities/home-community-based-services-1915c/index.html. Accessed 7 July 2020.
Centers for Medicare & Medicaid Services. (n.d.-c). *Supplemental Security Income (SSI) disability & Medicaid coverage.* https://www.healthcare.gov/people-with-disabilities/ssi-and-medicaid/. Accessed 7 July 2020.
Centers for Medicare & Medicaid Services. (n.d.-d). *What marketplace health insurance plans cover.* https://www.healthcare.gov/coverage/what-marketplace-plans-cover/. Accessed 7 July 2020.
Centers for Medicare & Medicaid Services. (n.d.-e). *Types of health insurance that count as coverage.* https://www.healthcare.gov/fees/plans-that-count-as-coverage/. Accessed 7 July 2020.
Centers for Medicare & Medicaid Services. (n.d.-f). *State Waivers list.* https://www.medicaid.gov/medicaid/section-1115-demo/demonstration-and-waiver-list/index.html?sl=yes&fcf=Autism&ap=a&auth_order=1915(c)&usid=&sb=status_order. Accessed 7 July 2020.
Centers for Medicare & Medicaid Services. (n.d.-g). *Community First Choice (CFC) 1915 (k).* https://www.medicaid.gov/medicaid/home-community-based-services/home-community-based-services-authorities/community-first-choice-cfc-1915-k/index.html. Accessed 7 July 2020.
Colorado Department of Health Care Policy and Financing. (2019). *Supported Living Services Waiver (SLS).* https://www.colorado.gov/pacific/hcpf/supported-living-services-waiver-sls. Accessed 7 July 2020.
Connecticut State Department of Education. (2016). *Transition bill of rights for parents of students receiving special education services.* https://portal.ct.gov/-/media/SDE/Special-Educat

ion/Trans_Bill_of_Rights_for_Parents_of_Students_Receiving_SpEd_Services.pdf. Accessed 7 July 2020.

Dicker, S., & Marion, R. (2012). Judicial spectrum primer: What judges need to know about children with autism spectrum disorders. *Juvenile and Family Court Journal, 63*(2), 1–19. https://doi.org/10.1111/j.1755-6988.2012.01074.x.

Disability Benefits 101. (2020). *Medi-Cal: The details*. https://ca.db101.org/ca/programs/health_coverage/medi cal/program2a.htm#MedicallyNeedy. Accessed 7 July 2020.

Disability Rights California. (2018). *Consumer information about the social security administration representative payee program*. https://www.disabilityrightsca.org/publications/consumer-information-about-the-social-security-administration-representative-payee. Accessed 7 July 2020.

Disability Rights California. (2019). *Response to proposed rule changes of Section 1557, the nondiscrimination provision of the Affordable Care Act (ACA)*. https://www.disabilityrightsca.org/post/response-to-proposed-rule-changes-of-section-1557-the-nondiscrimination-provision-of-the. Accessed 7 July 2020.

Douglas, M., Wrenn, G., Bent-Weber, S., Tonti, L., & Carneal, G. (2018). *Evaluating state mental health and addiction parity statutes: A technical report*. The Kennedy Forum. https://digitalcommons.psjhealth.org/cgi/viewcontent.cgi?article=2090&context=publications. Accessed 7 July 2020.

Employer Assistance and Resource Network. (n.d.). *State vocational rehabilitation agencies*. https://askearn.org/state-vocational-rehabilitation-agencies/. Accessed 7 July 2020.

Ermini v. Vittori, 758 F.3d 153, 165–166 (C.A.2). https://casetext.com/case/ermini-v-vittori-1. Accessed 7 July 2020.

Federal Reserve Bank of St. Louis. (2020). *Population level—Women*. https://fred.stlouisfed.org/series/LNU00000002. Accessed 7 July 2020.

Fernandez, B., Forsberg, V. C., & Rosso, R. J. (2018). *Federal requirements on private health insurance plans. congressional research service*. https://fas.org/sgp/crs/misc/R45146.pdf. Accessed 7 July 2020.

Foster, C. C., Agrawal, R. K., & Davis, M. M. (2019). Home health care for children with medical complexity: Workforce gaps, policy, and future directions. *Health Affairs, 38*(6), 987–993. https://doi.org/10.1377/hlthaff.2018.05531.

Francisco, S. M., & Martinis, J. G. (2017). *Supported decision-making teams: Setting the wheels in motion*. National Resource Center for Supported Decision-Making. https://www.supporteddecisionmaking.org/sites/default/files/Supported-Decision-Making-Teams-Setting-the-Wheels-in-Motion.pdf. Accessed 7 July 2020.

Godbolt, D. (2017). *Medicaid: America's largest health insurer*. Center for Global Policy Solutions. https://globalpolicysolutions.org/wp-content/uploads/2017/07/Medicaid-Final.pdf. Accessed 7 July 2020.

Goldman, T. R. (2013). Progress report: The Affordable Care Act's extended dependent coverage provision. *Health Aff Blog*. https://doi.org/10.1377/hblog20131216.035741.

Government of Massachusetts. (n.d.). *Learn about the responsibilities of a conservator of a protected person*. https://www.mass.gov/info-details/learn-about-the-responsibilities-of-a-conservator-of-a-protected-person. Accessed 7 July 2020.

Graham, J. R. (2017). *Autism speaks re: Public stakeholder listening session on strategies for improving parity for mental health and substance use disorder coverage*. https://www.hhs.gov/programs/topic-sites/mental-health-parity/achieving-parity/cures-act-parity-listening-session/comments/patients-and-advocates/autism-speaks/index.html. Accessed 7 July 2020.

H.B. 322, 54th Leg., 1st sess. (NM. 2019). https://www.nmlegis.gov/Sessions/19%20Regular/bills/house/HB0322.pdf. Accessed 7 July 2020.

In re Juan R., 2007 Ct. Sup. 22337, 22347. (Conn. Super. Ct. 2007). https://casetext.com/case/in-re-juan-r-no-w10-cp06-015101-a-dec. Accessed 7 July 2020.

Indiana Resource Center for Autism. (2016). *Indiana—The autism health insurance reform pioneer*. https://www.arcind.org/wp-content/uploads/2016/12/HistoryAutismMandateLawsFinal.pdf. Accessed 7 July 2020.

Internal Revenue Service. (2018). *IRS reminds those with disabilities of new ABLE Account benefits*. https://www.irs.gov/newsroom/irs-reminds-those-with-disabilities-of-new-able-account-benefits. Accessed 7 July 2020.

Internal Revenue Service. (2019). *Retirement savings contributions credit (saver's credit)*. https://www.irs.gov/retirement-plans/plan-participant-employee/retirement-savings-contributions-savers-credit. Accessed 7 July 2020.

Internal Revenue Service. (2020a). *FAQs for government entities regarding Cafeteria Plans*. https://www.irs.gov/government-entities/federal-state-local-governments/faqs-for-government-entities-regarding-cafeteria-plans. Accessed 7 July 2020.

Internal Revenue Service. (2020b). *Employer's tax guide to fringe benefits*. https://www.irs.gov/publications/p15b#en_US_2020_publink1000250341. Accessed 7 July 2020.

Kaiser Family Foundation. (2020). *Medicaid and CHIP income eligibility limits for children as a percent of the federal poverty level*. https://www.kff.org/health-reform/state-indicator/medicaid-and-chip-income-eligibility-limits-for-children-as-a-percent-of-the-federal-poverty-level/?currentTimeframe=0&sortModel=%7B%22colId%22:%22Location%22,%22sort%22:%22asc%22%7D. Accessed 7 July 2020.

Keith, K. (2018). *The short-term, limited-duration coverage final rule: The background, the content, and what could come next*. Health Aff Blog. https://doi.org/10.1377/hblog20180801.169759.

LaGuardia v. LaGuardia, No. E2004–00822-COA-R3-CV, 2005 WL 1566492, 4. (Tenn. Ct. App. Jul. 6, 2005). https://casetext.com/case/laguardia-v-laguardia. Accessed 7 July 2020.

Mann, C. (2014). *Clarification of Medicaid coverage of services to children with autism*. Center for Medicaid and CHIP Services Informational Bulletin. https://www.medicaid.gov/sites/default/files/Federal-Policy-Guidance/Downloads/CIB-07-07-14.pdf. Accessed 7 July 2020.

Martocchio v. Savoir, 2008 Ct. Sup. 12372, 12374. (Conn. Super. Ct. 2008). https://casetext.com/case/martocchio-v-savoir-no-ttd-fa-06-4006261-jul. Accessed 7 July 2020.

Medicaid and CHIP Payment and Access Commission. (2019). *Overview of the Affordable Care Act and Medicaid*. https://www.macpac.gov/subtopic/overview-of-the-affordable-care-act-and-medicaid/. Accessed 7 July 2020.

Medicaid and CHIP Payment and Access Commission. (n.d.-a). *Key CHIP design features*. https://www.macpac.gov/subtopic/key-design-features/. Accessed 7 July 2020.

Medicaid and CHIP Payment and Access Commission. (n.d.-b). *EPSDT in Medicaid*. https://www.macpac.gov/subtopic/epsdt-in-medicaid/#_edn1. Accessed 7 July 2020.

Medicaid and CHIP Payment and Access Commission. (n.d.-c). *Mandatory and optional benefits*. https://www.macpac.gov/subtopic/mandatory-and-optional-benefits/. Accessed 7 July 2020.

Mitchell, A. (2018). *Medicaid's Federal Medical Assistance Percentage (FMAP)*. Congressional Research Service. https://fas.org/sgp/crs/misc/R43847.pdf. Accessed 7 July 2020.

Mo. Rev. Stat. § 475.080. (2019). https://law.justia.com/codes/missouri/2019/title-xxxi/chapter-475/section-475-080/. Accessed 7 July 2020.

Musumeci, M., Kates, K., Dawson, L., Salganicoff, A., Sobel, L., & Artiga, S. (2020a). *The Trump Administration's final rule on Section 1557 non-discrimination regulations under the ACA and current status*. Kaiser Family Foundation. https://www.kff.org/racial-equity-and-health-policy/issue-brief/the-trump-administrations-final-rule-on-section-1557-non-discrimination-regulations-under-the-aca-and-current-status/. Accessed 6 May 2021.

Musumeci, M., Watts, M. O., & Chidambaram, P. (2020b). *Key state policy choices about Medicaid home and community-based services*. Kaiser Family Foundation. https://www.kff.org/report-section/key-state-policy-choices-about-medicaid-home-and-community-based-services-issue-brief/. Accessed 7 July 2020.

National Alliance on Mental Illness. (n.d.). *What is mental health parity?* https://www.nami.org/Your-Journey/Individuals-with-Mental-Illness/Understanding-Health-Insurance/What-is-Mental-Health-Parity. Accessed 7 July 2020.

National Conference of Commissioners on Uniform State Laws. (2018). Uniform Guardianship, Conservatorship, and other Protective Arrangements Act. In *Annual National Conference of*

Commissioners, San Diego, California, 14–20 July 2017. https://www.guardianship.org/wp-content/uploads/2018/09/UGCOPPAAct_UGPPAct.pdf. Accessed 7 July 2020.
National Conference of State Legislatures. (2018). *Autism and insurance coverage|State laws*. https://www.ncsl.org/research/health/autism-and-insurance-coverage-state-laws.aspx. Accessed 7 July 2020.
National Council of State Legislature. (2020). *Termination of child support*. https://www.ncsl.org/research/human-services/termination-of-child-support-age-of-majority.aspx. Accessed 7 July 2020.
National Resource Center for Supported Decision-Making. (n.d.-a). *Texas*. https://supporteddecisionmaking.org/state-review/texas. Accessed 7 July 2020.
National Resource Center for Supported Decision-Making. (n.d.-b). *Rhode Island*. https://supporteddecisionmaking.org/state-review/rhode-island. Accessed 7 July 2020.
Neale, B. (2017). *RE: Implications of the Cures Act for special needs trusts*. Center for Medicaid and CHIP Services. https://www.medicaid.gov/sites/default/files/federal-policy-guidance/downloads/smd17001.pdf. Accessed 7 July 2020.
North Carolina Judicial Branch. (n.d.). *Guardianship*. https://www.nccourts.gov/help-topics/guardianship/guardianship. Accessed 7 July 2020.
O'Keeffe, J., Saucier, P., Jackson, B., Cooper, R., McKenney, E., Crisp, S., & Moseley, C. (2010). *Understanding Medicaid home and community services: A primer*. U.S. Department of Health & Human Services. https://aspe.hhs.gov/report/understanding-medicaid-home-and-community-services-primer-2010-edition. Accessed 7 July 2020.
Olmstead v. L. C, 527 U.S. 581. (1999). https://casetext.com/case/olmstead-v-l-c. Accessed 7 July 2020.
Roux, A., Rast, J., Anderson, K., & Shattuck, P. (2016). *National autism indicators report: Vocational rehabilitation*. Life Course Outcomes Research Program, A.J. Drexel Autism Institute, Drexel University. https://drexel.edu/autismoutcomes/publications-and-reports/publications/National-Autism-Indicators-Report-Vocational-Rehabilitation/. Accessed 7 July 2020.
Roux, A., Rast, J., Anderson, K., & Shattuck, P. (2017). *National autism indicators report: Developmental disability services and outcomes in adulthood*. Life Course Outcomes Research Program, A.J. Drexel Autism Institute, Drexel University. https://drexel.edu/autismoutcomes/publications-and-reports/publications/National-Autism-Indicators-Report-Developmental-Disability-Services-and-Outcomes-in-Adulthood/. Accessed 7 July 2020.
Roux, A. M., Rast, J. E., & Shattuck, P. T. (2020). State-level variation in vocational rehabilitation service use and related outcomes among transition-age youth on the autism spectrum. *Journal of Autism and Developmental Disorders, 50*(7), 2449–2461. https://doi.org/10.1007/s10803-018-3793-5.
Salzman, L. (2010). Rethinking guardianship (again): Substituted decision making as a violation of the integration mandate of title II of the Americans with Disabilities Act. *University of Colorado Law Review, 81,* 157–245. https://lawreview.colorado.edu/wp-content/uploads/2013/11/10Salzman-FINAL_s.pdf. Accessed 7 July 2020.
Shattuck, P. T., Narendorf, S. C., Cooper, B., Sterzing, P. R., Wagner, M., & Taylor, J. L. (2012). Postsecondary education and employment among youth with an autism spectrum disorder. *Pediatrics, 129*(6), 1042–1049. https://doi.org/10.1542/peds.2011-2864.
Sowers, M., Claypool, H., & Musumeci, M. (2016). *Streamlining Medicaid home and community-based services: Key policy questions*. Kaiser Family Foundation. https://www.kff.org/medicaid/issue-brief/streamlining-medicaid-home-and-community-based-services-key-policy-questions/. Accessed 7 July 2020.
Special Needs Alliance. (2013). *Your special needs trust ("SNT") defined*. https://www.specialneedsalliance.org/the-voice/your-special-needs-trust-snt-defined-2/. Accessed 7 July 2020.
Special Needs Alliance. (2015). *Representative payee for Social Security benefits*. https://www.specialneedsalliance.org/the-voice/representative-payee-for-social-security-benefits/. Accessed 7 July 2020.

Special Needs Alliance. (2020). *ABLE Accounts and SNTs: How to choose?* https://www.specialneedsalliance.org/blog/able-accounts-and-snts-how-to-choose/. Accessed 7 July 2020.

Special Needs Answers. (2020). *The pros and cons of ABLE accounts*. https://specialneedsanswers.com/the-pros-and-cons-of-able-accounts-15004. Accessed 7 July 2020.

Suleman v. Egenti, No. 1791, 2016 WL 1436597, 13. (Md. Ct. Spec. App. 2016). https://casetext.com/case/suleman-v-egenti. Accessed 7 July 2020.

Thach, N. T., & Wiener, J. M. (2018). *An overview of long-term services and supports and Medicaid: Final report*. U.S. Department of Health and Human Services. https://aspe.hhs.gov/system/files/pdf/259521/LTSSMedicaid.pdf. Accessed 7 July 2020.

Thinking Person's Guide to Autism. (2017). *Why supported decision making is a better choice than conservatorship*. https://www.thinkingautismguide.com/2017/05/why-supported-decision-making-is-better.html. Accessed 7 July 2020.

U.S. Administration for Community Living. (2017a). *History of the DD Act*. https://acl.gov/about-acl/history-dd-act. Accessed 7 July 2020.

U.S. Administration for Community Living. (2017b). *State protection and advocacy systems—FY 2015 program performance report*. https://acl.gov/programs/protection-and-advocacy-systems/state-protection-advocacy-systems-fy-2015-program-4. Accessed 7 July 2020.

U.S. Administration for Community Living. (2019). *State protection and advocacy systems*. https://acl.gov/programs/aging-and-disability-networks/state-protection-advocacy-systems. Accessed 7 July 2020.

U.S. Bureau of Labor Statistics. (2018). *Employment situation news release*. https://www.bls.gov/news.release/archives/empsit_01052018.htm. Accessed 7 July 2020.

U.S. Defense Health Agency. (2019a). *Eligibility*. https://www.tricare.mil/Plans/Eligibility. Accessed 7 July 2020.

U.S. Defense Health Agency. (2019b). *Continued health care benefit program*. https://tricare.mil/Plans/SpecialPrograms/CHCBP. Accessed 7 July 2020.

U.S. Defense Health Agency. (2020a). *Autism care demonstration*. https://tricare.mil/autism. Accessed 7 July 2020.

U.S. Defense Health Agency. (2020b). *Covered services: Autism spectrum disorder*. https://www.tricare.mil/CoveredServices/IsItCovered/AutismSpectrumDisorder. Accessed 11 May 2021.

U.S. Department of Defense, Notice. (2014, June 16). Comprehensive autism care demonstration. *Federal Register, 79*(115), 34291–34296. https://www.govinfo.gov/content/pkg/FR-2014-06-16/pdf/2014-14023.pdf. Accessed 7 July 2020.

U.S. Department of Education. (2016). *Frequently-asked questions about pre-employment transition services*. https://www2.ed.gov/programs/rsabvrs/pets-faq.html. Accessed 7 July 2020.

U.S. Department of Education. (2017). *Vocational rehabilitation state grants*. https://www2.ed.gov/programs/rsabvrs/index.html. Accessed 7 July 2020.

U.S. Department of Health and Human Services. (2017). *Pre-existing conditions*. https://www.hhs.gov/healthcare/about-the-aca/pre-existing-conditions/index.html. Accessed 7 July 2020.

U.S. Department of Labor. (2010). *The Mental Health Parity and Addiction Equity Act of 2008 (MHPAEA)*. https://www.dol.gov/sites/dolgov/files/EBSA/about-ebsa/our-activities/resource-center/fact-sheets/mhpaea.pdf. Accessed 7 July 2020.

U.S. Department of Labor. (n.d.-a). *Young adults and the Affordable Care Act: Protecting young adults and eliminating burdens on businesses and families FAQs*. https://www.dol.gov/agencies/ebsa/about-ebsa/our-activities/resource-center/faqs/young-adult-and-aca. Accessed 7 July 2020.

U.S. Department of Labor. (n.d.-b). *ERISA*. https://www.dol.gov/general/topic/health-plans/erisa. Accessed 7 July 2020.

U.S. Department of Labor. (n.d.-c). *Fiduciary responsibilities*. https://www.dol.gov/general/topic/health-plans/fiduciaryresp. Accessed 7 July 2020.

U.S. Department of Health and Human Services. (2021). *Section 1557 of the Patient Protection and Affordable Care Act*. https://www.hhs.gov/civil-rights/for-individuals/section-1557/index.html. Accessed 11 May 2021.

U.S. Department of Veterans Affairs. (2020a). *02.18.06 PSYCHOLOGICAL TESTING.* In: CHAMPVA Operational Policy Manual. https://www.vha.cc.va.gov/system/templates/selfservice/va_ssnew/help/customer/locale/en-US/portal/554400000001036/content/554400000009345/02.18.06-PSYCHOLOGICAL-TESTING. Accessed 11 May 2021.
U.S. Department of Veterans Affairs. (2020b). *CHAMPVA benefits.* https://www.va.gov/health-care/family-caregiver-benefits/champva/. Accessed 7 July 2020.
U.S. Health Resources and Services Administration. (2018). *Early periodic screening, diagnosis, and treatment.* https://mchb.hrsa.gov/maternal-child-health-initiatives/mchb-programs/early-periodic-screening-diagnosis-and-treatment. Accessed 7 July 2020.
U.S. Rehabilitation Services Administration. (2015). *Technical assistance circular RSA-TAC-15–02.* https://www2.ed.gov/policy/speced/guid/rsa/subregulatory/tac-15-02.pdf. Accessed 7 July 2020.
U.S. Social Security Administration. (2012). SI 00820.102 Cafeteria benefit plans. In *Program operations manual system.* https://secure.ssa.gov/poms.nsf/lnx/0500820102. Accessed 7 July 2020.
U.S. Social Security Administration. (2017). SI 01715.010 Medicaid and the Supplemental Security Income (SSI) program. In *Program operations manual system.* https://secure.ssa.gov/poms.nsf/lnx/0501715010. Accessed 7 July 2020.
U.S. Social Security Administration. (2018). SI 01120.203 exceptions to counting trusts established on or after January 1, 2000. In *Program operations manual system.* https://secure.ssa.gov/poms.nsf/lnx/0501120203. Accessed 7 July 2020.
U.S. Social Security Administration. (2020a). *Supplemental Security Income (SSI) income.* https://www.ssa.gov/ssi/text-income-ussi.htm. Accessed 7 July 2020.
U.S. Social Security Administration. (2020b). *Supplementary Security Income (SSI) eligibility requirements.* https://www.ssa.gov/ssi/text-eligibility-ussi.htm#disabled-adult. Accessed 7 July 2020.
U.S. Social Security Administration. (2020c). *Supplemental Security Income (SSI) resources.* https://www.ssa.gov/ssi/text-resources-ussi.htm. Accessed 7 July 2020.
U.S. Social Security Administration. (2020d). *Spotlight on deeming parental income and resources.* https://www.ssa.gov/ssi/spotlights/spot-deeming.htm. Accessed 7 July 2020.
U.S. Social Security Administration. (2020e). SI 01130.740 achieving a better life experience (ABLE) Accounts. In *Program operations manual system.* https://secure.ssa.gov/apps10/poms.nsf/lnx/0501130740. Accessed 7 July 2020.
U.S. Social Security Administration. (2020f). *Spotlight on trusts.* https://www.ssa.gov/ssi/spotlights/spot-trusts.htm. Accessed 7 July 2020.
U.S. Social Security Administration. (n.d.-a). *Medicare information.* https://www.ssa.gov/disabilityresearch/wi/medicare.htm. Accessed 7 July 2020.
U.S. Social Security Administration. (n.d.-b). *Frequently Asked Questions (FAQs) for representative payees.* https://www.ssa.gov/payee/faqrep.htm. Accessed 7 July 2020.
Watts, M. O., Musumeci, M., & Chidambaram, P. (2020). *Medicaid home and community-based services enrollment and spending.* Kaiser Family Foundation. https://www.kff.org/report-section/medicaid-home-and-community-based-services-enrollment-and-spending-issue-brief/. Accessed 7 July 2020.
Wit v. United Behavioral Health, 2019 WL 1033730, 48. (N.D. Cal. 2019). https://casetext.com/case/wit-v-united-behavioral-health-8. Accessed 7 July 2020.
Wynn, S. (2016). *The Social Security Administration's representative payee program.* American Bar Association. https://www.americanbar.org/groups/law_aging/publications/bifocal/vol_37/issue_3_february2016/ssa-rep-payee-program/. Accessed 7 July 2020.

Alison Morantz, J.D., Ph.D., is the James and Nancy Kelso Professor of Law at Stanford University; the Director of the Stanford Intellectual and Developmental Disabilities Law and Policy Project; and a Senior Fellow of the Stanford Institute for Economic Policy Research. Her research focuses on the rights and welfare of individuals with I/DD, and the law and economics of protective labor regulation. A former anti-discrimination advocate, she has been the principal investigator of research projects funded by the National Science Foundation, the Department of Labor, and the National Institute of Occupational Safety and Health.

Lorri Unumb is a Lawyer, a Professional Speaker, a Mother of three boys, and an internationally renowned Autism Advocate. She began her career as an Appellate Attorney with the United States Department of Justice and then as a Full-time Professor at George Washington University Law School. Following her son's diagnosis with autism, she began volunteering for autism causes, writing ground-breaking insurance legislation for South Carolina ("Ryan's Law") that passed in 2007 and served as the catalyst for the national autism insurance reform movement. She served for a decade as the national head of state government affairs for Autism Speaks, testifying more than 100 times on health insurance issues in legislatures throughout the United States and beyond and leading the initiative that resulted in 50 states requiring meaningful coverage for autism. Lorri founded the annual Autism Law Summit and is a Co-author of the law school textbook "Autism and the Law." In 2010, she founded the Autism Academy of South Carolina, a nonprofit ABA center now known as The Unumb Center for Neurodevelopment. Lorri currently serves as CEO of The Council of Autism Service Providers, an international nonprofit trade association. For her local, national, and international advocacy efforts, Lorri has been recognized with the NASCAR Foundation's Betty Jane France Humanitarian Award; the Miss South Carolina Pageant Woman of Achievement Award; the Professional Women in Advocacy "Excellence in a State Campaign" Award; and the Civitan International World Citizenship Award. She has been profiled on CNN and in Town & Country magazine, from whom she received one of the three 2009 "Women Who Make a Difference" awards. Lorri is also profiled in the American Academy of Pediatrics 2013 book "Autism Spectrum Disorders: What Every Parent Needs to Know." She is a Phi Beta Kappa graduate of the University of South Carolina (Journalism, 1990; Political Science 1990; Law 1993).

Chapter 20
Clinicians as Advocacy Allies for People with ASD

Alison Morantz

Introduction

At each stage of the life cycle—whether the focus is on obtaining medical care or therapy, receiving a free and appropriate public education, attaining a college degree, pursuing a rewarding career, maximizing personal autonomy and financial security, or accessing the community—state and federal laws provide protections and resources that can, in theory, help individuals with Autism Spectrum Disorder (ASD) lead their best lives. Yet translating theory into practice poses formidable challenges. In clinical settings, some individuals with ASD may struggle to communicate their needs and priorities in ways that others will heed and understand, thereby limiting their capacity to shape the treatment decisions that affect their lives. Outside clinical settings, persuading judges or other legal decision-makers that an applicant qualifies for a particular program or benefit, or of the need for a specific service or accommodation, can be difficult if adjudicators lack a nuanced understanding of the challenges the individual faces. In both settings, the ability of individuals with ASD and their families to engage in meaningful *advocacy*—broadly defined here as the capacity to communicate limitations, needs, desires, or priorities to decision-makers in ways that can favorably influence the adjudication of legal entitlements and the delivery of services and supports—often requires considerable knowledge, resources, and a strong circle of support.

For their part, clinicians may feel ill-prepared to help individuals with ASD and their families confront the myriad practical challenges that effective advocacy entails. They may conceptualize their role as limited to either or both of two tasks: providing families with an initial ASD diagnosis; and providing the medical care, therapy, or treatment that was the focus of their clinical education. Lacking training or expertise

A. Morantz (✉)
Stanford University, Stanford, CA, USA
e-mail: amorantz@law.stanford.edu

F. R. Volkmar et al. (eds.), *Handbook of Autism Spectrum Disorder and the Law*,
https://doi.org/10.1007/978-3-030-70913-6_20

in the intricacies of disability law, many clinicians have only a vague and superficial knowledge of the systems that self-advocates, families, and their allies must navigate in their efforts to obtain needed services and supports.

Yet in practice, the success of medical treatments and the success of advocacy efforts are closely intertwined. For example, the inability of an adult with ASD to self-advocate in a clinical setting by conveying her felt experiences and preferences to her nurse or physician may affect her adherence to a particular medical or therapeutic intervention in ways that lessen its benefit. A similarly close relationship between effective advocacy and long-term outcomes exists outside of clinical settings. For example, if the parents of a school-age child with ASD cannot secure funding for home-based Applied Behavior Analysis (ABA), or cannot ensure that an Individualized Education Plan (IEP) includes a robust array of school-based services (such as occupational therapy or speech therapy) to facilitate educational progress, the child is unlikely to thrive even if she attends regular therapy sessions with a skilled psychologist. Likewise, an adult with ASD who cannot secure stable housing, access community supports, or find steady employment may fail to reach his potential even if he is under an expert psychiatrist's care.

Encouraging more effective advocacy by patients and their families may feel daunting to many clinicians, especially those burdened with high patient caseloads. This reluctance is understandable. Yet two factors counsel in favor of clinicians becoming more knowledgeable about—and playing more active roles in—advocacy efforts in clinical and non-clinical domains. First, when it comes to ASD, an ounce of effective advocacy is worth a pound of crisis management. By investing a little more time upfront to overcome barriers to effective service delivery, clinicians can substantially improve their patient outcomes in a holistic fashion, while reducing the frequency of unexpected crises or setbacks that can reverse months or even years of clinical gains. Secondly, although learning to support the advocacy efforts of individuals with ASD and their families requires a significant upfront investment of time, once a clinician learns the "rules of the game" in a particular domain, helping other patients in the same domain becomes far less time-consuming.

This chapter is divided into five sections. The first section presents general principles that can help clinicians think beyond the "medical model" of developmental disabilities, thereby strengthening their therapeutic alliance with their patients and clients with ASD. The second section describes advocacy challenges that can arise in clinical settings and suggests that Supported Decision-Making (SDM) can be used to mitigate these challenges. The third section shifts the focus to adjudicatory hearings and appeals, describing the myriad challenges individuals with ASD and their families face in enforcing their rights under state and federal law. The fourth section contains concrete guidance on how clinicians can become effective "advocacy allies" in these formal legal settings. The fifth and final section lists additional resources upon which clinicians may draw, so they can help individuals with ASD and their families parlay treatment gains into a higher quality of life.

Thinking Beyond the Medical Model

In the past century, popular and professional understandings of ASD have undergone several cataclysmic shifts. From the 1940s through the 1960s, the dominant theory of autism's pathogenesis—introduced by Leo Kanner (1943) in the early 1940s and popularized in the U.S. by Bruno Bettleheim (1967)—held that a lack of parental (and particularly maternal) warmth during early childhood caused autism, a proposition commonly known as the "refrigerator mother theory." Bettelheim's recommended solution was to forcibly remove autistic children from their emotionally frigid parents. By the 1970s, in part due to the work of Bernard Rimland (1964), the refrigerator mother theory gave way to a model of autism that emphasized the role of biology, including genetic and environmental factors, in causing the condition (Cohmer, 2018). Yet another critical transformation in thinking came in the 1960s and 1970s with the pioneering work of Ivar Lovaas, who used behavioral principles to develop a comprehensive method of treating children with ASD known as Applied Behavior Analysis (ABA) (Smith & Eikeseth, 2011). The publication of Lovaas's landmark study (1987) demonstrating that almost half of children subjected to intense ABA treatment in early childhood (before age 4) achieved "normal" intellectual and educational functioning by first grade, compared to just 2% of those who did not receive such treatment, raised hopes that autism could be effectively treated and even "cured." Like Lovaas and the home-based ABA industry that his early research helped to spawn, most autism-focused advocacy organizations around the turn of the twenty-first century prioritized the goal of identifying genetic or environmental biomarkers that could point the way toward effective cures, and perhaps even help to eradicate ASD.

Despite their markedly different assumptions and emphases, all of these medical pioneers shared the belief that the deviation from "normal" brain function that an autism diagnosis implied was pathological and maladaptive, and thus that the focus of treatment should be to change the neurobiology—or, at least, the behavior—of individuals with ASD to align as closely as possible with that of their non-autistic peers. In other words, researchers did not question the medical model that views autism as a complex brain disorder; their goal was rather to amass the knowledge and expertise necessary to prevent or cure it.

The term "neurodiversity," which gained currency around the turn of the millennium and is closely associated with the autism rights movement, challenged the supremacy of the medical model. Rather than conceptualizing autism as a "disease" to be cured or eradicated, the neurodiversity paradigm views it as a distinct neurological profile that confers strengths as well as weaknesses, and as such, should be valued and supported (Armstrong, 2015; Silberman, 2015). This perspective is typically grounded in the broader "social model" of disability, which emphasizes the critical role that societal norms, attitudes, and institutions play in turning "impairments," nonstandard physical or neurological characteristics, into disabilities. From this perspective, the disability itself is in large part "caused by a contemporary social organization that takes little or no account of people who have impairments and thus excludes them from participation in the mainstream of social activities" (Oliver, 1996: 22). From a neurodiversity standpoint, the goal of therapy should be to help people with ASD obtain the skills, opportunities, services, and supports that maximize their quality of life, regardless of how closely their behavior resembles that of their non-autistic peers (Sinclair, 1993). Noting that autistic people historically have had little influence over the decisions that affect their lives, many activists have additionally emphasized the importance of giving self-advocates a greater voice in their own treatment and in broader policymaking on ASD-related issues, versus a status quo in which (non-autistic) professionals typically make decisions on their behalf (Dawson, 2003, 2004). This perspective is sometimes encapsulated by the slogan "Nothing about us without us" (Autistic Self Advocacy Network [ASAN], 2020a).

Applicable to a wide range of disabilities, the idea of "person-centered thinking" usefully captures many of the principles associated with the neurodiversity/autism rights perspectives. Described as a "philosophy behind service provision that supports positive control and self-direction of people's own lives," person-centered thinking emphasizes:

- The importance of being listened to and the effects of having no positive control.
- The role of daily rituals and routines.
- How to discover what is important to people.
- How to respectfully address significant issues of health or safety while supporting choice.
- How to develop goals that help people get more of what is important to them while addressing issues of health and safety (D.C. Dept. on Disability Services, n.d.).

Yet in many real-world settings, individuals with ASD and their families struggle to communicate their needs and desires in ways that are persuasive to decision-makers, limiting the extent to which person-centered thinking can be put into practice. In light of this reality, the remainder of this chapter identifies barriers to effective advocacy and suggests how clinicians can help to overcome them.

Supporting Advocacy Efforts in Clinical Settings

Because the autism spectrum encompasses individuals with a wide range of impairments and support needs, it is difficult to generalize about the difficulties individuals can face in ensuring that their needs and priorities are taken into account. Some patients may rely on augmentative and alternative communication technology to convey their thoughts and desires; others may not use any conventional language system. Some may have difficulty in grasping the nature of the alternatives presented, including their attendant risks and benefits, in real time. Still others may struggle to make choices, or to communicate their preferences clearly, in the physical settings where clinical consults or care team meetings are typically held. Given these realities, it can be very difficult for individuals with ASD to contribute meaningfully to decisions that affect their treatment.

In recent years, the concept of Supported Decision-Making (SDM) has gained increasing prominence as a method to mitigate barriers to effective self-advocacy in a wide range of settings. In recognition of the fact that "good communication is essential for accurate diagnosis, for negotiating treatment plans and for adherence ... [and] is key to patient safety" (Kripke, 2016: 445), the essential aim of SDM in clinical settings is to "enable people with intellectual or developmental disabilities to name a trusted person [or persons] to communicate with doctors, understand health care information, make informed decisions about health care, and/or carry out daily health-related activities" (ASAN, 2020b). Importantly, even if some individuals with I/DD cannot fully grasp the nature or consequences of the available alternatives in certain domains, they may still be able to convey preferences regarding which individual(s) are permitted to provide them with decision-making support. For individuals with communication challenges, SDM practitioners also stress the importance of using individualized communication supports and attending to nonverbal forms of communication, such as body language and facial expressions (National Council on Disability, 2019: 76).

As of this writing, SDM has not yet become a standard part of clinical training and practice, and some implementation problems have yet to be resolved. Among the unsettled questions are the extent to which the technique can, and ethically should, be used with individuals who lack legal capacity to make decisions on their own behalf. For example, adults with ASD sometimes are stripped of legal capacity through the creation of guardianship or power of attorney arrangements. Moreover, until recently, minors were often categorically presumed to lack the capacity to make medical decisions on their own behalf (Lang & Paquette, 2018). Thus the use of SDM with individuals under guardianship, or among minors with I/DD, raises special complexities. Another potential consideration is the fact that trusted supporters, especially if they are parents or caregivers, may not always be available when needed, may not monitor symptoms proactively, and may not relay information accurately (Kripke, 2016).

In response to widespread inconsistencies and perceived injustices in medical professionals' treatment of patients with ASD, the Autistic Self Advocacy Network and the Quality Trust for Individuals with Disabilities have developed model legislation, "An Act Relating to the Recognition of a Supported Health Care Decision-Making Agreement for Adults with Disabilities," in an effort to place SDM on firmer statutory footing in health care settings. The model law seeks to address a number of important nuances in the implementation of Supported Health Care Decision-Making Agreements, such as the conditions under which supporters can be disqualified because of conflicts of interest; the rights and responsibilities of supporters; and the ability of health care providers to withhold treatment if they believe that the patient's consent was coerced or based on misinformation (ASAN, 2014a, 2014b).

In short, although the use of SDM in clinical treatment settings is still at a relatively early stage and some details have yet to be fully worked out, the technique holds considerable promise as a tool to promote effective self-advocacy among individuals with ASD.

Legal Advocacy Challenges in Adjudicatory Hearings and Appeals

The civil rights of individuals with ASD are protected by an extensive array of federal and state laws. For example, several major federal statutes—including the Americans with Disabilities Act (ADA), the Individuals with Disabilities Education Act (IDEA), and Section 504 of the Rehabilitation Act of 1973 (Section 504)—help facilitate equal access to public education, higher education, and competitive integrated employment. Meanwhile, broad federal entitlement programs overseen by federal agencies and administered at the state level—such as Medicaid, SSI, SSDI, and Vocational Rehabilitation—provide health insurance, cash benefits, and a variety of services and supports that can improve standard of living. Individuals with ASD also can benefit from discrete state and federal laws that address specific problems, such as the inadequacy of behavioral health care benefits available from private insurers, or the difficulty of accumulating savings without losing eligibility for federal entitlement programs.

Yet navigating this dense legal thicket is often bewildering for individuals with ASD and their families. First of all, given the highly fragmented nature of the system—which encompasses dozens of different laws and programs administered or enforced by a range of public and private entities—it is difficult for families even to identify the full range of resources that are available.

A second barrier to effective advocacy is the fact that individuals with ASD and their families are often required to enforce their legal rights at the same time they are experiencing considerable anxiety, uncertainty, and upheaval. In the aftermath of an ASD diagnosis,

> [Parents are] force[d] to rearrange their schedules and often to quit their jobs or restructure their time … [they] are often not able to take time to focus on how to process the news of the diagnosis. They are immediately caught up in whirlwind of therapists and intensive interventions and are reminded over and over again of the critical window of opportunity for helping their children. (de Wolfe, 2014: 78)

In these stressful and tumultuous circumstances, it may be difficult for parents to muster the resources and emotional energy necessary to challenge, let alone reverse, unfavorable eligibility determinations or denials of services. Later in the life cycle, individuals with ASD and/or their family members may similarly be required to engage in vigorous advocacy in the midst of major life transitions or crises, such as immediately upon leaving the public school system, or in the wake of catastrophic disruptions in service delivery. For these reasons, having to locate an attorney and mount an appeal can feel overwhelming to those most directly affected by a discriminatory practice or an adverse decision by an insurer, provider, or administrative agency.

Yet another barrier to effective advocacy is that the process for challenging adverse determinations is often cumbersome and opaque; the procedural requirements of different laws often vary widely, and even a single law's provisions can change across state lines. A brief procedural overview of six preeminent federal laws affecting the civil rights and entitlements of individuals with ASD—Medicaid, SSI, SSDI, the IDEA, the ADA, and Section 504 of the Rehabilitation Act—helps to illustrate this point.

In most cases pertaining to the IDEA, SSI, and SSDI, consumers initially must challenge adverse official determinations through administrative hearings (Rothstein & Johnson, 2014: 251; Ryther & Samuels, 2019; Yell, 2019: 63). Only after exhausting these remedies may the complainant seek judicial review of the adverse determination in a state or federal court (Rothstein & Johnson, 2014: 251; U.S. Social Security Administration [SSA], 2019).

The requirements for exhaustion of administrative remedies and the provision of judicial review are more variable in the Medicaid context, as states have considerable discretion over the design of the program. Complainants are generally required to challenge adverse decisions through the administrative hearing process before proceeding to state court (McCormick, 2019), but the specific procedural requirements depend on the case law and administrative law of each state.[1] Federal law does not guarantee Medicaid complainants the right to any judicial review (Medicaid and CHIP Payment and Access Commission [MACPAC], 2018), and in some jurisdictions, the only explicit form of administrative review may be an appeal to the director of the Medicaid Agency (MACPAC, 2018; Oklahoma Department of Human Services, 2015).

Section 504 of the Rehabilitation Act, which helps to protect the rights of students (among others) with ASD—particularly in postsecondary educational settings, to which the IDEA does not apply—provides a different configuration of procedural mechanisms to enable claimants to enforce their rights. As with the IDEA, the right to file Section 504 claims in court is generally guaranteed (Rothstein & Johnson, 2014: 305; Yell, 2019: 115). Yet the exhaustion requirement is somewhat more complex. Under federal law, exhaustion of administrative remedies is uniformly required if the subject matter of the complaint is covered by the IDEA (*Fry v. Napoleon Comm. Schools*, 2017), but not if the subject matter falls outside the IDEA's scope (Rothstein, 2019). Additionally, the procedural requirements for administrative hearings under Section 504 are less extensive and robust, and contain fewer explicit procedural safeguards than those provided under the IDEA (Council for Exceptional Children, 2002; Howey, 2019; U.S. Department of Education, n.d.; U.S. Department of Education, Office of Civil Rights, 2020).

[1] This requirement is generally waived for complainants who sue the state in federal court (McCormick, 2019).

The IDEA and Section 504 also differ in other ways that can affect families' capacity to advocate effectively on behalf of school-age children with ASD. For example, only the IDEA gives parents the right to obtain an Independent Educational Evaluation (IEE) at the district's expense if they disagree with the results of a school district's evaluation, although a district can circumvent this obligation by successfully challenging the IEE's necessity during an administrative hearing (Yell, 2019: 62).

The ADA, which is often used to protect the rights of individuals with ASD in the workforce and in higher education, sets forth yet another array of enforcement procedures. In the employment setting (Title I), plaintiffs have the right to file a claim in court as long as this right has not been waived by a contractual provision requiring disputes to be resolved through mandatory arbitration. However, they must first exhaust administrative remedies by filing a charge with the Equal Employment Opportunity Commission (EEOC) (U.S. Department of Justice, Civil Rights Division [DOJCRD], 2013; Yell, 2019: 129). The portions of the ADA that apply to public educational institutions (Title II) do not require plaintiffs to exhaust administrative remedies before filing claims in court (Yell, 2019: 130); however, the case law is unsettled as to whether complainants filing court actions against private educational institutions (through Title III) must first exhaust administrative remedies (Joseph et al., 2019). Moreover, in each of these contexts, complainants have the option of filing complaints with one or more federal agencies (DOJCRD, 2017; Yell, 2019: 130–132).

One particularly important source of variation among these federal laws is the availability (or lack thereof) of "cost-shifting" provisions that enable prevailing plaintiffs to recover attorney's fees. Both the IDEA and Section 504 allow courts to award attorney's fees to prevailing claimants in administrative or judicial proceedings (Osborne & Russo, 2014: 241–243; Weber, 2012: 645), although only Section 504 has been interpreted as allowing such awards to include expert witness fees (Council of Parent Attorneys & Advocates, 2013; Weber, 2012: 642, 646). The ADA likewise includes a cost-shifting provision that encompasses both judicial and administrative proceedings (42 U.S.C. § 12205). On the other hand, the federal regulations governin Medicaid administrative hearings contain no cost-shifting requirements (42 C.F.R. §§ 431.200–431.250), and the extent to which prevailing consumers can recover attorney's fees in administrative and/or judicial proceedings varies by state (Mo. Rev. Stat. § 536.087; Cal. Welf. & Inst. Code § 10962). For example, in several states' Medicaid hearings, the benefits at issue were categorized in such a way that prevailing claimants were deemed ineligible to recover attorney's fees (*Braddock v. Mo. Dep't of Mental Health*, 2006; *Good v. Iowa Dep't of Human Servs.*, 2019). Claimants who successfully challenge a denial of SSI or SSDI benefits by the Social Security Administration (SSA) likewise cannot typically recover attorney's fees at the administrative hearing stage (SSA, 2017). However, if a claimant successfully appeals an adverse decision to federal court, they may recover attorney's fees under the provisions of the Equal Access to Justice Act (28 U.S.C. § 2412).

How Clinicians Can Support Advocacy in Adjudicatory Hearings and Appeals

As discussed in the prior section, the barriers to effective advocacy facing individuals with ASD and their families in formal adjudicatory proceedings are formidable and multifaceted. Even in the best of circumstances, the civil rights enforcement and service delivery systems that in theory are available to provide assistance are highly fragmented, making it difficult for (self-)advocates even to identify which legal channels to pursue. These practical difficulties can become particularly acute during times of crisis or transition. The six federal laws discussed above—the IDEA, the ADA, Medicaid, Section 504 of the Rehabilitation Act, SSI, and SSDI—differ markedly in the scope, forum(s), sequence, and financial accessibility of their respective enforcement procedures; even the same federal law can vary significantly across state lines. In light of these complexities, there is no straightforward or uniform answer to the question of how clinicians can best assist families in adjudicatory hearings and appeals. The precise tasks that clinicians are expected to complete, and the manner in which they must carry them out, are highly contextual and case-specific.

Nevertheless, a few generalizations can be made. First, clinicians are typically asked to render a professional opinion on one of two questions: whether a claimant's ASD diagnosis brings him/her within the scope of a particular law; and whether a claimant's functional impairments justify the level of services, supports, or accommodations that an agency or employer is being asked to provide. Second, clinicians are usually called upon to render these opinions in writing in the form of checklists, questionnaires, or letters of support, and sometimes may be asked to attend a proceeding by phone or in person. Third, clinicians usually, but not always, perform these tasks at the request of attorneys or other professionals representing individuals with ASD or family members. Fourth, patients and family members often have little if any familiarity with the advocacy challenges they are about to confront, let alone the clinician's role in helping to achieve a favorable result.

Finally, it is safe to assume that in most contexts, clinicians play an essential role in persuading (or dissuading) the decision-maker of the merit of the individual's claim. Moreover, a well-substantiated diagnosis and thoughtful treatment plan help to align resources with expectations, providing a roadmap that the individual with I/DD, his/her family members, and other allies can use to obtain the supports necessary for a high quality of life. As the Social Security Administration notes in its guidance to medical professionals:

> [M]edical evidence is the cornerstone for the determination of disability .... SSA regulations place special emphasis on evidence from treating sources because they are likely to be the medical professionals most able to provide a detailed longitudinal picture of the claimant's impairments and they may bring a unique perspective to the medical evidence that cannot be obtained from the medical findings alone .... [T]imely, accurate, and adequate medical reports from treating sources accelerate the processing of the claim because they can greatly reduce or eliminate the need for additional medical evidence to complete the claim. (SSA, n.d.-a.)

The same observation holds true for most, if not all, civil domains in which clinicians are frequently called upon to render professional opinions.

The following four practices can help clinicians effectively support advocacy efforts across a wide range of adjudicatory settings.

Sympathetically Acknowledge the Magnitude of the Advocacy Challenge Facing the Patient/Client and Their Family, Express a Desire to Help, and Set Clear Expectations Upfront

Although the "refrigerator mother theory" of ASD's etiology described earlier was largely discredited by the 1980s, individuals with ASD and their families may nonetheless come away from interactions with medical professionals feeling intimidated, shamed, or blamed. For children or adults with ASD, the medical model's implicit assumption that autistic traits constitute a "disorder" that needs to be "fixed" can trigger feelings of inadequacy and low self-esteem. Meanwhile, parents may fear that medical professionals are judging them (or may even judge themselves) for failing to deliver enough services to cure or alleviate their child's condition, even if they do not blame themselves for causing it. These negative feelings not only constitute barriers to effective treatment, but also can interfere with the sense of trust and empowerment that successful advocacy demands.

To overcome these psychological barriers, clinicians can begin by familiarizing themselves with the concept of neurodiversity and the social model of disability. Not only are these perspectives far less stigmatizing than the conventional medical model, but in viewing ASD in a more holistic and accepting fashion that acknowledges societal barriers to inclusion, they draw attention to the accommodations, services, and supports that can help individuals with ASD lead full and rewarding lives.

More specifically, clinicians should aim to accomplish three goals when discussing the enforcement of legal rights with patients with ASD and their parents: (1) *conveying empathy* for the enormous time and effort that ongoing advocacy requires of patients with ASD and their families; (2) *communicating a willingness to help* by fulfilling a designated role within a particular adjudicatory proceeding; and (3) *setting clear boundaries and expectations* about the scope, timing, and cost of the task(s) the clinician is willing to perform.

The last point is particularly important, especially for medical professionals with large caseloads who may be unable to devote significant time to any individual patient. Knowing at the outset how much time a clinician can devote to an advocacy-related task enables the individual with ASD, together with his/her attorney and/or allies, to make informed choices about how best to prepare for an upcoming adjudication. For example, if a clinician can only devote twenty minutes to completing a checklist, and is not willing to draft a letter of support or attend a hearing in person or telephonically, conveying this information upfront gives the advocacy team an opportunity to approach other clinicians or rethink their litigation strategy. Discussing the clinician's expected role and his/her time constraints upfront also can create opportunities for creative problem-solving. For example, even if a clinician does not have enough time to draft a complete letter of support, he or she may be willing to review, edit, and cosign a letter drafted by another care provider.

Finally, clinicians should be sensitive to the fact that in most adjudicatory settings, the preeminence of the medical model is taken for granted, and eligibility determinations are focused narrowly on patients' deficits and limitations, not their strengths. Alerting patients and families to this reality upfront can help them prepare emotionally for what lies ahead, and lessen the risk that they feel stigmatized or shamed by the adjudicatory process itself.

Refer the Patient/Client and Their Family to Local Advocacy Resources

Although it is not always formally required, legal representation is crucial in most judicial or administrative adjudications. Yet as discussed earlier, some important federal laws (such as those governing Medicaid, SSI, and SSDI) do not guarantee plaintiffs who prevail in administrative proceedings the right to recover litigation fees and costs. Even if attorneys' fees are technically recoverable in the wake of a successful appeal to state or federal court, finding an attorney who is willing to accept a contingency fee arrangement (in which the attorney is entitled to fees only if the appeal is successful) may prove difficult. Many families, especially those who cannot afford to pay an upfront retainer or to pay an attorney on an hourly basis, may fail to secure any legal representation. Moreover, individuals with ASD or family members who opt to represent themselves (or are forced to do so because they cannot find an attorney) may struggle to learn enough about the applicable legal standards to advocate effectively on their own behalf.

Clinicians can play a critical role in referring patients with ASD and their families to local and online resources that can help them secure legal representation, or alternatively, to gain at least the basic knowledge necessary to advocate on their own behalf. The final section of this chapter lists a few helpful websites and national organizations, which can be augmented to include experienced attorneys, agencies, and legal clinics in the surrounding area. Providing patients and families with a list of advocacy-focused organizations and resources, ideally as a routine part of the intake process, can help them better understand and anticipate the advocacy challenges that await them.

Understand the "Clinical-Legal" Mindset

In most adjudicatory contexts, as noted above, clinicians are asked to opine on one of two questions: (1) whether the patient's disability qualifies him/her for legal protection or support; or (2) the nature and extent of the services, supports, or accommodations to which the patient is entitled. When called upon to opine on the first question,

> Many providers erroneously assume that simply confirming medical diagnoses is sufficient to document disabilities. 'Disability' is an administrative/legal determination made by an agency [or court,] not a medical diagnosis .... The role of clinicians and others is to provide documentation, or evidence, of disability. In other words, medical professionals are asked to provide the facts—diagnoses and functional limitations—that are necessary to determine disability. That is why a simple statement such as "my patient is disabled" is not sufficient. (O'Connell et al., 2007: 6)

This excerpt succinctly captures the essence of the "clinical-legal" mindset. Establishing that a patient meets the criteria for an ASD diagnosis under the DSM is rarely, if ever, adequate to establish his/her eligibility for legal accommodation or support. Rather, the adjudicator (typically a hearing officer, judge, or arbitrator) evaluates the scope, quality, and credibility of evidence presented by qualified clinician(s) to determine whether the claimant meets the eligibility criteria laid out in the pertinent statute.

Similar logic applies to adjudications regarding what type of accommodation(s), service(s), or support(s) an employer, agency, or other entity is required to provide. Here again, a clinician's mere assertion that the patient's ASD diagnosis and/or symptoms give rise to particular needs is legally insufficient. If the clinician cannot document and substantiate the particular way(s) in which ASD manifests in the particular individual and the functional impairments to which it gives rise, and then clearly link these facts to the necessity for a particular form of accommodation or relief, advocacy is unlikely to achieve its intended result.

Although exceptions are plentiful, the focus of the administrative or judicial proceeding often varies depending on whether the law at issue affects a patient's civil rights, or his/her entitlement to an accommodation or public benefit. For civil rights laws such as the ADA, IDEA, and Section 504, demonstrating that an individual with ASD is entitled to legal protection is frequently straightforward; often, the more formidable challenge lies in persuading the adjudicator to grant the requested accommodations or services. This is not the case for public benefit programs—such as Medicaid, SSI, and SSDI—in which demonstrating the patient's threshold eligibility for services often poses the most significant evidentiary hurdles. In adjudications involving Medicaid-funded programs, *both* of these questions (threshold eligibility and entitlement to services) are frequently in dispute.

Ground All Supporting Documentation or Testimony in Clinical-Legal Reasoning

Regardless of whether the issue being adjudicated is the patient's threshold eligibility for support or the nature and scope of that support, providing effective documentation or testimony to support the patient's advocacy team typically includes the following steps:

- Identifying the specific clinical-legal issue(s) to be resolved. In most contexts, as noted above, the primary advocacy challenge is either demonstrating threshold eligibility, or proving the patient's entitlement to particular services, supports, or accommodations. In some contexts, however, an adjudicator may be asked to resolve both of these questions in a single proceeding.
- Understanding the legal standard(s) to be applied. To provide effective support to the advocacy team, a clinician must understand the standards the adjudicator will apply to resolve the clinical-legal issue, and ensure that any documentation produced is sufficiently detailed and comprehensive to meet those standards. Yet in so doing, the clinician must bear in mind that the applicable standards can vary widely between different state and federal laws.

  For example, to qualify as "disabled" under SSI or SSDI, an individual with ASD not only must meet the basic diagnostic criteria ("Medical documentation of … [q]ualitative deficits in verbal communication, nonverbal communication, and social interaction; and [s]ignificantly restricted, repetitive patterns of behavior, interests, or activities"), but also must exhibit "extreme limitation" in one or "marked limitation" in four respective areas of mental functioning: "[u]nderstand[ing], remember[ing], or apply[ing] information"; "[i]nteract[ing] with others"; "[c]oncentrat[ing], persist[ing], or maintain[ing] pace"; or "manag[ing] oneself" (SSA, n.d.-b). Medicaid, in contrast, allows states considerable discretion to specify the diagnostic tools, the relative importance of adaptive functioning measures, and definition of "institutional" level of care that are used to make eligibility determinations (Zaharia & Moseley, 2008). Under the IDEA, a child not only must have a "developmental disability significantly affecting verbal and nonverbal communication and social interaction, generally evident before age three," such as ASD, but the disability must be shown to "adversely affect[] [the] child's educational performance" (34 C.F.R. § 300.8(c)(1)). Title I of the ADA takes yet another approach: the job applicant or employee not only must prove that (s)he has a "physical or mental impairment that substantially limits one or more major life activities" (or alternatively, has a record of or is regarded as having such an impairment); but also that (s)he is qualified to perform the "essential functions" of the job "with or without reasonable accommodation" (42 C.F.R. §§ 12102(1), 12111(8)).

  The same logic applies to determinations regarding an eligible individual's claim to a particular mixture of services, supports, or accommodations. Because different federal laws use different criteria to assess the merits of the claim and the array of benefits or accommodations to which the claimant is entitled, clinical documentation must be carefully drafted to meet the relevant legal standards.

- Compiling a checklist of criteria necessary to meet the applicable legal standard. Once the clinician understands the precise question(s) to be resolved and the legal standard(s) to be applied, the next step is to compile a checklist of the criteria that must be met for the claimant to prevail. For example, in the case of Social Security eligibility described above, the Listing of Impairments and associated documentation (available online) enumerates the specific criteria that a claimant with ASD must meet to qualify as "disabled" for purposes of SSI or SSDI (SSA, n.d.-b). The contents of the required "checklist" can vary widely depending on the law or regulation at issue and the specific issue being resolved. Importantly, clinicians must address *all* of the relevant criteria in their documentation (or testimony) to persuade an adjudicator of the patient's threshold eligibility and/or right to requested services.
- Substantiating each item on the checklist with supporting facts and documentation. Unlike a "doctor's note," which often simply asserts that an individual has a particular medical condition that necessitates a particular type of accommodation, clinical assertions carry no weight in adjudicatory settings unless they are backed up with supporting facts. For example, a clinician seeking to persuade a hearing officer in an SSI hearing that a patient with ASD has an extreme limitation in his/her capacity to "interact with others" must substantiate that claim by describing in some detail the patient's history of interaction with family members, coworkers, and care providers; and explaining how specific aspects of his/her disability—such as disruptive behaviors, unusual responses to sensory stimuli, cognitive rigidities, deficits in theory of mind, a diminished capacity to read social cues, restricted interests or activities, and/or verbal and nonverbal communication skills—have severely impeded his/her functional capacity to interact with others in a broad range of settings, including the workplace.
- Getting the right signatures. In most adjudicatory proceedings, different clinicians' opinions are accorded different evidentiary weights. To support a disability claim before the SSA, for example, federal regulations specify that documentation of a medical impairment must come from an "acceptable medical source," a category that is limited to physicians, licensed or certified psychologists, and qualified speech and language pathologists (O'Connell et al., 2007: 18). Moreover, "[b]y law, the statement of a treating [acceptable medical] source carries more weight than any other evidence, including the report of an outside examiner" (O'Connell et al., 2007: 18).

Although the SSA's clinician credentialing requirements are unusually explicit and detailed, similar principles apply in other adjudicatory settings. Rightly or wrongly, opinions and testimony submitted by certain clinicians (usually licensed physicians and psychologists) are granted more deference than others; and the opinions of treating clinicians who know their patients well and can describe their history in detail are generally accorded more weight than those of consulting clinicians. For this reason, if a document is drafted by a clinician who does not provide ongoing care, or who lacks an advanced clinical degree, it may be helpful for the document to be edited and cosigned by a treating medical provider and/or one with the "best" formal credentials.

Conclusion

Engaging in successful advocacy—that is, communicating an individual's limitations, needs, desires, or priorities to decision-makers in ways that can favorably influence the distribution of legal entitlements or the delivery of services and supports—is a vitally important, yet often very difficult, challenge for individuals with ASD and their families. Yet even clinicians who want to assist their patients or clients with this daunting task may not have the training or experience to do so effectively. This chapter outlines two distinct ways in which clinicians can become skilled advocacy allies. First, they can strengthen their therapeutic alliance with their patients or clients by understanding the concept of neurodiversity and the limitations of the medical model, and learn how SDM principles can be used to give people with ASD a greater "voice" in their own health care. In formal adjudicatory settings, clinicians likewise can play crucial supporting roles if they master the "clinical-legal" mindset, and understand how decision-makers in each case will evaluate the documentation or testimony they are asked to provide. Although becoming a proficient advocacy ally may require an upfront investment of time—especially among clinicians with little relevant training—it becomes far more manageable with increasing experience, and is an essential tool in improving the health, economic security, and long-term welfare of individuals with ASD.

Additional Resources

Perspectives on Neurodiversity/Autism Rights Movement

- *Don't Mourn for Us by Jim Sinclair*: Though primarily directed toward parents, this essay reflects many of the tenets of the autism rights movement and can help inform clinicians' interactions with individuals with ASD and their families (Sinclair, 1993).
- *NeuroTribes: The Legacy of Autism and the Future of Neurodiversity by Steve Silberman*: This book traces the history of ASD diagnosis and treatment before outlining the concept of neurodiversity (Silberman, 2015).
- *What Can Physicians Learn from the Neurodiversity Movement? by Dr. Christina Nicolaidis*: This article explains the clinical and non-clinical relevance of the neurodiversity movement and encourages physicians to incorporate a social understanding of disability, explained above, into their practice (Nicolaidis, 2012).

- *The Myth of the Normal Brain: Embracing Neurodiversity by Dr. Thomas Armstrong*: This article frames disability as a condition that carries with it both strengths and weaknesses, and encourages physicians to think beyond the medical model of "curing disease" (Armstrong, 2015).

Resources on the Use of Supported Decision-Making (SDM) in Health Care Settings

- *National Resource Center for Supported Decision-Making*: The Center's online website, found at https://www.supporteddecisionmaking.org/, provides informational and planning resources related to SDM, as well as descriptions of every state's guardianship and SDM laws (National Resource Center for Supported Decision-Making, n.d.).
- *University of California Davis, Center for Excellence in Developmental Disabilities (CEDD)*: CEDD offers an extensive online list of resources explaining SDM, its implementation, and its relationship to other decision-making arrangements for people with ASD. These resources can be found at https://health.ucdavis.edu/mindinstitute/centers/cedd/sdm.html (University of California Davis, Center for Excellence in Developmental Disabilities, 2020).
- *Autistic Self Advocacy Network (ASAN) Model Legislation*: As discussed above, ASAN has drafted model legislation providing guidance on the implementation of SDM in health care settings (ASAN, 2014a, 2014b).
- *Supported Decision-Making Teams: Setting the Wheels in Motion by Suzanne Francisco and Jonathan Martinis*: This resource provides planning materials and additional information related to SDM, financial planning, and other services for people with ASD (Francisco & Martinis, 2017).
- *WITH Foundation*: The WITH Foundation provides grants to organization developing programs to encourage the use of SDM in clinical settings and elsewhere. For example, they have supported advocacy projects and training related to SDM, including those listed here: https://withfoundation.org/previous-grant-recipients/ (WITH Foundation, 2020).

Resources for Medical Providers on Documenting Disability for Patients with ASD

- *Documenting Disability: Simple Strategies for Medical Providers by James O'Connell et al.*: This report offers tips to medical providers on how best to document disability for the purposes of obtaining SSI and SSDI (O'Connell et al., 2007).
- *Documenting Disabilities for Medical Providers by the National Health Care for the Homeless Council*: A collection of online informational modules and videos

for providers about how to document patients' disabilities, mostly in the context of SSI/SSDI claims. These resources can be found at https://nhchc.org/online-courses/documenting-disability/ (National Health Care for the Homeless Council, 2019).

Legal Representation and Resources for Individuals with ASD, Family Members, and Allies

- *Protection and Advocacy Systems (P&As)*: Each state is required to have its own protection and advocacy organization to provide legal support, training, and support to people with disabilities, including ASD. A comprehensive list of the state organizations can be found on the U.S. Administration for Community Living's website, https://acl.gov/programs/aging-and-disability-networks/state-protection-advocacy-systems (U.S. Administration for Community Living, 2019).
- *LawHelp.org*: LawHelp provides legal assistance for people of low and moderate incomes, connecting individuals with free legal aid in their communities and providing state-specific legal information as well as necessary forms for services related to many areas, including disability (LawHelp.org, 2020).
- *Legal aid organizations*: Many organizations across the country provide free legal services to low-income families on issues related to public benefits, housing, and other matters of direct service. A list of legal aid organizations by state can be found on the Legal Services Corporation's website, https://www.lsc.gov/grants-grantee-resources/our-grantees (Legal Services Corporation, n.d.).
- *Law school clinics*: In these clinics, law students provide free legal aid to low-income individuals and/or other disadvantaged groups, oftentimes including individuals with disabilities. A complete list of clinics can be found on the American Bar Association's website, https://www.americanbar.org/groups/center-pro-bono/resources/directory_of_law_school_public_interest_pro_bono_programs/definitions/pi_pi_clinics/ (American Bar Association, 2020).

Self-Advocacy Organizations Run by and for Individuals with ASD

- *Autistic Self Advocacy Network (ASAN)*: ASAN, whose motto is "Nothing about us without us," engages in legal and political advocacy to protect the rights of people with ASD. ASAN's website can be found at https://www.autisticadvocacy.org/ (ASAN, 2020a).
- *Self Advocates Becoming Empowered (SABE)*: SABE is a nonprofit organization whose voting membership is made up of individuals with disabilities. Its mission is to ensure that people with disabilities receive equal treatment and

are given the same rights, responsibilities, and opportunities to empower themselves as everyone else. See https://www.sabeusa.org/ (Self Advocates Becoming Empowered, 2020).

- *Autistic Women & Nonbinary Network (AWN)*: AWN is a nonprofit advocacy organization that provides "community, support, and resources for Autistic women, girls, transfeminine and transmasculine nonbinary and genderqueer people, trans people of all genders, Two Spirit people, and all others of marginalized genders." Founded in 2006, the organization seeks to encourage broader discourse on the intersection of gender and disability. AWN's website can be found at https://www.awnnetwork.org/ (Autistic Women & Nonbinary Network, 2020).

References

28 U.S.C. § 2412. (2018). https://www.govinfo.gov/app/details/USCODE-2018-title28/USCODE-2018-title28-partVI-chap161-sec2412. Accessed 7 July 2020.

34 C.F.R. § 300.8. (2020). https://www.ecfr.gov/cgi-bin/text-idx?SID=f2af09c10e0e612c119166b3ab6928df&mc=true&node=se34.2.300_18&rgn=div8. Accessed 7 July 2020.

42 C.F.R. §§ 431.200–431.250. (2020). https://www.ecfr.gov/cgi-bin/text-idx?node=pt42.4.431&rgn=div5#sp42.4.431.e. Accessed 7 July 2020.

42 U.S.C. § 12102(1). (2010). https://www.govinfo.gov/app/details/USCODE-2010-title42/USCODE-2010-title42-chap126-sec12102. Accessed 7 July 2020.

42 U.S.C. § 12111(8). (2010). https://www.govinfo.gov/app/details/USCODE-2010-title42/USCODE-2010-title42-chap126-subchapI-sec12111. Accessed 7 July 2020.

42 U.S.C. § 12205. (2018). https://www.govinfo.gov/app/details/USCODE-2018-title42/USCODE-2018-title42-chap126-subchapIV. Accessed 7 July 2020.

American Bar Association. (2020). *Public interest clinics*. https://www.americanbar.org/groups/center-pro-bono/resources/directory_of_law_school_public_interest_pro_bono_programs/definitions/pi_pi_clinics/. Accessed 7 July 2020.

Armstrong, T. (2015). The myth of the normal brain: Embracing neurodiversity. *AMA Journal of Ethics, 17*(4), 348–352. https://doi.org/10.1001/journalofethics.2015.17.4.msoc1-1504.

Autistic Self Advocacy Network. (2014a). *Model legislation: An Act relating to the recognition of a Supported Health Care Decision-Making Agreement for adults with disabilities*. https://autisticadvocacy.org/wp-content/uploads/2014/07/ASAN-Supported-Decisionmaking-Model-Legislature.pdf. Accessed 7 July 2020.

Autistic Self Advocacy Network. (2014b). *Questions and answers on the model Supported Health Care Decision-Making Agreement Act*. https://autisticadvocacy.org/wp-content/uploads/2014/07/ASAN-Q-and-A-on-model-legislature.pdf. Accessed 7 July 2020.

Autistic Self Advocacy Network. (2020a). *Nothing about us without us*. https://autisticadvocacy.org/. Accessed 7 July 2020.

Autistic Self Advocacy Network. (2020b). *Healthcare transition toolkit*. https://autisticadvocacy.org/policy/toolkits/healthtransition/. Accessed 7 July 2020.

Autistic Women & Nonbinary Network. (2020). *Neurodiversity is for everyone*. https://awnnetwork.org/. Accessed 7 July 2020.

Bettleheim, B. (1967). *The empty fortress: Infantile autism and the birth of the self* (p. 1967). Free Press.

Braddock v. Mo. Dep't of Mental Health, 200 S.W.3d 78. (Mo. Ct. App. 2006). https://casetext.com/case/braddock-v-missouri-dept-of-mental-hlt. Accessed 7 July 2020.

Cal. Welf. & Inst. Code § 10962. (2019). https://leginfo.legislature.ca.gov/faces/codes_displaySection.xhtml?sectionNum=10962&lawCode=WIC. Accessed 7 July 2020.
Cohmer, S. (2018). Infantile autism: The syndrome and its implications for a neural theory of behavior (1964), by Bernard Rimland. *The embryo project encyclopedia*. https://embryo.asu.edu/pages/infantile-autism-syndrome-and-its-implications-neural-theory-behavior-1964-bernard-rimland. Accessed 7 July 2020.
Council for Exceptional Children. (2002). *Understanding the differences between IDEA and Section 504*. LD OnLine. https://www.ldonline.org/article/6086/. Accessed 7 July 2020.
Council of Parent Attorneys and Advocates. (2013). *Reinstate prevailing parents' right to expert witness fees*. https://www.copaa.org/page/ExpertWitness. Accessed 7 July 2020.
Dawson, M. (2003). *No autistics allowed: Autism Society Canada speaks for itself—An open letter*. https://www.sentex.ca/~nexus23/naa_js.html. Accessed 7 July 2020.
Dawson, M. (2004). *No autistics allowed one year later: Autism Society Canada builds a Ghetto*. https://www.sentex.ca/~nexus23/naa_one.html. Accessed 7 July 2020.
D.C. Department on Disability Services. (n.d.). *Person-centered thinking philosophy*. https://dds.dc.gov/page/person-centered-thinking-philosophy. Accessed 7 July 2020.
de Wolfe, J. (2014). *Parents of children with autism: An ethnography*. Palgrave Macmillan.
Francisco, S. M., & Martinis, J. G. (2017). *Supported decision-making teams: Setting the wheels in motion*. National Resource Center for Supported Decision-Making. https://www.supporteddecisionmaking.org/sites/default/files/Supported-Decision-Making-Teams-Setting-the-Wheels-in-Motion.pdf. Accessed 7 July 2020.
Fry v. Napoleon Community Schools, 580 U.S. __ (2017). https://www.oyez.org/cases/2016/15-497. Accessed 7 July 2020.
Good v. Iowa Dep't of Human Services, 924 N.W.2d 853. (Iowa 2019). https://casetext.com/case/good-v-iowa-dept-of-human-servs. Accessed 7 July 2020.
Howey, P. (2019). *Key differences between Section 504 and IDEA*. Wrightslaw. https://www.wrightslaw.com/howey/504.idea.htm. Accessed 7 July 2020.
Joseph, B., Magrisso, J., & Schuster, S. (2019). Private rights of action—Remedy for existing violation of Title III. In *Public accommodations under the Americans with Disabilities Act: Compliance and litigation manual*. Thomson Reuters Westlaw. Available via Westlaw Edge. Accessed 7 July 2020.
Kanner, L. (1943). Autistic disturbances of affective contact. *Nervous Child, 2*, 217–250.
Kripke, C. (2016). Supported health care decision-making for people with intellectual and cognitive disabilities. *Family Practice, 33*(5), 445–446. https://doi.org/10.1093/fampra/cmw060.
Lang, A., & Paquette, E. T. (2018). Involving minors in medical decision making: Understanding ethical issues in assent and refusal of care by minors. *Seminars in Neurology, 38*(5), 533–538. https://doi.org/10.1055/s-0038-1668078.
LawHelp.org. (2020). *Helping people find solutions to their legal problems*. https://www.lawhelp.org/. Accessed 7 July 2020.
Legal Services Corporation. (n.d.). *Our Grantees*. https://www.lsc.gov/grants-grantee-resources/our-grantees. Accessed 6 May 2021.
Lovaas, O. I. (1987). Behavioral treatment and normal educational and intellectual functioning in young autistic children. *Journal of Consulting and Clinical Psychology, 55*(1), 3–9.
McCormick, H. (2019). Exhausting administrative remedies—Generally. In *Medicare and Medicaid claims and procedures*. Thomson Reuters Westlaw. Available via Westlaw Edge. Accessed 7 July 2020.
Medicaid and CHIP Payment and Access Commission. (2018). *Elements of the Medicaid appeals process under fee for service, by state*. https://www.macpac.gov/publication/elements-of-the-medicaid-appeals-process-under-fee-for-service-by-state/. Accessed 7 July 2020.
Mo. Rev. Stat. § 536.087. (2019). https://law.justia.com/codes/missouri/2019/title-xxxvi/chapter-536/section-536-087/. Accessed 7 July 2020.

National Council on Disability. (2019). *Turning rights into reality: How guardianship and alternatives impact the autonomy of people with intellectual and developmental disabilities.* https://ncd.gov/sites/default/files/NCD_Turning-Rights-into-Reality_508_0.pdf. Accessed 7 July 2020.

National Health Care for the Homeless Council. (2019). *Documenting disability for medical providers.* https://nhchc.org/online-courses/documenting-disability/. Accessed 7 July 2020.

National Resource Center for Supported Decision-Making. (n.d.). *Everyone has the right to make choices.* https://supporteddecisionmaking.org/. Accessed 7 July 2020.

Nicolaidis, C. (2012). What can physicians learn from the neurodiversity movement? *AMA Journal of Ethics, 14*(6), 503–510.

O'Connell, J. J., Zevin, B. D., Quick, P. D., Anderson, S. F., Perret, Y. M., Dalton, M., & Post, P. A. (Ed). (2007). *Documenting disability: Simple strategies for medical providers.* Health Care for the Homeless Clinicians' Network, National Health Care for the Homeless Council. https://nhchc.org/wp-content/uploads/2019/08/DocumentingDisability2007.pdf. Accessed 7 July 2020.

Oklahoma Department of Human Services. (2015). *Requesting a fair hearing, procedures and appeals from hearing decisions.* https://www.okdhs.org/aboutus/ogc/Pages/hearappeals.aspx. Accessed 7 July 2020.

Oliver, M. (1996). *Understanding disability: From theory to practice.* Palgrave Macmillan.

Osborne, A. G., & Russo, C. J. (2014). *Special education and the law: A guide for practitioners* (3rd edn.). Corwin.

Rimland, B. (1964). *Infantile autism: The syndrome and its implications for a neural theory of behavior.* Appleton-Century-Crofts.

Rothstein, L. (2019). Section 504 and the ADA—Procedural issues. In *Disabilities and the law.* Thompson Reuters Westlaw. Available via Westlaw Edge. Accessed 7 July 2020.

Rothstein, L., & Johnson, S. F. (2014). *Special education law* (5th edn.). Sage.

Ryther, P., & Samuels, B. (2019). Exhaustion of administrative remedies. In *Social Security disability claims: Practice and procedure.* Thompson Reuters Westlaw. Available via Westlaw Edge. Accessed 7 July 2020.

Self Advocates Becoming Empowered. (2020). *Self advocates becoming empowered.* https://www.sabeusa.org/. Accessed 26 June 2020.

Silberman, S. (2015). *Neurotribes: The legacy of autism and the future of neurodiversity.* Penguin Random House.

Sinclair, J. (1993). Don't mourn for us. *Our Voice, 1*(3). https://www.autreat.com/dont_mourn.html. Accessed 7 July 2020.

Smith, T., & Eikeseth, S. (2011). O. Ivar Lovaas: Pioneer of applied behavior analysis and intervention for children with autism. *Journal of Autism and Developmental Disorders, 41,* 375–378. https://doi.org/10.1007/s10803-010-1162-0.

University of California Davis, Center for Excellence in Developmental Disabilities. (2020). *Supported Decision Making (SDM).* https://health.ucdavis.edu/mindinstitute/centers/cedd/sdm.html. Accessed 7 July 2020.

U.S. Administration for Community Living. (2019). *State protection & advocacy systems.* https://acl.gov/programs/aging-and-disability-networks/state-protection-advocacy-systems. Accessed 7 July 2020.

U.S. Department of Education. (n.d.). *About IDEA.* https://sites.ed.gov/idea/about-idea/. Accessed 7 July 2020.

U.S. Department of Education Office of Civil Rights. (2020). *Frequently asked questions about Section 504 and the education of children with disabilities.* https://www2.ed.gov/about/offices/list/ocr/504faq.html. Accessed 7 July 2020.

U.S. Department of Justice Civil Rights Division. (2013). *Filing a complaint with the equal employment opportunity commission.* https://www.ada.gov/filing_eeoc_complaint.htm. Accessed 7 July 2020.

U.S. Department of Justice Civil Rights Division. (2017). *ADA designated investigative services.* https://www.ada.gov/investag.htm. Accessed 7 July 2020.

U.S. Social Security Administration. (2017). *Your right to representation.* https://www.ssa.gov/pubs/EN-05-10075.pdf. Accessed 7 July 2020.
U.S. Social Security Administration. (2019). *Federal court review process.* https://www.ssa.gov/appeals/court_process.html. Accessed 7 July 2020.
US. Social Security Administration. (n.d.-a). *Consultative examinations: A guide for health professionals.* https://www.ssa.gov/disability/professionals/greenbook/ce-evidence.htm. Accessed 7 July 2020.
U.S. Social Security Administration. (n.d.-b). *Appendix 1 to subpart P of Part 404—Listing of impairments.* https://www.ssa.gov/OP_Home/cfr20/404/404-app-p01.htm. Accessed 7 July 2020.
Weber, M. C. (2012). Procedures and remedies under Section 504 and the ADA for public school children with disabilities. *Journal of the National Association of Administration Law Judiciary, 32*(2), 610–647.
WITH Foundation. (2020). *Previous grant recipients.* https://withfoundation.org/previous-grant-recipients/. Accessed 7 July 2020.
Yell, M. L. (2019). *The law and special education* (5th edn.). Pearson.
Zaharia, R., & Moseley, C. (2008). *State strategies for determining eligibility and level of care for ICF/MR and Waiver program participants.* Rutgers Center for State Health Policy. https://www.nasddds.org/uploads/documents/NASDDDS-EligibilityReportFinal.pdf. Accessed 7 July 2020.

Alison Morantz is the James and Nancy Kelso Professor of Law at Stanford University; the Director of the Stanford Intellectual and Developmental Disabilities Law and Policy Project; and a Senior Fellow of the Stanford Institute for Economic Policy Research. Her research focuses on the rights and welfare of individuals with I/DD, and the law and economics of protective labor regulation. A former anti-discrimination advocate, she has been the principal investigator of research projects funded by the National Science Foundation, the Department of Labor, and the National Institute of Occupational Safety and Health.

Chapter 21
Psychological Assessment of Autism Spectrum Disorder and the Law

Lino Faccini and Catherine Burke

Screening, Identification, and the Comprehensive Evaluation of Autism Spectrum Disorders

Autism Spectrum Disorders (ASD) are neurodevelopmental disorders that can be evident as early as 20–24 months of age, but fully manifested before adulthood and are characterized by persistent difficulties with communication, socialization, repetitive behaviors, and particular sensitivities to sensory stimulation. A 2014 Center for Disease Control report estimated that ASDs occur in 1 in 59 children. As a result, the comprehensive assessment of this disorder is essential for the identification, intervention, and providing individuals with a good quality of life. For many individuals, this means being evaluated to establish the condition/disability, eligibility for special educationservices, or adult services from a government agency. When legal disputes arise, the comprehensive evaluation of an ASD could be needed for an impartial administrative special education service appeal or social security Administrative Law/Medicaid fair-hearing (when applying for adult services), as well as to resolve family law matters. An additional reason for the recognition and proper assessment of an ASD is that an individual with this disorder is seven times more likely, than neurotypical peers, to come in contact with the criminal justice system (Curry et al., 1993). As a result, the recognition and proper assessment of an ASD could better inform a court and possibly lead to a lesser sentence due to diminished capacity or mitigation, or for treatment options instead of incarceration. The purpose of this chapter is to identify and describe the identification and comprehensive assessment of an ASD to establish if an individual has the condition, and then to use the evaluation for situations related to educational, ADA accommodations, family law and

L. Faccini (✉)
New York, NY, USA

C. Burke
Division of Law and Psychiatry, Yale School of Medicine, New Haven, USA

F. R. Volkmar et al. (eds.), *Handbook of Autism Spectrum Disorder and the Law*,
https://doi.org/10.1007/978-3-030-70913-6_21

mental health law disputes, and to address competency and criminal responsibility issues for the courts.

For a detailed description of the diagnosis of ASD, please see Chap. 2. Chapter 22 also includes a discussion of assessment, as it relates to risk assessment.

General Principles for Testing in ASD

It is important to point out some general testing considerations that even experienced psychologists may not be familiar with if they do not specialize in ASD. Aside from standard considerations when administering assessments, such as reading level, there are some considerations when selecting tools to evaluate people with ASD. People with co-occurring ADHD may require accommodations to make it through longer self-assessments and care should be taken not to disrupt the standardization of the instrument. Some rating scales, for instance, can be read aloud and the test taker can verbally or gesturally indicate the response.

Language comprehension may be an issue, even among adults who present as very capable. It is important to ensure comprehension during interviews. Asking "do you understand?" is likely insufficient because an adult with ASD may say yes when they do not or may not realize that they do not comprehend. It may be helpful to say "Tell me what that means in your own words" or "Can you tell me what that means to you?". Many adults with autism also require additional structure in order to participate in an evaluation. A list of the steps to be covered, for instance, may make the difference between someone refusing participation and someone completing one.

Interviewees with ASD may have difficulty responding to questions that contain even a small amount of ambiguity. Questions may be interpreted in a literal and concrete manner. If examiners do not ask precisely the right question, they may not understand the information they require. He is prone to misinterpretation when speakers are not precise in their language. In his responses, he may have difficulty knowing what is important to say and what is irrelevant.

Malingering

Little is known about malingering, or feigning symptoms of psychiatric illness in order to obtain secondary gain, of ASD symptoms or malingering, more generally, by people with ASD. There is a possibility, particularly in evaluations to obtain disability benefits or for criminal cases, that the individual is faking or exaggerating symptoms. There are no measures for malingering that have been validated in ASD, and it is possible that measures standardized on general populations are inappropriate for people with ASD because they assume knowledge of social or communication constructs. Additionally, malingering measures tend to consist of orally administered questions, which may be challenging for those with receptive communication deficits.

If a proper, comprehensive evaluation of ASD were conducted, it should be quite difficult for a person to "fake" the disorder in a convincing manner. A comprehensive evaluation includes multiple data sources, which would highlight inconsistencies in reporting and observed characteristics when results were integrated. Furthermore, a trained evaluator has some knowledge of which signs of ASD tend to go together (for instance, one would not expect hand flapping in a highly verbal person), which may make it conspicuous when symptoms are fabricated.

Establishment of the Disability

ASD can be detected as early as approximately 18 months, and reliably by the age of two (Lord et al., 2006). The importance of identifying the disability early is so that services can be provided, and deficits and related needs addressed. The process of establishing the disability can include monitoring, developmental screening, and then a comprehensive diagnostic evaluation. Developmental monitoring involves observing a child for how they attain developmental milestones such as moving, speaking, learning, and socializing. Parents as well as pediatricians would routinely observe, interact, and question the parents/family to ascertain how and when milestones are met. In addition, the American Academy of Pediatrics recommends general developmental screenings, during regular well visits, at the intervals of 9, 18, and then 30 months; in particular, a screening for an ASD should occur during the 18 months and 24 months well visit. During the 18 and 24 month visits, especially if an ASD is suspected or delayed developmental milestones, then a pediatrician might ask the parents to complete a Modified Checklist for Autism Test-Revised with Follow-Up (M-CHAT-R/F developed by Robins et al., 2014). The M-CHAT-R/F is a screening measure where a parent can answer yes-or-no questions regarding their toddler's functioning/social developmental milestones, and the need for a follow-up with additional interview questions if a number of areas present concerns. If a toddler is suspected to be at risk for an ASD, or a developmental delay, then a referral for a more comprehensive evaluation can be made.

Comprehensive Evaluation of an ASD for Establishing the Disability and Obtaining Educational Services

A diagnosis of an ASD can only be made by a qualified practitioner after the completion of a comprehensive evaluation by a trained specialist such as a developmental pediatrician, psychiatrist, or child psychologist. The child may be evaluated by an entire team of early intervention professionals including the previously mentioned practitioners, as well as speech-language pathologists, occupational therapists, and other professionals.

The comprehensive diagnostic evaluation of an ASD would indicate if the individual does have an autism spectrum disorder along with adaptive functioning deficits. In addition, other areas such as academic, communicative, and any other co-occurring disorders, and deficits in independent self-care and management would also be part of the evaluation. This type of evaluation differs from screening and monitoring assessments in that it is comprehensive, and employs a multimethod procedure utilizing multiple informants across settings, as advocated by Volkman et al. (2014); Wilkonson (2010). Wilkonson (2010) asserted that the core of a best practice evaluation of an ASD would entail an assessment of the following areas: a records review, medical screening and/or evaluation, developmental and medical history, direct observation of the individual, parent or caregiver interview, parent and teacher ratings of social competence, a cognitive and academic assessment, and a communication and language assessment. Also, an assessment of behavioral and psychiatric disorders would be important, since they would help determine if these problems or disorders could better account for the symptom picture, and adaptive functioning deficits, or if they are co-occurring with the ASD. Incidentally, this type and scope of evaluation would also apply in answering questions regarding custody evaluations or treatment decisions when these types of situations arise in family court.

Measures of core autism symptomatology, intellectual ability, and adaptive skills are key to diagnostic evaluations. Please see Chap. 2 for a discussion of how these domains are assessed. In addition, an academic assessment is essential to be able to show a profile of strengths and weaknesses to identify that the deficits directly impact one's academic achievement, serving as an argument for special educationservices, and to aid in educational planning. For instance, a number of unusual learning profiles are common among students with ASD, including reading comprehension problems (see Ricketts et al., 2013), and students may require explicit instruction in particular academic areas, such as writing (Pennington & Delano, 2012). A thorough assessment of academic function is needed in some cases in order to pinpoint areas requiring additional support. Commonly used tests that assessment academic achievement includes the Woodcock–Johnson Psychoeducational Battery-Tests of Achievement IV (WJTA IV, Schrank et al., 2014) and the Wechsler Individual Achievement Test II (WIAT II, Wechsler, 2005).

Often, core communication deficits underly learning problems, and communication is an essential area to assess for its own sake, as well as its impact on academic learning. An assessment of communication and language is also essential to understand the strengths and weaknesses of expressive and receptive skills so that communications are tailored to the individual's abilities to facilitate actual understanding versus feigned understanding or acquiescence. Measures of both basic comprehension and use of language, as well as social and pragmatic applications, are appropriate. For a comprehensive assessment of expressive and receptive language, as well as the social and pragmatic aspects of language, the Comprehensive Assessment of Spoken Language 2 (CASL 2, Carrow-Woolfolk, 2017) is a commonly used option.

Finally, an assessment of maladaptive behavior is often needed in school settings. One tool that can be used is the Aberrant Behavior Checklist 2 (ABC, Aman &

Singh, 1994), for ages 5 to adults, to assess such problem behaviors as irritability, social withdrawal, stereotyped behaviors, inappropriate speech, and hyperactivity-noncompliance; also, these problem behaviors can suggest psychiatric conditions that can be further explored for instance, irritability as part of depression, ADHD, PTSD, and Bipolar Disorder, and hyperactivity-noncompliance for depression, ADHD, and Bipolar Disorder.

In summary, the essential task of the comprehensive evaluation is to clearly determine the extent and severity of symptoms of an ASD, that the symptoms/difficulties are not better accounted for by an intellectual disability, language, or psychiatric disorders, or if they all co-occur, and that there is a direct impact of the ASD (either alone or in conjunction with the co-occurring disorders) on the significantly impaired daily adaptive functioning before adulthood. Additionally, for school-aged children, it would recommend a classification, services, and/or school placement to provide an appropriate education. For adults, the comprehensive evaluation would help substantiate the presence of an ASD and adaptive functioning deficits before the age of 22, and serve as evidence to meet the eligibility criteria for that state's adult developmental disability agency to obtain services and/or residential placement.

Assessment of ASD for Special Education Services

Currently, there is a substantial increased demand for evaluations for special education, since ASD is the fastest growing developmental disability in the US (CDC, 2015). A majority of these evaluations are completed for determining eligibility for special education. In regard to obtaining special education services under the Individuals with Disabilities Education Act (IDEA, 1990), six elements are delineated to provide toddlers, children, and adolescents with an ASD an appropriate evaluation, free and appropriate education, individualized educational plan, parent as well as teacher participation in educational planning, learning in the least restrictive environment and other procedural safeguards. Regarding IDEA, "where a school professional believes that a student between the ages of 3 and 21 has a disability that has substantial impact on the student's learning or behavior, the student is entitled to an evaluation in all areas related to the specific disability (APA, 2018). The comprehensive assessment of an ASD is one of several evaluations completed by a multidisciplinary school team of professionals. In addition to satisfying the criteria to enter early intervention and then special education, other situations where a comprehensive evaluation of an ASD is needed to include the parents' requesting an independent evaluation if they don't agree with the school's evaluation, as evidence that a student continues to meet the criteria for services when a school seeks to "declassify" a student as no longer eligible for special education services, and for impartial due process hearings when there is a disagreement in the educational classification, services, or progress made with services.

In regards to legal disputes regarding special education, Hill (2009) reviewed case law regarding an ASD and violations to IDEA for the years 2007 until 2008.

For instance, 83% of these type of cases were heard by district courts and 16% by circuit courts. When reviewing these type of cases by state, Hill (2009) found 11% of the courts in Connecticut and New York involved an ASD and IDEA violations, while for Massachusetts and Pennsylvania, 5% and 18 percent, respectively. Of these cases, for an individual with an ASD, the case involved a violation of an appropriate evaluation in 27% of the cases, a violation in developing an appropriate Individual Educational Plan in 80%, a violation regarding placement in the least restrictive setting occurred in 59% of the cases, failure to provide services 59%, failure to provide an appropriate Functional Behavioral Assessment/Behavioral Intervention Plan in 20%, and that the provided services resulted in no progress occurred in 14% of the cases. A comprehensive evaluation of an ASD is fundamental in addressing or at least informing most of these areas that involve legal disputes of IDEA assurances. As a result, without an appropriate and thorough evaluation of one's autism spectrum disorder, associated difficulties and disorders, the remaining educational tasks of developing an appropriate IEP, how to design learning methodologies to maximuize learning and progress, and the designation of a least restrictive setting is compromised and may result in arbitration or a legal dispute.

Assessment of an ASD, and Obtaining Americans with Disability Act Accommodations

The Americans with Disabilities Act (ADA) was initially signed into civil law in 1990 and then amended in 2008 to include a broader definition of disability, and to prohibit discrimination against individuals with disabilities. The overall intent of the ADA was to make society as a whole more accessible to people with disabilities. The definition of a disability under the ADA includes the following areas: "a physical or mental disability that substantially limits one or more major life areas; having a record of such impairments, or regarded as having such impairments" (Job Accommodation Network, 2012). As a result, certain accommodations, or protections, can be made including the following: accommodations regarding employment (the structuring of jobs, worksites/stations, equipment, providing interpreters), public services (such as transportation and other local and state government services), public accommodations (regarding access to stores, restaurants, private transportation, etc.), telecommunications, and such miscellaneous services as prohibiting abuse, or retaliation against individuals or others attempting to help assert their rights.

In addition, an individual with a disability and substantial functional limitations can qualify for educational accommodations (throughout academic placement including college) under a 504 Accommodation Plan. If the individual's with autism condition and social adaptive functioning do not qualify for special education services, then an evaluation for a 504 accommodation may be completed. The evaluation for 504 accommodations is substantially similar to a comprehensive evaluation of autism in establishing that the individual has autism, associated social adaptive functioning, and most importantly that the functional limitations directly impact their educational and/or vocational performance. In addition to the accommodations identified above, there are educational accommodations that an individual with autism could qualify for (to assist with overcoming barriers that their disability poses to learning or functioning in a job) which includes having pictorial schedules with transition times identified, providing information through multimedia, allowing for extra breaks or more time taking exams, the use of calculators/special computer programs, aids to help improve focus or manage different sensory tasks or situations, etc. In addition, similar to those individuals with autism who qualified for special education, a parent can request an impartial hearing with legal representation when there is a question about the disability that is identified, results of the evaluation, placement, or accommodation(s) granted. Typical issues that could prompt an impartial hearing include a parent believing that their input into the development of the 504 plan was relatively ignored, their requests for various accommodations were denied, the 504 plan was not being followed, or that it was "working" and a change in accommodations is requested.

Assessment of ASD, Mental Health Law, and Eligibility for Adult Services

While youngsters are entitled to educational services under IDEA, when an individual is transitioning into adult services, they must apply and qualify for Medicaid funding and services provided through a government agency. Mental Health and Social Security Disability law informs the Developmental Disability Services agency regarding the qualifying conditions (i.e. developmental disabilities such as an ASD), the functional limitations required, the documentation that must be submitted with the application, review procedures that inform the applicant of findings, and finally the right and procedure for applying for an Administrative Law Medicaid Fair Hearing. For instance, according to the Mental Hygiene Law Section 1.03(22) of NYS, the criteria includes "the presence of a developmental disability (autism being one "qualifying condition"), the disability has occurred before the person reached age 22, be expected to continue indefinitely, or permanently, and cause a substantial handicap (scores which lie at or below 2 standard deviations below the mean) to a person's ability to function in normal society." A comprehensive evaluation of an ASD, provided that it clearly identifies an ASD, and connects the adaptive functioning deficits to the ASD in at least two areas of adaptive functioning (i.e. among communication, daily living, and socialization for instance), all before the age of 22 (although the age may vary by state to state); as a result, the comprehensive evaluation would satisfy as providing the necessary documentation for eligibility.

Due to the increase in the need for the comprehensive evaluation of an ASD, practitioners who specialize in ASD are in great demand, and may charge substantial fees and have waiting lists for evaluations. Often, ASD experienced clinicians are not available or not enlisted for these assessments, and the resulting evaluations do not follow best practice procedures and may miss or overdiagnose cases. In addition, the comprehensive assessment of an ASD is usually outside the scope of practice of a school psychologist, and other than during the initial evaluation for early intervention, the family must usually secure a comprehensive evaluation independent of the school when applying for state developmental disability services. Once again, clinical experience of presenting at Administrative Law Medicaid Fair Hearings usually involves educating the family regarding what constitutes a comprehensive evaluation of an ASD, how mental health law delineates criteria to satisfy, and how to obtain such an evaluation. An overwhelming majority of Fair Hearing cases involve the families providing less than comprehensive evaluations as support for an ASD; this is especially so since a youngster may have been classified since a very early age without an additional comprehensive evaluation. Another frequent issue regards someone applying for adult services as an older adult. Although usually diagnosed in childhood, individuals who are higher functioning and who may not have cognitive or language deficits, may go undetected in their youth. These situations are especially difficult since corroborating developmental reports or even informants may not still be available or provide contradictory information (Fombonne, 2012; Tantam, 2003). In these cases, the practitioner could identify information consistent with an ASD when the individual is in novel situations, during developmental crises, or in situations where the person is overwhelmed (Tantam, 2003) in trying to corroborate the condition.

ASD and Forensic Evaluations for Court

The number of individuals with autism who have come into contact with the legal system has increased significantly in recent years (Murphy, 2016). The impact of legal involvement among people with ASD can be pervasive and irreversible and, due to the nature of the disorder, people with autism can be at a significant disadvantage when facing the legal system. Research has demonstrated that people with this diagnosis can lack the ability to form mens rea (Katz & Zemishlany, 2006), struggle to understand their Miranda rights (Salseda et al., 2011), lack the competency to stand trial (Mayes, 2003), and perform significantly lower than their neurotypical counterparts in their fitness to plead to legal charges (Brewer et al., 2016). Research has found that ASD-related impairments can impact nearly every aspect of a person's experience in the legal system, beginning with their initial interactions with police (Freckelton, 2011).

Miranda v. Arizona (1966) was a landmark case that resulted in a law that mandated police to advise suspects of their rights prior to interrogation. Suspect rights include the right to remain silent, the right to an attorney, the right to a court-appointed attorney if the suspect cannot afford one, and the advisement that anything that the suspect says can be used against them in a court of law. The ruling mandated that confessions should only be admissible in court if the suspect waived *Miranda* rights "knowingly, voluntarily, and intelligently" (*Miranda v. Arizona*, 1966). Many autism-related deficits may decrease a suspect's understanding of *Miranda* rights and thereby nullify the waiver of these rights (Salseda et al., 2011). Furthermore, although people on the spectrum are no more susceptible to suggestibility than neurotypical individuals, the presence of autism can render a suspect increasingly vulnerable to other interrogative techniques and can increase the likelihood of an ill-given confession (North et al., 2008; Maras & Bowler, 2012). This lack of understanding and susceptibility to interrogative techniques can have devastating consequences and significantly diminish the person's ability to successfully navigate the legal system, once charges have been filed.

After being formally accused of a crime, a suspect must be deemed competent to stand trial to ensure the defendant autonomy and the dignity and accuracy of the judicial process (Hoge, 2016). Competency includes understanding several aspects of the legal system, including criminal charges, implications of being a defendant, adversarial nature of proceedings, and the role of court personnel, in addition to the ability to work with an attorney and make important decisions related to the court process (Hoge, 2016). Typical ASD-related deficits may render a person incompetent to stand trial and create numerous barriers navigating the legal system. Impairments in communication can create a significant barrier for a defendant's ability to consult with and assist their own attorney (Mayes, 2003). Defendants with poor abstract reasoning may be unable to differentiate between legal concepts such as plea bargaining and standing trial. Defendants with rigid thought processes may become so fixated on one aspect of the case that they are unable to assist their attorney to defend the totality of their charges.

Given the possible impairments in numerous competencies among people with autism, defendants who are identified as having ASD should be referred for forensic evaluation as early in the legal process as is feasible. Forensic psychologists rely on several assessments to gauge different competencies related to the criminal justice process. However, no assessment tool focused on evaluating competency has been specifically validated for people with ASD. Furthermore, the most commonly utilized tool in competency evaluations has been heavily criticized for lacking normative data and guidelines for even neurotypical defendants (Ryba et al., 2007). Given the unique impairments present in autism, utilizing assessments validated on neurotypical samples will likely inaccurately represent the understanding and performance of someone on the spectrum. Defendants should be referred to clinicians well-trained in both forensics and ASD evaluation.

Once the evaluation begins, both ASD and co-occurring disorders should be assessed for, then the focus of the evaluation turns to examining the degree that the symptoms of the disorder(s) are directly related, or functionally linked, to the commission of the crime. An example where the presence of an ASD, ADHD, and Bipolar Disorders were assessed in a psychiatric evaluation occurred in the case of Trevon Lucas (identified in Xuan & Weiss, 2014). Trevon Lucas threatened to kill and abduct a youth who he had played on an online game. The psychiatrist opined that because of his disorders, Mr. Lucas could not understand the significance of his behavior, especially since the violence was triggered by a manic episode from taking Modafinil (Provigil). However, since the psychiatric evaluation didn't functionally link the specific symptoms of the Asperger's, ADHD and Bipolar Disorders to Mr. Lucas' appreciation of wrongfulness and the commission of the criminal actions, the request for consideration of diminished capacity was denied. Although the court doesn't need to grant diminished capacity, a more cohesive conceptualization where the symptoms were functionally linked with the commission of the crime may have been more convincing.

Overall, there are a number of possible functional relationships between an ASD and crime that should be examined during a court evaluation. The first possibility involves that the full symptom picture of an ASD along with adaptive functioning deficits is functionally unrelated to the crime. For example, the media giving an enormous amount of coverage to rare offenses usually involves a lot of speculation that when someone with an ASD commits a crime it is a direct result of the ASD (Howlin, 2004). Hence, without a clear presentation involving specific symptoms and how they are directly related to the commission of the crime, it is an erroneous assumption that there exists a functional relationship between the ASD and the crime.

An example of this type of erroneous conclusion has occurred in situations with individuals with an ASD who have engaged in mass shootings. Allely and Faccini (2018) completed threat assessment analyses of four individuals with an ASD who engaged in mass shootings. Despite all having a diagnosis of an ASD, the symptoms or features of the ASD were not functionally linked to the commission of the mass shootings. Instead, these individuals engaged in the Path toward Intended Violence, and this path was suggested as the proximal and critical factor accounting for the shootings. The Path to Intended Violence (Calhoun & Weston, 2003) consists of six steps or behaviors, namely having a *grievance* (due to a sense of injustice, loss, destiny, need for fame, or revenge), *ideation* (thinking that violence is the only alternative, discussing one's thoughts with others, or modeling oneself after other assailants), *research/planning* (gathering information regarding one's target, or stalking the target), *preparations* (assembling one's costume, weapon, equipment, transportation, or engaging in "final act" behaviors), *breach* (evaluating security, devising sneaky or covert approaches), and *attack* (as cited in Faccini, 2010). Additionally, Allely and Faccini (2018) suggested that the presence of an ASD or psychiatric disorders, for the small sample of individuals with an ASD who engaged in a mass shooting, were not proximal or critical, and may only serve as more distantly related risk factors.

An example of core features of an ASD interacting with Psychopathology was exemplified in the case of Mr. G, presented in Faccini (2015). Mr. G's ASD was exhibited as a *heightened, fixated preoccupation, and interest* in trains, train schedules, and routes. At an early age, he started playing with trains and cars and then memorized the routines and timetables of particular trains. Also, he would spend his days watching trains, going on train rides, etc. Furthermore, he exhibited difficulties with *central coherence* exemplified when he took control of trains, he viewed this as just running the route, as volunteering, or as a means of getting his foot in the door toward employment without appreciating the social or legal consequences of his actions. In addition, Mr. G presented with *psychopathology* involving unresolved multiple traumas (the victim of 2 serious assaults), and an inconsistently treated cyclothymic mood disorder. Basically, Mr. G's heightened and fixated preoccupation and difficulties with central coherence contributed to him being involved in every aspect related to trains. However, when the traumas occurred, Mr. G escaped what he perceived as a threatening, cold, and unpredictable world into the safety of the train and subway system. Although his life was now restricted to everything trains, he felt safe, a sense of belonging and identity. He regarded the train system as provided him with a complete existence. After the traumas, Mr. G would ride the trains all day, every day. Also, due to his fixation and expert level of knowledge regarding trains, he repeatedly applied for a job with the train system. Since Mr. G wasn't hired, he eventually developed a depression, and eventually engaged in repeated train-related offenses across at least five US states. Essentially, Mr. G's autism-based deficits interacted with psychopathology (unresolved traumas and a cyclothymic disorder) contributing to criminal arrests.

In conclusion, the psychological assessment of autism was presented as completing a comprehensive diagnostic assessment, identifying any particular symptoms or "core features" that are important and critical, as well as the presence of other disorders, which directly impact adaptive functioning. Secondarily, comprehensive evaluations are needed for obtaining special education services, as well as subsequently transitioning into adult developmental disability services; as a result, the practitioner will need to be mindful of the special education and mental health law requirements to assist in framing the evaluation. Finally, psychological evaluations for the court should be ordered as soon as impairment is detected and should clearly functionally relate the core symptoms or features to the legal question or crime that was committed. Forensic assessments should be done by psychologists well-trained in both ASD and forensics. Also presented were the possibilities that there could be no functional relationship between the ASD and the crime, certain features of autism apply, or core symptoms or features of an ASD could interact with psychiatric disorders in accounting for the criminal activity. When there is a functional connection between an ASD and a crime, this clearly formulated conceptualization may support a claim for diminished capacity or mitigation in court cases.

References

Allely, C. S., & Faccini, L. (2018). A conceptual analysis of individuals with an Autism spectrum disorder engaging in mass violence. *Journal of Forensic and Crime Studies, 1*(1), 1–5.

Aman, M. G., & Singh, N. N. (1994). *Aberrant behavior checklist 2 (ABC-2).* Stoelting Company.

American Psychological Association. (2018). Regarding IDEA. www.americanpsychologicalassociation.org/advocacy/education/idea/index.apx. Accessed 23 July 2018.

Brewer, R. J., Davies, G. M., & Blackwood, N. J. (2016). Fitness to plead: The impact of autism spectrum disorder. *Journal of Forensic Psychology Practice, 16*(3), 182–197.

Calhoun, F. S., & Weston, S. W. (2003). *Contemporary threat management: A practical guide for identifying, assessing, and managing individuals of violent intent.* Specialized Training Services.

Carion-Woolfolk. (2017). *Comprehensive assessment of spoken language-2 (CASL-2).*Western Psychological Services.

Centers for Disease Control and Prevention. (2015). *Facts about ASD*. www.cdc.gov/ncddd/autism/facts.html. Accessed 1 July 2018.
Curry, K., Posluszny, M., & Kraska, S. (1993). *Training criminal justice personnel to recognize offenders with disabilities*. Office of Special Education and Rehabilitative Services News. In Print.
Eligibility Guidelines for the Office for People with Developmental Disabilities, New York State Mental Hygiene Law Section 1.03.
Faccini, L. (2010). The man who howled wolf: Diagnostic and treatment considerations for a person with ASD and impersonal repetitive fire, bomb and presidential threats. *American Journal of Forensic Psychiatry, 31*(4), 47–68.
Faccini, L. (2015). Autism, psychopathology, and deficient Eriksonian development contributing to criminal behavior. *American Journal of Forensic Psychology, 33*(1), 1–17.
Fombonne, E. (2012). Autism in adult life. *Canadian Journal of Psychiatry, 57*(5), 273–274.
Freckelton, I. (2011). Asperger's disorder and the criminal law. *Journal of Law and Medicine, 18*(4), 677–694.
Hill, D. A. (2009). Examination of case law 2007–2009 regarding Autism spectrum disorder violation of the individuals with disabilities educational act. https://www.tandfonlinr.com/doi/abs/10.1080.1045988/2010.542784. Accessed 1 July 2018.
Hoge, S. K. (2016). Competence to stand trial: An overview. *Indian Journal of Psychiatry, 58*(Suppl2), S187–S190
Howlin, P. (2004). *Autism and asperger's syndrome: Preparing for adulthood*. Routledge.
Individual with Disabilities Education Act (IDEA). (1990). https://en.wikipedia.org/wiki/Individuals_with_Disabilities_Education_Act. Accessed 24 July 2018.
Job Accommodation Network. (2012). *The American with disabilities acts: A brief overview*. https://asjan.org/articles/The-Americans-with-Disabilties-Act-A-Brief-Overview. Accessed 16 April 2020.
Katz, N., & Zemishlany, Z. (2006). Criminal responsibility in Asperger's syndrome. *Israel Journal of Psychiatry and Related Sciences, 43*(3), 166–173.
Lord, C., Risi, S., DiLavore, P. S., Shulman, C., & Pickles, T. A. (2006). Autism from 2 to 9 years of age. *Archives of General Psychiatry, 63*(6), 694–701.
Maras, K. L., & Bowler, D. M. (2012). Brief report: Suggestibility, compliance and psychological traits in high-functioning adults with autism spectrum disorder. *Research in Autism Spectrum Disorders, 6*(3), 1168–1175.
Mayes, T. A. (2003). Persons with autism and criminal justice: Core concepts and leading cases. *Journal of Positive Behavior Interventions, 5*(2), 92–100.
Miranda v. Arizona, 384 U.S. 436. (1966).
Murphy, D. (2016). Sense and sensibility: Forensic issues with autism spectrum disorders. In B. Barahona Correa, R.-J. van der Gaag (Eds.), *Assessment of autism spectrum disorder: Critical issues in clinical, forensic, and school settings* (pp. 247–266). Springer.
New York Consolidated Laws, Mental Hygiene Law. https://codes.findlaw.com/ny/mental-hygiene-law/. Accessed 22 July 2018.
New York State Office for People with Developmental Disabilities. OPWDD Eligibility Criteria for Services. https://www.opwdd.ny.gov/opwdd-services-supports/eligibility. Accessed 24 July 2018.
North, A. S., Russell, A. J., & Gudjonsson, G. H. (2008). High functioning autism spectrum disorders: An investigation of psychological vulnerabilities during interrogative interview. *The Journal of Forensic Psychiatry & Psychology, 19*(3), 323–334.
Pennington, R. C., & Delano, M. E. (2012). Writing instruction for students with autism spectrum disorders: A review of literature. *Focus on Autism and Other Developmental Disabilities, 27*(3), 158–167.
Ricketts, J., Jones, C. R., Happé, F., & Charman, T. (2013). Reading comprehension in autism spectrum disorders: The role of oral language and social functioning. *Journal of Autism and Developmental Disorders, 43*(4), 807–816.

Robins, D., Casagrande, K., Barton, M., Chen, C.-M., Dumont-Mathieu, T., & Fein, D. (2014). Validation of the modified checklist for Autism in toddlers, Revised, with Follow-up (M-CHATR/F). *Pediatrics, 133*(1), 37–45.

Ryba, N. L., Brodsky, S. L., & Shlosberg, A. (2007). Evaluations of capacity to waive Miranda rights: A survey of practitioners' use of the Grisso instruments. *Assessment, 14*(3), 300–309.

Salseda, L. M., Dixon, D. R., Fass, T., Miora, D., & Leark, R. A. (2011). An evaluation of Miranda rights and interrogation of autism spectrum disorders. *Research in Autism Spectrum Disorders, 5*, 79–85.

Schrank, F., Mather, N., McCrew, K., Wendling, B. S., & Woodcock, R.W. (2014). *Woodcock Johnson psychoeducational battery-tests of achievement IV*. Riverside Publishing.

Tantam, D. (2003). The challenge of adolescents and adults with Asperger Syndrome. *Child and Adolescent Psychiatric Clinics of North America, 12*, 143–163.

Volkman, F., Siegel, M., Woodbury-Smith, M., et al. (2014). Practice parameters for the assessment and treatment of children and adolescents with Autism spectrum disorders. *Journal of the American Academy of Child and Adolescent Psychiatry, 53*(2), 237–257.

Wechsler, D. (2005). *Wechsler individual achievement test* (2nd ed., WIAT-II). The Psychological Corporation.

Wilkonson, L. A. (2010). *A Best practice guide to assessment and intervention for Autism and Asperger's syndrome in schools*. Jessica Kingsley Publishers.

Xuan, Y., & Weiss, K. J. (2014). Diminished capacity or aggravating factor in sentencing? *The Journal of the American Academy and the Law, 42*(2), 242–243.

Lino Faccini Ph.D., is a school, clinical and forensic psychologist in New York.

Catherine Burke PsyD, is an Assistant Professor in the Law & Psychiatry Division at the Yale School of Medicine. Dr. Burke's expertise is in forensic assessment conducting evaluations for the legal system, including competency to stand trial, mitigation, risk assessment, and immigration, among others.

Chapter 22
Violence Risk Assessment in Autism Spectrum Disorder (ASD)

Alexander Westphal and Rachel Loftin

Research on the assessment of risk for violence in autism spectrum disorder (ASD) is very limited, despite acts of violence that have been linked to ASD in news stories. Few empirical studies exist alongside more numerous, but still limited, case reports on violence in ASD. In this chapter, we introduce the general topic of violence risk assessment, describe some of the risk factors for violence identified in the literature as having an association with ASD, and outline a structured framework for risk assessment of violence in a clinical context. The literature on the association between ASD and violence is covered elsewhere in this book.

The news media has made conjectural associations between ASD and premeditated acts of violent offending on multiple occasions. Even medical journals have published a number of clinical case reports on violence and ASD. The case reports are almost invariably about the most extreme cases and situations, giving the impression that sensational episodes of planned violence are common in ASD, or at least that such episodes make up a significant percentage of the violent acts committed by people with ASD. Additionally, they add legitimacy to the news stories.

However, planned acts of mass violence (sometimes known as predatory violence) are very rare in ASD. Impulsive acts of aggression (sometimes known as affective violence), which often target caregivers and family members are much more common. Impulsive violence is most common in those with ASD and intellectual disability, a group which forms a significant minority of the population with ASD (estimates range from 38% in a CDC analysis (Baio, 2012) to 47% in an Italian sample (Postorino

A. Westphal (✉)
Division of Law and Psychiatry, Yale University, New Haven, CT, USA
e-mail: alexander.westphal@yale.edu

R. Loftin
Department of Psychiatry and Behavioral Sciences, Northwestern University
Feinberg School of Medicine, Chicago, USA
e-mail: Rachel.loftin@northwestern.edu

F. R. Volkmar et al. (eds.), *Handbook of Autism Spectrum Disorder and the Law*,
https://doi.org/10.1007/978-3-030-70913-6_22

et al., 2016). Violence in this population is often attributed to communication deficits, and aggressive outbursts are often managed through behavioral interventions, such as functional communication training. In other situations, environmental manipulation, such as ensuring consistency on one's daily routines or minimizing overwheleming sensory stimulation, can help prevent aggressive outbursts. Risk assessment is not an appropriate tool for the ongoing management of impulsive violence because the risk is known in these situations, and programming and placement needs to be organized around the risk in an active and continuous fashion.

And risk assessment approaches are unlikely to pick up on acts of mass violence, because of their sporadic and rare nature (discussed in more detail below). This raises the question of when the process of risk assessment has utility. Risk assessment is most useful in a clinical context when someone has made threats or has concerning interests or behaviors, and providers need to know how seriously to take the risk and what they need to do to manage it.

Violence Risk Assessment in Typical Population

A lot is known about violence risk assessment in the population without ASD. The breadth of the field is described in a paper by Singh et al. (2014), who surveyed 2135 mental health professionals from 44 countries that had conducted at least one risk assessment during their careers. The majority (58%) used some sort of structured instrument to conduct a risk assessment, and over 400 instruments were described. Of these, approximately half were available to other clinicians; the remainder were developed for individual or institutional use. None, however, were designed for assessing risk in the population with ASD. Below we discuss some of the approaches to risk assessment in the population without ASD to provide context for further discussion.

Clinicians often approach risk assessment using "clinical judgement," creating risk profiles that are tailored to the individual on a case by case basis and result in a detailed, dynamic, and qualitative portrait of the individual and their risk. This approach integrates information about the "patient's personality, symptoms and environment with [the clinician's] understanding of the likely causes of violence" (Buchanan et al., 2015). Despite these benefits, clinical judgment approaches, used alone, have substantial limitations. By definition, they are unstructured and idiosyncratic, therefore not reproducible or transparent.

Clinical judgment approaches are often contrasted with "actuarial" approaches, sometimes called "non-discretionary approaches," which are based on a body of research that has identified risk factors across groups of subjects, and uses the results to make predictions about the risk of individuals. The results of actuarial assessments are quantitative, allowing them to be compared over time and populations. The use of actuarial approaches, alone, also has problems resulting mainly from applying facts derived from aggregate data to the individual. A fundamental problem with an exclusive, actuarial approach is the rarity of certain acts of violence. In principle, the more rarely an event occurs the more difficult it is to predict, which leaves the occasional true prediction lost in the noise of false positives. This problem is also at the core of a clinical predicament: If a positive prediction of violence on the measure is very likely a false positive, treating everyone who tests positive, for example, by admitting them to psychiatric hospitalizations, would be completely untenable. Further, a purely actuarial approach would inevitably miss people from lower risk categories who will act violently.

Structured Professional Judgment (SPJ) approaches combine clinical judgment and actuarial approaches into a predetermined interview structure, that is "discretionary in essence but relies on evidence-based guidelines to systematize the exercise of discretion" (Hart et al., 2016) There are risk assessment instruments that use SPJ to accomplish this task, for example, the HCR-20 (Webster et al., 1997).

The American Psychiatric Association Resource Document on Psychiatric Violence Risk Assessment (Buchanan et al., 2015) identifies the most important risk factors, including a history of prior arrests, substance abuse, exposure to trauma/abuse, antisocial personality, anger control issues, head injuries leading to loss of consciousness, as well as demographic factors, including age, gender, and employment status.

The MacArthur Violence Risk Assessment Study identified psychopathy as the most powerful predictor of violence. It also found identifies a mental health diagnosis, and several other well-established risk factors that include gender, prior violence, childhood experiences of physical abuse, and socioeconomic status (Monahan et al., 2005). The study also identified risk factors related to the symptoms of mental illness. The presence of delusions was not related to violence, even though a "suspicious attitude" was. Hallucinations, including "command" ones did not increase the risk of violence. Command hallucinations, however, in which the subject was commanded to act violently did increase the risk. Additionally, thoughts or fantasies about harming others also increased risk.

As discussed above, mental illness has been identified as a risk factor for violence. The relationship between mental illness and violence is a complex one, and is relevant to ASD in that a number of mental illnesses occur at higher rates in the population with ASD. However, it is also clear that conventional risk factors, including, but not limited to mental illness, may play out differently in ASD. In addition, factors which might not heighten risk in the general population may be very important in ASD, and need to be incorporated into any risk assessment. All of this said, the risk factors which have been established in the typical population are important to factor into the process of risk assessment for violence in ASD, and we recommend using a tool, such as the HCR-20, to capture them.

Violence Risk Assessment in ASD

There is some research on specific risk factors in ASD. This information comes from screening violent populations for ASD (e.g., Scragg & Shah, 1994), screening populations with ASD for violence (e.g., Mouridsen et al., 2008), and intervention studies for aggression (e.g., McCracken et al., 2002). The most descriptive information on risk factors in ASD does not come from systematic research, but rather from the case report literature (Im, 2016). When the case report literature is combined with the research, some recurrent themes emerge. These are discussed in more detail in the following sections.

In a total population-based record-linkage cohort (the Stockhom Youth Cohort) in Sweden, Heeramun et al. (2017) looked at convictions for violent crimes, and the associated risk and protective factors in 5,739 individuals with ASD aged between 15 and 27 years. They found that male sex and psychiatric conditions were the strongest predictors of violent criminality, along with parental criminal and psychiatric history and socioeconomic characteristics, mirroring the findings in the typical population. There was some evidence that a delayed diagnosis of autism was associated with a greater risk of violent crime. Better school performance and intellectual disability appeared to be protective.

Specific Risk Factors: Comorbid Psychiatric Conditions

In particular, research has helped to identify comorbid conditions that increase the risk for violence in ASD. Långström et al. (2009) found higher rates of violence in people with ASD and comorbid psychiatric conditions (67.7 vs 21.5%) in a study ($n = 422$) of recently hospitalized teenagers and adults with the diagnosis. Specifically, they found that comorbid schizophrenia or other psychosis increased the risk for violence (25.8 vs 9.2%), as did substance use disorder (16.1 vs 0.5%) and personality disorder (9.7 vs 1.5%). On the other hand, depressive disorder appeared to be protective (0.0 vs 3.8%). They identified limitations of the findings: "Notably, the prevalence of psychiatric comorbid diagnoses could reflect not only true comorbidities but also that ASDs may be difficult to diagnose, requiring nuanced appreciation of both symptoms, onset, and course of illness" (p. 5). They concluded that "assessment and management of co-occurring psychopathology may be helpful to reduce violence risk in individuals with ASD" (p. 11) make sure makes sense.

In the Stockholm Youth Cohort study mentioned above, Heeramun et al. (2017) found that although individuals with ASD, particularly those without intellectual disability, initially appeared to have a higher risk of violent offending (adjusted relative risk = 1.39, 95% CI = 1.23–1.58), these "associations markedly attenuated after co-occurring attention-deficit/hyperactivity disorder (ADHD) or conduct disorder were taken into account (adjusted relative risk = 0.85, 95% CI = 0.75–0.97)." The case report literature adds other risk factors, including mood disturbances, in particular mania, and paraphilias, however, these have not been evaluated by research studies.

Specific Risk Factors: Social-Cognitive Deficits

Case reports of violence in ASD suggest deficits in social cognition, or the ways in which people process and store information about other people, is a risk factor for violence. Social cognition includes two dimensions of empathy: affective and cognitive. Affective empathy includes sharing another's emotional state (emotional resonance; Blair, 2005), while "theory of mind" refers to understanding why people behave in certain ways and predicting future behavior (Baron-Cohen, 2000).

Both the affective and cognitive aspects of social cognition are implicated in some case reports involving people with ASD who commit violent crimes. Among clinicians and researchers, it is generally believed that people with ASD have intact affective empathy, while they demonstrate specific deficits in cognitive empathy (see Jones et al., 2010; Lockwood et al., 2013; Schwenck et al., 2012). In contrast to the expected pattern of intact affective empathy and impaired cognitive empathy in ASD, the typical profile of someone with antisocial personality disorder or psychopathy is the opposite, limited affective empathy and well-developed cognitive empathy, which is required to manipulate others. However, these profiles are likely more complex than it appears, as there are very few studies involving violent offenders with ASD, and some studies with more general ASD populations also find a difference in affective empathy within an individual with ASD based on the positive or negative valence of the stimuli.

It is easy to see why reduced affective empathy is associated with violent offending. Offenders who experience less emotional empathy are, by definition, less affected by others' suffering and, thus, may be more capable of performing acts of severe aggression (Winter et al., 2017). The skills to recognize and consider another person's perspective (cognitive empathy or theory of mind) is also directly related to social behavior, and deficits in this area may make one more likely to commit violence against another person (e.g., Heleniak & McLaughlin, 2019). An example of cognitive empathy is a perpetrator with ASD who experiences surprise that their violent actions upset their family members (who were not the direct victims). People with intact theory of mind would have no difficulty predicting that outcome and others' responses to their action would, quite likely, be considered before the person took action.

The literature also mentions moral reasoning as a deficit that may contribute to offending risk in people with ASD (Constantino, 2016). Moral reasoning is defined as the process by which a person deems an action worthy of praise or criticism. This reasoning process requires, by definition, capacity to consider another's internal states, intentions, and beliefs. Interestingly, given the high social cognitive demands of moral reasoning, some studies have found intact moral reasoning in samples of people with ASD (e.g., Blair, 2008). Others, such as Buon and colleagues, found subtle difficulties with moral judgments among people with ASD (2013).

To further complicate the picture, social cognitive problems often exist in people who do not have ASD and may also be related to violence as well. For instance, homicide offenders with schizophrenia demonstrate marked social cognitive deficits (Engelstad et al., 2019). The presence of other psychiatric conditions along with ASD can also exacerbate social cognitive difficulties. Psychotic traits in a person with ASD may decrease performance on cognitive theory of mind tasks (Gillespie et al., 2017), and worsening of ADHD symptoms can limit social attention required for many social cognitive functions.

ASD is a complex disorder that includes a range of presentations. There is not yet enough information to conclude whether there is a distinct social-cognitive profile among people with ASD who commit violent crimes. Rather, it is important to understand the functioning of the individual and how their unique pattern of strengths and deficits in social cognition affects the behavior associated with their case.

Specific Risk Factors: Social Exclusion

Not much is known about the role of social exclusion (loneliness, ostracism and romantic rejection) in violent offending by people with ASD. However, social isolation is thought to be a key risk factor in general (Fazel et al., 2018), and social isolation is common in ASD, as difficulty forming relationships is diagnostic of the condition. It is known that social relationships are critical to mental health and social well-being (Wang et al., 2017). Isolation can exacerbate co-occurring mental health conditions, such as depression and psychosis and can even have a negative impact on insight (White et al., 2000).

Bullying, intentional and repetitive exposure to situations that are deliberately hurtful and over which the victim has no power to stop or control the situation (Olweus, 2013), is suggested by some researchers (e.g., Constantino, 2016) as a risk factor for violence in ASD. In general populations, bullying may increase risk of violent behaviors including suicide (see Kim et al., 2009). Certainly, people with ASD are at risk of both perpetration and, more often, victimization of bullying, and bullying is particularly problematic in school settings (Maiano et al., 2016).

Involuntary social isolation may occur after someone repeatedly tries but fails to make friends or develop romantic relationships. Most autistic people who feel isolated remain lonely, meet people in person, or seek to join online communities that offer a sense of shared community, such as interest-related online communities and self-advocacy networks. A small subset, however, may join groups that offer a sense of identity and belonging through extremist ideology. One example is the INCEL movement, or "involuntary celibate." INCEL is an online community across several platforms that include men who are unsuccessful at finding sexual partners and assert that women and feminism are the reason they cannot find a partner. Members have been described as "self-radicalized," buying into a misogynistic belief system about the origin of their challenges, and a handful of instances of mass violence have now been committed by people who identify as INCELs (Emba, 2019), including by people who were also identified as having ASD.

In contrast, social affiliations and prosocial experiences are highly protective and mitigate against a range of risks. It is important, therefore, to understand an individual's integration into the community and the quality of his relationships in order to fully evaluate risk.

Specific Risk Factors: Executive Functioning Deficits

The case reports often cite executive functioning deficits as contributors to violence risk in ASD. The term "executive function" refers to the set of cognitive skills necessary for goal-directed problem solving, including working memory, inhibitory control, and set shifting/flexibility (Carlson et al., 2013). In ASD, deficits in executive function are considered common and significant contributors to the social communication deficits that are characteristic of the disorder (i.e., Happé et al., 2006; Kenworthy et al., 2008; Klin et al., 2003).

Difficulty inhibiting impulsive responses is a feature in a handful of psychiatric disorders. ADHD co-occurs with ASD quite commonly in the general population, while psychotic disorders commonly co-occur in cases of violent offending. In the population-based study in Sweden discussed above, Heeramun and colleagues (2017) found that people with ASD, when co-occurring ADHD and conduct disorder are controlled, are at no greater risk for criminal violence.

Behavioral rigidity, the result of executive dysfunction that inhibits normal flexibility when changing activities and adjusting to situational requests, is often noted in ASD (Happé et al., 2006). Challenges to rigidity can cause reactive aggression, as described in "Other Risks Associated with Affective Violence Risk" section below. Additionally, stressful life events are commonly cited as a risk factor for violence (Silver & Teasdale, 2005). It seems reasonable to assume that people with ASD, who tend to be particularly sensitive to change and who may have very limited problem solving or coping capacities, might be differentially impacted.

It seems reasonable to assume that the executive function of emotion regulation directly relates to violence because one's ability to regulate negative emotions can restrain that person from violence (McNulty & Hellmuth, 2008). In ASD, poor emotion regulation has been linked to uncontrolled outbursts and aggression, as well as self injury (Mazefsky & White, 2014). However, research investigations of emotion regulation and its relationship to violence in ASD are limited to bullying perpetration among adolescents with ASD (Rieffe et al., 2012), and the extent to which emotion regulation impacts *planned* acts of violence is not clear.

Specific Risk Factors: Circumscribed Interests, Routines, Rituals

Circumscribed interests are a common feature of autism, yet they remain poorly understood. The term "circumscribed interests" refers to the tendency for people with ASD to have interests that are intense. Little research has been done since a 2007 article outlining the need for more study (Klin et al., 2003) in this area. The authors reported most people with autism (88% of elementary-age participants with intact IQ) in their sample demonstrated circumscribed interests. Intense interests are not necessarily a problem, but they can greatly interfere with development of other skills and interests, as well as developmental of self-help skills and socialization.

Even less is known about how circumscribed interests may contribute to violence risk, although they appear to play a role, as offenders are more likely than nonoffenders to be interested in violent content (Woodbury-Smith & Dein, 2014). The mere topic of a person's interest may not provide information about whether that interest is violent, however. An interest in a specific war, for instance, may be limited to dates or facts about historical figures for some, while others may be focused on weapons of war and their destructive capabilities. Of course, even an interest in an extremely violent topic may not lead to offending.

Like circumscribed interests, insistence on particular routines is a core feature of ASD that is frequently present but not necessary for diagnosis. For some, the routine may include following a specific route to work each day and becoming upset if forced to detour. Others' routines may have a more compulsive quality, such that the person feels under pressure to complete the activity in a certain sequence or a certain number of times. This may include closing all of the bedroom doors any time they are home or making sure that items are arranged "just so" in their bedroom before going to sleep. When another person interferes with an expected routine or compulsion, the person with ASD can experience distress and may strike out.

Specific Risk Factors: Sensory Issues

Atypical responses to sensory input are a common feature of ASD which, in turn, can pose a risk for aggression (Murphy, 2010). A person may be diagnosed with ASD without demonstrating sensory processing differences, but most experience and under or over-response to sensory stimuli. When individuals are hypersensitive to stimuli, a smell, sound, sight, or touch that may not be upsetting to a typically developing person is perceived as highly distressing. In an attempt to stop the sensory input, the person with ASD person may push, hit or demonstrate other forms of aggression. A hyposensitive individual may be too rough, such as slamming into others, in an attempt to seek sensory stimulation. For example, Mawson et al. (1985) describe a man who assaulted a crying child at a railway station by placing his hands over the child's mouth to stop the sound of crying.

Assessment of Risk Factors

Given that ASD presents risk factors for violence that may be either unique to ASD, or modified by it, a framework for approaching risk assessment in this population is warranted. We recommend a Structured Professional Judgment (SPJ) approach (discussed earlier in the chapter), an approach which combines clinical judgment and actuarial approaches into a predetermined interview structure. The overall purpose of the approach is to generate an assessment of risk made on the basis of clinical interview, collateral interviews, and a history and record review, with the purpose of identifying and assessing both standard and ASD-related risk factors.

In terms of risk factors that are shared with the typical population, it is important to review school discipline records and speak with the family about types of violence which may not have been reported to the authorities, including domestic abuse and bullying, in addition to reviewing prior offenses. Information on substance use is also needed, an underappreciated risk in ASD. ADHD and social anxiety, which both occur at a high rate in people with ASD, are often linked to increase use of substances. There are many reports of people with ASD who use illegal drugs or marijuana (which is legal in many countries, as well as in parts of the US) to manage social anxiety or inattention.

The presence of an intellectual disability or developmental disability is an important consideration. Cognitive or intellectual profiles may not be a direct predictor of risk, but the unusual profiles that often occur in ASD have implications for information processing that may be related to social perceptions, language comprehension, and other challenges that can indirectly lead to violence.

Assessing for commonly co-occurring psychiatric conditions is necessary, as it is in non-ASD populations. Assessment of these often relies on self-report measures, such as rating scales or symptom checklists. This can be problematic because such measures rely on the individual having insight into his challenges, which people with ASD often do not, and willingness to report. The combination of self-report measures, clinical interview, and input from caregivers or close relatives can be helpful in determining whether co-occurring psychiatric conditions are present. Notably, many people with ASD use affect or tone of voice that does not match their internal state and, as such, caution should be used when applying observations from the mental status exam to diagnosis. Data from the MSE should be considered alongside other data points and not the sole determinant of co-occurring diagnoses.

In their practice guidelines, the American Academy of Psychiatry and the Law (AAPL, 2015) specifies:

> It is important to develop a diagnostic formulation that explains the evaluee's symptoms and signs and their relevance to the psycholegal question at issue. If symptoms and signs allow a diagnosis that is in accordance with the current categories of the Diagnostic and Statistical Manual of Mental Disorders (DSM) or the International Classification of Diseases (ICD), it should be so assigned. In North America, the DSM is the most frequently used reference, is familiar to attorneys and courts, and should therefore be used wherever possible.

More information about assessing for co-occurring conditions is in Chap. 2 of this book. To supplement the standard clinical interview and mental status exam, a number of rating scales and direct assessments of psychiatric conditions are available. Unfortunately, few of these tools have been validated for use in this population, and there is a real need for tools designed specifically for assessing comorbidity in ASD. There may also be a question of how well some people with ASD can respond to questions that require self-reflection (Pearl et al., 2016). Until better options are available, it is a reasonable approach to use existing assessment tools but to consider their limitations with this population in their interpretation.

Assessment of ASD-associated traits. Assessment of social-cognitive effects of ASD and other psychiatric problems, including perspective taking, empathy, and moral reasoning, can be challenging. Information about ASD-related symptoms should be collected using a variety of approaches: direct assessment, caregiver interview, rating scales, records review, and clinical interview. Caregiver interview is often a good source of information about a number of social risk factors.

The "gold standard" evaluation for ASD includes a few components: developmental history, IQ, adaptive, and a direct assessment of autism features, such as the Autism Diagnostic Observation Schedule, Second Edition (ADOS-2; Lord et al., 2012). See Chap. 2 for more information about the comprehensive evaluation process.

Additional information, beyond what is elicited during the ADOS-2 and a thorough development history, is helpful in understanding the specific areas of challenge. Use of other tools, such as the Social Responsiveness Scale (SRS-2; Constantino, 2012), a measure of the presence and severity of ASD-associated social impairment, can be useful in collecting information relevant to a forensic evaluation. SRS-2 scores are broken into five domains, including social cognition. The Empathy Quotient (EQ; Baron-Cohen & Wheelwright, 2004), a self-report measure of empathy, also adds valuable information that is often difficult to elicit in traditional clinical interviews.

Evaluation of social engagement is also important. People with ASD vary widely in their degree of social motivation and interest in relationships. Some are content to not have friendships, while others have several close friends. A person who does not desire friendships would not be very affected by a solitary life. In contrast, a person who wants contact but is alone may experience great distress. It is important to assess for the degree of social isolation of an individual, relative to the degree to which the person is impacted by isolation. Teasing apart the personal impact of social isolation can be challenging because people who have experienced social failures may learn to deny wanting friends in the first place, in order to reduce embarrassment or mitigate against the pain of loneliness. The evaluator may need to speak to caregivers and review the history, in addition to asking ADOS-2 questions that directly pertain to friendship, to gauge the degree of isolation.

Assessment of executive function deficits. A range of executive functioning deficits have been reported to occur in ASD. For some individuals, a complete neuropsychological evaluation may be appropriate to fully assess all domains of executive functioning. Cognitive flexibility and emotional regulation are, perhaps, of most relevance to violence risk assessment, as these are noted most often in the case reports.

To evaluate cognitive flexibility, anecdotes from caregivers, observations during the evaluation of the individual and history can all provide valuable information about cognitive flexibility and emotion regulation. Rating scales, such as the *Behavior Rating Inventory of Executive Function* (BRIEF), can be used to collect information from both caregivers and clients. Direct assessments, including card sort tasks and other specialized psychological tests, can be collected as well. Some rating scales provide information about emotion regulation.

Clinicial interviews and review of records may be particularly useful for assessing emotion regulation. In particular, records from functional behavior assessments and school discipline reports may provide crucial information about emotion regulation.

Restricted Interests. Information about restricted interests normally comes through interviews. Caregivers tend to be aware of most restricted interests (with the exception of any the individual deliberately kept private), and people with ASD are often very eager to share information about their interests when they are asked. There are exceptions, of course. Some people with ASD who have been ridiculed for an interest or have developed embarrassment about it may be less forthcoming. In some criminal cases in which a person with ASD is a defendant, the internet search history is available. This would likely provide information about the areas of interest. Tools like the Repetitive Behavior Scale, Revised (RBS-R) can be helpful to collect global information, but they tend not to provide sufficient detail about the types of interests for risk assessment. In particular, it is important to elicit information about interests related to violence, such as weapons and acts of extreme violence (mass shootings, for instance).

Sexual Compulsions/Frustration. Interviews may be helpful in learning about sexual compulsions and/or frustration. Many people with ASD are willing to discuss sexual content and may do so with less embarrassment than typically developing people. Thus, caregivers will sometimes have information about an individual's sexual history. Others, however, are less forthcoming and may not disclose sexual behaviors. In those situations, direct interviews will be challenging, and family members may be completely unaware of any sexual behaviors or desires. Depending upon the nature of the situation, a more in-depth sexual risk evaluation may be warranted. In that case, it is important that the evaluator is experienced and trained in ASD. As was the case with restricted interests, the internet search history, which may be part of the discovery in certain cases, can shed light onto sexual interests or, at least, types of pornography viewed.

Other Risks Associated with Affective Violence Risk. There are some risk factors that have little relevance to planned acts of violence but are important to consider in situations in which affective violence is a concern. Insistence on routines and upset when routines are interrupted or challenged can lead to outbursts of aggression. Typically the best way to assess this risk is through a functional behavior assessment (FBA), which is an assessment of a target behavior to learn more about the behavior, why it occurs and what factors maintain the behavior. A formal FBA may not be necessary. Sometimes informal collection of behavioral data (such as an antecedent, behavior, consequence chart on which caregivers note each time the target behavior is observed) can provide sufficient information. This charting can help identify what appears to trigger the behavior (antecedent), what the behavior looked like (behavior) and what was the result of the behavior (consequence).

Responses to sensory stimulation can also trigger affective violence. At times, it is quite obvious when sensory hypersensitivity triggered an outburst, as the cause and effect may be quite obvious. In other instances, the sensory stimulation may be more subtle and overshadowed by other environmental factors and, thus, easy to overlook. A FBA may be helpful in these instances to separate out the variables when they are not immediately obvious. It can also be helpful to analyze the environment for potential sensory triggers. In the chart below, we list components of a thorough risk assessment of someone with ASD.

Components of Evaluation of Violence Risk in ASD:

Component	Measurement
ASD assessments	Direct assessment of core features (such as the ADOS-2), developmental history, self and caregiver ratings (SRS-2, EQ, etc.)
Records review	Criminal records (including discovery documents, if available), school records, medical records, employment records
Clinical interview	Mental status evaluation, social history
Caregiver/Informant interview	Development, social history, psychiatric symptoms, subjective report of social cognitive and restricted and repetitive behaviors
Ratings of comorbid psychiatric symptoms	Measures of ADHD, mood, psychosis, and other areas as appropriate
Functional behavior assessment (affective aggression cases)	

Conclusions

There are a number of risk factors either are unique to ASD or express themselves in different ways. Risk assessment in ASD is a complex task that needs to reflect these ingredients. At this stage there is no simple instrument which brings it all together, and the only option is to draw from existing tools that are either designed for populations without ASD, or are specialized ASD assessment tools that have not been neither been validated in forensic populations nor designed for risk assessment. We have made a number of recommendations for this, summarized in the chart above. Most of these tools require specialized training, so consultation from an autism-focused clinician may be essential. Without question, further risk factors will be identified as more is understood about ASD, and the very substantial task of understanding the relative weights and interactions of the various risk factors remains.

References

Allen, D., Evans, C., Hider, A., Hawkins, S., Peckett, H., & Morgan, H. (2008). Offending behaviour in adults with Asperger syndrome. *Journal of Autism and Developmental Disorders, 38*(4), 748–758. https://doi.org/10.1007/s10803-007-0442-9.

American Psychiatric Association. (2013). *Diagnostic and statistical manual of mental disorders (DSM-5®)* (5th ed.). American Psychiatric Publishing.

Andrews, D. A., & Bonta, J. L. (1995). *LSI-R: The level of service inventory revised user's manual.* Multi-Health Systems.

Baio, J. (2012). Prevalence of autism spectrum disorders: Autism and developmental disabilities monitoring developmental disabilities monitoring network, 14 Sites, United States, 2008. *Morbidity and Mortality Weekly Report. Surveillance Summaries. Centers for Disease Control and Prevention, 61*(3), 1–9.

Baron-Cohen, S. (2000). Theory of mind and autism: A fifteen year review. *Understanding Other Minds: Perspectives from Developmental Cognitive Neuroscience, 2,* 3–20.

Baron-Cohen, S., & Wheelwright, S. (2004). The empathy quotient (EQ). An investigation of adults with Asperger syndrome or high functioning autism, and normal sex differences. *Journal of Autism and Developmental Disorders, 34,* 163–175.

Ben-Porath, Y., & Tellegen, A. (2008). *Minnesota multiphasic personality inventory-2 restructured form: Manual for administration, scoring, and interpretation.* University of Minnesota Press.

Bjørkly, S. (2009). Risk and dynamics of violence in Asperger's syndrome: A systematic review of the literature. *Aggression and Violent Behavior, 14*(5), 306–312. https://dx.doi.org/10.1016/j.avb.2009.04.003.

Bjørkly, S. (2013). A systematic review of the relationship between impulsivity and violence in persons with psychosis: Evidence or spin cycle? *Aggression and Violent Behavior, 18*(6), 753–760.

Blair, R. J. R. (2005). Responding to the emotions of others: Dissociating forms of empathy through the study of typical and psychiatric populations. *Consciousness and Cognition, 14*(4), 698–718.

Blair, R. J. R. (2008). Fine cuts of empathy and the amygdala: Dissociable deficits in psychopathy and autism. *The Quarterly Journal of Experimental Psychology, 61*(1), 157–170.

Bronfenbrenner, U. (1979). *The ecology of human development: Experiments by nature and design* (p. 330). Harvard University Press.

Buchanan, A., Binder, R., Norko, M., & Swartz, M. (2015). Resource document on psychiatric violence risk assessment. *Focus, 13*(4), 490–498.

Buon, M., Dupoux, E., Jacob, P., Chaste, P., Leboyer, M., & Zalla, T. (2013). The role of causal and intentional judgments in moral reasoning in individuals with high functioning autism. *Journal of Autism and Developmental Disorders, 43*(2), 458–470.

Calvert, S. L., Appelbaum, M., Dodge, K. A., Graham, S., Nagayama, G. C., Hamby, S., Fasig, L. G., Citkowicz, M., Galloway, D. P., & Hedges, L. V. (2017). The American Psychological Association Task Force assessment of violent video games: Science in the service of public interest. *American Psychologist, 72*(2), 126.

Carlson, S., Zelazo, P., & Faja, S. (2013). Executive function. In *The Oxford handbook of developmental psychology, vol. 1: Body and mind* (Vol. 1). Oxford University Press.

Centers for Disease Control and Prevention. (2020, January 28). *The social-ecological model.* https://www.cdc.gov/violenceprevention/publichealthissue/social-ecologicalmodel.html.

Cleckley, H. M. (1964). *The mask of sanity: An attempt to clarify some issues about the so-called psychopathic personality.* C.V. Mosby Co.

Constantino, J. N. (2012). *Social responsiveness scale-revised (SRS).* Western Psychological Services.

Constantino, J. N. (2016). 30.2 Autism traits and their potential contributions to violence. Abstract from the annual conference of the *American Academy of Child & Adolescent Psychiatry.*

Croen, L. A., Zerbo, O., Qian, Y., Massolo, M. L., Rich, S., Sidney, S., & Kripke, C. (2015). The health status of adults on the autism spectrum. *Autism: The International Journal of Research and Practice, 19*(7), 814–823.

de Jong, S., van Donkersgoed, R., Renard, S., Carter, S., Bokern, H., Lysaker, P., van der Gaag, M., Aleman, A., & Pijnenborg, G. H. M. (2018). Social-cognitive risk factors for violence in psychosis: A discriminant function analysis. *Psychiatry Research, 265,* 93–99.

Dziobek, I., Fleck, S., Kalbe, E., Rogers, K., Hassenstab, J., Brand, M., Kessler, J., Woike, J. K., Wolf, O. T., & Convit, A. (2006). Introducing MASC: A movie for the assessment of social cognition. *Journal of Autism and Developmental Disorders, 36*(5), 623–636.

Emba, C. (2019). Yes, God cancels people, and we can, too. *The Washington Post.* Retrieved October 7, 2019, from https://www.washingtonpost.com/opinions/2019/09/19/virtues-our-cancel-culture/?.

Engelhardt, C. R., Mazurek, M. O., Hilgard, J., Rouder, J. N., & Bartholow, B. D. (2015). Effects of violent-video-game exposure on aggressive behavior, aggressive-thought accessibility, and aggressive affect among adults with and without autism spectrum disorder. *Psychological Science, 26*(8), 1187–1200.

Engelstad, K. N., Rund, B. R., Torgalsbøen, A. K., Lau, B., Ueland, T., & Vaskinn, A. (2019). Large social cognitive impairments characterize homicide offenders with schizophrenia. *Psychiatry Research, 272,* 209–215.

Exelmans, L., Custers, K., & Van den Bulck, J. (2015). Violent video games and delinquent behavior in adolescents: A risk factor perspective. *Aggressive Behavior, 41*(3), 267–279.

Falco, MA. (2012, December 19). *Groups: Autism not to blame for violence.* CNN Health. https://www.cnn.com/2012/12/17/health/connecticut-shooting-autism/index.html.

Fazel, S., Smith, E. N., Chang, Z., & Geddes, J. R. (2018). Risk factors for interpersonal violence: An umbrella review of meta-analyses. *The British Journal of Psychiatry, 213*(4), 609–614.

Ferguson, C. J., & Wang, J. C. (2019). Aggressive video games are not a risk factor for future aggression in youth: A longitudinal study. *Journal of Youth and Adolescence, 48*(8), 1439–1451.

Frazier, J. A., Doyle, R., Chiu, S., & Coyle, J. T. (2002). Treating a child with Asperger's disorder and comorbid bipolar disorder. *American Journal of Psychiatry, 159*(1), 13–21.

Gillespie, S. M., Mitchell, I. J., & Abu-, A. M. (2017). Autistic traits and positive psychotic experiences modulate the association of psychopathic tendencies with theory of mind in opposite directions. *Scientific Reports, 7*(1), 1–9.

Gioia, G. A., Isquith, P. K., Guy, S. C., & Kenworthy, L. (2000). *Behavior rating inventory of executive function: BRIEF*. Psychological Assessment Resources.

Glancy, G. D., Ash, P., Bath, E. P., Buchanan, A., Fedoroff, P., Frierson, R. L., Harris, V. L., Friedman, S. J. H., Hauser, M. J., Knoll, J., & Norko, M. (2015). AAPL practice guideline for the forensic assessment. *The Journal of the American Academy of Psychiatry and the Law, 43*(2), S3-53.

Happé, F., Booth, R., Charlton, R., & Hughes, C. (2006). Executive function deficits in autism spectrum disorders and attention-deficit/hyperactivity disorder: Examining profiles across domains and ages. *Brain and Cognition, 61*(1), 25–39.

Hare, R. D. (1981). Psychopathy and violence. In *Violence and the violent individual* (pp. 53–74). Spectrum.

Hart, S. D., Douglas, K. S., & Guy, L. S. (2016). The structured professional judgement approach to violence risk assessment: Origins, nature, and advances. In *The Wiley handbook on the theories, assessment and treatment of sexual offending* (pp. 643–666). Wiley.

Hart, S. D., Webster, C. D., & Belfrage, H. (2013). *HCR-20V3: Assessing risk of violence—User guide.* Mental Health. Law, and Policy Institute, Simon Fraser University.

Harris, G. T., Rice, M. E., & Quinsey, V. L. (1993). Violent recidivism of mentally disordered offenders: The development of a statistical prediction instrument. *Criminal Justice and Behavior, 20*(4), 315–335.

Heeramun, R., Magnusson, C., Gumpert, C. H., Granath, S., Lundberg, M., Dalman, C., & Rai, D. (2017). Autism and convictions for violent crimes: Population-based cohort study in Sweden. *Journal of the American Academy of Child & Adolescent Psychiatry, 56*(6), 491–497.

Heleniak, C., & McLaughlin, K. A. (2019). Social-cognitive mechanisms in the cycle of violence: Cognitive and affective theory of mind, and externalizing psychopathology in children and adolescents. *Development and Psychopathology*, 1–16.
Helverschou, S., Rasmussen, K., Steindal, K., Søndanaa, E., Nilsson, B., & Nøttestad, J. (2015). Offending profiles of individuals with autism spectrum disorder: A study of all individuals with autism spectrum disorder examined by the forensic psychiatric service in Norway between 2000 and 2010. *Autism, 19*(7), 850–858.
Hodgins, S. (1992). Mental disorder, intellectual deficiency, and crime: Evidence from a birth cohort. *Archives of General Psychiatry, 49*(6), 476–483.
Im, D. S. (2016). Template to perpetrate: An update on violence in autism spectrum disorder. *Harvard Review of Psychiatry, 24*(1), 14–35. https://doi.org/10.1097/HRP.0000000000000087.
Jones, A. P., Happé, F. G., Gilbert, F., Burnett, S., & Viding, E. (2010). Feeling, caring, knowing: Different types of empathy deficit in boys with psychopathic tendencies and autism spectrum disorder. *Journal of Child Psychology and Psychiatry, 51*(11), 1188–1197.
Kenworthy, L., Yerys, B. E., Anthony, L. G., & Wallace, G. L. (2008). Understanding executive control in autism spectrum disorders in the lab and in the real world. *Neuropsychology Review, 18*(4), 320–338. https://doi.org/10.1007/s11065-008-9077-7.
Kim, Y. S., Leventhal, B. L., Koh, Y. J., & Boyce, W. T. (2009). Bullying increased suicide risk: Prospective study of Korean adolescents. *Archives of Suicide Research, 13*(1), 15–30.
Klin, A., Jones, W., Schultz, R., & Volkmar, F. (2003). The enactive mind, or from actions to cognition: lessons from autism. *Philosophical Transactions of the Royal Society of London. Series B: Biological Sciences, 358*(1430), 345–360. https://doi.org/10.1098/rstb.2002.1202.
Krug, E. G., Mercy, J. A., Dahlberg, L. L., & Zwi, A. B. (2002). The world report on violence and health. *The Lancet, 360*(9339), 1083–1088.
Långström, N., Grann, M., Ruchkin, V., Sjöstedt, G., & Fazel, S. (2009). Risk factors for violent offending in autism spectrum disorder: A national study of hospitalized individuals. *Journal of Interpersonal Violence, 24*(8), 1358–1370.
Lazaratou, H., Giannopoulou, I., Anomitri, C., & Douzenis, A. (2016). Case report: Matricide by a 17-year old boy with Asperger's syndrome. *Aggression and Violent Behavior, 31,* 61–65.
Lockwood, P. L., Bird, G., Bridge, M., & Viding, E. (2013). Dissecting empathy: High levels of psychopathic and autistic traits are characterized by difficulties in different social information processing domains. *Frontiers in Human Neuroscience, 7,* 760. https://doi.org/10.3389/fnhum.2013.00760.
Lord, C., Rutter, M., et al. (2012). *(ADOS™-2) Autism diagnostic observation schedule™* (2nd ed.). WPS.
Maiano, C., Normand, C., Salvas, M., Moullec, G., & Aime, A. (2016). Prevalence of school bullying among youth with autism spectrum disorders: A systematic review and meta-analysis. *Autism Research, 9*(6), 601–615.
Mawson, D. C., Grounds, A., & Tantam, D. (1985). Violence and Asperger's syndrome: A case study. *The British Journal of Psychiatry, 147*(5), 566–569.
Mazefsky, C. A., & White, S. W. (2014). Emotion regulation: Concepts & practice in autism spectrum disorder. *Child and Adolescent Psychiatric Clinics of North America, 23*(1), 15–24.
McCracken, J. T., McGough, J., Shah, B., Cronin, P., Hong, D., Aman, M. G., Arnold, L. E., Lindsay, R., Nash, P., Hollway, J., & McDougle, C. J. (2002). Risperidone in children with autism and serious behavioral problems. *New England Journal of Medicine, 347*(5), 314–321.
McNulty, J. K., & Hellmuth, J. C. (2008). Emotion regulation and intimate partner violence in newlyweds. *Journal of Family Psychology, 22*(5), 794. https://doi.org/10.1037/a0013516.
Monahan, J., Steadman, H. J., Robbins, P. C., Appelbaum, P., Banks, S., Grisso, T., Heilbrun, K., Mulvey, E. P., Roth, L., & Silver, E. (2005). An actuarial model of violence risk assessment for persons with mental disorders. *Psychiatric Services, 56*(7), 810–815.
Mouridsen, S. E., Rich, B., Isager, T., & Nedergaard, N. J. (2008). Pervasive developmental disorders and criminal behaviour: A case control study. *International Journal of Offender Therapy and Comparative Criminology, 52*(2), 196–205.

Murphy, D. (2010). Extreme violence in a man with an autistic spectrum disorder: Assessment and treatment within high-security psychiatric care. *The Journal of Forensic Psychiatry & Psychology, 21*(3), 462–477.
Murphy, D. (2013). Risk assessment of offenders with an autism spectrum disorder. *Journal of Intellectual Disabilities and Offending Behaviour, 4*(1–2), 33–41.
Murray, K., Johnston, K., Cunnane, H., Kerr, C., Spain, D., Gillan, N., Hammond, N., Murphy, D., & Happé, F. (2017). A new test of advanced theory of mind: The "Strange Stories Film Task" captures social processing differences in adults with autism spectrum disorders. *Autism Research, 10*(6), 1120–1132.
Murrie, D. C., Warren, J. I., Kristiansson, M., & Dietz, P. E. (2002). Asperger's syndrome in forensic settings. *International Journal of Forensic Mental Health, 1*(1), 59–70.
Olweus, D. (2013). School bullying: Development and some important challenges. *Annual Review of Clinical Psychology, 9,* 751–780.
Palermo, M. T. (2004). Pervasive developmental disorders, psychiatric comorbidities, and the law. *International Journal of Offender Therapy and Comparative Criminology, 48*(1), 40–48.
Pearl, A., Edwards, E. M., & Murray, M. J. (2016). Comparison of self-and other-report of symptoms of autism and comorbid psychopathology in adults with autism spectrum disorder. *Contemporary Behavioral Health Care.*
Peñuelas-Calvo, I., Sareen, A., Sevilla, J., & Fernández-Berrocal, P. (2019). The "Reading the Mind in the Eyes" test in autism-spectrum disorders comparison with healthy controls: A systematic review and meta-analysis. *Journal of Autism and Developmental Disorders, 49*(3), 1048–1061.
Postorino, V., Fatta, L. M., Sanges, V., Giovagnoli, G., De Peppo, L., Vicari, S., & Mazzone, L. (2016). Intellectual disability in autism spectrum disorder: Investigation of prevalence in an Italian sample of children and adolescents. *Research in Developmental Disabilities, 48,* 193–201.
Pouw, L. B., Rieffe, C., Oosterveld, P., Huskens, B., & Stockmann, L. (2013). Reactive/proactive aggression and affective/cognitive empathy in children with ASD. *Research in Developmental Disabilities, 34*(4), 1256–1266.
Rieffe, C., Camodeca, M., Pouw, L., Lange, A., & Stockmann, L. (2012). Don't anger me! Bullying, victimization, and emotion dysregulation in young adolescents with ASD. *European Journal of Developmental Psychology, 9*(3), 351–370.
Schwenck, C., Mergenthaler, J., Keller, K., Zech, J., Salehi, S., Taurines, R., Romanos, M., Schecklmann, M., Schneider, W., Warnke, A., & Freitag, C. M. (2012). Empathy in children with autism and conduct disorder: Group-specific profiles and developmental aspects. *Journal of Child Psychology and Psychiatry, 53*(6), 651–659.https://doi.org/10.1111/j.1469-7610.2011.02499..
Scragg, P., & Shah, A. (1994). Prevalence of Asperger's syndrome in a secure hospital. *The British Journal of Psychiatry, 165*(5), 679–682.
Serin, R. C. (1991). Psychopathy and violence in criminals. *Journal of Interpersonal Violence, 6*(4), 423–431.
Silver, E., & Teasdale, B. (2005). Mental disorder and violence: An examination of stressful life events and impaired social support. *Social Problems, 52*(1), 62–78.
Silver, J., Simons, A., & Craun, S. (2018). *A study of the pre-attack behaviors of active shooters in the United States between 2000 and 2013.*
Singh, J. P., Desmarais, S. L., Hurducas, C., Arbach-Lucioni, K., Condemarin, C., Dean, K., Doyle, M., Folino, J.O., Godoy-Cervera, V., Grann, M., & Ho, R. M. Y. (2014). International perspectives on the practical application of violence risk assessment: A global survey of 44 countries. *International Journal of Forensic Mental Health, 13*(3), 193–206. https://doi.org/10.1080/14999013.2014.922141.
Skeem, J. L., Mulvey, E. P., Appelbaum, P., Banks, S., Grisso, T., Silver, E., & Robbins, P. C. (2004). Identifying subtypes of civil psychiatric patients at high risk for violence. *Criminal Justice and Behavior, 31*(4), 392–437.
Søndenaa, E., Helverschou, S. B., Steindal, K., Rasmussen, K., Nilson, B., & Nøttestad, J. A. (2014). Violence and sexual offending behavior in people with autism spectrum disorder who have undergone a psychiatric forensic examination. *Psychological Reports, 115*(1), 32–43.

Steadman, H. J., Silver, E., Monahan, J., Appelbaum, P., Robbins, P. C., Mulvey, E. P., Grisso, T., Roth, L. H., & Banks, S. (2000). A classification tree approach to the development of actuarial violence risk assessment tools. *Law and Human Behavior, 24*(1), 83–100.
Swanson, J. W., Holzer, C. E., III., Ganju, V. K., & Jono, R. T. (1990). Violence and psychiatric disorder in the community: Evidence from the Epidemiologic Catchment Area surveys. *Psychiatric Services, 41*(7), 761–770.
Swartz, M. S., Swanson, J. W., Hiday, V. A., Borum, R., Wagner, H. R., & Burns, B. J. (1998). Violence and severe mental illness: The effects of substance abuse and nonadherence to medication. *American Journal of Psychiatry, 155*(2), 226–231.
Szycik, G. R., Mohammadi, B., Münte, T. F., & Te Wildt, B. T. (2017). Lack of evidence that neural empathic responses are blunted in excessive users of violent video games: An fMRI study. *Frontiers in Psychology, 8*, 174.
Tarasoff, V. (1976). Regents of the University of California, 17 Cal. 3d 425, 551 P. 2d 334, 131 Cal.
Ttofi, M. M., Farrington, D. P., & Lösel, F. (2012). School bullying as a predictor of violence later in life: A systematic review and meta-analysis of prospective longitudinal studies. *Aggression and Violent Behavior, 17*(5), 405–418.
Wang, J., Lloyd-Evans, B., Giacco, D., Forsyth, R., Nebo, C., Mann, F., & Johnson, S. (2017). Social isolation in mental health: A conceptual and methodological review. *Social Psychiatry and Psychiatric Epidemiology, 52*(12), 1451–1461.
Webster, C. D., Douglas, K. S., Eaves, D., & Hart, S. D. (1997). *HCR-20. Assessing risk for violence.* Version 2. Mental Health, Law, and Policy Institute, Simon Fraser University.
White v. United States of America, 780 F.2d 97 (D.C. Cir. 1986).
White, R., Bebbington, P., Pearson, J., Johnson, S., & Ellis, D. (2000). The social context of insight in schizophrenia. *Social Psychiatry and Psychiatric Epidemiology, 35*(11), 500–507.
Winter, K., Spengler, S., Bermpohl, F., Singer, T., & Kanske, P. (2017). Social cognition in aggressive offenders: Impaired empathy, but intact theory of mind. *Scientific Reports, 7*(1), 1–10.
Woodbury-Smith, M., & Dein, K. (2014). Autism spectrum disorder (ASD) and unlawful behaviour: Where do we go from here? *Journal of Autism and Developmental Disorders, 44*(11), 2734–2741.

Dr. Alexander Westphal is on Faculty at the Yale School of Medicine within the Department of Psychiatry. Westphal is dual fellowship trained in Child and Adolescent Psychiatry and Forensic Psychiatry.

Rachel Loftin is an Autism Specialist trained in school and clinical psychology. She maintains a private practice that offers diagnosis and assessment, therapy, and consultation on educational and legal cases. She is an Adjunct Faculty in the psychiatry departments of Northwestern and Yale University. She was previously an Associate Professor in the Department of Psychiatry at Rush University Medical Center, where she was the clinical director of the autism program. Dr. Loftin completed fellowship training in developmental disorders at Yale.

Chapter 23
Autism and Operational Policing

Nick Chown, Dennis Debbaudt, Luke Beardon, Kleio Cossburn, and Jack Scott

Review and Analysis of the Literature on First Responder Training in Autism

Very little has been written about training in autism for first responders. In fact, one can truthfully state that this lack of training literature reflects the lack of training in autism for first responders. Although first responders include fire fighters, ambulance personnel, first aiders, and others, it is likely that the majority of difficulties experienced by autistic people in a first response situation involve contact with police officers. The section on police training is focused on the UK and USA, as much of the published research on the topic comes from those places. The situation in other countries varies, but the UK and USA seem to be largely representative of what happens in much of the English-speaking world.

The most recent review of current police training in autism in the UK is by Diana Hepworth of the University of Salford whose paper 'A critical review of current police training and policy for autism spectrum disorder' was published in 2017.

N. Chown (✉)
Birmingham, UK

D. Debbaudt
Debbaudt Legacy Productions, LLC, Port St. Lucie, FL, USA
e-mail: ddpi@flash.net

L. Beardon
Sheffield Hallam University, Sheffield, UK
e-mail: L.Beardon@shu.ac.uk

K. Cossburn
Staffordshire, UK

J. Scott
Florida Atlantic University, Boca Raton, FL, USA
e-mail: jscott@fau.edu

F. R. Volkmar et al. (eds.), *Handbook of Autism Spectrum Disorder and the Law*,
https://doi.org/10.1007/978-3-030-70913-6_23

This is a thorough review and analysis of the training in autism as it relates to autistic *suspects* and only touches upon the involvement of autistic individuals in the criminal justice system (CJS) as victims and witnesses. Nevertheless, despite its narrow focus—from the perspective of this review and analysis of the literature on first responder training—it makes some 'key' points which we will refer to. Hepworth (2017: 1) concludes, as others have done before her, that 'The current criminal justice response in England and Wales is unequipped to deal with offenders with (autism)'. While she has focused on suspects, what training in autism there is, and there isn't much, is of a general nature, so it is correct to conclude that the CJS in England and Wales is unequipped to deal with autistic individuals in whatever capacity they come into contact with it. This is of great concern given the implications that potentially vulnerable people may be exposed to unlawful and excessive force, breach of their human rights, in addition to anxiety and stress over and above that which any person coming into contact with the police can face. The importance of training for police officers has been emphasised by various researchers (Artingstall, 2007; Blackhurst, 2012; Chown, 2010; Chown et al., 2018; Crane et al., 2016; Debbaudt, 2007; Hepworth, 2017; Kelly & Hassett-Walker, 2016; Krameddine et al., 2013; Laan et al., 2013; Teagardin et al., 2012).

More recently Crane et al. (2016: 1) reported that 37% of the 242 officers who responded to a question on police training had received training in autism and that nearly half the officers who had received autism training expressed satisfaction with the training received. This is remarkably consistent with the second author's finding back in 2010 that only 38% of the police officer respondents to his survey had received any formal training in autism and is further indication of little or no improvement in the last few years. Previous research has indicated that officers tend to overestimate their competence when asked (Modell & Mak, 2008). This factor might have led to the responses to the question about satisfaction with the training giving a false impression of its effectiveness. Over a quarter of the respondent officers to the Crane et al. survey were dissatisfied with their autism training. The top three areas of discontent with their training were: (1) lack of focus on the criminal justice system context, (2) that it was too simplistic, and (3) lack of practical relevance to operational policing, which implies that the training received was inappropriate and unlikely to have enhanced the officers' ability to interact with autistic members of the public. The researchers identified a need for operational policing-specific training. The autistic adults and parents who had responded to their survey were 'largely dissatisfied with their experience of the police and echoed the need for police training on (autism)'.

So what is the current situation regarding police officer training in England and Wales? Sarah Artingstall (2007) concluded a decade ago that training for police officers in autism was limited. Artingstall wrote that only one of the 30 participants in her survey of police officers had received specific training in autism, and went on to state that it is likely that the knowledge of autism participants appeared to have 'was gained through personal experience rather than through their experience as a police officer' (2007: 24). Nearly 50% of the officers stated that they had no knowledge of any autism-specific communication strategies. It hardly needs pointing out that relying on personal experience rather than strategies appropriate for autism is a recipe for unfortunate outcomes. Teagardin et al. (2012) write that in the absence of training to enable an officer to identify and respond appropriately to autistic individuals the officer may make a situation worse, resulting in avoidable trauma, injury, or death. The first author reported a couple of years later that 'Not one respondent in (his) study had received training from the police service fitting (the respondent) to interact effectively with persons on the autism spectrum' (Chown, 2010: 256). This situation has apparently not changed significantly since then as Hepworth (2017: 213) advises that 'Currently, frontline police officers in England and Wales receive very little training about (autism): a two-hour online "mental health" training session is provided to new recruits, which includes a sub-section on (autism)'. Freedom of Information Act requests submitted by the fourth author to UK police forces in 2018 shows that the situation is even worse than reported by Hepworth as only 10 of the 46 forces[1] have an e-learning package. We echo Hepworth's concern that training in autism is delivered under the umbrella of mental health when autism is a developmental disability. It would be entirely appropriate for autism training to cover the common comorbidities—which can include mental health issues—but the present approach risks perpetuating the myth that autism is itself a mental health issue. We would add to Hepworth's concerns that a two-hour online training session is wholly inadequate to cover mental health. To limit autism to a subsection of a two-hour module is, in effect, likely to achieve little more than a tick in this particular box. Although online training has its place, it cannot replace in-person training involving experienced trainers with a thorough understanding of their subject. We also recommend that all autism training involves an autistic adult in addition to the trainer as they are the only people with lived experience of autism. The combination of a top-quality trainer and an autistic adult experienced in describing their experiences is unbeatable in our view, and in a different league to a short online training module. Hepworth has made the following two recommendations relevant in a first response situation which we support.

1. Only about one-quarter of the 43 forces in England and Wales have adopted an autism alert/attention card scheme to increase the confidence of autistic individuals and increase the likelihood of disclosure. Hepworth recommends that this scheme be made obligatory for all forces, and rolled out nationally. Although there are issues regarding the fear of negative stereotyping, such a scheme would be entirely voluntary as far as autistic individuals are concerned. It is hoped that over time the stereotyping of autism will reduce to negligible levels so that nobody will be unwilling to disclose; however, this is a long-term objective if not actually wishful thinking given the vagaries of human nature.
2. While we do not agree with Hepworth that all autistic individuals have difficulty understanding the police caution, we do agree that an autism-friendly version of the caution should be developed so that autistic suspects understand their rights.

[1] The 46 forces comprise the 43 English regional forces together with British Transport Police, the Police Service of Northern Ireland, and Police Scotland.

The Situation in the USA

In their study of the knowledge and perceptions of persons with disabilities of police officers in the USA, Modell and Mak found that 80% of the officer respondents to their survey were unable to identify characteristics of autism accurately. Amazingly, a further finding was that in excess of 35% of the officers listed ‘Rain Man’ as their response to the question asking what autism means to them (Modell & Mak, 2008). Although the Modell and Mak research related to disabilities generally, they were particularly concerned at the lack of police officer knowledge of autism and recommended that the entire criminal justice system would benefit from training on autism (Modell & Mak, 2008).

Five years after the Modell and Mak study was reported on, Laan et al. (2013) analysed existing training in the Southeastern United States relating to autism and other conditions. These researchers conducted interviews with training coordinators from each of the seven states[2] in the region and compared training materials from each state to existing training guidelines. They reported that police officer training in each state in this region was inconsistent with the existing guidelines. Training time allocated to training in relation to ‘mental disorders’ varied from 0.52 to 2.82% in each state. Only two states advised that more than 1% of training time was allocated to ‘mental disorders’. There is no indication in the report of how much time was allocated to autism in the six states that did cover autism in their ‘mental disorders’ training (one state did not cover autism). To determine how consistent each state’s training was with then-existing guidelines for police autism training,[3] Laan and his colleagues compared the training with a checklist the authors based on recommendations made by the third author of this chapter. The results of this analysis were that only 7% of the recommended topics were delivered ‘on average’ by the training in an autism-specific manner. Over 50% of the topics were delivered by training that was not specific to autism and the remaining topics were not covered at all. There was no data to enable us to evaluate the method(s) of training delivery or the time allocated to autism training. However, the subject coverage in relation to autism would not in our opinion have any significant effect on an officer’s ability to recognise autism and respond appropriately in an interaction with an autistic person irrespective of the time allowed and delivery.

More recently, the fourth author and a colleague reported on training in autism for police officers, firefighters, and emergency medical technicians in New Jersey (Kelly & Hassett-Walker, 2016). Their objective was to compare the training delivered in New Jersey with the requirements of a 2008 state law making autism awareness training mandatory for police, fire, and emergency medical service personnel. The Act required that first responders employed prior to its enactment should receive training within three years of the Act. The researchers undertook a questionnaire

[2] The seven states are Alabama, Arkansas, Florida, Georgia, Mississippi, South Carolina, and Tennessee.

[3] Laan, Ingram, and Glidden also compared the training delivered by the seven states against the guidance for mental disorder training issued by the Police Executive Research Forum.

Table 23.1 Type of training received in relation to 'special needs'

Type of training	Number	Percent
Read and sign	9	6.1
Video-based training	20	13.6
Internet-based training	35	23.8
Speaker/instructor	36	24.5
Combination training (i.e. speaker with video, read, and sign, internet)	42	28.6
Other	5	3.4
Total	147[a]	100.0

[a]Respondents ($n = 85$) who had received no 'special needs' training did not respond to this question

survey of law enforcement agencies, fire services, and emergency medical service (EMS) units in each county. Of the respondents who advised the nature of their service 44.1% were police, 16.6% were fire, and 25.6% were voluntary EMS units. The types of training received in relation to 'special needs' are set out in Table 23.1. Over 50% of respondents considered the training to have been either 'effective' or 'highly effective' and over 90% of respondents stated that the training was at least 'somewhat effective'. However, about half the training reported on amounted to no more than reading a document or watching a video. Furthermore, it was reported that a significant percentage of emergency service personnel had not been trained despite the training being a legal requirement. The response to the 2008 law was seen to be patchy and, in many cases, wholly inadequate to achieve the purposes of the legislation. The authors recommended that (a) speaker-based training should be used, (b) emergency services personnel with an immediate family relationship with autistic people are an 'untapped resource and engaging emergency service personnel to train other emergency service personnel brings a personal bond and validity to the training' (ibid.: 551). To this we would add that the involvement of autistic individuals in the delivery of training is essential as these people are the only ones with lived experience of autism.

An experimental training programme developed by Teagardin et al. (2012) was trialled with 82 frontline officers (either patrol officers or detectives) from the Ventura County, California Law Enforcement Department. To ensure that prior knowledge of autism did not bias their findings, the authors ensured that none of their participants had an autistic relative. This study used a randomised, waitlist-controlled, between-groups design. This meant that participants were randomly assigned to either a first round of training or to a second round. The second group acted as the control group. Pre- and post-test questionnaires were completed by all participants undergoing training. The autism training was undertaken during scheduled training sessions. The training consisted of a 13-min video entitled 'Law Enforcement: Your Piece to the Autism Puzzle'.[4] The video is said to have explained what autism is and how to recognise and respond to autism. Teagardin and her colleagues report

[4] This video is available at: https://www.youtube.com/watch?v=sFB48E_xeGg.

that analysis of pre- and post-test scores indicated that both knowledge of autism and confidence to handle interactions with an autistic person increased as a result of the training. However, they add that 'the posttest scores for participants in the training group and control group … are still much lower than one would hope and do not suggest mastery of the training material' (2012: 1116). However good a video is, it is our firm view that 13 min of training is woefully insufficient for trainees to learn how to recognise and respond appropriately to autism. But in this case many of the trainees did not even master the 13 min of training. The third author—who is a specialist in producing videos for autism training purposes—has analysed the video used by Teagardin et al. and we report on his analysis later on.

Krameddine et al. trialled an experimental one-day training programme for police officers that improves interactions with *mentally ill individuals* and is cost-effective. Their approach involves scripted role-play training involving police officers and actors and feedback from experienced officers, a mental health professional, and the role players. The primary goal of the training is to 'improve empathy, communication skills, and the ability of officers to de-escalate potentially difficult situations' (2013: 1). The authors state that their training programme led to improved recognition of mental health issues, a decrease in physical interactions with the mentally ill, and cost savings. They propose that their approach be adopted by other police forces. The question has to be whether this approach would also be effective for autism training. We heartily approve of having a full day's training, although we also know of the many training demands on police officer time which may cause senior officers to regard this as impractical. We think that a role-playing approach could work with autism as long as actors play the part of the autistic victim, witness or suspect and undergo thorough training involving autistic individuals. We strongly advocate autistic participation in all training but please do not ask an autistic professional to 'act autistic' in a training session as a retired police officer colleague of the first and second author was asked to do. We also suspect that a substantial training time commitment for autism would pay off financially for police forces and recommend that a trial—involving training and longitudinal follow-up—be undertaken to test this hypothesis.

Recommendations for Practice in the Criminal Justice System

Given the already heavy training burden on police officers, the issue of mainstreaming autism awareness within the police service through training delivery should be approached sensitively. Some guidance on mainstreaming autism awareness through training emerged from the survey. A sensitive approach to the issue should take into account the following points made by respondents to a survey undertaken by the second author. We have referred to first responders in what follows even though the survey involved police officers because the principles and best practice outlined applies just as much to other first responders.

1. An efficient and effective means of mainstreaming training in a specific area such as autism is to embed such training within existing training programmes (including probationer training) rather than by developing stand-alone courses;
2. There is value in having a variety of delivery mechanisms as people learn best in different ways, and wholly computer-based training was criticised;
3. First responders do not need to be experts in autism. There may be a tendency to 'over deliver' training when all that is required is a sufficient (basic) understanding;
4. Training should encompass the range of disabilities (developmental, learning, etc.) and mental illness that first responders may come across in the course of their duties;
5. Training should incorporate the best advice on tactics to be used;
6. Trainees should have the opportunity to interact with autistic individuals.

Crane et al. echoed previous calls for a national approach to police training in autism from the Independent Commission on Mental Health and Policing (Adebowale, 2013) and the Department of Health (2010). They recommend that police autism training needs to be 'evidence-based, informed by those personally affected by (autism), and tailored to specific policing roles, to ensure its suitability for improving job performance across the wide range of police settings' (2016: 23). We echo Crane et al. and wonder how many more echoes of this nature will be required before Government takes action to ensure that the specific needs of autistic people coming into contact with the CJS are no longer largely ignored?

Audiovisual Training for Autism

After viewing the video used in the 2012 Teagardin et al. training experiment, the low test scores indicating poor mastery of the subject matter are understandable: the video was poorly produced and hardly memorable. The use of actors to portray autistic individuals engaged in a highly stereotypical manner was egregious and misleading. The generic autism tips as on-screen graphics and heard in narration were limited to seconds on screen after each scenario, not during the scenarios. This made the tips less memorable. Some of the tips, advice, and visual depictions were directly copied from earlier video productions and not cited as such in the credits. The use of police officers and high school students as actors also added to the poor production results. The scenarios were stiff, poorly acted, and had an amateur feel. The on-screen cast did not reflect American diversity nor indicate that females can also be autistic. While one hopes it was not intentional, nevertheless, the producers left a visual impression that only white males are autistic or mothers, neighbours, store clerks, or police officers. However, the last three and a half minutes of this video before its rolling credits at least provided a short dose of reality through unscripted interview and video images of officers with their autistic children. This video appears to have been produced about ten years ago but would have been two or three years old when chosen for this project. Teagardin et al. could have reviewed higher quality productions for their experiment.

When produced in documentary style, audiovisual illustrations, can and will lift live classroom training to the level of memorable. Avoiding or minimising the use of actors, allowing officers and others to use their own words and ideas by following a general outline of a scenario will produce results more reflective of reality, or a documentary feel. These videos can also illustrate the words on a screen or in on-screen narration. Using the images of the words to help make the point more memorable is the point. Viewing talking heads without illustrating their words produces the opposite result.

Law enforcement departments in the USA are increasingly using officer perspective (body cam) video to document field interactions. There are now a growing number of these videos documenting actual interactions between frontline police officers and autistic individuals. High-risk contacts discussed in other sections of this chapter including missing children and adults, suspicious persons, and use of force contacts are now memorialised on video and are extremely useful for discussion and learning in training. To these can be added open-source bystander videos, typically within local news reports, that also paint pictures of real-life situations, which enable production of memorable autism and policing related audiovisual training tools.

Online training should never replace in-person training with a qualified instructor in tandem with autistic individuals. High-quality audiovisual tools will enhance learning when provided in short duration and followed by discussion and commentary. They also become valuable for making clear to the audience that each autistic person is unique and may act or react differently from the next autistic person. Is the goal to make training memorable to the learner? If so, pictures tell a thousand words!

Information and Advice for First Responders to an Autistic Person

Sensory Needs

It is likely that the autistic person will have sensory sensitivities—both hyper and hypo sensory issues (i.e. over or under sensitive in some or all of the sensory domains). While the following is not an exhaustive list it is a start to what first responders should take into consideration:

1. Where possible avoid touch as even a light touch may cause pain where a person is hypersensitive. Touching may cause a 'flight or fright' reaction; don't assume that means the person is guilty of an offence.
2. In line with the above avoid handcuffs if at all possible.
3. Avoid bright, direct lighting.

4. Avoid spithoods which could cause immense distress or panic.
5. Keep all noise to a minimum—however insignificant it may seem, many noises may be amplified to the autistic person and cause all sorts of issues.
6. It may be advisable to ensure that any autistic person in custody has his own area rather than a shared area.
7. Allow as much personal space as possible in all situations.
8. If a person appears to need to 'stim' (e.g. rock) then give them time and space to do so.
9. Understand that there may be certain foods that a person cannot tolerate; the person may also only be able to eat while isolated from others.

It is almost impossible to cover all sensory issues that might crop up, so it is highly recommended that the person themselves is consulted from as early a point as possible to ascertain what sensory issues may be impacting on him/her. A sensory questionnaire can be found on Beardon's Blog which may prove a useful tool.

Behaviour and Anxiety

The behaviour of an autistic individual at times of duress is highly likely to differ from that of a neurotypical individual. If that behaviour is only understood within a neurotypical context, it is very probable that it will be misinterpreted. At times of increased anxiety the individual may well present behaviours necessary to avoid a 'meltdown', or indeed may already be suffering from a meltdown. Many autistic people experience meltdowns, and there is a direct correlation between levels of anxiety and increased risk of having a meltdown. The public often finds it hard to tell meltdowns and temper tantrums apart, but they are different things. A meltdown is an intense response to a situation an autistic person finds overwhelming—and very often the person has little or no control over their behaviour at this time, which is an extremely important point to make. To cope with such a situation the autistic person may need to engage in repetitive body movements (stimming) or a whole range of other behaviours that could include:

- Self-injury
- Screaming/shouting
- Inability to talk
- Harming or attempting to harm others
- Covering eyes/ears
- Fleeing.

Interrupting a meltdown may increase levels of anxiety exacerbating the situation (though of course one might be forced to intervene if there are safety concerns). Some possible scenarios that could lead to incorrect initial perceptions on the part of first responders include:

1. *Refusal to engage*—sometimes when under duress the autistic response is essentially to shut off from external stimuli as much as is possible. To the 'untrained eye' the person may appear to be refusing to respond, or excessively rude, or even having something physically wrong with them. But it may be a coping mechanism to reduce their anxiety. In some cases the individual may not even physically be able to hear if their senses are overloaded (see point 6).
2. *Seemingly excessive reaction to proximity and/or touch*—at times of high anxiety sensory sensitivities may be greatly increased. This means that if someone is tactile sensitive, for example, then any touch (including very light touch) may be processed as intense pain. In some cases a 'natural' reaction to a perceived assault for some people would be to defend themselves. Even well-intentioned contact meant as reassurance might be perceived as painful. Sometimes an autistic individual can move from a state of anxiety to a state of panic simply because someone such as a first responder is too close to them.
3. *Already in a state of panic*—levels of arousal might be so high that the individual may be close to or at panic level before a responder even arrives; this may mean that any additional stressor could trigger a meltdown.
4. *Eye contact issues*—social practice assumes a good way of gaining attention is to insist on eye contact and that eye contact reciprocity will lead to a greater sense of trust. Although some autistic people do not have difficulty looking other people in the eye, many do and this difficulty can be exacerbated at times of stress. A first responding police officer may easily misinterpret this as deliberate evasion, a guilty reaction, or disrespect. Of course, as with any other individual, an autistic person can deliberately evade, react guiltily or show disrespect but it is far more likely than not looking the officer in the eye is an aspect of their autism.
5. *Flight risk*—An autistic person may try and run away from a situation involving a first responder. Unless an officer has an understanding of autism they will assume that this is a guilty reaction. It could be a guilty reaction of course but the officer should not assume this as it may be an autistic reaction. The autistic person may have great difficulty with social interaction and experience high levels of anxiety. Their natural response may be to get away from a highly stressful situation without thought as to the impression this creates, nor to the potential consequences of their own actions.
6. *Sensory processing*—Autistic individuals may only be able to process sensory information through one sensory channel at a time. This is known as single attention (Murray et al., 2005). They may be unable to process auditory information, for example, because they are focusing on visual information. A lack of ability to hear, and subsequently respond to, verbal requests may come across as defiance and/or non-compliance.
7. *Shutdown*—A shutdown is caused by the same factors that cause a meltdown but instead of losing behavioural control the individual stops reacting to the situation as a means of avoiding it.
8. *Lack of or 'odd' facial expression/non-verbal communication*—some autistic people demonstrate either no facial expression (i.e. the 'same' face irrespective

of the situation) or a facial expression seemingly at odds with the situation (e.g. smiling when in distress). The misinterpretation of facial expressions could put the autistic individual at risk. First responders should be aware that facial expressions, 'body language', and other non-verbal cues are not always an indication of an emotional state or intent.

9. *Expressive versus receptive language*—for most people, expressive language skills are a reasonable indicator of receptive skills (comprehension). In other words there might be an assumption that an eloquent person will have equally good comprehension skills. This may not be the case with an autistic person who may display very good expressive language skills but have huge problems with understanding what is being said to them; conversely, they may not speak but have a good understanding when being spoken to.
10. *Feeling obliged to respond*—remaining with the poor comprehension theme, some individuals will have learnt (usually by being directly taught) that a rule in verbal exchanges is that they must respond if asked a question. This places the individual at a huge disadvantage if they feel obliged to respond despite not understanding the question. In an interview situation this clearly could create numerous problems for an autistic individual.
11. *Literal interpretation*—an autistic person often has a very specific way of understanding language. They may assume a direct correlation between the words being spoken and their meaning (sometimes referred to as literal interpretation). However, many people do not use language in this way, even if they might think they do. Language is full of contradictions and ambiguities and some people's use of language is more accurate than others. For example the instructions: 'Freeze! Don't move! Take your hands out your pockets and turn around slowly…' have a clear meaning for most people. But to an autistic person in a stressful situation it might appear that the person is quite literally contradicting himself or herself and they will not know how to react to what they hear as a confusing set of commands.
12. *Processing language*—Processing time may be considerably longer for autistic individuals than for neurotypical people individuals. This means that after each sentence, for example, an individual might need a few seconds to 'digest' what has been said in order to understand it. If this additional processing time is not allowed, either the person will fall further and further behind the communication—or they will simply miss chunks of it in order to keep up.
13. *Multiple concepts or questions at one time*—many autistic people can get confused when they are asked to deliberate over multiple concepts at the same time, or when more than one question is asked at the same time. It is good practice when communicating with an autistic person to ask questions that are clear and 'one dimensional' and to do so one at a time. In a similar vein, it can be confusing for an autistic person to be asked the 'same' question but in a different format, e.g. with a differing word order.
14. *Verbal rather than visual*—some autistic individuals prefer visual forms of communication, in which case written questions may be far preferable to verbal.

15. *Prosody*—this refers to the tone of voice, inflection, and stressors placed on words—which is often either misunderstood or not taken into account at all by an autistic person. In some cases the same sentence can have very different meanings dependent on the prosodic expression—in written language grammar along with italics provides the equivalent information. It is important for anyone communicating with an autistic person to take into account that their language (including prosody) needs to be as ambiguity-free as possible. For example, asking '**what** do you think happened' may mean something very different to 'what do **you** think happened' but the prosodic inflection may not be processed by the autistic person.

What Can First Responders Do?

Police officers and other first responders come into contact with all types of neurodiversity, not just autism. While clinicians often require hours to diagnose a neurodiverse condition, first responders may have very little time in which to 'size up' an individual with whom they are in contact. Even if all first responders received effective training in neurodiverse conditions they cannot be expected to identify any one of these conditions in a first response situation. This emphasises the importance of disclosure in such situations. It is appreciated that there are various reasons why an individual may not wish to disclose a diagnosis outside family and friends. However, we consider it important that police forces, other first response organisations, and those advocating for autism and other neurodiverse conditions do all they can to encourage disclosure in first response situations (even by those individuals who otherwise would not disclose) as first responders cannot reasonably be expected to react appropriately in every situation they may face in the absence of disclosure.

Major autism charities in the UK, like the National Autistic Society, have produced information cards that autistic people can carry and share with first responders. These cards explain that the person they are speaking to is autistic. They also highlight the potential of communication difficulties the autistic person may have during unfamiliar situations. Debbaudt (2002) has developed some guidelines to assist first responders when an individual is known to be autistic which are embedded in the following and added to:

1. Approach in a quiet, non-threatening manner; if possible keep the approach down to one person, and avoid speech as much as possible.
2. Turn sirens and flashing lights off.
3. Talk calmly in a moderated voice if need be.
4. Allow plenty of time for communication to be digested—avoid overwhelming the individual with verbal instructions.
5. Avoid giving multiple instructions at the same time.
6. Do not interpret limited eye contact as deceit or disrespect.
7. Avoid metaphorical questions that cause confusion when taken literally.

8. Avoid body language that can cause confusion. Be alert to a person modelling your body language.
9. Understand the need to repeat questions.
10. Understand that communications will take longer to establish.
11. Use simple and direct instructions and allow for delayed responses to questions, directions, and commands.
12. Avoid putting the person into any situation in which he feels threatened—this might include the back of a police van, for example.

When a person is arrested they are being deprived of their liberty and an officer needs to explain why, in the form of a police caution. The police caution can be complicated to understand so instead of asking a suspect if they understand which may produce a 'yes' or 'no' response, ask them to explain in their own words what they understood; this could help to identify vulnerable suspects. It is worth noting that in the UK the Police and Criminal Evidence Act, 1984 (PACE), states that a person should be treated as vulnerable when a custody officer has any doubt about their mental state. Easy read custody sheets that help bridge the gap between a custody officer and a suspect while they await an appropriate adult have been piloted in a UK force with positive outcomes for autistic people. Moreover, they take away the uncertainty of what will happen while they are in custody (Parsons & Sherwood, 2016).

Predictability

Autistic people may require high levels of predictability in order to feel safe and secure. If possible ensure that the autistic person understands what is going to happen, when, and in what order. Keep to any timings that you have identified. Make sure that the person has as much prior warning of any changes that are going to impact upon his situation as is possible.

Assumption of Prior Knowledge

Do not assume anything in terms of what the autistic person might or might not know. While there are some things that one might assume is common sense, common knowledge, or obvious—one should not assume that such information is readily available to the autistic person, particularly when in a heightened state of anxiety. In a similar vein, it is useful to keep checking that any information given (particularly verbal) is understood and retained by the autistic individual.

Low Arousal

At all times it is worth noting that all actions and interactions should be as least provocative as possible. As throughout this chapter it is not possible to include everything that will be of use to all autistic individuals, but the following is likely to benefit most:

- Voices should be calm, clear, precise, even in tone;
- Keep facial features neutral;
- Keep body movement to a minimum;
- Avoid irritating noises such as chairs scraping across the floor, ticking of clocks, etc.;
- Avoid sudden movements;
- Keep change to a minimum—any changes of circumstance should be clearly explained in advance;
- Back up verbal communication with written instructions whenever possible.

Interviews[5]

Debbaudt (2002) highlights susceptibility in autistic people during interviews; in particular, when leading questions are asked. As a result of the susceptibility of some autistic people they may feel that they do not need legal advice and confess to an offence that they did not commit. This is especially true if the questions were not responded to correctly due to misinterpretation. It is good practice to summarise from time to time during an interview to check understanding. If the person is quiet or confused consider asking them to write their responses down. Allow them extra time to process information. Additionally, direct support from another person, either a family member or an appropriate adult should be considered a reasonable adjustment. An autistic person may also agree to receiving a police caution for a crime they have not committed due to the anxiety of going to court and being cross-examined. It is also paramount that the person understands that accepting a police caution results in a criminal record and will affect any criminal conviction checks in the future. It is also noteworthy that in the UK you can only appeal against your conviction, sentence, or both at a magistrates' court if you pleaded not guilty at your trial (https://www.gov.uk/appeal-against-sentence-conviction/magistrates-court-verdict). Therefore, a custody officer's risk assessment for an autistic person should include assigning an appropriate adult to ensure procedures are followed and understood by the detainee. An appropriate adult should be additional to legal representation and should be present during the interview (PACE, 1984). However, it is only when vulnerabilities

---

[5] Content from Beardon, L. et al. (2018). First responders and autism. In *The Encyclopedia of Autism Spectrum Disorders* (F. Volkmar, Ed.). Springer-Verlag. Is used here with permission from Springer Nature.

are suspected or declared that such provision will be arranged emphasising the importance of disclosure when in police custody. Officers should consider taking statements from an autistic victim of a crime in surroundings familiar to them. Explain what being a witness entails and offer support if a case goes to trial.

Autism and High-Risk Law Enforcement Contacts

This section will identify three predictable high-risk contacts that less independent autistic children, adolescents, and adults will have with law enforcement professionals throughout their lifetimes and describe safety and risk strategies that can help minimise and manage these risks. These three contacts are for suspicious persons, aggressive persons, and missing, vulnerable children, and adults. Each contact comes with a tragic potential for injury or death. The first two hold the potential for use of force and are fraught with communication and proximity dilemmas. The third, tragically, is too often a cause of death for the less independent and vulnerable child, young person, or adult.

Less Independent Persons

These high-risk contacts typically involve children and adults that are less independent. The term less independent is used to describe children and adults who have difficulty in areas involving basic life skills such as safely crossing a street, negotiating a financial transaction, recognising dangerous risks, and then taking steps to manage or avoid them.

Less independent autistic individuals may also have a diagnosis of intellectual disability and limited, difficult to understand verbal abilities. They may also be nonverbal and use alternative forms of communication such as sign language, Picture Exchange Communications Systems (PECS), or computer tablets that can speak for them. If verbal, their communications may be understood only by people who know them well. Less independent individuals should be accompanied by a responsible adult whenever and wherever they travel in the community. They will likely be dependent on a responsible adult for the basic necessities of life including their personal safety.

Suspicious Persons

Without disclosure, officer observations and descriptions of the behaviour and body language of less independent autistic persons have ranged from persons presenting as under the influence of phencyclidine (PCP), methamphetamine, or alcohol, having a mental health episode, preparing to commit a crime, or acting suspiciously. Asking police officers to accurately conduct a quick field diagnosis of a person's autism may go beyond reasonable expectations. Disclosure will help by avoiding the need for 'diagnostic' guesswork.

When police officers suspect that the person they are interacting with may be autistic they should ask family members, care providers, or neighbours who may be with them or nearby if there are any vulnerabilities or disabilities that the officers might need to be aware of, for example, epilepsy, autism, other neurodiversity, sensory issues. If the individual is on their own they should be asked the same question.[6] Disclosure of autism may also come during an emergency call from a parent, caregiver, teacher, or neighbour.

Suspicious person reports can include parent or caregiver actions that may be misinterpreted or appear as assault. For example, a father picking up and carrying away his crying, kicking, red-faced, and teary-eyed child from a store or park may appear to observers as a possible child abduction. Another example would be a caregiver using a comforting strong yet suspicious looking hug with a struggling, visibly upset man or woman in a public place. Additionally, when the person displays unusual behaviour in a community setting where they are not known, including sitting on someone's lawn chair or swing, climbing trees, looking into windows of homes, and running into traffic. Others may be observed in or on dangerous structures—for instance, river or lake break-walls, fences, cement walls, bridges, or overpasses. Their fascination with water may find them swimming or splashing in mall fountains or in store restroom turning faucets on and off or flushing toilets continuously.

Inappropriate or unexpected social skills such as unwarranted laughing or crying, walking on one's toes and flapping hands while staring into space, turning lights on and off repetitively accompanied by a close in focus on the same lights, becoming mesmerised by a ceiling fan for endless periods of time and repeated flicking of small objects such as thread, twigs, or toys a few inches in front of one's eyes are examples of behaviours that can concern observant citizens. All these observations are precisely the sorts of situations that may result in a suspicious person report to the police. When police respond, a lack of disclosure and proximity only add to suspicion and potential for a volatile interaction.

Domestic Violence Calls

Autism-related domestic violence calls for assistance may be generated from homes or from any community setting including, educational premises, recreational centres, hospitals, and entertainment venues. The less independent child or adult's capability to recognise social proximity boundaries—including Covid-19 era expectations—only increases the risks for attending police officers as well as for the autistic individual themselves.

---

[6] It is unethical and inappropriate to ask a person if they are autistic under normal circumstances.

Often described in the autism community with terminology such as 'meltdown' (correct, as cognitive and/or sensory overload is involved) or 'tantrum' (incorrect, because anger is not usually involved), these contacts are perhaps the highest risk situation for the frontline police officer and come with the potential to result in use of force physical confrontations between police and autistic citizens. The risks for all involved are multifaceted: families agonise about making an emergency call and parents fear that responding police will be quick to use force due to a lack of understanding of autism and of the behaviours of their child or adult. Even when all protocols are followed, police personnel may need to defend against immediate scrutiny in professional and social media and subsequent civil litigation. Calls from caregivers seeking assistance to control behaviour that has escalated from manageable to an aggressive point beyond their control should be considered high-risk contacts.

Police informational topics should include how a physical outburst might well be related to the autistic person's sensory sensitivities, inability to deal with interruptions in the daily routine, or emotional lability. This often presents itself in individuals with autism—their emotions can change quickly and they can become upset, scared, or anxious very quickly. They may also be extremely anxious one minute, and then calm the next, or vice versa.

The distressed, less independent autistic person may be unaware of the effect their behaviour has on other people or the situation at hand. It may be difficult for them to predict the consequences of their actions or appreciate that their actions could be misinterpreted as suspicious or aggressive. Being approached by someone may cause an autistic person to flee, failing to obey an order to stop. Some autistic people react by crumpling to the ground or rocking back and forth They may avoid eye contact. When responding police officers know, suspect, or are told that a person is autistic, they will be able to interpret displays of unusual and confusing behaviours as evidence of autism. These behaviours should not then be seen as intentional failure to respond to questions, cooperate with commands, or as a reason for use of increased force. The person may be slow to comply, or be completely unable to comply, even with simple requests. Processing a request, command, or question and replying with an answer or response, even under the best of circumstances, may take the autistic person longer than one may expect, perhaps as much as fifteen to twenty seconds or more.

Escalated behaviour may be in the form of rocking, pacing, grunting, noisemaking, utterances, running into walls, head-banging, or hiding under mattresses or other large objects. They may also bite, scratch, and pull hair. These behaviours may be a form of self-stimulation or a sensory reaction to objects and influences in the environment.

While there may be situations that require quick action—such as a person near traffic, on a bridge, near water sources, or other dangerous places—be prepared to invest extra time, keep communication simple and free of jargon, idioms, and slang. Scan the immediate and background area. What do you see and hear that might be hurtful for an autistic person with sensory sensitivities? Are you able to eliminate or minimise sensory such things as flashing lights, sirens, squawking radios, or personal communication devices, canine partners, members of the public, or police personnel? Use your discretion. If you have determined that the person is not a threat, have established geographic containment (person cannot escape from the location), invest the extra time necessary to allow them to de-escalate themselves without physical intervention. It will often be best for an officer to back off from the autistic individual and keep quiet until they have calmed down sufficiently for interaction.

Escapism and Vulnerable Missing Persons

While independent adults may escape from and wander away from homes and caregivers, a majority of missing person calls will involve children; the reporters will be family members, educators, and caregivers. Florida, with a very large number of home swimming pools, has more drowning deaths and nonfatal hospitalisations for water-related injuries among children one to four years of age than any other US state. According to the Florida Bureau of Vital Statistics, autistic children made up 10% of all deaths by drowning in Florida for children ages one to fourteen (Jones, 2019). When one considers that the prevalence of autism in the population is about 2%, this should spark outrage.

Escape by the less independent autistic child or adult from safety and responsible supervision often occurs at night when caregivers are asleep. Escape can also occur when caregivers become injured or incapacitated, ill, or distracted, perhaps when using a restroom, taking a call, or caring for a sibling or another client.

Florida-based and US online research survey results indicate that escapism-related drowning of less independent autistic individuals, and some autistic children, is a leading cause of concern and contact with police and public safety professionals in America. They may be unusually attracted to water sources and frequently be found in or near rivers, lakes, ponds, swimming pools, and fountains. In addition to water sources, some individuals may also be attracted to vehicles and wander into traffic. Their attempts to enter nearby homes, dwellings, or vehicles of persons that do not know them have been met by force and calls to police. Children and adults have wandered onto train tracks and elevated places such as rooftops, trees, and on or under bridges. They may seek refuge in underbrush, alleys, and dumps in order to rest. Searchers and rescuers are well advised to look under discarded mattresses and inside discarded furniture and appliances. In urban settings, the person may seek refuge in abandoned buildings or vacant homes.

Further highlighting autism-related elopement in America is the involvement of the Federal Bureau of investigation (FBI). The FBI initiated their Child Abduction Rapid Deployment (CARD) units in 2005. There is now a CARD team agent in nearly every one of the FBI's 56 field offices. As part of their mission, the FBI-CARD teams respond to mysterious disappearances of children, in particular children of tender years—12 and under.

In recent years these units of highly trained and experienced agents have responded to incidents involving missing autistic children. FBI-CARD team members were among hundreds of law enforcement and search and rescue personnel that assisted in the search for Maddox Ritch,[7] who walked away from a park in Gastonia on 22 September 2018. His body was found five days later partially submerged in a creek near the park.

Since then, a special agent on the FBI team that assisted in the search for Maddox has developed a one-page Autism Checklist questionnaire for investigators to use when a child with autism goes missing. FBI Special Agent James Granozio works in the Bureau's Charlotte Field Office and also leads one of the FBI's four regional Child Abduction Rapid Deployment (CARD) Teams. 'He was a little boy that was just running around having a good time. And he died', Granozio said in a 2020 fbi.gov news interview titled, Every Minute Counts: CARD Team Develops Checklist to Aid Searches for Missing Autistic Children. 'So we all wanted to know what we could learn from it to hopefully prevent it from happening again'.[8] The FBI-CARD Autism Checklist template includes autism-specific insight gathered from responding to a growing number of missing autistic children. The Autism Checklist is available through FBI field offices to any requesting law enforcement agency.

In light of the importance of the drowning risk in autism, and differences in attention given to drowning deaths by professionals and the media in the USA and UK, we discuss the autism drowning risk in detail later on.

For each of these high-risk contacts, the first step for families, school officials, or other caregivers must be to call the emergency number immediately, certainly upon discovery of a missing child or adult, and use the word autism to describe the individual. In cases of missing persons, families, and care providers should resist the temptation to conduct a search before calling the police.

When an autism report is made to the emergency call centre, alert dispatchers to expect to follow-up calls from citizens who report suspicious persons near roadways or vehicles, in neighbourhoods, on property, or attempting to enter homes or unlocked vehicles.

Mandatory Reporting

Parents and families may take measures at home to ensure safety that could appear to police, social service professionals, and other mandatory reporters as evidence of parental neglect or abuse. Left unexplained, homes that feature higher fences in yards, extra locks and alarms, motion and sound sensors could easily be seen as suspicious, neglectful, or abusive. While these are typical precautions taken by autism families to alert and protect against a dangerous escape, search and rescue, law enforcement will need to rule out parental neglect or direct criminal involvement as a cause for the disappearance and for referral to child and adult protective services for investigation. In cases involving autistic children, occurrences of this have been low in frequency.

[7] https://www.fbi.gov/contact-us/field-offices/charlotte/news/press-releases/fbi-joins-search-for-boy-missing-from-gastonia-park.

[8] https://www.fbi.gov/news/stories/fbi-checklist-aids-searches-for-missing-autistic-children.

Yet, troubling recent (2018, 2019, and 2020) US incidents of parents being charged with murder for killing their children prior to reporting them to authorities as missing. While not directly a reason for mandatory reporting, falsely or truthfully reporting a vulnerable autistic child as missing will cause law enforcement and public safety to unleash search and rescue responses. The investigation should include interviews of non-offending family members, neighbours, and persons known to the missing child or adult. Search coordinators will muster foot patrol, tracking animals and technology, aircraft, boats, and assistance from outside policing agencies as well as professional and volunteer search and rescue personnel. Additionally, awareness outreach to citizens at large through television, radio, and print news outlets and social media that seek information and additional eyes and ears are efforts that can last multiple, deeply emotional days. Beyond the waste of time and resources, false reporting is troubling for the emotional toll it reaps on a community. Falsely reporting a vulnerable child or adult as missing should be added to the broader topic of filicide of autistic children and adults.

Disclosure

Since each autistic individual is unique and may act or react differently the responsibility of providing information for autistic persons, family members, and care providers looms large. For law enforcement professionals, having knowledge that autistic people may have different independence levels becomes essential when they prepare for these high-risk field interactions. This begs the question: how can autistic individuals, families, and caregivers provide this actionable intelligence? In a word: disclosure.

Disclosure of person-specific information can be achieved very simply by means of an autism alert card. While most of these cards are of a generic nature, some UK police forces have introduced a system for producing cards which contain person-specific information such as details of sensory sensitivities and advice on communication requirements. Disclosure enables more informed interactions with law enforcement professionals.

Other simple and highly effective disclosure options might include autism awareness magnets, decals, and vehicle licence plates. Neighbourhood traffic signs that alert drivers to the possible presence of autistic children are in use in the USA and Canada.[9] Identification (ID), name, or phone number, may be included in an autism tag or bracelet, an autism information card, information printed or on quick response (QR) codes (scanned by smart phones) on radio frequency identification devices

[9] Signage relating to elopement and wandering can be a valuable risk management measure. However, the risks of elopement and wandering are not restricted to autism and most autistic people are no more likely to elope or wander than are neurotypical individuals. We therefore recommend that where there is a known high risk of elopement and wandering in a particular area a more generic form of signage be installed such as: 'Please be aware that there may be vulnerable children in the area and slow down'.

(RFID) tags placed in shoes, jackets, and backpacks, sewn into garments, imprinted on undergarments, or on a non-permanent ID tattoo. Second generation RFID tagging for alert and disclosure capabilities: digital information including contact advice and photos coupled with increased capacity reader/receivers may open up enhanced drone, aircraft, and ground tracking and recovery operations.

Police officers may hear such idiomatic terms for being autistic as 'on the spectrum', 'aspie', 'spectrumite', and terms often associated with autism such as 'stimming' (self-stimulatory behaviours). Police and other public safety professionals should be taught that hearing these words amounts to a disclosure of autism and a direct cue to put autism training room knowledge about how to interact with autistic individuals into action.

Person-Specific Information.

In response to a growing number of missing person reports and sudden high-risk contacts with police and public safety personnel, every autism community advocacy group should be encouraged to advise families, friends, educators, and care professionals to develop a person-specific autism safety plan. An essential part of these voluntary plans is sharing autism emergency contact information including the name of the person at risk, current photograph, complete physical description, home and mobile phone numbers for all emergency contact persons. Parents and responsible adults should determine what sensory, medical, or dietary issues and requirements to disclose.

Each plan should be created and designed for a specific person. The plan development team should be led by the autistic individual as much as possible and include parents, family members, and legally responsible adults. To keep the plan fresh and add or replace information, the team should plan to meet at least quarterly, monthly, or more as needed.

Ask safety-related questions to decide what information to provide police and public safety professionals such as:

Does the person have an inclination to escape care and wander dangerously?
What are the attractions and locations where the person may be found?
Do they display behaviours or characteristics that may attract attention?
What are favourite topics of interest to pursue and calm the person?
What are topics to avoid that may cause fear, anger, or outbursts?
What are recommended approach and de-escalation techniques?
What is the best method of communication?
Does the person wear ID jewellery or disclosure tags or technology?
Does the person carry a handout card? If so, where? Wallet? Backback? Pocket. Elsewhere?
Does the person wear communications technology to track their location, such as radio frequency (RF) or global positioning system (GPS)?

Parents and responsible adults may create a handout guide to nearby properties with water sources and dangerous locations highlighted. Information should be legible, printed out, and copied for distribution to all caregivers: family, educational, child or adult care, and transportation, therapeutic, and recreational service providers. Copies should be kept in vehicle glove compartments, under sun visors, in care providers and child or adults purses, wallets, and backpacks. If possible and as backup, transfer information to digital formats such as PDF or jpeg and transfer to thumb drives RFID chips, mobile devices, and tablets.

Sharing Information with Police and Public Safety

Emergency call centres are now offering voluntary registration programmes in regions of the USA and Canada. For families that participate, person-specific information can be uploaded and accessed quickly by way of mobile computer, tablet, or dispatch. Law enforcement professionals also report that having access to person-specific information, for example someone's likes, dislikes, and favourite topics, before an interaction occurs with an autistic child or adult, will greatly enhance their ability to provide a safer, more informed response.

Parents, family members, educators, and service providers are the best providers of safety information and advice. For example, wandering away into potentially dangerous situations is a safety risk many families have experienced or prepared for. Other autistic individuals may have a high tolerance for pain or lack of fear of real danger, information that can well inform a high-risk situation. Combined with wandering, these and the risks described may affect families in their relationships with their neighbours, and during excursions outside of the home. Mums and dads may very well know what triggers their son or daughter's behaviours. They may also have well-developed techniques designed to deal with or avoid those triggers, or they may know ways to de-escalate their child's behaviour. This knowledge base is enhanced through sharing.

Sharing information in a variety of settings—proactively through the emergency call centre, in real time through technology and printed information may very well be the difference between an ill-informed and well-informed response by police and public safety professionals. All stakeholders—families, clinicians, law enforcement, and community members—share responsibility for ensuring the safety of those autistic people unable to do this for themselves.

With the twenty-first century increase in diagnostic prevalence of autism,[10] there is no better time than the present to get together with our police and public safety partners and share information that can save lives. Policing and public safety professionals understand well that their preparation will serve them well when they are

[10] We do not believe that there has been a particularly noteworthy increase in autism over the years. In our view increases in the numbers of identified individuals is much more likely to be as a result of improving diagnostic practice rather than an actual increase of autism.

put into high-risk situations that increase their anxiety and challenge their ability to process information quickly. The autism community and advocacy organisations must help autistic persons, family members, and care providers to share effective, generic, and person-specific autism safety information with police and public safety professionals.

Drowning Deaths and Autistic Children in the USA versus the UK

One particular risk that first responders must be aware of is drowning. Drowning deaths for children and youth in the USA have received considerable attention in recent years. Certainly, well publicised deaths such as those of Avonte Oquendo and Kevin Willis, autistic boys who both wandered and drowned have done much to raise awareness of this issue. Their deaths were honoured in Kevin and Avonte's Law,[11] recently passed by the US Congress (March, 2018). These deaths represent a portion of the deaths of autistic children due to unintentional injury and, all too often, elopements[12] that end in drowning.

The elevated risk of autistic children is very well established. Studies by Mouridsen et al. (2008), Shavelle et al. (2001), Pickett et al. (2006), and Gillberg et al. (2010), and many others, all provide data for significantly greater chances of an early death for autistic individuals, with medical conditions predominant but unintentional injury a strong contributing factor.

Obtaining conclusive data on autism drowning deaths is not easy. Death records simply may not record the fact that a child had autism, rendering systems such as the National Vital Statistics System less than reliable. Guan and Li (2017) in a study looking at the nature of autism drowning deaths resorted to newspaper accounts for relevant details of the deaths. This is, in one way, illustrative of the accurate data problem that accompanies any effort to get a true number of autism drownings. Locally, the fifth author has sent letters to County Medical Examiners in an effort to determine the number of autism deaths. One medical examiner provided a list of 10 autism deaths in 10 years, while the medical examiner in an adjacent county reported that they would not have recorded most of these types of deaths. In the absence of solid data, the true number of autism drowning deaths will remain a mystery but

[11] Among other matters, this law amends the Violent Crime Control and Law Enforcement Act of 1994 to promote initiatives intended to reduce the risk of injury or death relating to the wandering or elopement of autistic children and adults, and those with other developmental disabilities or dementia.

[12] Although colloquially used in relation to running-off to get married, the definition of 'elopement' includes an act or instance of an individual putting themselves at risk by leaving a safe premises or other safe area. It is important to appreciate that autistic children and adults, and those with other developmental disabilities or dementia, may lack age-appropriate self-preservation and personal safety judgement skills.

elopements are the pathway to these drowning deaths and we do have some good data on this problem.

Rice and colleagues (2016) in *The Journal of Pediatrics*, reported that 37.7% of autistic children and intellectual disability were reported by their parents to have eloped in the past year. Even those autistic children without intellectual disability eloped at a rate of 32.7%. Most elopements end with the child returned home safely but a young child, typically lacking self-preservation skills, alone in a risk-filled world is at extraordinary risk. It is not surprising then that so many elopements do result in injury or death.

The issue of autism drowning does not now appear to be a major topic of inquiry in the UK. In the USA, people often reside within close proximity to water. Depending on where in the country one lives, pools, spas, canals, lakes, and the ocean may pose ever-present risks, all of them dangerous for the unsupervised child with weak self-preservation skills. The patterns of residential development in the UK do not seem to feature so much water so close to residences but, that being said, England is an island with a considerable coastline and many rivers and streams and lakes. Most European countries have some sort of universal swim instruction for children. This is rare in the USA with only a very few examples to be found including Broward County (Fort Lauderdale area) Florida, and Juneau, Alaska as exceptions. Early swim instruction may be reducing drowning deaths for autistic children in counties with universal or near universal swim instruction.

Parent reporting of elopement is sometimes delayed in the USA as parents may fear negative consequences for such reporting including investigation for child negligence or being stigmatised as a poor parent by the community. A careful review of the factors that may facilitate or impede parent reporting of elopements in the UK in contrast to the USA will be helpful. Further, consider an interesting and troubling finding in the USA from a 2011 report by the Interactive Autism Network by Paul Law. He reported that.... 'Despite the difficulties families have faced, 51% reported they had never received any advice or guidance about their child's elopement behaviour from a professional, with only 14% receiving such advice from a paediatrician or other physician and only 19% receiving such advice from a mental health professional'. It was as if elopement behaviour was a hidden topic, at least in 2011 for many professionals who should have been actively sharing this information with parents but who did not. This situation, to the degree that it was that way has now certainly changed, with so much more awareness of elopement in the USA. It has become a topic of conversation within the autism community when it may well have been previously suppressed or kept quiet. It could be that elopement and the horrible sequela of elopement in terms of drowning, is not a frequently discussed topic of conversation within the UK autism community at this time.

It may be the case that children in the UK simply do not elope as often as do those in the USA. Or it may be that research and information on wandering are viewed in an entirely different manner in the UK. The US scholars, Solomon and Lawlor (2018: 9, authors' italics) point out that 'prevention of "wandering" puts people with autism at potential *other* risks besides drowning, exposure, and traffic injuries' given that walking out can be about the exploration of an individual's world and sense of self. This chapter focuses on physical safety and the dangers of elopement in relation to *less independent* autistic individuals.

So, it is possible that there is both less research on wandering in the UK, less safety-related research on autism wandering and, perhaps less appreciation for the risks associated with autism wandering incidents. Full consideration, obviously, requires a comprehensive review of the UK autism literature by someone immersed in this literature. But we have to believe that the nature of autism will be the same in any country and with it the propensity for children with autism to wander or elope. The consequence of elopements, unless the child is found in the shortest possible time period, will not be good. If elopement is not being reported much in the UK and if drowning as a result of elopement is not an issue, we suspect that careful, comprehensive investigations into why there is such a contrast to the USA are certainly warranted.

Conclusion: The Autism Imperative for the Police Service and Academic Researchers

Although there has not been a great deal of research into contacts between police officers and autistic people, there is sufficient research to demonstrate that, generally speaking, police officers do not have the necessary understanding of autism for such contacts to go as smoothly as one would be entitled to expect interaction between the police and members of the public to go. Even allowing for misreporting, the news media regularly report incidents where contact between police officers and autistic members of the public have apparently gone badly wrong. Such incidents can involve physical and/or psychological injury to the autistic person, and often unnecessary anxiety and stress (over and above the anxiety and stress that any contact with law enforcements can involve). It has even been reported that hospitalisation after such contacts occurs on a sufficiently frequent basis for researchers to refer to it (Turcotte et al., 2018). It is high time that researchers investigated the circumstances surrounding incidents that have gone wrong to ascertain why problems with police/public interaction appear to be such a regular occurrence.

Clearly, the responsibility for ensuring that interactions between law enforcement and autistic members of the public go as smoothly as one could reasonably expect such interactions to go cannot lie with the autistic individuals alone. With that in mind, and taking note of the general lack of training provided for operational police officers as reported in the literature, the obvious hypothesis regarding why police/public interactions appear to go wrong so regularly is that police officers do not have the necessary understanding of autism to know how to handle such interactions. There is plenty of 'evidence' from the incidents themselves, in addition to media and academic reporting of incidents, to demonstrate the need for police officers to understand autism.

There is a training resource available to police services that is clearly not being used. We are in contact with various police officers and retired police officers with a familial connection with autism who represent a potential training resource. Many of these officers have sought to raise the profile of autism within the service through personal action and via setting up organisations such as National Police Autism Association (NPAA) in the UK. But, more importantly, some officers have a personal connection with autism. The NPAA website includes the following: 'There are police officers with autism? Really? Yes, really. Officers with Asperger syndrome (a form of autism without intellectual impairment) can be found at all levels of the police service'.[13] It is clear from this wording that it must come as a surprise to many people that any police officer could be autistic. This misunderstanding associated with the wider nature of autism needs correction. But, continuing our focus on autism training for police officers, what better resource is there than their autistic colleagues who understand operational policing and autism? Despite the efforts of individuals, the media, academia, and statutory legal training requirements in parts of the USA, the great majority of US policing agencies do not train their officers in autism sufficiently to make a positive difference to the outcome of many interactions with autism. The situation is no better in the UK.

We have stated our hypothesis that police/public interactions involving autistic people go wrong so regularly is that police officers do not have the necessary understanding of autism to know how to handle such interactions. And we have suggested that there is sufficient academic and other evidence to demonstrate that our hypothesis is correct. If, indeed, we are correct, the next question to ask is why police forces are not taking action to remedy this situation. Our subsidiary hypothesis is that the extent of the training demands on police officer time make it very difficult to ensure that officers receive training in all areas of relevance to operational policing. It has been reported that: '… most officers received between 400 and 770 h of total training, of which only 3 to 12 h are focused on mental health disorders' (Gardner et al., 2019: 1278). Ignoring the fact that autism is not a mental health disorder, these figures provide a stark indication of the extent of police training and imply that the addition of new training requirements will not be easy to achieve. One of the authors has personal experience of the difficulty involved in getting a police force to undertake new training, especially where the training is not seen as an operational priority. We have some sympathy with police forces in this regard and hence we have sought creative solutions to the clear and present problem of lack of police officer understanding of autism. Our proposal is that autism should be embedded within existing officer training as appropriate, that existing training officers receive a high level[14] of autism training, and that the delivery of autism training content to new recruits and operational officers be led by autism-trained officers complemented by officers with a personal and/or familial connection with autism who have also received a high level of autism training before they deliver any training.

[13] https://www.npaa.org.uk/faq/?doing_wp_cron=1535133367.9983890056610107421875.

[14] By 'high level' of autism training we mean the equivalent of the Sheffield Hallam University/National Autistic Society Post Graduate Certificate in Autism and Asperger Syndrome.

In conclusion, here is a brief reflection on reasons why autism appears not to be an operational priority for so many police forces on both sides of the Atlantic, and what might be required to make a 'case' for autism training to senior police management. Because the research is still limited, the task at this juncture is to develop some further hypotheses and advocate for more study. It is our opinion that attitudes towards autism do not predispose anyone towards autism, and there is no reason to suppose that, generally speaking, police officers will be any more receptive to the autism imperative than anyone else, i.e. this is not a police issue per se but a societal issue. We might describe this as systemic discrimination against autism. It is our view that the accusation of systemic racism against the Metropolitan Police Service in London following the death of Stephen Lawrence may have unfairly branded the police service as being more racist than society in general.

We see a parallel between racism and autism discrimination and see the police as generally being representative of the society from which their officers are drawn. We therefore believe that societal change is required in response to the autism imperative. In the meantime, a 'case' must be made to convince senior police management that action in response to this imperative is required now. In his song '400 Years', the late Jamaican reggae artist Peter Tosh[15] wrote of freeing Black people from the oppression they have suffered since their ancestors were taken from Africa. The killing of George Floyd in Minneapolis in May 2020 is only the latest in a long line of instances involving the killing of black people by police officers in the USA. In their report of an investigation of the lived experiences of Black men in contact with the police, Brooks et al. (2016: 347) wrote of 'law enforcement bias, extreme mistreatment of Black people, the need for cultural competency, and training restructuring'. These researchers call for implementation of 'new procedures that specifically address the systemic cultural misunderstandings and bias' (ibid.: 358) associated with racism. For ethnic minority individuals who are autistic there is a risk of 'double discrimination' when interacting with police officers. We call for research into the experiences of those at risk of this. In the meantime, we stress that autism knows no racial boundaries and encourage law enforcement to be aware that their actions may doubly discriminate if they fail to treat all members of the public equally.

One of us has worked with the senior management team of a major UK police force. His experience indicates that the best way of making a case for change is to demonstrate the potential damage to a force's reputation when an incident goes badly wrong and the force is the subject of media and other criticism. We think that such a case should not be difficult to make given the many incidents that have put law enforcement in the public spotlight and the knowledge that such incidents will continue to occur until something is done. As part of this 'case' we recommend that autism (including the risk of double discrimination when an autistic person is from an ethnic minority) should be embedded within existing national and force-level officer

[15] Peter Tosh was a member of the original Wailers alongside Bob Marley and Bunny Wailer (Neville O'Riley Livingston).

training courses and be delivered by officers who fit a combination of the following profiles:

Profile A

1. be an officer already involved in the delivery of training;
2. have received an agreed high level of training in autism.

Profile B

1. have a personal and/or familial connection with autism;
2. have received an agreed high level of training in autism;
3. have received 'train the trainer' training.

This recommended approach will help police forces to serve and protect autistic members of the public, protect the forces themselves against potential damage to their reputations as a result of interactions with autistic people that hit the headlines, and enable the delivery of training in autism without adding additional training courses.

References

Adebowale, V. (2013). *Independent commission on mental health and policing report*. Independent Commission on Mental Health and Policing.

Artingstall, S. (2007). What do the police know and understand about ASD? *Good Autism Practice (GAP), 8*(2), 21–30.

Beardon L., Chown N., & Cossburn K. (2018). First responders and autism. In Volkmar F. (Eds) *Encyclopedia of Autism Spectrum Disorders*. New York, NY: Springer. https://doi.org/10.1007/978-1-4614-6435-8_102159-1.

Blackhurst, J. (2012). The involvement of the police in the lives of people with Asperger syndrome: What are the perspectives of both parties? *Good Autism Practice (GAP), 13*(1), 22–30.

Brooks, M., Ward, C., Euring, M., Townsend, C., White, N., & Hughes, K. L. (2016). Is there a problem officer? Exploring the lived experience of black men and their relationship with law enforcement. *Journal of African American Studies, 20*(3–4), 346–362.

Chown, N. (2010). 'Do you have any difficulties that I may not be aware of?' A study of autism awareness and understanding in the UK police service. *International Journal of Police Science & Management, 12*(2), 256–273.

Crane, L., Maras, K. L., Hawken, T., Mulcahy, S., & Memon, A. (2016). Experiences of autism spectrum disorder and policing in England and Wales: Surveying police and the autism community. *Journal of Autism and Developmental Disorders, 46*(6), 2028–2041.

Debbaudt, D. (2002). *Autism, advocates and law enforcement professionals: Recognizing and reducing risk situations for people with autism spectrum disorders*. Jessica Kingsley.

Debbaudt, D. (2007). Autism spectrum and law enforcement training. *The Best of the OARacle: A Compilation of Articles from, 2002–2007*, 58.

Debbaudt, D. (2008). *Autism & field response instructors guide NYPD*. ADD DoH, 2010 reference.

Gardner, L., Campbell, J. M., & Westdal, J. (2019). Brief report: Descriptive analysis of law enforcement officers' experiences with and knowledge of autism. *Journal of Autism and Developmental Disorders, 49*(3), 1278–1283.

Gillberg, C., Billstedt, E., Sundh, V., & Gillberg, I. C. (2010). Mortality in autism: A prospective longitudinal community-based study. *Journal of Autism and Developmental Disorders, 40*, 352–357.
Guan, J., & Li, G. (2017). Characteristics of unintentional drowning deaths in children with autism spectrum disorder. *Injury Epidemiology, 4*, 32.
Hepworth, D. (2017). A critical review of current police training and policy for autism spectrum disorder. *Journal of Intellectual Disabilities and Offending Behaviour, 8*(4), 212–222.
Home Office. (1984). *Police and criminal evidence act*. HMSO.
Jones, K. T. (2019). *Personal communication with Jack Scott*.
Kelly, E., & Hassett-Walker, C. (2016). The training of New Jersey emergency service first responders in autism awareness. *Police Practice and Research, 17*(6), 543–554.
Krameddine, Y., DeMarco, D., Hassel, R., & Silverstone, P. H. (2013). A novel training program for police officers that improves interactions with mentally ill individuals and is cost-effective. *Frontiers in Psychiatry, 4*, 9.
Laan, J. M., Ingram, R. V., & Glidden, M. D. (2013). Law enforcement training on mental disorders and autism spectrum disorders in the southeastern United States. *Journal of Global Intelligence & Policy, 6*(10), 51–67.
Modell, S. J., & Mak, S. (2008). A preliminary assessment of police officers' knowledge and perceptions of persons with disabilities. *Intellectual and Developmental Disabilities, 46*(3), 183–189.
Mouridsen, S. E., Brønnum-Hansen, H., Rich, B., & Isager, T. (2008). Mortality and causes of death in autism spectrum disorders: An update. *Autism, 12*(4), 403–414.
Murray, D., Lesser, M., & Lawson, W. (2005). Attention, monotropism and the diagnostic criteria for autism. *Autism, 9*(2), 139–156.
Parsons, S., & Sherwood, G. (2016). Vulnerability in custody: Perceptions and practices of police officers and criminal justice professionals in meeting the communication needs of offenders with learning disabilities and learning difficulties. *Disability & Society, 31*(4), 553–572.
Pickett, J. A., Paculdo, D. R., & Shavelle, R. M. (2006). Letter to the editor. *Journal of Autism and Developmental Disorders, 36*, 287–288.
Rice, C. E., Zablotsky, B., Avila, R. M., Colpe, L. J., Schieve, L. A., Pringle, B., & Blumberg, S. J. (2016). Reported wandering behavior among children with autism spectrum disorder and/or intellectual disability. *Journal of Pediatrics, 174*, 232–239.
Shavelle, R. M., Strauss, D. J., & Pickett, J. (2001). Causes of death in autism. *Journal of Autism and Developmental Disorders, 31*(6), 569–576.
Solomon, O., & Lawlor, M. C. (2018). Beyond V40.32: Narrative phenomenology of wandering in autism and dementia. *Culture, Medicine, Psychiatry, 42*, 206–243.
Teagardin, J., Dixon, D. R., Smith, M. N., & Granpeesheh, D. (2012). Randomized trial of law enforcement training on autism spectrum disorders. *Research in Autism Spectrum Disorders, 6*(3), 1113–1118.
Turcotte, P., Shea, L. L., & Mandell, D. (2018). School discipline, hospitalization, and police contact overlap among individuals with autism spectrum disorder. *Journal of Autism and Developmental Disorders, 48*(3), 883–891.

Dr. Nick Chown is a former Insurance Loss Adjuster and a Corporate Risk Manager who is now a Book Indexer and an Autism Researcher. His book Understanding and Evaluating Autism Theory was published by Jessica Kingsley Publishers. Nick also co-edited Neurodiversity Studies: A New Critical Paradigm published by Routledge. His team of independent autism researchers have co-authored reports on support for autistic students in further and higher education and developed a framework for participatory and emancipatory autism research. He has been a member of the Editorial Board of the Journal of Autism and Developmental Disabilities and currently is a Reviewer for the Disability & Society journal.

Dennis Debbaudt was an investigative agency owner and an Investigative Reporter in Michigan and Florida from 1977 through 2014. He first reported on autism contacts with law enforcement in 1993. He has presented direct training throughout the US and globally since 1995. Dennis has produced over sixty autism-related reports in print and video including Autism, Advocates and Law Enforcement Professionals, Jessica Kingsley Publishers, Contact with Individuals with Autism: Effective Resolutions, FBI Law Enforcement Bulletin, Autism: Managing Police Field Contacts, International Association of Chiefs of Police, and the Autism & Law Enforcement training video. Dennis is the proud parent of Brad, an autistic adult.

Dr. Luke Beardon starting as a volunteer aged fourteen in the autism field in a whole range of positions, from a hands-on support worker all the way through to his current role as a Senior Lecturer in Autism at Sheffield Hallam University's Autism Centre where he is the Course Leader for the Post-Graduate Certificate in Autism and Asperger Syndrome. With multiple autism-related awards, inspirational teaching awards, four books to his name, and several other publications, Luke is passionate in trying to make the world a better place for the autistic community through teaching and other forms of knowledge transfer.

Kleio Cossburn served as a Police Officer with Cheshire Constabulary until her retirement. Since leaving the police force, she has graduated with a Masters degree in Criminology and Criminal Justice from Keele University and a Post-Graduate Certificate in Autism from Sheffield Hallam University. Kleio's research draws on her experience as a former police officer, as well as her knowledge of autism.

Dr. Jack Scott serves as the Executive Director of the Florida Atlantic University Center for Autism and Related Disabilities. This state-funded agency provides supports for over 6,000 families in a five-county region of southeast Florida. He is an Associate Professor in the Department of Exceptional Student Education teaching courses on applied behavior analysis, inclusion, and autism. Jack has special research interests in safety for persons with autism, elopement and water risks faced by children with ASD, and the intersection of autism and the police. Jack is a Board Member of the Autism Society of American and chairs the ASA Panel of Professional Advisors.

Chapter 24
Preventing Criminal Sexual Behavior

Eileen T. Crehan and Laurie Sperry

Introduction

There is no reason to believe that autistic people are more likely than non-autistic people to perpetrate sex crimes. While it is possible for an autistic person to have a pedophilic sexual orientation or to have psychopathic personality traits, it is rare, and there is no clear evidence to suggest that such problems occur at a higher rate in ASD than in the general population. When they do, either inadvertently or because they are a rare case of someone with both ASD and co-occurring psychopathy or pedophilia, it is important that clinicians have the proper tools to work with them.

When considering people with ASD as offenders, the social context is vitally important. ASD as a diagnosis that is characterized by deficits in social learning (Mogavero, 2016). A lack of understanding of appropriate and legal behavior is problematic for anyone but especially for those who struggle with social communication. Discussions about sexual behavior oftentimes include vague language or nonverbal cues, which are difficult for autistic individuals to interpret, or take place with peers, which may be less common for autistic adolescents. A comprehensive understanding of how autistic traits may impact sexuality education access and interpretation is vital to avoid legal issues while enabling the autistic person to pursue romantic and intimate relationships in a way that leads to personal satisfaction.

E. T. Crehan (✉)
Eliot-Pearson Department of Child Study & Human Development, Tufts University, 105 College Avenue, Medford 02155, MA, USA
e-mail: eileen.crehan@tufts.edu

L. Sperry
Autism Services and Programs, 4940 Ward Rd, Wheat Ridge, CO 80033, USA
e-mail: drsperry@asapsperry.com

F. R. Volkmar et al. (eds.), *Handbook of Autism Spectrum Disorder and the Law*,
https://doi.org/10.1007/978-3-030-70913-6_24

ASD-specific challenges in social communication, non-social interests, and social learning create barriers to addressing important social, developmental needs of transition age and older youth (Brown-Lavoie et al., 2014). For autistic individuals, the complexity of written and unwritten expectations wrapped up in many sexual behaviors provides layers of challenges to understand and exhibit lawful behavior. For instance, the line between pursuing a romantic interest and stalking is rarely clearly defined or explicitly taught (see Chap. 14 for more information about Stalking). Movies and television often send messages that persistence in pursuing a romantic interest will pay off. But how many calls is too many? What sorts of mediums are appropriate to use in pursuing a romantic interest (e.g., text messages vs. sexting)? If someone is not responding to your advances but not directly saying "stop," how do you know WHEN to stop? Similarly, direct guidance to establish boundaries for masturbating and viewing pornography is rarely discussed, except in response to a problem behavior (Curtis, 2017). These behaviors may be problematic in schools and limit opportunities for inclusive education and can also carry significant long-term stigma and legal complications especially once individuals reach adulthood.

The majority of autistic individuals have the same sexual urges and desire for companionships, platonic or romantic, as their neurotypical peers. Yet rates of sexual relationships have been reported as lower, particularly for individuals with autism and intellectual disability (Strunz et al., 2017). Clearly, the gap between desire to engage romantically with others and success in forming relationships could be mitigated from supports. From another perspective, this unmet desire for relationships may open up the potential for maladaptive behaviors. In the absence of pedophilia or another problematic paraphilia, sexual needs may be met in the context of a consensual intimate relationship. Without this type of relationship available, individuals who may not otherwise offend may revert to other ways of getting sexual needs met. This could present in appropriate ways (for instance, masturbating in private or using sex toys) or inappropriate and even illegals ones (such as seeking out illegal pornographic material or masturbating in public). For many reasons, increased education about sexuality and relationships is key to promoting healthy sexual and intimate patterns of behavior.

A common difficulty in forensic situations involving autistic individuals is separating their intention from the perception of others. When criminal sexual behavior is exhibited by the neurotypical offender, it may have been caused by an intent to harm or offend. Due to challenges with perspective taking, the offender with ASD may not realize the impact of their behavior on others or the actual harm it caused. Especially for work settings, explicitly defining comments that are acceptable is one easy way to avoid legal trouble. This would include avoiding comments about a coworker's appearance that could be interpreted as sexual harassment and establishing guidelines for this (e.g., it may be safest to not comment on the physical appearance of coworkers and instead, comment on their work-related efforts). Reaching to touch an interesting looking piece of jewelry or tactically appealing shirt material that is close to a woman's chest is another example to proactively define and establish as outside the bounds of appropriate workplace behavior.

It is also possible that when traits or behaviors, which have always been present, occur in a sexual context, the interpretation is negative or classified as criminal. This phenomenon of understanding behaviors that appear paraphilic in the context of a person's profile and functional behavior is referred to as counterfeit deviance (Griffiths et al., 2013). For instance, someone may have a special interest in a particular cartoon character, and they collect items related to this cartoon. Online, they find pornographic images relating to this cartoon character, or pornographic videos with pictures of this character in the background and so they save these images and videos. Problems arise if there are pornographic images with children in them among the images collected. The rates at which apparent offending by autistic people are, in fact, counterfeit deviance is an area in need of further study, especially as, historically, ASD has not consistently been differentiated from other developmental disorders which do not include the same social communication or sensory profiles. Compounding this issue is that illegal sexual behaviors can have long-standing negative implications. For instance, sending or receiving sexual images with a minor can result in being added to the registered sex offender list. This can severely limit work options, due to legal history and type of charge, and living situations, such as proximity to schools, recreation centers, churches, or other facilities that provide care for children. There are many ways in which criminal sexual behavior could have a long-lasting impact on perpetrators and survivors alike.

A decrease in criminal sexual behavior benefits everyone. While training and awareness after a crime has been committed may be helpful, a model which provides tailored delivery of information that would prevent the crime in the first place is highly preferable. At this time, providing education and training relating to sexual behavior is a low risk, potentially high-impact intervention and perhaps our best opportunity to decrease sexual behaviors that are deemed inappropriate or even criminal without understanding these incidents in the context of an autism spectrum disorder. The goal of this chapter is to describe ways to close this gap, to describe the state of sexuality and relationship education (SRE) currently, and to provide suggestions for next times for providers and research areas.

Sexuality and Relationship Education Programs

Health promotion campaigns are generally part of middle and high school programs, including education about cigarettes, drugs, and self-care. These are widely accepted to be efficacious, with the educational component against cigarettes resulting in demonstrated decreases in smoking rates across the globe in the short term after the campaigns are run (Siegel & Biener, 2000; Warner, 1977). Sexual health impacts all middle and high school students, even more than drugs and alcohol.

SRE programs can include a range of topics, commonly include the reproductive cycle, puberty and development, contraception, sexually transmitted infection prevention, safe relationships, and pregnancy. Sex education programs are known to increase positive sexual behaviors, such as contraception use and delayed age of first sexual encounter, and decrease risky sexual behaviors as shown by decreased rates of sexually transmitted infections (Goesling et al., 2014; Mueller et al., 2008; Weaver et al., 2005). Yet SRE in general education settings is often insufficient, delayed, or omitted altogether due to time constraints or lack of perceived need for certain topics to be covered (Buston et al., 2002; Scales, 1980). Many programs emphasize disease and pregnancy prevention and not the development of healthy relationships, despite adolescents' expressed need for more guidance in this area (Anderson, 2015). Empirically derived SRE programming is scarce, with many schools, individuals, families, and mental health providers eager for resources (Ballan, 2012). There are no federal guidelines for sexuality education in the United States, and specific content, timing, and educational approaches vary widely. The lack of appropriate programming is felt even more acutely in neurodiverse populations, such as ASD.

Autistic individuals are less likely to receive SRE and even when they do, the presentation format is not consistently accessible (Brown-Lavoie et al., 2014). For instance, a student in special education courses may be mainstreamed temporarily for SRE in health class to fulfill a school/state requirement, but little to no adjustment in the delivery method is made to accommodate the student's unique learning style. Further, due to time in other therapy or services, autistic students may miss sexuality education entirely. For instance, sex education may be offered during physical education or health, and these "electives" are often periods during which specialist services may be offered. In the intellectual disability literature, studies have shown that access to sex education is diminished when compared to same-age peers (Ramage, 2015). For mainstreamed students, the curriculum may be more accessible but (a) the language may be indirect or not literal enough to be useful or (b) critical relationship development components may be skipped. This skill area is often one highlighted by autistic individuals and their families as needed, but remains unaddressed.

Sexuality and Relationship Educations Programs for ASD

The combination of social communication impairments and inappropriate or inaccessible SRE programming means that in addition to violating the autonomy of that person over their own development and sexuality, individuals with ASD are vulnerable to manipulation (Brown-Lavoie et al., 2014), abuse (Mandell et al., 2005), and legal challenges related to the inappropriate conceptualization of sexual behaviors (Allen et al., 2008). Further, individuals with autism are at increased risk for bullying (Humphrey & Symes, 2010), poorer mental health outcomes, including depression and anxiety (Joshi et al., 2014), increased likelihood of inappropriate sexual behavior (Stokes & Kaur, 2005), and decreased likelihood of experiencing positive romantic relationship success, despite desiring a relationship (Jobe & White, 2007). There is an unmistakable need to mitigate the risk of these outcomes for autistic individuals while promoting healthy sexual development. Designing a SRE program specifically with the needs of autistic individuals in mind can partly fulfill these needs. There are emerging efforts in this area and a selection of programs are described below. Many more programs exist which have not yet been carefully studied but show clinical promise (e.g., Corona et al., 2016; Hatton & Tector, 2010; Tissot, 2009; Wolfe et al., 2009). Replications of these studies would help work toward evidence-based pieces to use with autistic teens and adults with varying intellectual and language abilities.

Developed in the Netherlands, the Tackling Teenage Training (TTT) is an 18-session, one-on-one sexuality course designed specifically for adolescents ages 11–19 on the autism spectrum (Dekker et al., 2015). The TTT is delivered by a mental health professional and engages the caregiver by inviting them to help the adolescent complete sets questions and home practice activities. To our knowledge, it is the only randomized control trial (RCT) of an ASD-specific sex education program. This program resulted in improvements in knowledge and social communication and decreases in negative sexual behavior (Visser et al., 2017). Typically covered topics in the TTT include not only the physical components of sexuality, such as safe sex and changes during puberty, but also the social and emotional components of relationship development and maintenance. These components include relationship and identity development skills (e.g., differentiating between love and friendship), the implications and nonverbal behaviors associated with forming a good "first impression," defining appropriate boundaries around masturbation and fantasies, and values around sex and intimacy. The results of this RCT are promising and the tailored topics and one-on-one presentation structure are a true strength of this program. SRE programs are frequently offered in group formats. Although this structure allows for cost efficiency and better access to a high demand service/program, individual sessions allow space for teenagers to build a comfortable rapport with the therapist and ask personal questions. However, individual sessions can bring their own challenges in terms of insurance coverage in the United States, that can undermine their accessibility.

There is a TEACCH (the highly regarded statewide autism program in North Carolina), approach to SRE which is offered clinically but as of yet, there is not a randomized controlled trial of a TEACCH sexuality education program. Primary curriculum areas for the clinical program include social rules and safety, body changes during puberty, masturbation, and interpersonal issues (Van Bourgondien, 2016). A strength of this program is its adaptations for individuals with varying levels of cognitive abilities. This is a great example of applying established ASD-specific teaching methods and integrating SRE goals.

Dr. Hénault (2005) provides a comprehensive overview of Asperger's and sexuality. This title also includes teaching exercises to use as part of the sociosexual education curricula. As with the TEACCH model, the tools in Hénault's book utilize best practices but the program itself has yet to be empirically tested. Distinct conversations around finding appropriate peers to date and to be friends with, also covered in the Young Adults PEERS curriculum (Laugeson, 2017), could help to understand boundaries which are at risk for being violated later in life. Also, this approach to mindfully thinking about romantic interests may provide an appropriate outlet for sexual interests and behavior.

A Need for Updated Curricula

Inclusion of updated information in SRE programs is not a distinct need for autism-specific programs but given some of the propensity of autistic people to spend inordinate amounts of time online relative to other leisure pursuits, keeping information updated would allow SRE programs to be aware of new and potential areas of concern. For example, sexting and internet dating are common components of the development of adult (and younger!) romantic relationships. In a study of adults, about 40% of respondents engaged in sexting (Gordon-Messer et al., 2013). Studies differ on whether the act of sexting has negative sexual or psychological effects (Klettke et al., 2014). Regardless, if someone does not understand the rules around sexting (e.g., local age of consent, when and to whom to send sexts), it could easily lead to legal trouble.

Another critical area for improvement in sexuality education curricula broadly and especially within autism is the heteronormative nature of these programs in the United States. Nonheterosexual orientations and nonbinary gender identities are rarely covered in sexuality education programs and are controversial in some states. Even more concerning is that students are discouraged from discussing LBGTQA+ related topics in class (Kosciw & Gay, 2014). Although this must be addressed for all students, building materials in this area may be of particular salience to the ASD community. The findings on rates of sexual orientation in ASD populations have been mixed, with some studies finding similar rates of identities between neurotypical and ASD groups (Kellaher, 2015), and others finding that individuals with ASD are more likely to identify as nonheterosexual (Byers et al., 2013; Dewinter et al., 2017; George & Stokes, 2018).

In studies of individuals with gender dysphoria, the incidence of ASD is six to seven times higher than in the general population (de Vries et al., 2010). From studies of transgender children and adolescents in samples without a diagnosis of ASD, data suggest that feeling as if you "do not belong" in your own body is related to a host of negative outcomes, such as social isolation (Meyer, 2014), increased risk of suicide, not finishing school (CDC, 2016), and substance abuse (Jordan, 2000). These identity issues can be complex for all individuals to work through. This complexity is only compounded by a lack of relevant education and support in this area generally, and even further by social communication impairments in ASD. In the TTT, a session is dedicated to terms and behaviors in the context of gender identity and sexual orientation. There is room for the development of additional materials utilizing evidence-based which target LGBTQA+ issues, such as coming out for the first time (Mustanski et al., 2013). The more access teenagers have to relevant information on sexuality, the less taboo topics are, which results in safer sex behaviors (Bay-Cheng, 2003).

Even relative to sex education programs for ASD, sex education programs across diagnostic groups need to be improved in response to the increased use of technology. For instance, in a 2012 study, Mitchell et al. published findings indicate that 2.5% of teens age 10–17 were sending nude or partially nude images to their peers. In many states, sexting and distribution of child pornography laws are creating long-term implications for adolescents who engage in this behavior; clear instruction about this type of behavior must become an emphasized portion of health education courses. Guidelines are even more necessary for individuals who are less able to read social situations via text.

ASD-Specific Considerations for Adaptations

For autistic adults who understand societal boundaries and behaviors with more nuance, communication around sensory needs and aversions should be practiced. For instance, if someone has always enjoyed receiving physical pressure, they can share this with a partner. If they do not enjoy the sensation of holding hands or the "wet" feeling of open-mouthed kissing might be unpleasant, brainstorming ways to communicate these likes and dislikes to partners can be extremely helpful. This is a skill which all individuals pursuing intimate relationships could use but becomes more salient for individuals with strong sensory needs or aversions.

Restricted interests and repetitive behaviors are somewhat unique to autistic populations and discussion of these and the role they may play in sexual behaviors is important to consider. At a basic level, some repetitive behaviors, such as putting one's hand in one's waistband, may appear sexual when an adult engages in these behaviors. Strong repetitive interests which align more with interests of young children may put some adults at risk of interacting with younger children or teens and if any intimate relationship is attempted. This could result in severe consequences for the adult and a traumatic experience for the child. Recognizing how some of these behaviors may cause difficult legal issues later in life is an important conversation to have with families and professionals caring for young people with autism. Especially if they have an accompanying intellectual disability, autistic individuals may not realize the impact of certain actions and it is the responsibility of their caregivers to help prepare for these situations.

Potential Areas of Focus

Targeted Skill Development

The complexity of defining appropriate dating and relationship behaviors makes this area both fascinating and challenging to study. In the absence of an evidence-based program, many practitioners turn to targeting specific skills or education areas.

In order to pursue relationships, people must have ways of meeting other people. Establishing that increasing in-person interaction with others may increase the likelihood of engaging in a romantic relationship will be an important first step. Meet-up groups that reflect the person's special interest guarantee a foundation of shared interests upon which to build friendships and potential intimate relationships. "Buddy Bands" for adolescents and age parameters for adults can be useful in establishing age ranges for acceptable romantic targets. This means that an age bandwidth is established. An adolescent who is 14 may have a "buddy band" of 2 years (+,−) spending time with friends who are no more than 2 years older (16) and no more than 2 years younger (12). This is especially helpful when people on the spectrum come of age and a sexual relationship with a minor can result in a charge of statutory rape. Proactive discussions about what someone is looking for in a partner as well as how to approach a romantic target, how to recognize rejection, and what to do when one is rebuffed should be practiced ahead of time. Especially if individuals are getting information from television and social media, reviewing typical timelines for relationship development and the behaviors that accompany each stage (e.g., what behaviors are appropriate/expected when you first start dating, when sexual intimacy occurs, timeframes for dating, living together, getting married).

Communication is another critical area of relationship building that is often impacted in ASD. Clear rules about what is appropriate to say out loud or internally at various levels of "closeness" with a person are helpful to do before problems arise. While many people may be aroused by an especially attractive person, they have learned that there is an internal dialogue that does not have to be spoken aloud. Practitioners and autistic clients should specifically define the settings and people with whom certain types or topics of communication are appropriate and clearly define rules to match those situations. For instance, interacting with colleagues at work: It is okay to compliment a colleague on their accomplishments at work, but it is NOT okay to compliment a person on their hair, makeup, outfit, or body. This can also be a good opportunity to brainstorm appropriate conversation topics (green topics) which are largely acceptable to most people, under most circumstances. In addition to verbal communication, establish eye gaze guidelines around where to look and how long to look, such as Neck up, Knees down: In between the neck and the knees is the "no go zone." This can be a good time to clarify where certain behaviors (e.g., kissing, masturbation, watching pornography) can take place, as well as less clearly obvious sexual behaviors, such as scratching or adjusting genitalia. Defining clear rules and boundaries around nonverbal communication is also critical. Concepts such as how does nonverbal communication exist in the larger context of an interaction and how congruous (or not) verbal and nonverbal communication are (Thompson, 2015).

Need for Prosocial Examples

Oftentimes families and schools become more interested in sexuality education after a negative incident, such as a student masturbating at school. Ideally, this information would be taught early and often for students who learn best with repetition. Having prosocial examples of behavior relating to intimate relationships should be incorporated into training programs, either through autistic group leaders, guest speakers, or videos by self-advocates. Anecdotally, group leaders or therapists who can provide examples of behaviors and relationships being discussed in a program can help make material more accessible and visual.

Frequently, schools, therapists, or parents are addressing learning in the realm of sexuality, but they are doing so by piecing materials together in the absence of one established curriculum. To do this, they must apply knowledge about a student's learning style to adapt sexuality education curricula. Tarnai and Wolfe (2008) present examples of social stories to use for sex education topics. Social stories are commonly used as a teaching tool for ASD and the intersection of this tool and this topic shows promise. Similarly, a picture exchange communication system (PECS) can be used to illustrate good hygiene practices or the do's and don'ts of masturbation. Video modeling of dating situations is another easy intervention to try, although the precise effects of these tools on long-term learning has not been established.

Although there is not a known examination of this, repetition of material may dictate the efficacy of sex education programs because repetition is an effective learning strategy for many autistic individuals. Unfortunately, sex education in the United States is often a short-term presentation in middle school, which may be insufficient for people with autism. In contrast, countries such as the Netherlands have developmentally tiered a sexuality education program that begins as early as kindergarten, with lessons about boundaries and relationships development, and builds in complexity as the students move through school grades. Outcomes on metrics such as older age of first sexual encounter, lower rate of teenage pregnancies, and more positive experiences associated with first sexual experiences (Jones et al., 1985) suggest that this early start and scaffolding approach to sex education (in combination with other cultural factors) may have positive long-term effects for all students, with or without autism.

Treatment

Lack of effective treatment programs for sexual offending is a significant challenge not only for autistic offenders but neurotypical individuals as well. Traditional sex offender treatment focuses on enhancing empathy for the victim and on recognizing cognitive distortions, among other goals. The program is based on learned socially deviant experiences whereas for those with autism the difficulties come from "a failure to benefit from any experience, rather than learning on the basis of socially deviant experiences." The focus of the treatment, i.e., recognizing cognitive distortions, and promoting empathy, is unlikely to be effective in individuals with ASD, even though it is effective in neurotypical individuals, who need behavioral rather than cognitive interventions (Bolton, 2006).

Specifically, the challenge for autistic offenders is not "cognitive distortions" because they are not aware of the social norms that such mechanisms serve to circumvent. Sex offender treatment programs are designed for the person with antisocial features, individuals who know very well the physical and psychological impact of sexual aggression on victims, but care little about it. The antisocial person is not only aware of the feelings and fears of the other person, they readily take advantage of these feelings and fears to manipulate the other person. They lack "emotional empathy."

In contrast, many autistic individuals struggle with "cognitive empathy," or noticing what others are feeling. If the true feelings of others are pointed out to them, they are then very concerned about the other person's feelings and will try to act appropriately. Thus the goal of treatment would likely be different for an autistic offender. For an individual with ASD, who does not present with a paraphilia or antisocial traits, traditional sex offender treatment program would pointless and damaging (Griffiths & Fedoroff, 2009). Effective treatment of an offender with ASD requires an individualized treatment program focusing on sexuality training and education on sociosexual boundaries and tools they can use to assess social situations.

An additional challenge is that treatment for criminal sexual behavior traditionally takes the form of group. Sugrue (2017) argues that this style of treatment (which can be effective with neurotypical individuals) is not suitable for individuals with ASD (Griffiths & Fedoroff, 2009; Ray et al., 2004). A specialized treatment which includes very explicit sex education with a focus on learning "specific responses to specific situations" is needed for individuals with ASD (Griffiths & Fedoroff, 2009). Moreover, repetition is also important in treatment with individuals with ASD due to their difficulty in understanding abstract concepts (Klin et al., 1995).

It is important to note that specific training on recognizing and supporting symptoms of ASD is critical for any type of treatment to be effective. For instance, taking the perspective of others and executive functioning can both be difficult for autistic people. Savvy group leaders should recognize this and spend extra time exploring theory of mind and the experience of survivors of a sexual crime with perpetrators. Group members may need more guidance on how and when to complete group assignments, or ways to adjust their schedules to avoid contact with survivors. Leaders of group or individual treatment programs should be well versed on how autism presents in adulthood.

Without a cache of ASD-specific programs from which to choose, modifying existing programs is the next most accessible step. An important first step would be to ensure that group staff understand what autism is and the way autistic symptoms may have played a role in the crime as well as treatment programming. The learning methods should be ASD-accessible. For instance, using visual supports to make resources and concepts less verbally based would be helpful. Presenting concrete rules is an effective teaching approach as well, especially if individuals have court ordered restrictions, as generalizing across settings can be challenging for autistic individuals.

Although not developed specifically for autistic offenders, the design of the Good Lives Model (GLM) has potential for practice with autistic populations. The GLM focuses on enhancing the capacities, interests, and motivations of the offender rather than operating from a risk reduction, compensatory paradigm. The model is based on the premise that humans share a basic set of needs that must be fulfilled and offending results when the individual lacks the skills to meet these needs. The GLM identifies risk factors that set the individual on a path to offending including criminogenic needs that confer increased risk of offending. Treatment is matched to ameliorate these barriers to fulfillment and cultivate prosocial behaviors (Ward & Stewart, 2003).

In the GLM, an individual develops a Good Life Plan which serves as a guiding vision for the offender's life. The aim of the plan is to reduce offending behavior by differentially reinforcing adaptive behavior that cannot co-occur with the problem behavior. Within the Good Life Plan, primary reinforcers are identified and skills are developed so the individual can obtain those reinforcers. Primary goals are developed to match the individual's vision of a good life. Secondary and instrumental goals help identify the skills necessary to achieve this plan and its related goods (Willis et al., 2013). Incompatible goals associated with offending are identified and addressed. Triggers for offending behavior are faced rather than avoided. For example, rather than only avoiding interactions with the person who pressed charges, the GLM would focus on enhancing the skills necessary to have intimate relationships and friendships with other adults. The GLM was originally developed for use with sex offenders (Ward et al., 2007), but there is a growing body of research to examine its use with other groups of offenders. People with ASD would benefit from participation in social skills training based on the GLM which specifically focused on the development of a Good Life Plan, training on the actionable items that help achieve that plan, and someone to monitor adherence to the plan.

People on the autism spectrum often seem unaware of problematic behaviors until someone points them out. This is not the same as denying responsibility for one's actions. Rather, it is learning social rules post hoc by breaking them. Considering the impact of an ASD diagnosis with respect to treatment adherence and adjusting the strategies used to change behavior based on the learning characteristics of people on the spectrum can make the difference between failing in treatment and successfully completing treatment. Individuals with intellectual and developmental disabilities convicted for sex offenses, as pointed out so persistently by Dorothy Griffiths, do not necessarily require "rehabilitation"; it requires "habilitation." Offending, based on blindness to social norms, or the social implications of what is looked at online, or what is said in online communications, calls for treatment that supplants the intuitive socialization and sexuality learning processes experienced by typically developed individuals. This must be in a program that can present this explicitly to those with autism in a way they can understand it. "Habilitation" uses active education and training about social norms and appropriate behaviors. It must be adapted to take into account the learning capabilities of the individual and the difficulty of those with ASD in generalizing how social rules apply across situations.

Resources for Women

Careful approaches to supplying program for men and women on the spectrum is critical, although the sexual needs and behaviors of women with autism are less studied than those of men. We do know that autistic men are more likely to masturbate than women on the spectrum (Pecora et al., 2016). This pattern holds true in non-autistic populations as well (Hogarth & Ingham, 2009) and many women learn about sexual pleasure first through partnered activity, which may be less accessible or later experienced for autistic individuals. Especially given the higher prevalence of autism in boys, research must remember to support the needs and pro-sexual goals of autistic women. Furthermore, there is a need for more support and provider training for women with autism seeking sexual health services in a medical setting (e.g., getting pap smears, birth control, etc.).

SRE Adaptations for Other Populations

Sex education has been adapted in the intellectual disability (ID) world. These programs may benefit individuals with ID and ASD. The use of pictures and visuals and planning activities, such as the who-what-where-when of a date (Couwenhoven, 2007), demonstrates how effective teaching tools can be used to present sexuality education material in a variety of ways. Many books such as *Sexuality: Your Sons and Daughters with Intellectual Disabilities* (Schwier & Hingsburger, 2000) cover the complexity of balancing safety, consent, and the individual rights of people with disabilities. Whether preventing criminal behavior or promoting positive sexual development, the ID sex education materials and models offer a blueprint for mobilizing a community to pursue tailored programming. Puberty and relationship development are some of the rare truly ubiquitous experiences in the world. Enabling access to accurate and helpful information on these topics should be an inalienable right.

Measurement of Efficacy

A limitation of studying SRE is the lack of tools available to measure the impact of these programs. Sex education modules may seem effective because oftentimes teenagers with an Asperger's profile may ceiling out on knowledge tasks relating to the reproductive cycle or disease prevention. The Socio-Sexual Knowledge and Attitudes Test-Revised (*Socio-Sexual Knowledge and Attitudes Test-Revised (SSKAAT-R)*, n.d.) is a tool designed for individuals with developmental disabilities that assess knowledge of reproduction, safety, self-care, and anatomy. Although the images are somewhat dated at this time, this can be a good tool to establish what knowledge a person does or does not have. However, knowledge-based tasks demonstrate that facts have been memorized when it is the application of the material (e.g., how to interact with a potential romantic partner, how to identify when you can and cannot masturbate) that is important. Individuals and families express a need for materials that also teach contextual social and emotional skills, namely relationship development.

In a small sample, vignettes were developed to assess the applied component of sexuality and relationship education. After a group SRE program for individuals with "high functioning autism" (developed using materials from Davies & Dubie, 2011), scores on the SSKAAT-R did not change significantly as they were high initially but did shift on these vignettes (Burns et al., 2017). This early step into more applicable tools deserves further study. Clinically, many in the ASD community seek topics such as boundaries, identity development, partner identification, and knowing the when and the where of sexual behavior. It is the social application of knowledge relating to boundaries, consent, expressing romantic interest, etc., that can be challenging due to communication (e.g., when someone is nonverbal or when someone interprets language very literally). This gets further complicated when thinking about the assessment of accused sexual behavior; Mogavero (2016) makes a case for the special consideration of this population in the assessment and intervention during criminal investigations.

Consequences of Lack of Treatment

From a behavior analytic perspective, prison is an ineffective consequence for problematic sexual behaviors. Punishment is a consequence that occurs after a problem behavior with the intent of reducing the likelihood the problem behavior will occur in the future. In a study of the general prison population across 30 states, 75% of all prisoners were rearrested within five years (Durose & Cooper, 2005). This cycle sets the stage for criminals to become savvier as the result of the prison education they receive from their confederates. Research has shown that the certainty of punishment is a stronger deterrent than the length of punishment (Killias et al., 2009). Given this information, proactive education about boundaries and expectations and legal issues for social and sexual behaviors in combination with explicit information about what happens when these are violated would be the best way to prevent or at least reduce the rate of criminal sexual behavior.

Gaps

There is a significant need, both in terms of health promotion and avoidance of criminal behaviors, for increased development and study of programming in this area and for replication of existing studies. The benefits of this work will be felt by individuals, families, and communities in mental health, physical health, and financial domains. Specifically, longitudinal examination of the impact of evidence-based programs and the role they play in criminal prevention would bolster the case for delivery of these models. Funding in this area has long been hard to come by and this may be an area where combining efforts from legal professionals and mental health/service providers would provide a more comprehensive resulting product. Furthermore, best practices for delivery models of sexuality information have yet to be established. Should parents and caregivers provide this information? Would school staff be better equipped in teaching methods that would make the training more effective? Or should these lessons be taught and reviewed by someone outside a student's daily circle, such as a therapist, to avoid any embarrassment? Like most topics, the answer likely lies at the intersection of these possibilities, but the delivery method of this information must be studied to develop best practices, in the context of culture and religion in particular.

Better understanding of potentially problematic behavior and pitfalls for autistic individuals could inform preventative work; proactive prevention work obviously would benefit both potential offenders and victims/survivors. Unfortunately, adolescents with disabilities are often deliberately excluded from studies of adolescent sexuality (O'Sullivan & Thompson, 2014). There is frustratingly little information about the development of criminal sexual behavior. Understanding the ASD profile could help researchers identify areas to study. For instance, young adults with ASD are typically delayed five years in their development and can often engage in behavior seen as inappropriate, including touching others. This age difference is a significant one when autistic adolescents and young adults more easily befriend children at their developmental (and not chronological) age. This could easily become problematic when engaging in sexual behaviors. Child sexual experimentation is seen as part of normal development. A child "discovers" their genital areas and tends to repeat the act of touching and rubbing because it creates a sense of pleasure. Boys often touch or hold their penis in public. Boys and girls often engage in "child on child" sexual experimentation. They begin mimicking adult affectionate behaviors such as kissing, hugging, and holding hands. Preschool staff have reported observing children looking or showing each other's genitals (Wurtele & Kenny, 2011). These early childhood sexual experiences do not appear to correlate to particular effects on adult adjustment (Leitenberg et al., 1989; Okami et al., 1997). Some consider these behaviors beneficial in terms of typical sexual development into a healthy adults (LeVay et al., 2015).

Although exploratory behaviors are normal, this quickly becomes problematic as children age and as the age gap between the individuals increases. "Age discordant sex play" is a familiar concept in the sexual therapy literature (Bruce et al., 2012; Lee et al., 2003; O'Sullivan & Thompson, 2014). The Arc advises that "Sex Offenses by a person with I/DD are often not the result of

> sexual deviance … Often, sex offenses are the result of counterfeit deviance" and "ignorance of what is considered appropriate," and that persons with developmental disabilities "may engage in acceptable sexual behaviors but with someone who is not an appropriate age—this is called 'age discordant sex play'."

Therefore, when it comes to reports or allegations of an autistic individual involved in sexual contact with minors that might, but for the age differential, fall into the category of "child sexual experimentation," it is essential to determine whether this might more accurately be considered to be a case of age discordant sex play, rather than molesting behavior. This is just one example of where a better understanding of criminal sexual behavior in the context of ASD could help inform programming from both the preventative and treatment angle.

Where to Begin

While promising sexuality education programs are being rigorously tested and becoming more widely distributed, there are existing guidelines currently available in the literature. In their review of sex education for autistic individuals, Tullis and Zangrillo (2013) summarize five areas that have been highlighted in the limited literature; namely (1) reproductive education, contraception, social rules of privacy, complex social skills, (2) dating and marriage, (3) technology and sexual education, (4) dating, and (5) marriage. Travers and Tincani (2010) also elegantly lay out areas that would benefit from research energy, as well as ways to select which skills to teach and prioritize in the Individualized Education Program (IEP) context. They include body awareness, social development romantic relationships and intimacy, masturbation and modifying behavior to meet social norms, and reproductive and parenting rights of individuals with ASD.

Apart from the development of sexuality education programs for autistic individuals, there is a need for further assessment of ASD and criminal sexual behavior to help determine best interventions. In this vein, tracking the long-term impact of programs we are testing now can help continue to move the field forward. This would include both measuring decreases in criminal sexual behavior and increases in the prosocial impact of these programs including ratings of satisfaction with sexual behavior or relationships. Dissemination is another significant hurdle in understanding the impact of sexuality education programming. Studied curricula must be made accessible to schools, families, individuals, and providers on a more regular basis. There are few domains of functioning which affect such a large portion of the population as sexuality and navigating one's own body, desires, and identity in a comfortable way should be accessible to all.

Conclusions and Next Steps

Sexuality and relationship education programming and resources for non-autistic children are not well studied or understood, and efforts in this area for autistic populations are even more limited. As a field, we still need to answer some foundational dissemination and educational questions; who would best provide sexuality education programming? How often should this be offered? What materials should we teach by what age? Some models such as the one in the Netherlands may offer a good start to build out and study the implementation of sexuality education programs for ASD, pulling from developmentally appropriate practices. Second, we need to better understand which topics or behaviors must be covered that are of particular importance to the ASD community. This will allow us to develop best practices to provide comprehensive information using evidence-based teaching methods.

One limitation in this area is funding. The "sensitivity" of this topic and the range of opinions on what is important to teach or not teach prevents this type of work from being financially viable, despite the critical need. When considering the legal implications, presenting an SRE program would cost substantially less than paying for a misplaced individual as they navigate the legal system. Legal groups, autistic advocacy groups, and child health organizations seeking to fund the study of these programs will help continue to move this science forward.

Once an evidence-based approach to these topics is better defined, we need to disseminate this information around best practices as care providers are saying that they want more training and resources in this area (Saxe & Flanagan, 2016). As the needs of autistic adults are being more widely recognized as an area deserving focus and services, SRE should be a priority in the pursuit of fulfilling personal relationships, of developing identity, of managing and understanding one's own body, and for safety.

What Can I Do?

1. Apply learning approaches which have been effective with your child or student previously. Do they learn best with videos? Repetition? Visuals? Utilize this information to present SRE materials.
2. Be direct and clear when sharing information about sexuality to decrease shame or fear around questions. Do not use indirect phrases. Rely on explicit rules when you can, including any relevant contextual information (e.g., you should not kiss romantic partners at school but can kiss them at the end of a date if they say it is ok).
3. Talk about uncomfortable topics. Oftentimes, the uncomfortable topics are the ones which could have the most negative outcomes if not discussed, and are the hardest to get safe information on. The use of porn is a great example of this; online pornography is often accessed by teens but when this behavior goes unchecked, can lead to legal trouble especially for someone with a developmental disability. Rules about where and when, legal age of the viewer and a discussion about images that are always illegal, should be established.
4. Consider sensory sensitivities and preferences and imagine what those will look like in a public context. Discuss the person's sensory profiles and teach them how to communicate this to their romantic partner (if relevant) in appropriate settings, as well as defining when to not discuss or engage in these behaviors due to legal risks.

Resources to Explore

Books

Asperger's Syndrome and Sexuality: From Adolescence Through Adulthood, 2005 by Isabelle Hénault.

Intimate Relationships and Sexual Health: A Curriculum for Teaching Adolescents/Adults with High-Functioning Autism Spectrum Disorders and Other Social Challenges, 2011 by Catherine Davies & Melissa Dubie.

PEERS for Young Adults with Autism Spectrum Disorder and Other Social Challenges, 2017 by Elizabeth Laugenson.

Web-Based Resources

Sex ed resources curated and developed with self-advocates: Sex Ed for Self-Advocates https://researchautism.org/sex-ed-guide/.

Spark Webinar by Eileen T. Crehan: *Talking about the birds and the bees in ASD: Sexuality and sexuality education programming*. https://sparkforautism.org/discover_article/talking-about-the-birds-and-the-bees-in-asd/.

Where to get more information regarding minority gender identity or sexual orientation:

PFLAG has historically championed causes for lesbian, gay, bisexual, transgender and questioning people and their website links to useful information and local chapters.

https://www.pflag.org/.

This site provides links for parents and service providers for transgender children:

https://www.genderspectrum.org/quick-links/books-and-media/.

LGBTQ: The Survival Guide for Lesbian, Gay, Bisexual, Transgender, and Questioning Teens, 3rd edition, 2018 by Kelly Huegel Madrone.

References

Allen, D., Evans, C., Hider, A., Hawkins, S., Peckett, H., & Morgan, H. (2008). Offending behaviour in adults with Asperger syndrome. *Journal of Autism and Developmental Disorders, 38*(4), 748–758. https://doi.org/10.1007/s10803-007-0442-9.

Anderson, S. (2015). Sex education programs focused on "protection" and "prevention" with little attention given to supporting people to develop healthy, positive sexual relationships. *Research and Practice in Intellectual and Developmental Disabilities, 2*(1), 98–100. https://doi.org/10.1080/23297018.2015.1021740.

Ballan, M. S. (2012). Parental perspectives of communication about sexuality in families of children with autism spectrum disorders. *Journal of Autism and Developmental Disorders, 42*(5), 676–684. https://doi.org/10.1007/s10803-011-1293-y.

Bay-Cheng, L. Y. (2003). The trouble of teen sex: The construction of adolescent sexuality through school-based sexuality education. *Sex Education, 3*(1), 61–74. https://doi.org/10.1080/1468181032000052162.

Bolton, W. (2006). Developmental theory and developmental deficits: The treatment of sex offenders with Asperger's syndrome. In J. Hiller, H. Woods, & W. Bolton (Eds.), *Sex, mind, and emotion*. Routledge.

Brown-Lavoie, S. M., Viecili, M. A., & Weiss, J. A. (2014). Sexual knowledge and victimization in adults with autism spectrum disorders. *Journal of Autism and Developmental Disorders, 44*(9), 2185–2196. https://doi.org/10.1007/s10803-014-2093-y.

Bruce, D., Harper, G. W., Fernández, M. I., Jamil, O. B., & Adolescent Medicine Trials Network for HIV/AIDS Interventions. (2012). Age-concordant and age-discordant sexual behavior among gay and bisexual male adolescents. *Archives of Sexual Behavior, 41*(2), 441–448. https://doi.org/10.1007/s10508-011-9730-8.

Burns, A., Crehan, E. T., & Loftin, R. (2017). *Problem solving in sexuality education.* International Meeting for Autism Research.

Buston, K., Wight, D., Hart, G., & Scott, S. (2002). Implementation of a teacher-delivered sex education programme: Obstacles and facilitating factors. *Health Education Research, 17*(1), 59–72. https://doi.org/10.1093/her/17.1.59.

Byers, E. S., Nichols, S., & Voyer, S. D. (2013). Challenging stereotypes: Sexual functioning of single adults with high functioning autism spectrum disorder. *Journal of Autism and Developmental Disorders, 43*(11), 2617–2627. https://doi.org/10.1007/s10803-013-1813-z.

CDC. (2016). *Sexual identity, sex of sexual contacts, and health-risk behaviors among students in grades 9–12: Youth risk behavior surveillance.* U.S. Department of Health and Human Services.

Corona, L. L., Fox, S. A., Christodulu, K. V., & Worlock, J. A. (2016). Providing education on sexuality and relationships to adolescents with autism spectrum disorder and their parents. *Sexuality and Disability, 34*(2), 199–214. https://doi.org/10.1007/s11195-015-9424-6.

Couwenhoven, T. (2007). *Teaching children with down syndrome about their bodies, boundaries, and sexuality* (1st ed.). Woodbine House.

Curtis, A. (2017). Why sex education matters for adolescents with autism spectrum disorder. *AJN The American Journal of Nursing, 117*(6), 11. https://doi.org/10.1097/01.NAJ.0000520233.91525.1f.

Davies, C., & Dubie, M. (2011). *Intimate relationships and sexual health: A curriculum for teaching adolescents/adults with high-functioning autism spectrum disorders and other social challenges* (A. Publishing, Ed.; Pap/Cdr edition). AAPC Publishing.

de Vries, A. L. C., Noens, I. L. J., Cohen-Kettenis, P. T., van Berckelaer-Onnes, I. A., & Doreleijers, T. A. (2010). Autism spectrum disorders in gender dysphoric children and adolescents. *Journal of Autism and Developmental Disorders, 40*(8), 930–936. https://doi.org/10.1007/s10803-010-0935-9.

Dekker, L. P., van der Vegt, E. J. M., Visser, K., Tick, N., Boudesteijn, F., Verhulst, F. C., Maras, A., & Greaves-Lord, K. (2015). Improving psychosexual knowledge in adolescents with autism spectrum disorder: Pilot of the tackling teenage training program. *Journal of Autism and Developmental Disorders, 45*(6), 1532–1540. https://doi.org/10.1007/s10803-014-2301-9.

Dewinter, J., De Graaf, H., & Begeer, S. (2017). Sexual orientation, gender identity, and romantic relationships in adolescents and adults with autism spectrum disorder. *Journal of Autism and Developmental Disorders, 47*(9), 2927–2934. https://doi.org/10.1007/s10803-017-3199-9.

Durose, M. R., & Cooper, A. D. (2005). *Recidivism of prisoners released in 30 states in 2005: Patterns from 2005 to 2010* (p. 31).

George, R., & Stokes, M. A. (2018). Sexual orientation in autism spectrum disorder. *Autism Research: Official Journal of the International Society for Autism Research, 11*(1), 133–141. https://doi.org/10.1002/aur.1892.

Goesling, B., Colman, S., Trenholm, C., Terzian, M., & Moore, K. (2014). Programs to reduce teen pregnancy, sexually transmitted infections, and associated sexual risk behaviors: A systematic review. *Journal of Adolescent Health, 54*(5), 499–507. https://doi.org/10.1016/j.jadohealth.2013.12.004.

Gordon-Messer, D., Bauermeister, J. A., Grodzinski, A., & Zimmerman, M. (2013). Sexting among young adults. *Journal of Adolescent Health, 52*(3), 301–306. https://doi.org/10.1016/j.jadohealth.2012.05.013.

Griffiths, D., & Fedoroff, J. P. (2009). Persons with intellectual disabilities who sexually offend. In F. M. Saleh, A. J. Grudzinskas, J. M. Bradford, & D. J. Brodsky (Eds.), *Sex offenders: Identification, risk, assessment, treatment, and legal issues* (pp. 352–374). Oxford University Press.

Griffiths, D., Hingsburger, D., Hoath, J., & Ioannou, S. (2013). "Counterfeit deviance" revisited. *Journal of Applied Research in Intellectual Disabilities: JARID, 26*(5), 471–480. https://doi.org/10.1111/jar.12034.

Hatton, S., & Tector, A. (2010). Sexuality and relationship education for young people with autistic spectrum disorder: Curriculum change and staff support. *British Journal of Special Education, 37*(2), 69–76. https://doi.org/10.1111/j.1467-8578.2010.00466.x.

Hénault, I., & Attwood, T. (2005). *Asperger's syndrome and sexuality: From adolescence through adulthood* (1st ed., 1st Printing ed.). Jessica Kingsley.

Hogarth, H., & Ingham, R. (2009). Masturbation among young women and associations with sexual health: An exploratory study. *The Journal of Sex Research, 46*(6), 558–567. https://doi.org/10.1080/00224490902878993.

Humphrey, N., & Symes, W. (2010). Responses to bullying and use of social support among pupils with autism spectrum disorders (ASDs) in mainstream schools: A qualitative study. *Journal of Research in Special Educational Needs, 10*(2), 82–90. https://doi.org/10.1111/j.1471-3802.2010.01146.x.

Jobe, L. E., & White, S. W. (2007). Loneliness, social relationships, and a broader autism phenotype in college students. *Personality and Individual Differences, 42*(8), 1479–1489. https://doi.org/10.1016/j.paid.2006.10.021.

Jones, E. F., Forrest, J. D., Goldman, N., Henshaw, S. K., Lincoln, R., Rosoff, J. I., Westoff, C. F., & Wulf, D. (1985). Teenage pregnancy in developed countries: Determinants and policy implications. *Family Planning Perspectives, 17*(2), 53–63. https://doi.org/10.2307/2135261.

Jordan, K. M. (2000). Substance abuse among gay, lesbian, bisexual, transgender, and questioning adolescents. *School Psychology Review, 29*(2), 201–206.

Joshi, G., Faraone, S. V., Wozniak, J., Petty, C., Fried, R., Galdo, M., Furtak, S. L., McDermott, K., Epstien, C., Walker, R., Caron, A., Feinberg, L., & Biederman, J. (2014). Examining the clinical correlates of autism spectrum disorder in youth by ascertainment source. *Journal of Autism and Developmental Disorders, 44*(9), 2117–2126. https://doi.org/10.1007/s10803-014-2063-4.

Kellaher, D. C. (2015). Sexual behavior and autism spectrum disorders: An update and discussion. *Current Psychiatry Reports, 17*(4), 25. https://doi.org/10.1007/s11920-015-0562-4.

Killias, M., Scheidegger, D., & Nordenson, P. (2009). The effects of increasing the certainty of punishment: A field experiment on public transportation. *European Journal of Criminology, 6*(5), 387–400. https://doi.org/10.1177/1477370809337881.

Klettke, B., Hallford, D. J., & Mellor, D. J. (2014). Sexting prevalence and correlates: A systematic literature review. *Clinical Psychology Review, 34*(1), 44–53. https://doi.org/10.1016/j.cpr.2013.10.007.

Klin, A., Volkmar, F. R., Sparrow, S. S., Cicchetti, D. V., & Rourke, B. P. (1995). Validity and neuropsychological characterization of Asperger syndrome: Convergence with nonverbal learning disabilities syndrome. *Journal of Child Psychology and Psychiatry, 36*(7), 1127–1140. https://doi.org/10.1111/j.1469-7610.1995.tb01361.x.

Kosciw, J. G., Gay, L., & Straight Education Network. (2014). *The 2013 national school climate survey: The experiences of lesbian, gay, bisexual and transgender youth in our nation's schools.* http://arks.princeton.edu/ark:/88435/dsp01wd375z94x.

Laugeson, E. A. (2017). *PEERS® for young adults: Social skills training for adults with autism spectrum disorder and other social challenges* (1st ed.). Routledge.

Lee, J. K., Jennings, J. M., & Ellen, J. M. (2003). Discordant sexual partnering: A study of high-risk adolescents in San Francisco. *Sexually Transmitted Diseases, 30*(3), 234–240. https://doi.org/10.1097/00007435-200303000-00012.

Leitenberg, H., Greenwald, E., & Tarran, M. J. (1989). The relation between sexual activity among children during pre adolescence and/or early adolescence and sexual behavior and sexual adjustment in young adulthood. *Archives of Sexual Behavior, 18,* 299–313.

LeVay, S., Baldwin, J., & Baldwin, J. (2015). *Discovering human sexuality.* Sinauer Associates.

Mandell, D. S., Walrath, C. M., Manteuffel, B., Sgro, G., & Pinto-Martin, J. A. (2005). The prevalence and correlates of abuse among children with autism served in comprehensive community-based mental health settings. *Child Abuse and Neglect, 29*(12), 1359–1372. https://doi.org/10.1016/j.chiabu.2005.06.006.

Meyer, E. J. (2014). Supporting gender diversity in schools: Developmental and legal perspectives. In *Supporting transgender and gender creative youth*. Peter Lang.

Mitchell, K. J., Finkelhor, D., Jones, L. M., & Wolak, J. (2012). Prevalence and characteristics of youth sexting: A national study. *Pediatrics, 129*(1), 13–20. https://doi.org/10.1542/peds.2011-1730.

Mogavero, M. C. (2016). Autism, sexual offending, and the criminal justice system. *Journal of Intellectul Disabilities and Offending Behavior, 7*(3), 116–126. https://www.emerald.com/insight/content/doi/10.1108/JIDOB-02-2016-0004/full/html.

Mueller, T. E., Gavin, L. E., & Kulkarni, A. (2008). The association between sex education and youth's engagement in sexual intercourse, age at first intercourse, and birth control use at first sex. *The Journal of Adolescent Health: Official Publication of the Society for Adolescent Medicine, 42*(1), 89–96. https://doi.org/10.1016/j.jadohealth.2007.08.002.

Mustanski, B., Birkett, M., Greene, G. J., Hatzenbuehler, M. L., & Newcomb, M. E. (2013). Envisioning an America without sexual orientation inequities in adolescent health. *American Journal of Public Health, 104*(2), 218–225. https://doi.org/10.2105/AJPH.2013.301625.

Okami, P., Olmstead, R., & Abramson, P. R. (1997). Sexual experiences in early childhood: 18-year longitudinal data from the UCLA family lifestyles project. *Journal of Sex Research, 34,* 339–347.

O'Sullivan, L., & Thompson, A. (2014). Sexuality in adolescence. In D. Tolman & L. M. Diamond (Eds.), *APA handbook of sexuality and psychology: Vol. 1 person-based approaches*. APA Publications.

Pecora, L. A., Mesibov, G. B., & Stokes, M. A. (2016). Sexuality in high-functioning autism: A systematic review and meta-analysis. *Journal of Autism and Developmental Disorders, 46*(11), 3519–3556. https://doi.org/10.1007/s10803-016-2892-4.

Ramage, K. (Ed.). (2015). *Sexual health education for adolescents with intellectual disabilities: A literature review*. Saskatchewan Prevention Institute.

Ray, F., Marks, C., & Bray-Garretson, H. (2004). Challenges to treating adolescents with Asperger's syndrome who are sexually abusive. *Sexual Addiction and Compulsivity, 11,* 265–285. https://doi.org/10.1080/10720160490900614.

Saxe, A., & Flanagan, T. (2016). Unprepared: An appeal for sex education training for support workers of adults with developmental disabilities. *Sexuality and Disability, 34*(4), 443–454. https://doi.org/10.1007/s11195-016-9449-5.

Scales, P. (1980). Barriers to sex education. *The Journal of School Health, 50*(6), 337–341.

Schwier, K. M., & Hingsburger, D. (2000). *Sexuality: Your sons and daughters with intellectual disabilities* (1st ed.). Paul H. Brookes Pub Co.

Siegel, M., & Biener, L. (2000). The impact of an antismoking media campaign on progression to established smoking: Results of a longitudinal youth study. *American Journal of Public Health, 90*(3), 380–386.

Socio-Sexual Knowledge and Attitudes Test-Revised (SSKAAT-R). (n.d.). Retrieved November 25, 2018, from https://www.stoeltingco.com/socio-sexual-knowledge-and-attitudes-test-revised-sskaat-r.html.

Stokes, M. A., & Kaur, A. (2005). High-functioning autism and sexuality: A parental perspective. *Autism: The International Journal of Research and Practice, 9*(3), 266–289. https://doi.org/10.1177/1362361305053258.

Strunz, S., Schermuck, C., Ballerstein, S., Ahlers, C. J., Dziobek, I., & Roepke, S. (2017). Romantic relationships and relationship satisfaction among adults with Asperger syndrome and high-functioning autism: Romantic relationships among autistic adults. *Journal of Clinical Psychology, 73*(1), 113–125. https://doi.org/10.1002/jclp.22319.

Sugrue, D. P. (2017). Forensic assessment of individuals on the autism spectrum charged with child pornography violations. In L. A. Dubin, E. Horowitz, A. Gershel, G. Mesibov, & M. Sreckovic

(Eds.), *Caught in the web of the criminal justice system: Autism, developmental disabilities, and sex offenses*. Jessica Kingsley.

Tarnai, B., & Wolfe, P. S. (2008). Social stories for sexuality education for persons with autism/pervasive developmental disorder. *Sexuality and Disability, 26*(1), 29–36. https://doi.org/10.1007/s11195-007-9067-3.

Thompson, J. (2015). *Nonverbal communication and the skills of effective mediators: Developing rapport, building trust, and displaying professionalism*. Griffith University. https://research-repository.griffith.edu.au/bitstream/handle/10072/367994/Thompson_2015_02Thesis.pdf?sequence=1.

Tissot, C. (2009). Establishing a sexual identity: Case studies of learners with autism and learning difficulties. *Autism, 13*(6), 551–566. https://doi.org/10.1177/1362361309338183.

Travers, J., & Tincani, M. (2010). Sexuality education for individuals with autism spectrum disorders: Critical issues and decision making guidelines. *Education and Training in Autism and Developmental Disabilities, 45*(2), 284–293.

Tullis, C. A., & Zangrillo, A. N. (2013). Sexuality education for adolescents and adults with autism spectrum disorders: ASD and sexuality. *Psychology in the Schools, 50*(9), 866–875. https://doi.org/10.1002/pits.21713.

Van Bourgondien, M. (2016, April 13). *Sexuality in adolescents with autism and concrete learners.*

Visser, K., Greaves-Lord, K., Tick, N. T., Verhulst, F. C., Maras, A., & van der Vegt, E. J. M. (2017). A randomized controlled trial to examine the effects of the tackling teenage psychosexual training program for adolescents with autism spectrum disorder. *Journal of Child Psychology and Psychiatry, 58*(7), 840–850. https://doi.org/10.1111/jcpp.12709.

Ward, T., Mann, R. E., & Gannon, T. (2007). The good lives model of offender rehabilitation: Clinical implications—ScienceDirect. *Aggression and Violent Behavior, 12*(1), 87–107. https://www.sciencedirect.com/science/article/pii/S1359178906000462?via%3Dihub.

Ward, T., & Stewart, C. A. (2003). The treatment of sex offenders: Risk management and good lives. *Professional Psychology: Research and Practice, 34*(4), 353. https://psycnet.apa.org/record/2003-06801-003.

Warner, K. E. (1977). The effects of the anti-smoking campaign on cigarette consumption. *American Journal of Public Health, 67*(7), 645–650. https://doi.org/10.2105/AJPH.67.7.645.

Weaver, H., Smith, G., & Kippax, S. (2005). School-based sex education policies and indicators of sexual health among young people: A comparison of the Netherlands, France, Australia and the United States. *Sex Education, 5*(2), 171–188. https://doi.org/10.1080/14681810500038889.

Willis, G. M., Prescott, D. S., & Yates, P. M. (2013). The good lives model (GLM) in theory and practice. *Sexual Abuse in Australia and New Zealand, 5*(1), 3.

Wolfe, P. S., Condo, B., & Hardaway, E. (2009). Sociosexuality education for persons with autism spectrum disorders using principles of applied behavior analysis. *Teaching Exceptional Children, 42*(1), 50–61. https://doi.org/10.1177/004005990904200105.

Wurtele, S., & Kenny, M. (2011). Normative sexuality development in childhood: Implications for developmental guidance and prevention of childhood sexual abuse. *Journal of Multicultural Counseling and Development, 43,* 1–24.

Dr. Eileen T. Crehan is a Clinical Psychologist who specializes in autism spectrum disorder in adolescents and adulthood. In collaboration with an Autism Community Advisory Board, she leads a research lab at Tufts University which focuses on improving access to care, especially sexuality and relationship education, for autistic people across the lifespan. She consults with schools, medical providers, and care professionals on best practices for supporting and promoting healthy outcomes for and with autistic individuals. Prior to joining the faculty at Tufts, she was the Associate Clinic Director at the Autism Assessment, Research, and Treatment Services Center at Rush University Medical Center.

Dr. Laurie Sperry is a Board Certified Behavior Analyst-Doctoral and the Director of Autism Services And Programs in Wheat Ridge, Colorado. She has worked as a developer of the Neurodiverse Student Support Program at Stanford University, School of Medicine, Department of Psychiatry. Prior to joining Stanford, she was an Assistant Clinical Faculty at Yale University, Department of Psychiatry.

In 2006 she was added to the Fulbright Scholarship's Senior Specialist Roster for Autism. She moved to Australia in 2010 and worked at Griffith University in the Department of Arts, Education and Law. Her research focuses on people with ASD who come in contact with the criminal justice system to ensure their humane and just treatment. She has served as a Special Interest Group Chairwoman at the International Meeting for Autism Research (IMFAR) providing mentoring and leadership in the field of criminality and ASD. She has provided training to secure forensic psychiatric facility staff in England and presented at the International Conference for Offenders with Disabilities. She has published numerous articles and book chapters and was an expert panelist at the American Academy of Psychiatry and Law conference where she spoke on Risk Assessment, Management, and ASD. She has completed ADOS evaluations in prisons, has testified as an expert witness in sentencing hearings, has written amicus curiae briefs and has participated in cases that have been considered before state supreme courts.

Chapter 25
Violence Prevention

Marc Woodbury-Smith

Introduction

The term 'violence prevention' has a specific meaning in relation to public health initiatives to prevent relapse among those who have already engaged in violent acts (secondary prevention), as well as the prevention of violence where future risk has been identified (primary prevention) (World Health Organization, 2010; Butchart & Mikton, 2014; Sumner et al., 2015; Faculty of Public Health, 2016). In contrast, tertiary prevention refers to 'bigger picture' public health-driven strategies. Violence prevention is also conceptualised according to victim profile into intimate partner violence, elder abuse, child maltreatment and youth crime/gang-related violence (Faculty of Public Health, 2016). Of course, these specific categories may be less relevant to those with ASD, a proportion of whom may remain unmarried and without children, and most of whom will have no experience of gangs; unless, of course, they are 'recruited' as vulnerable and acquiescent individuals (Palermo, 2013; Allely & Faccini, 2017). This notwithstanding, considering the range of violent behaviours reported among people with ASD, and the many different factors hypothesised as relevant to risk (Box 1) (Dein & Woodbury-Smith, 2010; Woodbury-Smith & Dein, 2014; Im, 2016a), a framework divided along with primary, secondary and tertiary levels of prevention, provides a useful grounding for the categorization of therapeutic and other preventative strategies. Moreover, embedding violence prevention in relation to ASD in the broader theories of violence and public health-driven topics, offers full consideration to those more generic strategies that might also be appropriate for this population. Consequently, therefore, this chapter proceeds along the route of general theories of violence and the applicability of these to ASD, rather

M. Woodbury-Smith (✉)
Biosciences Institute, Newcastle University, Newcastle upon Tyne, UK
e-mail: marc.woodbury-smith@newcastle.ac.uk

F. R. Volkmar et al. (eds.), *Handbook of Autism Spectrum Disorder and the Law*,
https://doi.org/10.1007/978-3-030-70913-6_25

than taking the wholly theoretical (and often unsubstantiated) theories of violence in ASD, drawn from small case numbers, as the starting point.

Box 1
Circumscribed interests
Sensory preoccupations
Lack of empathy
Anger and frustration
Suggestibility and acquiescence
Social naivete
Desire for friendships
Mental health comorbidities

As Box 1 indicates, there are some individuals with ASD whose violent behaviour towards both self and others is intimately linked with their associated intellectual disability. There may be a relationship with developmental age, whereby egocentricity linked with poor problem-solving skills and a limited repertoire of sublimative responses necessitates the expression of unchecked emotion. This 'model' does little to describe the inherent complexity involved, but foregrounds the very idea that such violence is not mediated by 'higher' cognitive processes, such as moral decision-making, planning and judgement. This type of violence will not be discussed in this chapter, and the reader is referred to other resources. Simply put, this type of violence, often termed 'challenging behaviour', is a well-researched topic, and has been shown to be amenable to behavioural interventions coupled with supervision (Heyvaert et al., 2010; Lloyd & Kennedy, 2014; Strydom et al., 2020). The distinction is discussed in more detail in this volume (Chap. 22). In contrast, what unites other violent behaviours is that understanding the 'higher' cognitive elements, that is the socio-emotional developmental processes and conscious motivating factors, is important in the determination of strategies to address all levels of prevention (World Health Organization, 2002).

Theoretical-Driven Violence Prevention

Theories of violence: Violence has characterised the human condition in all of its known history. The psychoanalytic theories on violent behaviour are extensive, complex and largely divergent. At the risk of oversimplification, there is an overarching theme of instinctual drives that are aggressive in nature (Freud, 1961; Lorenz, 2002; Plaut, 1984). There is an element of abstractness in much of the theory that problematises its translation into the focus of this chapter, i.e. preventing violence. One notable exception is in the work of Karl Menninger (Menninger et al., 1963). He first proposed the idea that violence may be a result of the need to maintain the integrity of the self, and that acts of violence, therefore, have intrinsic meaning. It is not so far-fetched to imagine how an external 'insult' can disturb one's integrity, as these sorts of things happen to everyone at some point (Menninger, 2007). The inhibition of violence in these situations is multifactorial, and from an analytic perspective involves the psyche's defence mechanisms. These may be developed, such as humour or sublimation (e.g. we may simply laugh off an insult). In contrast, Klein and other object relations theorists focussed on the interaction between the mind and its environment through the internalisation of objects, and the use of defence mechanisms that are more primitive, such as projection and projective identification (essentially, sending the unwanted bits into someone else and acting towards them accordingly) (Grotstein, 1982). Also relevant in this level of abstract discussion is Freud's superego, the opinionated and critical guilt-provoking structure (Freud, 1961).

One further thread from psychoanalytic thought in relation to violence is attachment theory (Sroufe et al., 1999). Bowlby formulated a theory that captured the apparently 'pre-wired' relationships that exist between an infant and their primary caregiver(s) and the anxiety that can be provoked when these fundamental relationships go awry. Importantly, however, from the perspective of future relationships, Bowlby envisioned that these fundamental interpersonal experiences earmarked internal working models that would then dictate a person's future pattern of relationships. Simply put, insecure early relationships could result in insecure later relationships. Indeed, it has been widely demonstrated that among offender populations there is a disproportionate number who had insecure childhood attachments as well as other traumas (Ogilvie et al., 2014) (discussed subsequently). The implication for violence prevention lies in the therapeutic domain, where opportunities for individual and group behaviour focussed on developing positive internalised interpersonal models offers the possibility of reversing these fundamental abnormal 'blueprints' (World Health Organization, 2002; Faculty of Public Health, 2016).

From the perspective of ASD, there is very little in the way of scientific literature that has explored early patterns of attachment behaviour; those studies that do exist largely describe attachments as within normal limits (Rogers et al., 1991, but see Rutgers et al., 2007). This notwithstanding, the importance of early, predictably secure significant others cannot be understated, and much tertiary prevention from a public health perspective has focussed on strategies to ensure child–parent bonding is given the importance it deserves (World Health Organization, 2002; Faculty of Public Health, 2016). Attachment is a dyad, and if one element is missing, whether this is the parent or the infant, the processes involved in establishing secure attachment will likely be impacted. Consequently, it probably makes little sense trying to infer patterns of attachment in ASD from the existing schema of secure and insecure attachments, as there may be other, as yet unexplored, patterns of insecurity concomitant on a lack of typical responsiveness from the ASD infant. This requires further exploration as it, too, may have implications for the later emergence of violent behaviour.

Childhood trauma: Childhood adversity, in the form of negative life events during the formative years, is a well-established risk factor for the later development of mental health problems, poor resilience to everyday stressors and risk of later violence (Duke et al., 2010; Hughes et al., 2017), and the same is true for ASD (Im, 2016b;

Westphal, 2016). Considering particular significant life events such as physical abuse, sexual abuse and neglect, the strength of this relationship is increased (Hughes et al., 2017). For example, those who have experienced such abuse during their childhood are more likely to become perpetrators of such crimes in adulthood. Those who have witnessed such acts are also at a greater risk of adult violence. The nature of this relationship is unclear, although these early negative experiences do impact on brain development, and this in turn will influence behaviour at the level of executive functioning and the hypothalamic-pituitary-adrenal axis (Anda et al., 2006). The strengths of these relationships, along with the emerging evidence of a biological underpinning, are particularly relevant to violence prevention interventions. However, the myriad of different factors that mediate the relationship between early negative experiences and later crime is also apparent (Zielinski & Bradshaw, 2006), including socio-economic confounds, gender-specific effects (Jung et al., 2017) and the mediating impact of academic attainment (Lochner & Moretti, 2004) and personal resilience (Fergusson & Horwood, 2003). As with all the theories discussed so far, there is an underlying complexity that muddies the water when thinking about translation into treatment modalities.

Psychological theories: Psychological theories of violence are particularly important in violence prevention in terms of the different models of treatment that have developed from these theoretical underpinnings. The literature is vast, but Social Learning Theory and Social Control Theory are of particular importance, with both embedded in a person's interaction with their environment. **Social learning** foregrounds the very process of learning, and, in particular, the ways in which behaviour can be learned from others (Bandura, 1978; Burgess & Akers, 1966). The essence is a set of social norms that dictate how a person behaves in different situations, with these normative rules being 'learnt' from others' patterns of behaviour, and the reinforcement contingencies (including consequences) for those behaviours. In the current context, this may involve imitation of others, particularly if behaviour is associated with positive reinforcement (as may be the case for unpunished theft of objects). This may be further compounded if the person grows up around those with a pro-delinquent attitude. Such learning takes place across the developmental stages, with adolescence particularly important in line with Kohlberg's stages of moral development. Although simplistic, the model is probabilistic rather than deterministic. Nonetheless, violence prevention programmes have been developed based on this theory (for example, Esbensen, 2009; Sullivan & Jolliffe, 2014), that focus particularly on positive relationships during adolescence, although none of these programmes have been robustly evaluated. Whether or not social learning theory is relevant to understanding the motivation for violence in ASD is unknown, although opportunities for the modelling of social behaviour, both positive and negative, is more limited in this population.

In contrast, **Social Control Theory** is concerned with a person's bond with their environment, with a weak bond a risk factor for delinquent behaviour. Durkheim first talked about the connection between an individual and their environment in his concept of *anomie* (Marks, 1974), describing individuals who are disconnected from others and socially excluded. This idea was developed by Hirschi, who emphasised four elements to this connection, namely: attachment, commitment, involvement and belief (Hirschi, 1969). It is the very connectedness between people that is important, and without these 'bonds', a person is without any motivating factors to behave prosocially, and antisocial behaviour may result. This is, of course, not entirely distinct from social learning theory, as both theories give emphasis to the role of others in our prosocial behaviour. Consequently, programmes that are based on Social Control Theory also emphasise peer relationships during adolescence as a pivotal element of treatment (Sullivan & Jolliffe, 2014). Again, however, the relevance of this theory to ASD is unclear. Being disconnected from others by choice will not be interpreted by the person as social exclusion, and therefore emotionally syntonic rather than dystonic. Of course, it cannot be assumed that all people with ASD are socially isolated, nor that those who are, are so by choice.

Psychiatric disorders and violence: It was a long-held belief that schizophrenia was associated with an increased risk of violence. (Hodgins, 1998) This is of particular relevance given the inflated risk of schizophrenia among those with ASD (5% or more) (Lugo Marin et al., 2018; Zheng et al., 2018). However, research over a period of many decades has debunked a direct relationship between schizophrenia and violence in favour of the stronger evidence that the confound of substance abuse explains most of the association: while, therefore, schizophrenia is indeed associated with a greater risk of violence, much of the variance is due to the common comorbidity of substance abuse (Fazel et al., 2009). This is important in the context of ASD, which is generally associated with a lower risk of substance abuse, although it remains to be determined whether this association also holds for those who have a comorbid diagnosis of schizophrenia. Of course, there are also a myriad of other important factors, including aspects of the psychotic phenomenology itself (Hodgins et al., 1996; Hodgins, 1998). Among those studies of violence in ASD published up to now, schizophrenia and other mental illnesses do not feature strongly in the clinical descriptions, and are generally not put forward as mediators of illegal activity and violence.

There are also certain personality types that seem to have a higher propensity for violence. Most strikingly, of course, is psychopathy, a disorder characterised by impaired empathy, egocentricity and antisocial patterns of behaviour. Individuals who score above the Psychopathy Checklist—Revised (PCL-R) threshold for diagnosis of psychopathy are over-represented in prisons and this inflation is largely due to violent crimes (Kiehl & Hoffman, 2011). Moreover, this disorder is characterised by a stable pattern of socio-cognitive impairments (Gao et al., 2009); specifically, a reduced physiological response to the distress of others, and difficulties decoding the distress cues of others (Blair, 2003). Theory of mind, defined in broad terms as cognitive perspective taking, appears intact (Blair et al., 1996). These impairments, therefore, do not overlap with the socio-cognitive difficulties seen in people with ASD. Similarly, antisocial personality disorder, which strongly overlaps with psychopathy, is also associated with violence, although there are issues of tautology that do require consideration. For example, the diagnostic item "a disregard for social norms" itself earmarks law-breaking behaviour, and other similar diagnostic traits may be correlated with violent or other illegal behaviour. Nonetheless, the stability of ASPD from childhood into middle adulthood and beyond, and its known prognostic correlates, makes it a useful diagnostic construct (Black, 2015). There is no evidence in the literature that ASPD occurs with a higher prevalence among those with ASD, and cases describing the existence of both sets of traits in an offender are rare (although see, for example, Frick & Viding, 2009; Rogers et al., 2006; Woodbury-Smith et al., 2005 for a more detailed discussion). The same is true for psychopathy, and additionally there is no evidence of autism traits in this population.

In contrast, there is a strong association between ASD and ADHD (Joshi et al., 2017; Simonoff et al., 2008). Furthermore, ADHD is associated with ASPD and is independently associated with risk of violence and antisocial behaviour (Eyestone & Howell, 1994; Gunter et al., 2008). This strong association between ADHD and ASD, therefore, may mediate the risk of violence among those with ASD (Heeramun et al., 2017). In reality, the relationship between psychiatric disorders and violence is confounded by the oftentimes multiple comorbidities that exist in a number of people, and this relationship extends to those with ASD. Consequently, apportioning correlation, let along causality, will require longitudinal data on large cohorts (Heeramun et al., 2017). This is a not insignificant undertaking, but disentangling the role of one diagnosis versus another will be important when considering violence prevention strategies for those with ASD and other neurodevelopmental disorders. Moreover, whatever programmes of violence prevention are introduced, specialist mental health services for those with complex comorbidities will be crucial in delivering such interventions effectively.

The Relevance of Theories of Violence to ASD

The theories described above are, of course, based on population-level epidemiological data, and do not take into consideration those elements of development and behaviour that are unique to ASD. As indicated above, violent and aggressive behaviour in ASD will have a different etiology according to the level of intellectual capacity. Among those who are more able, research has examined the relationship between such factors as rigid thought, the nature of interests and core cognitive factors such as empathy and impaired theory of mind (Im, 2016a; King & Murphy, 2014; Woodbury-Smith & Dein, 2014). As discussed elsewhere in this volume, there is no strong evidence collectively that ASD is specifically associated with violent behaviour, although there may be a subgroup at higher risk (Rogers et al., 2006; Woodbury-Smith et al., 2005; Woodbury-Smith & Dein, 2014). The nature of risk in this subgroup is not well understood. There does seem to be a higher prevalence of ASD in secure psychiatric hospitals (Allely, 2018; King & Murphy, 2014), but this may be due to ASD's strong relationship to ADHD (Heeramun et al., 2017), itself implicated in criminality. Indeed, another consideration is that the nature of illegal behaviour is not necessarily violent. In the special hospital studies a range of transgressions is described, as evidenced by the themes across the different chapters in this volume.

There has been concern that some circumscribed interests, particularly those with a violent focus, raise the risk of violence, although the data are far from conclusive. Certainly, some case descriptions exist in which a person with a violent interest has engaged in violence. For example, Everall and Le Couteur (1990), Hare et al. (1999), Barry-Walsh and Mullen (2004) and Woodbury-Smith et al. (2010) have all described individuals whose convictions for an index offence of arson were preceded by an 'interest' in, or fascination with, fires. Similarly, another person in the sample described by Hare and his colleagues (1999), with an interest in knives, was subsequently convicted of unlawful wounding. In contrast, however, for other cases any relationship is unconvincing. For example, Tantam (1988a, 1988b) described an individual with probable Asperger Syndrome and a fascination with extreme politics, who dressed in a Nazi uniform before an unprovoked assault on a soldier. Indeed, in one study that attempted to establish links between violent interests and offending, for only 1 offender among 21 with ASD could a relationship be robustly established, and even in this case other factors were also relevant (Woodbury-Smith et al., 2010).

Through the study of development in ASD, other more nuanced aspects of social cognition have also emerged, impairments of which may mediate violent behaviour. This includes deficits in theory of mind and tolerance of uncertainty. Both have been shown to be impaired in ASD, but neither are specifically associated with violence. Indeed, as mentioned above, considering those with psychopathy as a specific group with a raised risk of violence, the literature suggests a preserved or even *superior* ToM ability in this population (Blair et al., 1996). Interestingly, in our own study comparing ASD offenders with ASD non-offenders, we found that unlike their non-offending ASD counterparts, the offenders had a relatively *preserved* ToM ability, suggesting this factor may itself earmark a subgroup whose cognitive profile underlies the risk of violence, particularly if coupled with other risk factors, such as those described in the theoretical literature above (Rogers et al., 2006; Woodbury-Smith et al., 2005).

Even if we do accept that people with ASD are over-represented among detainees in the criminal justice system, what is also unclear is whether it is ASD itself, or simply 'autism traits', that is linked to illegal behaviour and aggression. The difference is more than semantic, given the fact that autism traits are known to be continuously distributed in the population. Take the prison studies for example. In the US, Fazio et al. (2012) found that the mean AQ score (a measure of autistic traits, with a higher score indicative of greater vulnerability) in a maximum secure psychiatric population was 20 (SD = 6.4) (Fazio et al., 2012), which is higher than in the general population (16.94 [95% CI 11.6, 20.0]) (Ruzich et al., 2015). Similarly, in a study of Scottish prisoners, Robinson et al. (2012) also identified a mean AQ-20 score of 20.1 (SD = 7.3) in incarcerated prisoners (Robinson et al., 2012). This does suggest that the naturally occurring Gaussian distribution of this trait is shifted to the left among the prison population, favouring greater impairment. Perhaps, therefore, there is indeed an association between violent behaviour and autism, but this association goes beyond diagnostic classification. Alternatively, traits that *overlap with* ASD may drive the elevated AQ scores. The nature of risk in this wider group with 'autistic traits' will itself be complicated to unravel, but in consideration of violence prevention, this may present an important avenue of research to inform the wider tertiary level of violence prevention initiatives.

Violence Prevention Initiatives

What does this all mean, then, from the point of view of violence prevention initiatives? From a Public Health point of view, *primary* violence prevention has focussed on early intervention aimed at promoting safe and nurturing environments at home, including facilitating greater resilience among those who grow up in difficult environments (Butchart & Mikton, 2014; Sumner et al., 2015; World Health Organization, 2002, 2010). In line with the psychoanalytic and psychological theories presented above, this is an important element of facilitating the development of secure attachments and good self-esteem from an early age, and is typically delivered through parenting programmes, such as the Positive Parenting Programme (PPP) in the US. Such programmes vary in their delivery method, for example whether they take an individual or group approach, but in general terms all include elements of parent education and all engender positive interactions between parents and their children (World Health Organization, 2010).

Such programmes (discussed in more detail in World Health Organization, 2010 and references therein) are typically delivered in a small group setting making them economically feasible and easily deliverable. Moreover, there is now accumulating evidence for the effectiveness of such programmes, and therefore there has been much investment in setting up and implementing these programmes (Butchart & Mikton, 2014; Sumner et al., 2015). A number of key elements are believed to facilitate a positive outcome, including the delivery of a service that focusses on positive interactions between children and their caregivers, and non-punitive measures for wrongdoing. Actual delivery of therapy in the home as well as actual observation of and correction where appropriate of interactions are also associated with a better outcome, although this clearly requires an individualised approach and is less cost-effective. Of course, one consideration is that the effectiveness of these generic programmes in violence prevention has not been investigated specifically in ASD. However, bearing in mind that typical ABA interventions are based on the same principles, their efficacy might also be reasonably assumed in this population too.

It is important not to overlook the usefulness of such programmes for individuals with ASD. While there is no evidence to support the fact that early relationships among those with ASD are difficult, there is no reason why such factors may not be relevant in the small subgroup of people with ASD who have engaged in violent behaviour. Indeed, the difficulties of looking after young children have been well described in the literature in terms of the levels of carer stress in such families (e.g. Keenan et al., 2016). Identifying such families and offering support and guidance in the very least will mitigate stress and its consequences, which, for some, may be violent sequelae. Unfortunately, service provision is largely structured around diagnosis, and consequently there is always a risk that having a diagnosis of ASD will *exclude* a family from treatments. Equally, there is a risk that such programmes may be too generic and fail to take into consideration the impact of ASD on methods of delivery.

Beyond these primary prevention measures, secondary prevention from a public health point of view has focussed on factors such as alcohol and the availability of weapons as well as the management of mental health problems. It cannot be assumed that people with ASD are at low risk of alcohol use as this is not substantiated in the literature. It cannot also be assumed that weapons are not available to people with ASD due to an oftentimes higher level of supervision in the community. While supervision is often higher, the use of weapons among those with ASD who have engaged in violence is well described.

Primary and secondary violence prevention from a mental health point of view has been informed by a long history of empirical investigation that has accumulated robust data from large-scale longitudinal studies. A detailed consideration of this literature is out of the scope of this current chapter, but, in short, these studies all conclude that the risk of violence is increased in this population, with factors such as childhood trauma and substance and alcohol use clear correlates of violent and other unlawful behaviour in this population (Fazel & Danesh, 2002; Fazel et al., 2009, 2016). As mentioned previously, ADHD is also independently associated with violence (Gunter et al., 2008). In addition to management of specific mental illness, including good compliance with medication and support and supervision in the community, there is also evidence that management of ADHD symptoms can reduce violence (Lichtenstein et al., 2012). Furthermore, from a primary prevention perspective, better educational support and positive parenting may also reduce later violence in this population.

In terms of psychopathy and ASPD, although the research on treatment approaches is vast, the actual evidence of the superiority of one approach to management versus another is weak, confounded by such factors as small sample size, poor diagnostic characterisation, and bias introduced by the willingness of some, but not other, participants to take part in such programmes (Hecht et al., 2018; Kiehl & Hoffman, 2011; Klein Haneveld et al., 2018; Sewall & Olver, 2019). One programme, the Dangerous and Severe Personality Disorder (DSPD) programme in the UK, has been extensively evaluated (Barrett & Tyrer, 2012; Burns et al., 2011; Vollm, 2009). The individuals labelled as such are highly heterogeneous, but some data have reported risk reduction, albeit at great expense and with unknown implications for questions such as the longer-term safety in the community (Barrett & Tyrer, 2012; Burns et al., 2011).

Violence Prevention in ASD

In the preceding paragraphs, the general approach to primary and secondary prevention strategies has been described. Thinking more specifically about ASD, violence prevention can also be conceptualised in primary, secondary levels, although the caveat we introduce throughout this volume is that there is still very little understanding of the nature of the risk factors in this population. Primary prevention, by definition, will be based on addressing early life risk factors. In some cases, these may significantly overlap with those described above, but other factors, such as the nature of a person's interest and their identified pattern of social and communication vulnerabilities at a cognitive level, may also be relevant. In the absence of robust data, it seems reasonable to expect that individuals with certain sensory predilections, such as fire, or circumscribed interests that are potentially harmful, such as bomb-making, should be monitored, and their interests 'shaped' into something more appropriate. Similarly, individuals with certain comorbidities, such as ADHD, and those who are known to use substances and/or alcohol will also need more careful management of risk. For those who are deemed to lack empathy, and show little remorse or understanding of the impact of wrongdoing on others, a more careful approach will be needed. Programmes that 'teach' empathy are available, with variable efficacy. These involve elements such as cognitive reframing of scenarios, as well as reappraisal of past behaviours, and have been shown to improve empathic responsiveness, although sample sizes are small and selective.

Mass Violence

In the last decade or so, attention has been drawn towards a number of individuals who have engaged in mass violence for no apparent reason and without any 'red flags' (Allely, 2017). Such individuals do not clearly act in the context of affiliation with any known terrorist or right-wing organisation. What has been striking is that a number of these individuals have been diagnosed with ASD, and many others, perhaps unsurprisingly, present with social vulnerabilities. Such 'lone wolf terrorists' present a major challenge for existing paradigms of violence prevention, and also do not clearly align with wider terrorist activities that are usually associated in some way with membership of a larger group who share similar extreme ideologies. Several such cases, such as the perpetrator of the Sandy Hook massacre, have a clear history of an ASD diagnosis, but little in the way of 'warning signs' (see Conclusion Chap. 20).

Among such individuals, post hoc analysis of textual information (e.g. diaries, blogs etc) often finds evidence of extreme leanings, anger and frustration and disgruntlement with various aspects of society, but the event itself almost appears out of the blue. Understanding the motivation for such behaviour is confounded by the extreme rarity of such events, along with the fact that the perpetrator often dies during the act. This notwithstanding, the availability of powerful text mining methods in conjunction with deep learning machine intelligence will allow diaries, blogs and other documents written by such perpetrators to be examined in detail and facilitate a better understanding of motivation.

Conclusions

Violence prevention is a global challenge: it is estimated that 1.3 million deaths a year are mediated by a violent incident (Butchart & Mikton, 2014) and the World Health

Organization has declared that violence is predictable and therefore preventable (Butchart & Mikton, 2014). The lone wolf terrorist and other aspects of mass violence carried out by loners currently undermines this assertion, and presents a new challenge for scientific research, needed in order to fully realise a robust process of risk prediction. The fact that several individuals who have been the perpetrators of such crimes were known to have ASD reinforce the need for a wider programme of research that seeks a better understanding of the interface between ASD and the law.

In more general terms the nature of *prediction* is a major challenge, confounded by factors such as different risk factors for different types of violence, the many theoretical bases of violence, and the changing nature of patterns and types of violence over the years. Much of the focus has been on those types of violence that are particularly common, such as intimate partner violence, and that might not be entirely relevant to the ASD population. In contrast, other initiatives that focus on mass violence may be more relevant but only to a small number of individuals. Consequently, there is a need to develop more robust studies of violence in ASD in order to be able to usefully inform primary and secondary prevention in this population.

References

Allely, C. S. (2017). Violence is rare in autism: When it does occur, is it sometimes extreme? *Journal of Psychology, 151*(1), 49–68.

Allely, C. S. (2018). A systematic PRISMA review of individuals with autism spectrum disorder in secure psychiatric care: Prevalence, treatment, risk assessment and other clinical considerations. *Journal of Criminal Psychology, 8*(1), 58–79.

Allely, C. S., & Faccini, L. (2017). Rare instances of individuals with autism supporting or engaging in terrorism. *Journal of Intellectual Disabilities and Offending, 8*(2), 70–82.

Anda, R. F., Felitti, V. J., Bremner, J. D., Walker, J. D., Whitfield, C., Perry, B. D., ... Giles, W. H. (2006). The enduring effects of abuse and related adverse experiences in childhood: A convergence of evidence from neurobiology and epidemiology. *European Archives of Psychiatry and Clinical Neuroscience, 256*(3), 174–186.

Bandura, A. (1978). Social learning theory of aggression. *Journal of Communication, 28*(3), 12–29.

Barrett, B., & Tyrer, P. (2012). The cost-effectiveness of the dangerous and severe personality disorder programme. *Criminal Behaviour and Mental Health, 22*(3), 202–209.

Barry-Walsh, J. B., & Mullen, P. E. (2004). Forensic aspects of Asperger's syndrome. *The Journal of Forensic Psychiatry and Psychology, 15*(1), 96–107.

Black, D. W. (2015). The natural history of antisocial personality disorder. *Canadian Journal of Psychiatry, 60*(7), 309–314.

Blair, J., Sellers, C., Strickland, I., Clark, F., Williams, A., Smith, M., & Jones, L. (1996). Theory of mind in the psychopath. *The Journal of Forensic Psychiatry, 7*(1), 15–25.

Blair, R. J. (2003). Neurobiological basis of psychopathy. *British Journal of Psychiatry, 182,* 5–7.

Burgess, R. L., & Akers, R. L. (1966). A differential association-reinforcement theory of criminal behavior. *Social Problems, 14,* 128–147.

Burns, T., Yiend, J., Fahy, T., Fitzpatrick, R., Rogers, R., Fazel, S., & Sinclair, J. (2011). Treatments for dangerous severe personality disorder (DSPD). *Journal of Forensic Psychiatry and Psychology, 22*(3), 411–426.

Butchart, A., & Mikton, C. (2014). *Global status report on violence prevention 2014.* Retrieved from https://www.who.int/violence_injury_prevention/violence/status_report/2014/en/.

Dein, K., & Woodbury-Smith, M. (2010). Asperger syndomre and criminal behaviour. *Advances in Psychiatric Treatment, 16,* 37–43.
Duke, N. N., Pettingell, S. L., McMorris, B. J., & Borowsky, I. W. (2010). Adolescent violence perpetration: Associations with multiple types of adverse childhood experiences. *Pediatrics, 125*(4), e778–786.
Esbensen, F.-A. (2009). *Evaluation of the teens, crime and the community and community works program.* Retrieved from https://www.ojp.gov/pdffiles1/nij/grants/228277.pdf.
Everall, I. P., & Le couter, A. (1990). Firesetting in an adolescent boy with Asperger's syndrome. *British Journal of Psychiatry, 157,* 284–287.
Eyestone, L. L., & Howell, R. J. (1994). An epidemiological study of attention-deficit hyperactivity disorder and major depression in a male prison population. *Bulletin of the American Academy of Psychiatry and the Law, 22*(2), 181–193.
Faculty of Public Health. (2016). *The role of public health in the prevention of violence.* Faculty of Public Health: London, UK.
Fazel, S., & Danesh, J. (2002). Serious mental disorder in 23 000 prisoners: A systematic review of 62 surveys. *Lancet, 359,* 545–550.
Fazel, S., Hayes, A. J., Bartellas, K., Clerici, M., & Trestman, R. (2016). Mental health of prisoners: Prevalence, adverse outcomes, and interventions. *Lancet Psychiatry, 3*(9), 871–881.
Fazel, S., Langstrom, N., Hjern, A., Grann, M., & Lichtenstein, P. (2009). Schizophrenia, substance abuse, and violent crime. *The Journal of the American Medical Association, 301*(19), 2016–2023.
Fazio, R. L., Pietz, C. A., & Denney, R. L. (2012). An estimate of the prevalence of autsm spectrum disorders in an incarcerated population. *Open Access Journal of Forensic Psychology, 4,* 69–80.
Fergusson, D. M., & Horwood, L. J. (2003). Resilience to childhood adversity: results of a 21 year study. In S. S. Luthar (Ed.), *Resilience and vulnerability: Adaptation in the context of childhood adversities* (pp. 130–155). Cambridge University Press.
Freud, S. (1961). Civilization and its discontents. In J. Strachey (Ed.), *The standard edition of the complete psychological works of Sigmund Freud* (Vol. 21, pp. 1–182). Hogarth Press.
Frick, P. J., & Viding, E. (2009). Antisocial behavior from a developmental psychopathology perspective. *Development and Psychopathology, 21*(4), 1111–1131.
Gao, Y., Glenn, A. L., Schug, R. A., Yang, Y., & Raine, A. (2009). The neurobiology of psychopathy: A neurodevelopmental perspective. *Development and Psychopathology, 54*(12), 813–823.
Grotstein, J. S. (1982). The specturm of aggression. *Psychoanalytic Inquiry, 2*(2), 193–211.
Gunter, T. D., Arndt, S., Wenman, G., Allen, J., Loveless, P., Sieleni, B., & Black, D. W. (2008). Frequency of mental and addictive disorders among 320 men and women entering the Iowa prison system: Use of the MINI-plus. *Journal of the American Academy of Psychiatry and the Law, 36*(1), 27–34.
Hare, D. J., Gould, J., Mills, R., & Wing, L. (1999). *A preliminary study of individuals with autistic spectrum disorders in three special hospitals in England.* National Autistic Society.
Hecht, L. K., Latzman, R. D., & Lilienfeld, S. O. (2018). The psychological treatment of psychopathy: Theory and research. In D. David, S. J. Lynn, & G. H. Montgomery (Eds.), *Evidence-based psychotherapy: The state of the science and practice* (pp. 271–298). Wiley-Blackwell.
Heeramun, R., Magnusson, C., Gumpert, C. H., Granath, S., Lundberg, M., Dalman, C., & Rai, D. (2017). Autism and convictions for violent crimes: Population-based cohort study in Sweden. *Journal of the American Academy of Child and Adolescent Psychiatry, 56*(6), 491–497, e492.
Heyvaert, M., Maes, B., & Onghena, P. (2010). A meta-analysis of intervention effects on challenging behaviour among persons with intellectual disabilities. *Journal of Intellectual Disability Research, 54*(7), 634–649.
Hirschi, T. (1969). *Causes of delinquency.* University of California Press.
Hodgins, S. (1998). Epidemiological investigations of the associations between major mental disorders and crime: Methodological limitations and validity of the conclusions. *Social Psychiatry and Psychiatric Epidemiology, 33*(Suppl. 1), S29–37.
Hodgins, S., Mednick, S. A., Brennan, P. A., Schulsinger, F., & Engberg, M. (1996). Mental disorder and crime: Evidence from a Danish birth cohort. *Archives of General Psychiatry, 53*(6), 489–496.

Hughes, K., Bellis, M. A., Hardcastle, K. A., Sethi, D., Butchart, A., Mikton, C., … Dunne, M. P. (2017). The effect of multiple adverse childhood experiences on health: A systematic review and meta-analysis. *Lancet Public Health, 2*(8), e356–e366. https://doi.org/10.1016/S2468-2667(17)30118-4.

Im, D. S. (2016a). Template to perpetrate: An update on violence in autism spectrum disorder. *Harvard Review of Psychiatry, 24*(1), 14–35.

Im, D. S. (2016b). Trauma as a contributor to violence in autism spectrum disorder. *Journal of the American Academy of Psychiatry and the Law, 44*(2), 184–192.

Joshi, G., Faraone, S. V., Wozniak, J., Tarko, L., Fried, R., Galdo, M., … Biederman, J. (2017). Symptom profile of ADHD in youth with high-functioning autism spectrum disorder: A comparative study in psychiatrically referred populations. *Journal of Attention Disorders, 21*(10), 846–855.

Jung, H., Herrenkohl, T. I., Lee, J. O., Hemphill, S. A., Heerde, J. A., & Skinner, M. L. (2017). Gendered pathways from child abuse to adult crime through internalizing and externalizing behaviors in childhood and adolescence. *Journal of Interpersonal Violence, 32*(18), 2724–2750.

Keenan, B. M., Newman, L. K., Gray, K. M., & Rinehart, N. J. (2016). Parents of children with ASD experience more psychological distress, parenting stress, and attachment-related anxiety. *Journal of Autism and Developmental Disorders, 46*(9), 2979–2991.

Kiehl, K. A., & Hoffman, M. B. (2011). The criminal psychopath: History, neuroscience, treatment, and economics. *Jurimetrics, 51,* 355–397.

King, C., & Murphy, G. H. (2014). A systematic review of people with autism spectrum disorder and the criminal justice system. *Journal of Autism and Developmental Disorders, 44*(11), 2717–2733.

Klein Haneveld, E., Neumann, C. S., Smid, W., Wever, E., & Kamphuis, J. H. (2018). Treatment responsiveness of replicated psychopathy profiles. *Law and Human Behavior, 42*(5), 484–495.

Lichtenstein, P., Halldner, L., Zetterqvist, J., Sjolander, A., Serlachius, E., Fazel, S., … Larsson, H. (2012). Medication for attention deficit-hyperactivity disorder and criminality. *The New England Journal of Medicine, 367*(21), 2006–2014.

Lloyd, B. P., & Kennedy, C. H. (2014). Assessment and treatment of challenging behaviour for individuals with intellectual disability: A research review. *Journal of Applied Research in Intellectual Disabilities, 27*(3), 187–199.

Lochner, L., & Moretti, E. (2004). The effect of education on crime: Evidence from prison inmates, arrests, and self-reports. *The American Economic Review, 94*(1), 155–189.

Lorenz, K. (2002). *On aggression.* Routledge.

Lugo Marin, J., Alviani Rodriguez-Franco, M., Mahtani Chugani, V., Magan Maganto, M., Diez Villoria, E., & Canal Bedia, R. (2018). Prevalence of schizophrenia spectrum disorders in average-IQ adults with autism spectrum disorders: A meta-analysis. *Journal of Autism and Developmental Disorders, 48*(1), 239–250.

Marks, S. R. (1974). Durkheim's theory of anomie. *American Journal of Sociology, 80*(2), 329–363.

Menninger, K. A., Mayman, M., & Pruyser, P. (1963). *The vital balance.* Viking Press.

Menninger, W. W. (2007). Uncontained rage: A psychoanalytic perspective on violence. *Bulletin of the Menninger Clinic, 71*(2), 115–131.

Ogilvie, C. A., Newman, E., Todd, L., & Peck, D. (2014). Attachment & violent offending: A meta-analysis. *Aggression and Violent Behavior, 19*(4), 322–339.

Palermo, M. T. (2013). Developmental disorders and political extremism: A case of Asperger syndrome and the neo-nazi subculture. *Journal of Forensic Psychology Practice, 13*(4), 341–354.

Plaut, E. A. (1984). Ego instincts: A concept whose time has come. *The Psychoanalytic Study of the Child, 39,* 235–258.

Robinson, L., Spencer, M. D., Thomson, L. D., Stanfield, A. C., Owens, D. G., Hall, J., & Johnstone, E. C. (2012). Evaluation of a screening instrument for autism spectrum disorders in prisoners. *PLoS One, 7*(5), e36078.

Rogers, J., Viding, E., Blair, R. J., Frith, U., & Happe, F. (2006). Autism spectrum disorder and psychopathy: Shared cognitive underpinnings or double hit? *Psychological Medicine, 36*(12), 1789–1798.

Rogers, S. J., Ozonoff, S., & Maslin-Cole, C. (1991). A comparative study of attachment behavior in young children with autism or other psychiatric disorders. *Journal of the American Academy of Child and Adolescent Psychiatry, 30*(3), 483–488.

Rutgers, A. H., van Ijzendoorn, M. H., Bakermans-Kranenburg, M. J., Swinkels, S. H., van Daalen, E., Dietz, C., … van Engeland, H. (2007). Autism, attachment and parenting: A comparison of children with autism spectrum disorder, mental retardation, language disorder, and non-clinical children. *Journal of Abnormal Child Psychology, 35*(5), 859–870.

Ruzich, E., Allison, C., Smith, P., Watson, P., Auyeung, B., Ring, H., et al. (2015). Measuring autistic traits in the general population: A systematic review of the Autism-Spectrum Quotient (AQ) in a nonclinical population sample of 6,900 typical adult males and females. *Molecular Autism, 6,* 2.

Sewall, L. A., & Olver, M. E. (2019). Psychopathy and treatment outcome: Results from a sexual violence reduction program. *Personality Disorders, 10*(1), 59–69.

Simonoff, E., Pickles, A., Charman, T., Chandler, S., Loucas, T., & Baird, G. (2008). Psychiatric disorders in children with autism spectrum disorders: Prevalence, comorbidity, and associated factors in a population-derived sample. *Journal of the American Academy of Child and Adolescent Psychiatry, 47*(8), 921–929.

Sroufe, L. A., Carlson, E. A., Levy, A. K., & Egeland, B. (1999). Implications of attachment theory for developmental psychopathology. *Development and Psychopathology, 11*(1), 1–13.

Strydom, A., Bosco, A., Vickerstaff, V., Hunter, R., PBS Group a.s., & Hassiotis, A. (2020). Clinical and cost effectiveness of staff training in the delivery of Positive Behaviour Support (PBS) for adults with intellectual disabilities, autism spectrum disorder and challenging behaviour—Randomised trial. *BMC Psychiatry, 20*(1), 161.

Sullivan, C. J., & Jolliffe, D. (2014). Peer influence, mentoring and the prevention of crime. In B. C. Welsh & D. P. Farrington (Eds.), *The Oxford handbook of crime prevention* (pp. 207–225). Oxford University Press.

Sumner, S. A., Mercy, J. A., Dahlberg, L. L., Hillis, S. D., Klevens, J., & Houry, D. (2015). Violence in the United States: Status, challenges, and opportunities. *The Journal of the American Medical Association, 314*(5), 478–488.

Tantam, D. (1988a). Lifelong eccentricity and social isolation. I. Psychiatric, social, and forensic aspects. *British Journal of Psychiatry, 153,* 777–782.

Tantam, D. (1988b). Lifelong eccentricity and social isolation. II: Asperger's syndrome or schizoid personality disorder? *British Journal of Psychiatry, 153,* 783–791.

Vollm, B. (2009). Assessment and management of dangerous and severe personality disorders. *Current Opinion in Psychiatry, 22*(5), 501–506.

Westphal, A. (2016). Trauma and violence in autism. *Journal of the American Academy of Psychiatry and the Law, 44*(2), 198–199.

Woodbury-Smith, M., Clare, I. C., Holland, A., Kearns, A., Staufenberg, E., & Watson, P. (2010). Circumscribed interests among offenders with autistic spectrum disorders: A case-control study. *Journal of Forensic Psychiatry and Psychology, 21*(3), 366–377.

Woodbury-Smith, M., Clare, I. C. H., Holland, A. J., Kearns, A., Staufenberg, E., & Watson, P. (2005). A case-control study of offenders with high functioning autistic spectrum disorders. *The Journal of Forensic Psychiatry & Psychology, 16*(4), 747–763.

Woodbury-Smith, M., & Dein, K. (2014). Autism spectrum disorder (ASD) and unlawful behaviour: Where do we go from here? *Journal of Autism and Developmental Disorders, 44*(11), 2734–2741.

World Health Organization. (2002). *World report on violence and health.* World Health Organization.

World Health Organization. (2010). *Violence prevention: The evidence.* World Health Organization.

Zheng, Z., Zheng, P., & Zou, X. (2018). Association between schizophrenia and autism spectrum disorder: A systematic review and meta-analysis. *Autism Research, 11*(8), 1110–1119.

Zielinski, D. S., & Bradshaw, C. P. (2006). Ecological influences on the sequelae of child maltreatment: A review of the literature. *Child Maltreatment, 11*(1), 49–62.

Marc Woodbury-Smith is a Clinical Senior Lecturer in the Biosciences Institute at Newcastle University, UK and an Honorary Consultant Psychiatrist. He is also an Associate Investigator at the Centre for Applied Genomics at the Hospital for Sick Children in Toronto, Canada. He trained in psychiatry in Cambridge, UK and at the Yale Child Study Center, USA. As a psychiatrist specializing in developmental disabilities, he has worked clinically with children and adults with autism spectrum disorder (ASD) for more than 20 years, and has published widely on both basic sciences (genetics) and legal aspects of ASD. He is currently an Associate Editor of the Journal of Autism and Developmental Disorders.

Chapter 26
Service Provision in Forensic Settings

David Murphy

Introduction

Individuals with an Autism Spectrum Disorder (ASD) are recognised to represent a small and diverse proportion of those admitted to secure forensic settings, whether that be prisons or forensic psychiatric units with differing degrees of security. As has been highlighted throughout this book, individuals with an ASD present with a complex range of difficulties and needs that can challenge all stages of the criminal justice process, whether that is during initial contact and interview with law enforcement professionals, involvement with the legal process and attending court, through to receiving a custodial sentence or period of 'treatment' within forensic psychiatric services. Examining the available literature and supported by clinical experience of the author, this chapter outlines some key findings to date regarding; the prevalence of individuals with an ASD detained in secure forensic settings: how individuals with an ASD detained in non-specialist ASD forensic settings differ from other forensic populations in their presenting characteristics, cognitive profiles and self-reported difficulties: how staff who work in secure forensic settings view individuals with an ASD relative to other groups: an exploration of the experiences and quality of life of individuals with an ASD detained within secure forensic environments: a discussion of management issues and 'treatment' options open to individuals with ASD in such settings. A final summary outlines gaps in the current knowledge, along with suggestions for future research and improved clinical practice.

D. Murphy (✉)
Broadmoor Hospital, Crowthorne RG45 7EG, Berkshire, UK
e-mail: david.murphy@westlondon.nhs.uk

F. R. Volkmar et al. (eds.), *Handbook of Autism Spectrum Disorder and the Law*,
https://doi.org/10.1007/978-3-030-70913-6_26

What Is the Prevalence of Individuals with an ASD in Forensic Settings?

Obtaining an accurate estimate of how many individuals with an ASD engage in law breaking behaviours that result in contact with the Criminal Justice System (CJS) and who are subsequently detained within forensic settings has proved to be a difficult task. Examining the available literature suggests that studies vary significantly in their respective methodologies. Many studies also tend to be based on a single setting and selected populations, as well as there being some variation between studies in how ASD has been defined and assessed resulting in limited generalisability (Gómez de la Cuesta, 2010). Studies also tend to be based on individuals already convicted, with virtually nothing known about those individuals with an ASD who offend but who do not come into contact with the CJS and perhaps get diverted into the health care rather than forensic systems. For example, in a UK study, Allen et al. (2008) examined adults with an ASD across 98 different services in South Wales (with a general population of around 1.2 million). Within these services, 126 individuals with Asperger's syndrome were identified, 33 of whom had offended or whose behaviour could have resulted in contact with the CJS. Among these, 7 were reported as not having been processed/arrested, 5 had been imprisoned, 1 had been hospitalised and 3 were reported as living in the community. These findings suggest that offending among individuals with an ASD may not necessarily result in direct contact with the CJS. They also suggest that a wider inclusion of forensic and non-forensic services may be helpful in not only establishing prevalence, but also perhaps provide insights into the decision-making process of why some individuals with an ASD and who offend enter the CJS and others do not.

Whilst an accurate prevalence estimate of ASD within custodial settings remains unclear (Cashin & Newman, 2009), most of the studies completed to date in such environments suggest that individuals with an ASD tend to be over-represented compared to the general estimate of ASD in the population of 1% (Baird et al., 2006; Maenner et al., 2020). For example, within the UK, one study of a London prison identified high levels of ASD traits among male prisoners using the self-report questionnaire the Autism Spectrum Quotient—20—AQ—20 (Underwood et al., 2016). Of the 186 prisoners who were approached, 10% were said to be screened positive or displaying significant autistic traits (i.e. who scored 10 or more on the AQ 20) and within this group 2% were said to fulfil the diagnostic criteria for an ASD following a diagnostic assessment using the *Autism Diagnostic Observation Schedule*, 2nd Edition (Lord et al., 2012). Although likely to be an underestimate, based on this 2% estimate, the Ministry of Justice within the UK suggested that it was likely that approximately 1600 men and 120 women may have an ASD within prisons (Ministry of Justice, 2015). It was also suggested that the prevalence of ASD was likely to vary between different types of prisons, such as whether they are for remand or sentenced prisoners, high secure, mainstream or open prisons (Underwood et al., 2013). Some international studies also support the finding for an over-representation of individuals with an ASD within prisons. For example, within the United States, Fazio et al. (2012)

found following a screen using the 50 items AQ (Baron-Cohen et al., 2001) of prisoners detained within a maximum security state prison in the Midwest that of the 431 prisoners who agreed to complete the questionnaire (24% of those approached) 4.4% (19 individuals) produced scores above the 32 cut-off score suggestive of an ASD.

Likely to be a reflection of the relative stability of the patient population compared to prison settings, UK high-security psychiatric care (HSPC) hospitals were the focus of early prevalence estimates. For example, in a widely cited study, Scragg and Shah's (1994) examination of one HSPC hospital found after an initial screen of patient files followed by interviews with primary nurses and obtaining patient consent, that from 17 individuals identified from an initial screen (from a total 392 male patients), 9 met the diagnostic criteria for Asperger's syndrome (representing a prevalence rate of 2.3%). The conclusion from this study was that Asperger's syndrome was over-represented compared to the general population prevalence rate. However, a limitation of this study was that the diagnostic process used does not reflect the contemporary best practice of confirming a diagnosis of an ASD such as using the *Autism Diagnostic Observation Schedule* and the *Autism Diagnostic Interview Revised* (Lord et al., 1994). It is also important to highlight that not only has the admission criteria to HSPC changed over the 20 years since Scragg and Shah's study was completed (with a much higher focus on minimally restrictive practice and therefore a higher threshold for admission to HSPC), but also that the current total patient population of the HSPC hospital is approximately two-thirds of that examined by Scragg and Shah. Similar points can also be put against another prevalence study of ASD in all three of England's HSPC hospitals (Broadmoor, Rampton and Ashworth) completed by Hare et al. (1999). In this study, using a two stage survey methodology the patient population of all three HSPC hospitals, 31 individuals (2.4%) out of a total of 1305 patients (96% of the total population) were identified as having an ASD. During the initial stage, a nine item staff questionnaire was used to identify potential individuals with an ASD resulting in 240 individuals being identified as having severe social dysfunction and which led to inclusion in the second stage of the project. Of these 240 individuals, 25 could not be followed up for a range of reasons including being transferred from the hospitals. During the second stage, individual records were examined with all those with a confirmed diagnosis of an ASD automatically being included (around 10% of patients) and others being screened using the Handicaps, Behaviours and Skills (HBS) schedule (Wing & Gould, 1978) that included information relevant to impairments of social interaction, communication, imagination, repetitive, stereotyped activities and special interests, as well as with items on motor function, self-care, planning and organisation ability. Of these, 31 definite cases of ASD were identified, as well as a further 31 so-called 'equivocal cases', i.e. had significant features of an ASD, but not enough information to receive the diagnosis. Within the ASD group, 29 (93.5%) were male and 2 (6.5%) female. Within the equivocal group, 28 (90.3%) were male and 3 (9.7%) female. No significant group differences were found between groups in age at the time of assessment or in their respective length of stay in the hospital. Other observations included most individuals in all groups receiving the diagnosis of schizophrenia. Individuals within the ASD group also tended to have a high prevalence of neurological conditions such as epilepsy. In terms of offending, murder, manslaughter and violence were common in all groups, but sexual offending was low in the ASD group. Although most research on the prevalence of ASD within secure psychiatric environments has focused on men, one study of an English HSPC hospital found using another two stage assessment process (including an initial screen of the entire female population followed by a standard diagnostic interview, review of case notes and completing a basic social inference task—Dewey's stories) that around 6 (11%) of the total females detained (51) met ICD 10 criteria for an ASD. Five individuals (approximately 10%) were also rated as being 'uncertain', i.e. who displayed some, but not all features consistent with an ASD (Crocombe et al., 2006). In another prevalence study, Myers (2004), carried out a 'scoping exercise' in which 57 forensic and specialist settings, including four prisons, two secure accommodation units and the Carstairs high secure psychiatric hospital in Scotland were asked to provide information about the unit and how many individuals had been formally diagnosed with an ASD. It was found that whilst the prevalence of ASD appeared low (around 0.93% in prisons, 0.46% in secure units and 1.39% in mental health units), the true figure was unknown, with many prison staff raising concerns that the number of individuals formally identified probably fell short of the actual number.

In summary, whilst most studies to date suggest there is likely to be an over-representation of individuals with an ASD in forensic settings, various methodological issues such as being based on single samples, differences in the diagnostic methods used, completing research with shifting forensic populations, as well as ethical issues such as obtaining consent limit how much the results from many studies can be generalised more widely. Although a qualitative impression of the author working within HSPC, it also appears that the overall percentage of patients with an ASD may actually have slightly increased with around 4% of patients (out of a total of 198 patient) being identified as having an ASD in a recent study of patient incompatibilities and seclusions (Murphy et al., 2017). Clinical experience also suggests that there are several individuals who present with 'equivocal' features of ASD. If these individuals are included within studies the overall prevalence estimate of ASD in many secure environments will be significantly higher. Several individuals are seen by the author also present with many features consistent with an ASD (such as poor appreciation of other perspectives, need for routines and predictability, sensory sensitivity, emotional regulation difficulties) and likely comorbid psychosis, but who refuse to engage with formal assessments, as well as declining consent to speak with any family members to obtain a developmental history. Indeed, such individuals can be extremely difficult to interview and engage with, as well as often presenting with considerable mistrust of all 'authority' figures (Murphy, 2019). Whilst there is very little information regarding the socio-economic status or ethnicity of offenders with an ASD detained within forensic settings, clinical experience suggests that admissions to HSPC with an ASD come from all ethnic groups and socio-economic backgrounds. However, in terms of the latter, many individuals with ASD from lower socio-economic backgrounds appear to receive a diagnosis of ASD in adulthood rather than childhood and often following their involvement with the CJS.

How Individuals with an ASD Differ from Other Groups Detained in Forensic Settings?

Consistent with much of the prevalence research, most of the research to date that has examined how individuals with an ASD might differ from other groups detained in forensic settings has been completed in UK forensic psychiatric services. For example, the author found in a comparison study of individuals with an ASD, those with schizophrenia and those with a personality disorder detained in a HSPC hospital and broadly matched on age that those patients with an ASD were less likely to have a significant history of alcohol and illicit substance misuse. There was also a rough split within the ASD group of patients between those admitted under the personality disorder and the mental illness classifications of the Mental Health Act (1983)—an act of the UK parliament designed to give approved health professional the powers in certain circumstances to detain, assess and treat people with mental disorders in the interests of their health and safety or for public safety. Using a Violence Rating Scale—VRS (Gunn & Robertson, 1976), compared to patients with a personality disorder and a mental illness, patients with an ASD also had lower violence ratings for their index offence (the offence leading to their admission to the hospital) and lower total violence rating (the sum of the violence ratings for an individual's index offence and offending histories), i.e. were likely to have offences that were rated as having 'minimal' (mostly verbal aggression) or 'moderate' violence (was a physical assault that did not result in serious injury). Qualitatively, it was also noted that the offences of many individuals with an ASD were also unusual in both circumstances and actions. For example, one individual had an index offence related to sending a homemade explosive device to a probation officer after taking offence at being described as a possible sex offender, whilst another was related to taking hostage a health visitor following concerns with their physical health (Murphy, 2003). In terms of basic neuropsychological functioning, it was found that whilst individuals with an ASD had similar general levels of intellectual functioning (Wechsler Adult Intelligence Scale full-scale IQ) compared to those individuals with a personality disorder, both groups had significantly higher general levels of intellectual functioning than individuals with a schizophrenia (Murphy, 2003). In another study of examining social cognition within these groups, it has been found that individuals with an ASD and those with a schizophrenia performed at a similar level, but worse than those with a personality disorder in the revised eyes task (Baron-Cohen et al., 2001), i.e. made a similar amount of errors in correctly matching a mental state word to a photographic image of a pair of eyes, despite having significantly higher general levels of intellectual functioning (Murphy, 2006).

Although no comparison groups were included in the research, in another study of individuals with an ASD detained in HSPC, it has been found that no individuals were rated to have significant features of psychopathy as defined using the Hare Psychopathy Checklist-Revised—PCL-R (Hare, 2003). In this study, the Hare PCL-R profiles of 13 individuals with an ASD were examined and it was found that whilst there was some variation in the specific profiles between individuals, no individuals had PCL-R total scores above the suggested North American or British cut-off figures for psychopathy (35 and 25, respectively). However, of interest was the finding that in comparison to other patients in the hospital ($n = 112$, unpublished data), whilst the mean PCL-R total score for individuals with an ASD was similar to other non-ASD patients (15 vs. 15.8), the factor 1 mean total was higher (7.9 vs. 6.8), specifically for facet 2 (affective components). In contrast, the mean total score for factor 2 was lower (7 vs. 9.1), specifically facet 1 (interpersonal features such as glibness and superficial charm, grandiose sense of self-worth, pathological lying, conning and manipulative behaviours). Additional analyses also failed to find any significant relationship between an individual's PCL-R rating and their performance within the revised eyes task, the modified advanced theory of mind task (a social cognitive theory of mind test in which a story is read to an individual and they are asked to infer the meaning behind a story character's intentions and behaviours), as well as a number of other offence details including age at first conviction, age at index offence and the number of formal convictions (Murphy, 2007). Although a small study of a highly select group of individuals, this study appears to be consistent with other research in suggesting that psychopathy and ASD are not necessarily associated, but can sometimes be present for a minority (e.g. Rogers et al., 2006) and that where it is present individuals may represent a specific subgroup of offenders with an ASD (e.g. Alexander et al., 2016). In terms of clinical experience, those individuals with an ASD who present with features of psychopathy are a difficult group to assess and engage with any therapeutic interventions. Whilst the relationship is a complex one, 'extreme' empathy deficits and egocentricity, as well as repeat offending (typically interpersonal violence) and deliberate inconsistent answers to questions during interviews, in the context of relatively good reciprocal verbal communication abilities appears to be a characteristic.

Some characteristic features with emotional regulation have also been identified among HSPC patients with an ASD. In a study examining the self-reported experience and expression of anger has found a characteristic profile. In an examination of the State-Trait Anger Expression Inventory 2—STAXI 2 (Speilberger, 1999) profiles of male patients with an ASD it was found that individuals with offending behaviours linked to preoccupations (notably another individual) in comparison to those individuals whose offending was not directly linked to a preoccupation tended to have profiles suggesting high rates of 'suppressed anger' (i.e. significantly lower scores within the 'anger expression out' scale), as well as higher scores in the 'attention to detail' subscale of the Autism Spectrum Quotient questionnaire—AQ (Baron-Cohen et al., 2001). In contrast, those individuals with an ASD and whose offending behaviour was not linked to any direct preoccupation (such as interpersonal assaults) tended to have more complex psychiatric presentations, including active symptoms of a psychosis (Murphy, 2014). This finding appears to be consistent with a more recent suggestion that individuals with an ASD and a comorbid psychotic disorder may be more vulnerable to acting on active symptoms such as auditory hallucinations (Wachtel & Shorter, 2013).

In terms of the everyday management issues, a study of patient incompatibilities (i.e. where individuals may have had some form of interpersonal conflicts such as physical altercation or verbal threats resulting in the need for them to be separated) and seclusions found that individuals with an ASD in one HSPC hospital appear to have a disproportionately higher number of both compared to patients without an ASD. Examining the hospital data during a one-year time period found that for individuals with an ASD, 87.5% had at least one formal incompatibility with another patient compared to 50.5% of individuals without an ASD. Further examination of the proportion of ASD patients in the hospital (4.04%) and patients with an ASD on the incompatibilities list (6.80%) found a statistically significant difference. Examining the total incompatibility list found that of the 103 individuals listed, 20 (16.7%) involved at least one patient with an ASD, with the average number of incompatibilities listed for ASD patients being 2.8 versus 1 for patients without an ASD. In terms of seclusions, it was found that individuals with an ASD experienced both a higher number of long-term seclusions—LTS (a specific HSPC care option used within the context of the Mental Health Act (1983) implemented by respective clinical teams on wards when an individual's immediate interpersonal risks are deemed too high to be managed safely in ordinary location with others on a ward) and more hours spent in LTS compared to individuals without an ASD. In addition, of the six individuals with an ASD secluded, all had experienced more than two seclusions, putting them in the top 75% of secluded patients. Three of these individuals also experienced more than ten seclusions putting them in the top 25% of secluded patients in the hospital (Murphy et al., 2017). Clearly managing such complex individuals presents with significant challenges for nursing staff and clinical teams. However, they raise questions about whether a different approach to their care is required which includes a more detailed analysis of environmental, interpersonal and internal triggers for violence, as well as the development of alternative coping strategies for dealing with emotional dysregulation.

Further evidence of individuals with an ASD differing from other patient groups comes from an examination of individuals with an ASD detained in a UK low secure psychiatric care unit. Haw et al. (2013) examined the characteristics of patients with an ASD ($n = 45$) compared to other patients without an ASD ($n = 43$). In terms of basic demographic characteristics, Haw et al. found that on average the patients with an ASD were significantly younger at admission (27 years versus 33 years old) and significantly younger at the first contact with psychiatric services. Although most patients with an ASD tended to be admitted from other hospitals, some had been directly referred from prison and the courts. With regard to psychiatric comorbidity, whilst 27% of the patients with an ASD were considered to only have this diagnosis, psychosis was the most common psychiatric comorbidity and some form of intellectual disability. Within the ASD group, a comorbid personality disorder was found to be less likely. In terms of other personal characteristics, patients with an ASD were also less likely to have a significant history of alcohol and illicit substance misuse, with around 38% having a lifetime history of alcohol misuse compared to 56% of individuals without an ASD. Individuals with an ASD were also less likely to be under the influence of illicit substances at the time of their index offence (the offence leading to an individual's conviction prior to their detention). A lifetime history of physical violence to others was found to be 78% in those with ASD compared to

93% in those without an ASD. Self-injurious behaviour was found to be 38% in the ASD group compared to 56% in the non-ASD group. Consistent with the Murphy (2003) study, qualitative impressions of the index offence details of the ASD group suggested unusual circumstances and actions such as one individual sending razors blades in a letter to an organisation after being rejected for a job or another being said to have set light to his own clothes in response to being moved to a residential home that he did not want to live in. In another UK study of a low secure forensic intellectual disability unit forty two patients with an ASD in comparison to patients without an ASD, were found to have lower rates of both personality disorder and a history of illicit substance misuse. Patients with an ASD were also found to be less likely to be subject to criminal sections or restrictions orders of the UK Mental Health Act (1983). However, patients with an ASD did have significantly higher rates of self-harm. No differences were found in the length of stay or direction of care pathways (Esan et al., 2015).

In summary, the small number of studies that have been completed to date all suggest that individuals with an ASD differ from other individuals without an ASD in a number of cognitive, emotional regulation and clinical characteristics. Perhaps reflecting some of the difficulties associated with completing research in prison environments, most studies to date have also been completed with males detained in forensic psychiatric settings. In terms of any differences in presenting features and difficulties between low, medium and high secure ASD populations, to date there has not been any direct comparison research. However, from a HSPC perspective it is typical for individuals with an ASD to have histories of being detained in medium secure care and lower levels of security. As such, any specific differences are more likely to be present in terms of judgements regarding the individual's immediate risk to others (and the factors driving this such as a comorbid psychosis or deviant preoccupation, as well as protective factors) rather than any specific features linked to an ASD as such.

Views of Individuals with ASD Held by Staff Working in Secure Forensic Settings

Although there is a small body of research from which to draw any definitive conclusions, available studies suggest that most staff who work within non-specialist forensic settings feel unskilled to work with individuals who have an ASD and express the view that such individuals present with needs and difficulties that are not always addressed. For example, Myers (2004) examination of staff perceptions and experiences of individuals with an ASD within a range of forensic and non-forensic settings in Scotland suggested that many individuals with a learning disability and or an ASD were viewed as 'multiply disadvantaged'. Within prison settings Myers found that individuals with an ASD were considered by staff to be at risk of being exploited, bullied and ostracised by other prisoners. Prison staff were also said to express the view that prisons were poorly equipped to meet the needs of individuals with an ASD. In another study of a large English prison, McAdam (2009) found that only 35 (66%) of the 53 members of prison staff who completed a survey reported being aware of what ASDs were and around a half the sample specifically what Asperger's syndrome was. In addition, only a very small percentage of staff were said to be aware of the diversity in clinical presentations found between individuals and around 40% of staff reported being unaware of any of the individuals they worked with had an ASD. In terms of likelihood to re-offend, half of the staff group expressed the view that individuals with an ASD were unlikely to re-offend, whilst a small number thought individuals with an ASD were at increased risk for re-offending. Of interest was the finding that 80% of staff thought prisoners with an ASD experienced more stress compared to others. Other findings included 35% of staff endorsing the view that the prison hospital was the most appropriate location for such individuals and 6% that the segregation wing was the most appropriate location. Over a third of staff also endorsed the view that hospital admission was a more appropriate location.

Within UK HSPC settings two staff surveys into ASD have been completed. In an audit of one hundred nursing staff assessing their knowledge of autism and best practice, Misra et al. (2013), found that whilst most nursing staff reported being aware of what ASD was, the majority were also unfamiliar with best practice guidelines (such as the Autism Act, 2009) and expressed the view that they were unsure of how best to work with someone who had an ASD. In a more comprehensive staff survey, Murphy and McMorrow (2015), using a 15 item questionnaire, explored the views and experiences of two hundred and six hospital staff who had direct patient contact during their everyday working lives including psychologists, psychiatrists, nursing staff, occupational therapists and other clinical staff such as the hospital general practitioner, dentist and optician. Most staff reported knowing someone with an ASD outside of their work environment and most also reported working directly with a patient who they knew to have an ASD. In terms of everyday management, just over half the staff group reported making some form of adjustment to their clinical practice, interactions and the expectations of individuals with an ASD. A similar figure also expressed the view that individuals with an ASD would benefit from being managed in a different way compared to other patients in the hospital. Only a small percentage of the staff group (22.3%) thought that the difficulties of patients with an ASD were considered in their care and most (64%) thought that such patients were more vulnerable to bullying or intimidation than other patients. Most staff thought patients with an ASD definitely or mostly benefitted from the therapies on offer within the hospital. Other key findings from the survey included only a small number of staff (27%) believing they had adequate skills and knowledge to work with individuals with an ASD, with most staff expressing the wish for more training on ASD (92%) and that such training should be mandatory (76%). In terms of qualitative comments, some members of staff expressed the view that a specialist ASD service would be useful within the hospital.

What Are the Experiences of Individuals with an ASD Within Secure Settings?

Supporting some anecdotal accounts of prison (e.g. Attwood, 2018), two reviews to date by Allely (2015) and Robertson and McGillivray (2015) both explore the experience of prison environments by individuals with an ASD. Among the studies quoted include Myers (2004) examination of staff perceptions and experiences of individuals with an ASD within a range of forensic and non-forensic units in Scotland that found individuals with an ASD reported situations involving being exploited, bullied and ostracised by other prisoners. Other available studies include Patterson's (2007) detailed description of two men with an ASD detained within UK prisons. Using a combination of observation and interviews carried out over a four-month period Patterson found that whilst the offending, background circumstances and presenting difficulties of these two men differed, both reported significant difficulties linked to three key issues including behaviour in prison, adherence to prison regimes, relationships and empathy. Both individuals were said to have experienced difficulties with various aspects of prison life that could be directly attributed to their socio-communicative problems and behavioural rigidity associated with having an ASD. Consistent with these experiences are earlier accounts such as by Gordon (2002) who describes his personal account of a 25-year sentence in the UK prison system following the conviction for murder. After being initially misdiagnosed with schizophrenia and an antisocial personality disorder before receiving the diagnosis of Asperger's syndrome (said to have been a positive aspect of his prison experience), Gordon described experiencing significant interpersonal difficulties with prison staff and other inmates. Among the difficulties described by Gordon was being perceived by staff as unemotional and anti-social. Gordon also described the experience that in order to fit in with other inmates he would often attempt to copy their behaviour despite not knowing the meaning behind many actions and which in turn often led to interpersonal conflicts. In contrast, other studies such as that by Allen et al. (2008) following interviews with individuals with an ASD who had the experience of being detained in a range of secure facilities found that in general they did not perceive themselves as being more disadvantaged than individuals without an ASD within prisons and that they may actually have benefited from the structured and routine nature such settings provide, as well as opportunities for minimal social interference. However, among the negative experiences of prison life reported by individuals included limited staff awareness of what ASD was, missing family, difficulties with making friends in the prison, problems with sharing cells with others and difficulties interacting with prison staff.

Outside of the UK, among the limited number of studies available that has explored the experiences of individuals with an ASD in forensic settings is a study by Helverschou et al. (2017) of nine individuals with an ASD within the Norwegian CJS (including 8 men and 1 woman). Although negative experiences of the early stages within the CJS were described by most, those that went onto be imprisoned reported a generally good level of custodial care linked with the high levels of structure and routines in such settings, as well as opportunities for education and occupational activities. Relationships with other prisoners, however, were described as being some source of stress. Another useful study completed within the US prison system by Morris (2009) completed qualitative interviews with five inmates with an ASD (four male and one female, all Caucasian) within the Oregon Department of Corrections. Interviews were described as focusing on daily living, difficulties experienced in prison, the perceived benefits of prison and suggestions for positive institutional change. Among the positive aspects of prison life identified by individuals included low financial stress in comparison to the community, high structure and consistency of routines (with the exception of when there was a delay or cancellation in an activity), opportunities to reflect on life, feeling safe within some secure units, as well as improved opportunities for medical input such as receiving prescribed medications. In terms of the negative aspects to prison life, some individuals identified relationship problems with other inmates and staff as a source of stress, whether that was coping with the relational aggression between other inmates, difficulties with being able to understand interpersonal situations such as gossip (identified by the female prisoner) and with being able to read body language. Being unable to pursue personal interests was also described as problematic. More counselling opportunities were identified as a recommendation by several individuals.

In terms of the experiences of individuals with an ASD within forensic psychiatric settings, there are also a limited number of available studies from which to draw any clear conclusions. However, my impression of individuals with an ASD within a range of forensic psychiatric settings (including secure ASD units and secure generic non-specialist ASD settings) is that experiences vary. In a study by the author in which seven individuals with an ASD were interviewed about their experience of being detained in HSPC (Murphy & Mullens, 2017) it was found that although the group was small in number there was a diverse range of backgrounds, offending behaviours, experiences, as well as relative vulnerabilities and objective measures of functioning (including participation in occupational and therapeutic activities, number of problem incidents and views from staff). Although some individuals certainly expressed negative views and experiences of their care, as well as feeling that their difficulties were not always understood by others, these individuals were very much in the minority. Indeed, whilst most individuals described having negative experiences in custodial environments such as prisons (with the noise, lack of privacy and fear of bullying being identified as being particularly problematic), they were more positive about the forensic psychiatric system. Consistent themes reported by individuals included valuing the structure, predictability and routine of a hospital environment, as well as feeling safe and being cared for by highly trained and sympathetic staff. Many individuals also described benefitting from the therapies they had participated in such as dialectical behaviour therapy, mindfulness and different psychoeducation programmes, as well as being actively involved in a range of occupational and educational activities. Most individuals also confirmed that their ASD had not been diagnosed until admission to HSPC. Of interest were the views of two patients transferred to HSPC from a specialist ASD medium secure unit and who both reported negative views of their care there and experiences with other

ASD patients. Although it is not possible to generalise these individuals, they do highlight the possibility that even within specialist ASD units there can be negative experiences. Although the reasons for such different experiences need to be explored, impressions suggest some of those who do report negative experiences present with complex psychopathology including comorbid mental illness and probable personality disorder. This in turn may have implications on how staff view and manage such individuals, as well as an individual's relative insight and presence of any other factors that may influence experiences such as paranoid ideation. Some objective measures of hospital experience such as participation in activities, as well as any time spent in seclusion appear unrelated to the views held.

As highlighted by the reviews of Allely and Robertson and McGillivray, there is a need for more detailed research in this area and much to be learnt with regard to promoting positive individual experiences. However, it is also important to consider the diversity present within this group of individuals including the varied backgrounds of individuals, their profiles of cognitive strengths and the presence of possible comorbid conditions (whether psychiatric and other neurodevelopmental disorders), which in turn is likely to influence the relative experience of secure care. It is also significant to note that whilst a hospital environment appears to be preferred over a custodial environment, many individuals report that they like the structure and relative isolation of the latter, notably that there is rarely any pressure to engage with psychological interventions.

Interventions Available Within Forensic Settings

Within the UK over recent years, regardless of whether the forensic setting is a specialist ASD unit, generic forensic psychiatric settings or prisons, the management of individuals with an ASD has been significantly influenced by growing professional awareness and various pieces of government legislation. For example, the Autism Act (2009), followed by other pieces of legislation including Think Autism Strategy (2014), the Adult Autism Strategy: Statutory Guidance (2015) and Transforming Care (2017) have placed ASD on the agenda of most institutions and established a duty to provide appropriate ASD diagnostic assessments and staff training. Although not specifically targeted just at the needs of individuals with an ASD, the Equalities Act (2010) within the UK has also had some impact in ensuring 'reasonable adjustments' are made to make environments, procedures and opportunities more 'autism friendly'.

In an attempt to comply with these pieces of legislation, the author provides both general autism awareness training to staff within one HSPC hospital and bespoke ward-based training. During training in addition to providing information on what ASD is and how it might present, the SPELL guidelines are promoted, placing emphasis on a Structured approach, a Positive approach, Empathy, Low arousal and Links with other professionals (National Autistic Society, 2013). The aim of the SPELL approach is to encourage staff to work with an individual's strengths and to reduce the likelihood of problem behaviours by making the immediate environment and any interactions more autism-friendly. Although the impact of such training on the management of patients with an ASD remains to be established, as illustrated by a staff survey in HSPC (Murphy & McMorrow, 2015), there is the general view that training is valued and that it should be mandatory (Murphy & Broyd, 2019). These findings are particularly interesting in the context of the proposal by the UK government, where all relevant NHS staff have been suggested should receive some form of compulsory ASD awareness training (Department of Health, 2019).

In terms of prison settings, personal experience of assessing individuals with an ASD suggests that whilst there has been an increased awareness of ASD among many staff, as well as several prisons obtaining accreditation by the National Autistic Society (e.g. Lewis et al., 2013), there remains considerable uncertainty with regard to how best to therapeutically address an individual's needs, as well as individuals themselves reporting limited opportunities to engage with rehabilitation programmes (Robertson & McGillivray, 2015). At the time of writing there are no accredited group programmes available just for individuals with an ASD detained in forensic settings. Whilst some adapted versions of the Sex Offender Treatment Programmes designed for individuals with intellectual difficulties have been developed, outcomes for individuals with an ASD in these groups do not appear promising where they often function at a much higher level compared to others and present with different needs (Haaven, 2006). Indeed, some research also suggests that men with an ASD who have completed such groups may actually have higher recidivism rates (Heaton & Murphy, 2013). Participation in mainstream offender groups within prison settings may also be problematic, where individuals with an ASD may experience sensory overload and exclusion (Higgs & Carter, 2015). However, within forensic psychiatric settings, it remains debatable as to whether it is harmful to include individuals with an ASD in mainstream groups. There is an argument that individuals with an ASD benefit from participating in mixed groups by hearing different points of view and listening to other individuals' experiences. The qualitative reports by some individuals with an ASD seen by the author suggest that some mixed membership groups are useful, notably dialectical behaviour therapy that aims to promote positive coping and change unhelpful behaviours through recognising the cognitive and emotional triggers that increase stress. Key factors influencing outcomes with such groups appear to be facilitator awareness of the difficulties associated with having an ASD and sensitivity to make some adjustments, as well as other group members also being sensitive to such difficulties.

Evidence for individual psychological work addressing the offending behaviours of individuals who have an ASD also remains at an early stage of evaluation. Whilst cognitive behaviour therapy (CBT), as well as other psychological approaches, such as mindfulness that are adapted for any cognitive and communication difficulties, have been found to be useful interventions for adults who have an ASD in non-forensic contexts (e.g. Gaus, 2007; Hare, 2013; Spain et al., 2016), there has been limited exploration of how psychological therapies can address offence-specific behaviours in ASD (Melvin et al., 2017). Personal experience with several individuals has found that if a CBT approach is used to address risk or criminological issues among offenders with an ASD (such as improving victim empathy and an appreciation of consequences), there is a need to identify clear realistic goals and make specific further adaptations allowing for the presence of any cognitive, communication, sensory and emotional regulation difficulties, as well as any comorbid psychiatric disorder (Murphy, 2010). For many individuals a 'personalised' education plan about ASD can also be helpful as a way of improving their understanding of past and current difficulties. For example, one individual described being able to 'outthink' his ASD as a result of being aware of what his difficulties had been in the past. However, whilst many individuals with an ASD do respond to individual psychological interventions (such as developing general problem-solving skills, working on basic social inference skills, encouraging appropriate assertiveness, reducing individual social anxieties, shifting preoccupations and obsessive thoughts, negative ruminations, as well as developing perspective taking skills), it may be unrealistic to expect significant changes in cognitive style compared to other offenders who do not have an ASD. Engagement with those individuals who present with significant egocentricity, who take limited personal responsibility and reject their diagnosis can be particularly problematic. For example, Hare (2013) has suggested that a primary goal in CBT with ASD should be not to focus on cognitive changes, but more to concentrate on behavioural changes that increase an individual's ability to function in everyday life, whilst being aware of difficulties in challenging dysfunctional cognitions and beliefs that may be present. As with many individuals with an ASD, some specific therapeutic adaptations may also be required with the pace of therapy, providing individuals with sufficient time to process information and with what some therapists have described as a need to work on 'Asperger's time' (Jacobsen, 2003). Such adaptations with time to process information may be particularly prominent in forensic settings where comorbid psychosis may also be an issue. For many individuals with an ASD in forensic settings there is also a role for pharmacological interventions that can assist with anxiety and comorbid neurodevelopmental or psychiatric disorder. Other activities including occupational therapy and further education can also have a very positive impact on social inclusion, self-esteem, as well as opportunities to learn new skills.

As with all forensic cases, risk formulation and subsequent management are probably the most important aspect of care. For individuals with an ASD who offend there is growing recognition that many conventional risk assessment tools do not capture the difficulties associated with having an ASD (such as preoccupations, sensory sensitivities, emotional regulation problems, as well as perspective taking difficulties, etc.) that can be related to offending or help identify factors which may protect against re-offending. There remains a need for good practice guidelines or frameworks that clinicians can refer to when assessing and formulating, as well as managing risk for future re-offending within this group (Murphy, 2013; Shine & Cooper-Evans, 2016). The use of virtual reality technology with offenders who have an ASD detained in secure settings also offers significant potential, with the ability to simulate specific environments and high degree of experimental control (Benbouriche et al., 2014). Indeed, the cost–benefits of using such technology are high where it may be possible to familiarise an individual with new environments and change but without the resource costs associated with such visits.

Beyond detention, there also remains a lack of research examining what difficulties individuals with an ASD experience during the transition back to the community from prison. Leaving custodial settings back to the community can be difficult for many individuals, but it may be particularly difficult for individuals with an ASD who can experience particular issues dealing with change and the reduced structure (Royal College of Psychiatrists, 2006). Within the UK, where prison to community services are available it has been found that accessing these for many individuals with an ASD can be confusing and that success depends on a coordinated multi-agency approach including health, social care and justice (Prison Reform Trust, 2018). Perhaps because of the relatively low numbers, there is relatively little in the literature devoted to addressing the specific needs of women with an ASD within secure settings (Markham, 2019).

Summary and Future Developments

The assessment and management of individuals with an ASD detained within forensic settings will continue to evolve. Current evidence suggests that whilst individuals with an ASD may not necessarily be more likely to be referred to forensic services in comparison to individuals without an ASD, there is an accumulating body of evidence suggesting that individuals with an ASD detained in forensic settings are disproportionately represented relative to the general population estimate for ASD. It is also possible that the actual prevalence figure for ASD in forensic settings is higher, especially when individuals with atypical presentations are included as are those who are difficult to engage with assessments. Research to date also suggests that individuals with an ASD present with a range of different clinical presentations, risk profiles and needs in comparison to other patient groups. Some research within secure psychiatric settings including staff surveys and individual experiences, as well as specific care management issues such as incompatibilities with others and rates of seclusions, also suggests that individuals with an ASD present with specific issues that challenge mainstream services. In terms of psychological interventions, whilst clinical experience and patient self-reports suggest that individuals with an ASD held in HSPC do benefit from participation in some psychological interventions (e.g. Murphy & Mullens, 2017), there is a lack of research examining what interventions are useful in addressing the forensic and clinical difficulties of individuals with an ASD detained in custodial and secure hospital settings, as well as what factors are associated with positive outcomes (including how outcome is measured). Among the limited research devoted to this topic, are the difficulties experienced by staff attempting to engage individuals with an ASD in conventional offence focused interventions, noticeably those addressing the risk, needs and responsivity addressing deviant sexual behaviours (Higgs & Carter, 2015; MacDonald et al., 2017).

It is also significant to note that whilst the research completed to date has been helpful in identifying the specific difficulties and needs of individuals with an ASD in forensic settings, it is not without limitations (Allely, 2018; Robertson & McGillivray, 2015; Murphy, 2020). With many studies based on single samples and settings, there remains a need for large multi-site, collaborative studies that bring together different populations and services (Woodbury Smith & Dein, 2014). Among the many areas of research that remain to be adequately explored, two key topics are a high priority. The first is associated with obtaining an accurate estimate of how many individuals with an ASD are present in different forensic environments, including the factors that may have influenced the professional decision-making to direct an individual to one setting rather than another. With many studies relying on self-report screening questionnaires as means of identifying an ASD, this automatically excludes a large number of individuals who lack sufficient literacy skills to complete questionnaires, who refuse to cooperate with such assessments, as well as not being either honest in their responses or who lack sufficient self-awareness to complete a questionnaire meaningfully. In order to include these individuals there remains a need for a simple to use and sensitive ASD screening measure that can be used by different staff groups, applied across a range of forensic settings and not restricted to self-report questionnaires, i.e. based on observable behaviours (including those related to cognition, emotional regulation, need for predictability, preoccupations and sensory sensitivities). However, it is also significant to highlight that no screen substitutes a detailed diagnostic assessment including an individual's developmental history and current presentation, as well as ideally their performance in a range of social and non-social cognitive tasks. There is also the question of whether women with an ASD require a different assessment process (Bargiela et al., 2016). By obtaining a more inclusive estimate of the ASD population in forensic settings it will be helpful in guiding the development or commissioning of specialist services and interventions, as well as developing better links between custodial, mental health and neurodevelopmental/intellectual disability services. As was highlighted by Wing (1997) the appropriate management of individuals with an ASD within forensic environments is dependent on obtaining an accurate diagnosis and awareness of the associated difficulties.

The second area of research requiring considerably more attention is that devoted to understanding the diversity of presentations found among individuals with an ASD in forensic settings. Whilst most professionals are aware that the clinical presentations and profiles of relative strengths and weaknesses of cognitive abilities, among individuals with ASD can vary significantly despite sharing the same diagnosis, our understanding of how these different presentations influence engagement and subsequent outcome with interventions remains poor. A similar issue also remains with understanding how the diversity of presentations impact on any formulation and management of risk for re-offending. Although typologies of ASD offenders has been suggested based on the presence or absence of psychosis and psychopathy (e.g. Alexander et al., 2016), these alone can potentially oversimplify presentations and fail to include sufficient assessment of the complexity of underlying strengths and difficulties individuals can present with (notably within different aspects of social and non-social cognition, emotional regulation, sensory sensitivities). There may also be a need to recognise and address the difficulties associated with the presence of comorbidities such as attention deficit hyperactivity disorder and conduct disorder that have been linked with violent crime in ASD (Heeramun et al., 2017).

In addition, there is a need to understand how these different presentations seen among individuals with an ASD appear to respond differently to psychological interventions. Clinical experience suggests that some individuals with an ASD engage very well with psychotherapeutic interventions addressing a range of issues that are sensitive to their ASD whether in a one to one situation or group-based. In contrast, other individuals perhaps those with significant social cognition difficulties and extreme literal thinking, do not appear to benefit from 'insight orientated' psychological or occupational interventions (Murphy, 2010). For these individuals, behaviour and risk management seem best addressed by staff following the SPELL guidelines that aim to work with individual strengths, as well as reducing inconsistencies in how individuals are managed and promote social inclusion. By having a better understanding of the factors that contribute to the diversity of individual ASD presentations will also help inform risk management procedures and how best to monitor outcomes.

Finally, the most economically and clinically effective method of addressing the needs of individuals with an ASD in forensic settings remains in promoting an awareness of ASD among all professionals involved with their care. Although there is no specific research evidence examining how staff training can improve the outcomes of individuals with an ASD in forensic settings, prison and secure psychiatric care staff surveys consistently find most staff feel under skilled with regard to how they work with individuals who have an ASD and that training is valued. Whilst staff surveys may also be biased in only including those who value research, they nevertheless suggest staff training and skills are key factors in the management of individuals with an ASD. There is also the possibility that having staff with particular ASD sensitive qualities (including ASD knowledge and empathy) is particularly beneficial (Worthington, 2016). In terms of promoting positive outcomes for individuals with an ASD who offend and are detained within forensic settings, it also remains to be established whether secure specialist ASD services have better 'outcomes' for individuals than more generic secure units that aim to be ASD sensitive. As has been suggested by a study examining patient experiences in HSPC, some individuals with an ASD report a preference to be around mixed patient groups rather than just those with an ASD (Murphy & Mullens, 2017). With some UK prisons achieving accreditation with the National Autistic Society by becoming more ASD sensitive (Lewis et al., 2013) and other secure psychiatric settings set to follow, it may the case that non-specialist settings with staff who have a good awareness of ASD, make reasonable environmental or procedural adjustments that are sensitive to the difficulties associated with having an ASD, can have as good and if not better positive outcomes for many individuals.

References

Adult Autism Strategy. (2015). Available at www.gov.uk/government/publications/adult-autism-strategy-guidance.

Alexander, R., Langdon, P., Chester, V., Barnoux, M., Gunaratna, I., & Hoare, S. (2016). Heterogeneity within autism spectrum disorder in forensic mental health: The introduction of typologies. *Advances in Autism, 2*(4), 201–209.

Allely, C. (2015). Experiences of prison inmates with autism spectrum disorders and the knowledge and understanding of the spectrum amongst prison staff: A review. *Journal of Intellectual Disabilities and Offending Behaviour, 6*(2), 55–67.

Allely, C. (2018). A systematic PRISMA review of individuals with autism spectrum disorder in secure psychiatric care: Prevalence, treatment, risk assessment and other clinical considerations. *Journal of Criminal Psychology, 8*(1), 58 and 79.

Allen, D., Evans, C., Hider, A., Hawkins, S., Peckett, H., & Morgan, H. (2008). Offending behaviour in adults with Asperger's syndrome. *Journal of Autism and Developmental Disorders, 38,* 784–758.

Autism Act. (2009). Accessed at www.legislation.gov.uk/ukpga/2009/15/contents.

Attwood, W. (2018). *Asperger's syndrome and jail: A survival guide.* Jessica Kingsley.

Baird, G., Simonoff, E., Pickles, A., Chandler, S., Loucas, T., Meldrum, D., & Charman, T. (2006). Prevalence of disorders of the autism spectrum in a population cohort of children in South Thames: The special needs and autism project (SNAP). *Lancet, 368,* 210–215.

Bargiela, S., Steward, R., & Mandy, W. (2016). The experiences of late diagnosed women with autism spectrum conditions: An investigation of the female phenotype. *Journal of Autism and Developmental Disorders, 46*(10), 3281–3294.

Baron-Cohen, S., Wheelright, S., Skinner, R., Martin, J., & Clubley, E. (2001). The autism spectrum quotient (AQ): Evidence from Asperger syndrome/high functioning autism, males and females, scientists and mathematicians. *Journal of Autism and Developmental Disorders, 31*(1), 5–17.

Benbouriche, M., Nolet, K., Trottier, D., & Renaud, P. (2014, April 9–11). Virtual reality applications in forensic psychiatry. In *Proceedings of the virtual reality international conference.* Laval Virtual (VRIC 14).

Cashin, A., & Newman, C. (2009). Autism in the criminal justice detention system. *Journal of Forensic Nursing, 5,* 70–75.

Crocombe, J., Mills, R., & Wing, L. (2006). *Autism spectrum disorders in the high security hospitals of the United Kingdom.* The National Autistic Society.

Department of Health. (2019). *'Right to be heard' the Government response to the consultation on learning disability and autism training for health and care staff*. Published on 5th November. Available at https://assets.publishing.service.gov.uk/government/uploads/system/uploads/attachment_data/file/844356/autism-and-learning-disability-training-for-staff-consultation-response.pdf.

Equalities Act. (2010). Legislation.gov.uk. (2010). *Equality Act 2010.* Retrieved from https://www.legislation.gov.uk/ukpga/2010/15.

Esan, F., Chester, V., Gunaratna, I., Hoare, S., & Alexander, R. (2015). The clinical, forensic and treatment outcome factors of patients with autism spectrum disorder treated in a forensic intellectual disability service. *Journal of Applied Research in Intellectual Disabilities, 28*(3), 193 and 200.

Fazio, R. L., Pietz, C. A., & Denney, R. L. (2012). An estimate of the prevalence of autism spectrum disorders in an incarcerated population. *Open Access Journal of Forensic Psychology, 4,* 69–80.

Gaus, V. (2007). *Cognitive behavioural therapy for adult Asperger syndrome.* The Guildford Press.

Gómez de la Cuesta, G. (2010). A selective review of offending behaviour in individuals with autism spectrum disorders. *Journal of Learning Disabilities and Offending Behaviour, 1,* 47–58.

Gordon, R. (2002). Asperger syndrome: One prisoner's experience. *Prison Service Journal, 143,* 2–4.

Gunn, J., & Robertson, G. (1976). Drawing a criminal profile. *British Journal of Criminology, Delinquency and Deviant Social Behaviour, 16*(2), 156.
Haaven, J. (2006). Suggested treatment outline using the old me/new me model. In G. Blasingame (Ed.), *Practical treatment strategies for forensic clients with severe and sexual behaviour problems among persons with developmental disabilities.* Wood N. Barnes/Safer Society Press.
Hare, D. (2013). Developing psychotherapeutic interventions with people with autism spectrum disorders. In J. Taylor, W. Lindsay, R. Hastings (Eds.), *Psychological therapies for adults with intellectual disabilities.* Wiley.
Hare, D., Gould, J., Mills, R., & Wing, L. (1999). *A preliminary study of individuals with autistic spectrum disorders in three special hospitals in England.* National Autistic Society. Available at www.aspires-relationships.com/3hospitals.pdf.
Hare, R. (2003). *The psychopathy checklist revised.* Multi Health Systems.
Haw, C., Radley, J., & Cooke, L. (2013). Characteristics of male autistic spectrum patients in low security: Are they different from non-autistic low secure patients? *Journal of Intellectual Disabilities and Offending Behaviours, 4*(1/2), 24–32.
Heaton, K., & Murphy, G. (2013). Men with intellectual disabilities who have attended sex offender treatment groups: A follow up. *Journal of Applied Research in Intellectual Disabilities, 26*(5), 489–500.
Heeramun, R., Magnusson, C., Hellner Gumpert, C., Granath, S., Lundberg, M., Dalman, C., & Rai, D. (2017). Autism and convictions for violent crimes: Population based cohort study in Sweden. *Journal of the American Academy of Child and Adolescent Psychiatry, 56*(6), 491–497.
Helverschou, S. B., Steindal, K., Aage Nottestad, J., & Howlin, P. (2017). Personal experiences of the criminal justice system by individuals with autism spectrum disorders. *Autism, 22*(4), 460–468. https://doi.org/10.1177/1316685554.
Higgs, T., & Carter, A. (2015). Autism spectrum disorder and sexual offending: Responsivity in forensic interventions. *Aggression and Violent Behaviour, 22,* 112–119.
Jacobsen, P. (2003). *Asperger syndrome and psychotherapy.* Kingsley.
Lewis, A., Pritchet, R., Hughes, C., & Turner, K. (2013). Development and implementation of autism standards for prisons. *Journal of Intellectual Disabilities and Offending Behaviour, 6*(2), 68–80.
Lord, C., Rutter, M., DiLavore, P., Risi, S., Gotham K., Bishop, S., Luyster, R., & Guthrie, W. (2012). *Autism diagnostic observation schedule—2.* Pearson.
Lord, C., Rutter, M., & LeCouteur, A. (1994). Autism diagnostic interview revised: A revised version of a diagnostic interview for caregivers of individuals with possible pervasive developmental disorders. *Journal of Autism and Developmental Disorders, 24*(4), 659–685.
MacDonald, S., Clarbour, J., Whitton, C., & Rayner, K. (2017). The challenges of working with sexual offenders who have autism in secure services. *Journal of Intellectual Disabilities and Offending Behaviour, 8*(1), 41–54.
Maenner, M. J., Shaw, K. A., & Baio, J. (2020). Prevalence of autism spectrum disorder among children aged 8 years—Autism and developmental disabilities monitoring network, 11 sites, United States, 2016. *MMWR Surveillance Summaries, 69*(4), 1.
Markham, S. (2019). Diagnosis and treatment of ASD in women in secure and forensic hospitals. *Advances in Autism, 5*(1), 64–76.
McAdam, P. (2009). Knowledge and understanding of the autism spectrum amongst prison staff. *Good Autism Practice (GAP), 10*(1), 19 and 25.
Melvin, C., Langdon, P., & Murphy, G. (2017). Treatment effectiveness for offenders with autism spectrum conditions: A systematic review. *Psychology, Crime & Law, 23*(8), 748–776.
Mental Health Act. (1983). Amended 2007 and 2015. London, HMSO.
Ministry of Justice. (2015, August 7). Prison population figures. *Population Bulletin: Weekly.* Available at www.gov.uk/government/statistics/prison-population-figures-2015.
Misra, P., Patel, M., & Edwards, J. (2013). The need for a specialist service for offenders with autistic spectrum disorder in high secure psychiatric care. *European Psychiatry, 28,* 1.

Morris, A. (2009). *Offenders with Asperger's syndrome: Experiences from within prison* (Doctoral dissertation), Pacific University.

Murphy, D. (2003). Admission and cognitive details of male patients diagnosed with Asperger's syndrome detained in a special hospital: Comparison with a schizophrenia and personality disorder sample. *Journal of Forensic Psychiatry and Psychology, 14*(3), 506–524.

Murphy, D. (2006). Theory of mind in forensic patients with Asperger's syndrome, schizophrenia and a personality disorder. *Cognitive Neuropsychiatry, 11*(2), 99–111.

Murphy, D. (2007). Brief communication: Hare PCL-R profiles of male patients with Asperger's syndrome detained in high security psychiatric care. *Journal of Forensic Psychiatry and Psychology, 18*(1), 120–126.

Murphy, D. (2010). Extreme violence in a young man with an autistic spectrum disorder: Assessment and intervention within high security psychiatric care. *Journal of Forensic Psychiatry and Psychology, 21*(3), 462–477.

Murphy, D. (2013). Risk assessment in Autism spectrum disorders. *Journal of Learning Disabilities and Offending, 4*(1/1), 33–41.

Murphy, D. (2014). Self-reported anger among individuals with an autism spectrum disorder detained in high security psychiatric care. *Journal of Forensic Psychiatry and Psychology, 25*(1), 100–112.

Murphy, D. (2019). Interviewing individuals with an autism spectrum disorder in forensic settings. *International Journal of Forensic Mental Health, 17*(4), 310–320.

Murphy, D. (2020). Autism: Implications for high secure psychiatric care and move towards best practice. *Research in Developmental Disabilities, 100,* 103615. https://doi.org/10.1016/j.ridd.2020.103615.

Murphy, D., & McMorrow, K. (2015). View of autism spectrum conditions held by staff working in a high secure psychiatric hospital. *Journal of Forensic Practice, 17*(3), 231–240.

Murphy, D., & Mullens, H. (2017). Examining the experiences and quality of life of patients with an autism spectrum disorder detained in high secure psychiatric care. *Advances in Autism, 3*(1), 3–14.

Murphy, D., & Broyd, J. (2019). Evaluation of autism awareness training for staff in high secure psychiatric care hospital. *Advances in Autism, 6*(1), 35–47.

Murphy, D., Bush, E. L., & Puzzo, I. (2017). Incompatibilities and seclusions among individuals with an autism spectrum disorder detained in high secure psychiatric care. *Journal of Intellectual Disabilities and Offending Behaviour, 8*(4), 188–200.

Myers, F. (2004). *On the borderline? People with learning disabilities and or autistic spectrum disorders in secure, forensic and other specialist settings.* Scottish Development Centre for Mental Health, Scottish Executive Social Research. The Stationary Office Bookshop. 71 Lothian Rd. Edinburgh, Scotland.

National Autistic Society. (2013). *SPELL.* Available at www.autism.org.uk/spell.

Patterson, P. (2007). How well do young offenders with Asperger's syndrome cope in custody? Two prison case studies. *British Journal of Learning Disabilities, 36,* 54–58.

Prison Reform Trust. (2018). *Behaviour that challenges: Planning services for people with learning disabilities and or autism who sexually offend.* https://www.prisonreformtrust.org.uk/Portals/0/Documents/Behaviour%20that%20challenges.

Robertson, C., & McGillivray, J. (2015). Autism behind bars: A review of the research literature and discussion of key issues. *Journal of Forensic Psychiatry and Psychology, 26*(6), 719–736.

Rogers, J., Viding, E., Blair, J., Frith, U., & Happé, F. (2006). Autism spectrum disorder and psychopathy: Shared cognitive underpinnings or double hit? *Psychological Medicine, 36,* 1789–1798.

Royal College of Psychiatrists. (2006). *Psychiatric services for adolescents and adults with Asperger syndrome and other autistic spectrum disorders.*

Scragg, P., & Shah, A. (1994). Prevalence of Asperger's syndrome in a secure hospital. *British Journal of Psychiatry, 165,* 679–682.

Shine, J., & Cooper-Evans, S. (2016). Developing an autism specific framework for forensic case formulation. *Journal of Intellectual Disabilities and Offending Behaviour, 7*(3), 127 and 139.
Spain, D., O'Neil, L., Harwood, L., & Chaplin, E. (2016). Psychological interventions for adults with ASD: Clinical approaches. *Advances in Autism, 2*(1), 24–30.
Speilberger, C. (1999). *Manual for the state trait anger expression inventory—2*. Psychological Assessment Resources.
Think Autism: Fulfilling and rewarding lives. The strategy for adults with autism in England: An update. (2014). Available at https://Assets.publishing.service.gov.uk/government/uploads/system/uploads/attachment_data/file/299866/Autism_Strategy.pdf.
Transforming Care. Model service specifications supporting implementation of the service model. A resource for commissioners to develop service specifications to support implementation of the national service model for people with a learning disability and or autism who display behaviour that challenges, including those with a mental health condition. (2017). *HNS England*. www.england.hns.uk/wp-content/uploads/2017/model-service-spec-2017.
Underwood, L., McCarthy, J., Chaplin, E., Forrester, A., Mills, R., & Murphy, D. (2016). Autism spectrum disorder among prisoners. *Advances in Autism, 2*(3), 106–117.
Underwood, L., Forrester, A., Chaplin, E., & McCarthy, J. (2013). Prisoners with neurodevelopmental disorders. *Journal of Intellectual Disabilities and Offending Behaviour, 4*(1/2), 17–23.
Wachtel, L., & Shorter, E. (2013). Autism plus psychosis: A 'one-two punch' risk for tragic violence? *Medical Hypotheses, 81*(3), 404–409.
Wing, L. (1997). Asperger's syndrome: Management requires diagnosis. *Journal of Forensic Psychiatry, 2*(8), 253–257.
Wing, L., & Gould, J. (1978). Systematic recording of behaviours and skills of retarded and psychotic children. *Journal of Autism and Childhood Schizophrenia, 8*(1), 79–97.
Woodbury Smith, M., & Dein, K. (2014). Autism spectrum disorder (ASD) and unlawful behaviour: Where do we go from here? *Journal of Autism and Developmental Disorders, 44*(11), 2734–2741.
Worthington, R. (2016). What are the key skills that staff require to support adults on the autism spectrum effectively? British Psychological Society. Division of Forensic Psychology. *Forensic Update: A Compendium of the Main Articles in Issues, 121, 122 and 123,* 61 and 69.

Dr. David Murphy is a consultant forensic and clinical neuropsychologist based at Broadmoor high-secure psychiatric hospital. Clinical and research interests include the neuropathology and neuropsychology of mentally disordered offenders. Dr. Murphy also has extensive experience with the assessment and management of offenders with neurodevelopmental disorders. He has experience of working in a range of secure psychiatric settings and provided evidence in a number of high-profile cases for the courts.

Afterword

Moving Forward: A Translation, Research and Policy Agenda for the Next Decade

Rachel Loftin
Fred R. Volkmar
Alexander Westphal
Marc Woodbury-Smith

In this book, we sought to provide an overview of what is currently known about autism and the law. Drastic improvements in the medical care, education, and rights of autistic people have occurred since the diagnosis was first conceptualized in the 1940s. However, there is a long ways to go, and more research and better policies are required in countless areas. In this summary, we highlight the primary areas of need. First, in the Civil section, ASD is discussed as it affects one throughout the lifespan, and key research and social policy needs are highlighted in each phase. Then in the Unlawful Behavior section, a discussion of risk and ASD highlights the need to further research and proposes aims for future work.

Civil

The Civil section of this handbook provided an overview of the aspects of the law that pertain to the rights, entitlements, and well-being of people with ASD. While issues of tort law sometimes arise, they are not covered in this volume. Instead, space is devoted to legal processes affecting the largest number of people with ASD. Autistic people may require these laws at many points in life and a lifespan perspective is useful when considering what an individual requires at a given time. This long-term perspective is essential whether education, family law, employment law, or other types of civil cases are the focus. Understanding their rights and developing skills to

F. R. Volkmar et al. (eds.), *Handbook of Autism Spectrum Disorder and the Law*,
https://doi.org/10.1007/978-3-030-70913-6

self-advocate (or have someone to advocate on their behalf) are critical for autistic people to gain access to the available protections, accommodations, and services.

Throughout an autistic person's life, advocacy is key to obtaining needed services, accommodations, and support. It is apparent that providing a range of needed services can be cost-effective (see Järbrink & Knapp, 2001; Odom, 2001) and that appropriate services result in important, meaningful gains in all but the rarest cases. For the most part, however, available services and protections have not kept pace with the needs of the autism community (see Anderson et al., 2018; Eskow et al., 2015).

Despite some efforts from government agencies, numerous challenges are reported in the literature, from obstacles faced by immigrant families in Canada to receive services for autistic children (Rivard, 2019) to inequalities in access to diagnosis and treatment services in Australia (Mallitt & Jorm, 2018) to large-scale failure to plan for adults with autism in the United States (Anderson & Butt, 2018). Further, outside of the educational setting, therapies in the United States are funded through private insurance, state-funded insurance programs, and, in a few instances, state-funded centers. This means that the quality of service a family receives is often tied to their ability to pay for a top of the line health insurance policy or to privately fund the service itself.

What is needed? The path toward a meaningful quality of life in adulthood requires advocacy at many levels. In childhood, caregivers advocate in the medical and special education systems in order to obtain services. Navigating these systems can be challenging for parents and guardians, particularly for those who are outside of the dominant culture. Even today, with some advancements in access to care, racial disparities persist. In the United States, a recent national survey found that Black children are significantly less likely than White children to receive early diagnosis of ASD, and Hispanic children are diagnosed later than both Black and White children (Maenner, 2020). In turn, targeted therapies may not initiate until later, potentially causing the child to miss critical access to early intervention. Further, both Black and Hispanic children were more likely to be identified with intellectual disability, which may in part reflect the fact that they receive less access to early intervention (which can help increase scores on IQ tests, as well as adaptive skills). Despite significant progress against disparities in recent years (e.g., prevalence numbers are now equivalent for older White and Black children in the United States), more work is needed to improve access to diagnosis and treatment.

Differences in the identification for and the quality of special education provided can also differ by race, with negative impacts for Black and Hispanic students, even when controlling for income (see Grindhal et al., 2019). Thus, educational advocacy is likely even more crucial for caregivers of non-White students. Education law in the United States guarantees free and appropriate education for all students, but there has long been a debate about what constitutes free and appropriate. With recent supreme court decisions, special education programs in the United States are expected to provide "meaningful" educational benefit (Yell & Bateman, 2017). However, determining what is appropriate and meaningful for a given student is often challenging, and families and schools may be at odds in terms of what is meaningful in the cultural context. Ensuring access to quality, culturally sensitive education is necessary to help students with ASD develop to their fullest potential.

In increasing numbers, people with ASD are attending college and university, both competitive programs and those that were designed for students with special learning needs. Campus programs are beginning to offer specific programs to meet the needs of students with ASD, but such programs are not yet universally available, nor accessible to all students. Once again, advocacy at the college stage is crucial. For many autistic students and their caregivers, the college experience represents more than traditional education. Often, they are seeking not just academic instruction but also further instruction and assistance with social, executive functioning and mental health concerns (Anderson & Butt, 2017), but the specific needs of each student in regards to each of these areas are substantially different. Many young adults with ASD, even those who do quite well academically, leave for college without having had instruction and opportunities to develop independence and may not be able to manage on their own. The pragmatic language deficits of autistic college-age students also appear to play a significant role in adjustment and may require specific treatment and support to address (Trevisan & Birmingham, 2016). Thus, more comprehensive university programs that include adaptive, organizational, and social skills, as well as academics, are often needed to prepare one for adulthood. It will be important, in the coming years, to ensure that all students have access to higher education that can prepare them for adulthood and independence.

To further complicate the college experience, the onset of some psychiatric disorders peaks around college age, which means that the mental health needs of autistic college students may substantially change during their time on campus. Those students who remain at home and do not attend college, go to work or participate in formal adult programming may be hit particularly hard by psychiatric disorders, as they are often exacerbated by social isolation. While research on psychiatric comorbidity in autism is growing, more research is needed. Better information on the relationship between ASD and other psychiatric disorders, including diagnosis and treatment of co-occurring conditions, would improve the quality of life and outcomes for many people on the spectrum who struggle with other psychiatric challenges.

Unsupervised social freedom can be challenging for some individuals whose social skills are not yet well developed, and ASD-specific challenges may lead to behavioral and even disciplinary issues in college. Sexuality education, including a strong focus on teaching how to give and obtain consent, can be helpful in protecting an individual from abuse as well as inadvertently perpetrating a sexual offense. The (lack of) education that many autistic students receive is inadequate and leaves them vulnerable. In adolescence, as well as in college, there is a need for more comprehensive and systematic sexuality education instruction.

At the next major transition, moving into the workplace, new struggles arise. After the substantial hurdle of finding and securing employment, obtaining training and on-the-job supports may also require advocacy, as many workplaces are not equipped to assess for need and implement supports. And, of course, at numerous points of development, the autistic person and/or their caregivers must decide whether to disclose the diagnosis and how much, if any, of the specific areas that are affected are worth discussing. Workplace disclosure appears to promote better inclusion and acceptance (Lindsay et al., 2019) by helping minimize social distancing from the autistic person (O'Connor et al., 2019), as well as helping increase overall ASD awareness and the accommodations the employee receives. However, the threat of stigma and discrimination is real and must be weighed in decision making.

Misperceptions about the costs of hiring people with ASD, as well as underestimates of the potential benefits, prevent many employers from hiring autistic candidates (Solomon, 2020). Education of the general public, including potential employers, is key to improving options for autistic people. Bias can prevent people with ASD from obtaining gainful employment in the first place. In addition to expanding the opportunities for autistic people in the broader job market, opportunities in autism-specific employment can be profitable and enriching sources of competitive employment. Aspiritech, an American-based technology company that provides software testing and quality assurance is one excellent example. They employ 130 people, 115 of whom are "neurodivergent" (Aspiritech, 2019). With this model, they are able to create an environment that is sensitive to social, communication, and sensory differences in their employees. Tapping into the strengths of autistic workers can be a successful business model, as well as an invaluable asset in careers such as scientific research that require skills in many of the domains in which a subset of autistic people excel (Mottron, 2011).

When it comes to supporting older autistic adults, almost nothing is known, and the elderly autistic population remains quite neglected in the research literature (Bennett, 2016; Wright et al., 2019), with only a handful of articles available. This means that clinicians are operating with very little guidance about best practices with this population. A particular problem is finding primary care and geriatric physicians who are familiar with ASD and comfortable with autistic patients; in turn, providers may refuse to see patients because they feel ill-equipped. Telehealth models, such as Project ECHO, may be helpful in increasing primary care provider's confidence and willingness to work with people with ASD (Mazurek, 2019).

Unlawful Behavior

When considering the risk of unlawful behavior among individuals with ASD, we, as clinicians, recognize that for the vast majority of our patients the risk of the observed behavior will simply reflect those same risk factors relevant to the population-at-large. Simply put, in general terms there is nothing "special" about ASD that should *automatically* raise red flags, or, conversely, that is particularly protective against such risks. However, that being said, we also recognize that for a minority, their legal transgressions and the nature of the risk associated with these appear to be intimately linked with their diagnosis of ASD and its underlying vulnerabilities. We should always be alert to this possibility, but should not assume such a relationship. In evaluating risk in any individual, the challenge is often apportioning significance to a number of potentially important factors, which will vary from one individual to another; in this respect, risk is unique to that person. This will be true even for two individuals with virtually identical risk factors, as over time risk factors interact with each other, and with background stochastic variation, culminating in an unlawful event.

As reflected in the chapters in this volume, risk has been considered in its broadest sense, and in relation to a variety of issues. While this volume covers various topics and issues it is, of course, impossible to cover everything in one book. For example, below we will consider the more serious mass violence incidents, on a number of occasions purportedly carried out by individuals with an established or possible ASD diagnosis. Additionally, the criminal offense of arson has also been described in the literature in connection with ASD. There is already a body of literature describing the risk of arson among those with intellectual disability (ID), many of whom we assume will also have ASD, whether or not formally diagnosed as such. The nature of this risk is intimately linked with cognitive capacity and communication skills. Specifically, feelings of anger and frustration, with limited ability (and opportunity) to articulate these emotions, and compounded by social isolation and low self-esteem, are described as common characteristics associated with arson in this population (Hall, 2000).

Other problems exist, e.g., a small number of case studies and case series have documented fire-setting among individuals with ASD. This includes the study of Mouridsen et al. (2008), which suggested that arson was the only offense more frequent among cases with ASD compared to a community control sample. Does this suggest, then, that there may be a specific association between arson and ASD? Based on the accumulation of evidence, i.e., considering all the literature published so far, this seems very unlikely. However, this notwithstanding, arson is of particular relevance because the literature has described such incidents by people who have a particular circumscribed interest in, or preoccupation with, fire (Allely, 2019; Freckelton & List, 2009); i.e., there is a direct link between the core impairments of ASD and the legal transgression observed.

Unlawful behavior of lesser severity, such as theft and so-called "conventional" rule breaking (parking and driving offenses for example), certainly also occur, but in the general population these behaviors are relatively common, even among those who would otherwise see themselves as law-abiding people; understanding risk in these instances is arguably of lesser importance although educating police and first responders about autism clearly remains a high priority. There is no reason to believe that relevant risk factors for such behavior will differ in any way among those with ASD. Indeed, the rule abiding and rule-governed nature that characterizes the majority of people with ASD may result in such offenses being observed *less* frequently, but there are no data to support this assertion.

An important area of future research for which we currently have little understanding is the risk of mass violence among people with ASD. This includes actions carried out by lone individuals, some of whom may have an affiliation with a terrorist organization or extremist group, although for others they may be truly acting in a lone manner. Additionally, others who engage in mass violence may have been seen as vulnerable and recruited into a terrorist organization through the internet. Such individuals may be lonely, and have low self-esteem, and welcome the opportunity for "friendship." Consistent with the literature, they may also be highly suggestible, and acquiescent to the demands and expectations of dominant and convincing others who they may be deceived into thinking are friends. Recruitment into such organizations is known to specifically target vulnerable individuals, and people with ASD, who may spend more time using the internet as a platform to reach out to others socially, may be particularly at risk. So-called "lone wolf terrorism" by individuals with ASD has been described in both the scientific literature—by way of detailed study of single cases and small case series—and also in the popular media. This latter platform often presents a less balanced portrayal, foregrounding the ASD and de-emphasizing other aspects that may be equally important in understanding the behaviors described.

As clinicians and scientists, we have a responsibility to attempt to understand these outcomes for the population we work with, although as a forensic research agenda studying extremism and mass violence in this group will be problematic. First, if experts raise the profile of this behavior, a necessary prerequisite to understanding it more, the autistic community will justifiably feel inappropriately labeled. If approached insensitively it could result in a backlash against the scientific community, but, more importantly, a misunderstanding of ASD by society.

Studying this phenomenon from the point of view of ASD or any other neurodevelopmental disorder will require a much more sophisticated methodological approach than case descriptions. Understanding such behaviors will necessarily involve drawing on expertise from fields outside of the typical specialisms that have so far dominated this research, principally psychology and psychiatry. Specifically, drawing on expertise from the criminal justice system, from law and international relations and from security will be important. Interpretation of behavior by psychologists and psychiatrists is generally constrained by our own framework of understanding human behavior, which includes carving up phenomena into signs and symptoms, phenotypes and endophenotypes, or the substance for applied behavior analysis. However, approaching this issue in this way does not allow a diagnostic-agnostic consideration of what motivates people to engage in unlawful and, sometimes, incomprehensible acts.

Moreover, the small numbers of individuals who are likely to engage in such behavior, or be at risk of such an outcome, will require the development of robust methodologies that allow small "Ns" to be examined in a vigorous manner. We are in the fortunate position that the internet allows us access to voluminous information, including blogs, diaries, emails, and other textual information posted by alleged perpetrators. Although on the other hand for some situations, e.g., cases in juvenile courts or cases that involve nondisclosure agreements, available cases may not be available for review. Methods do exist to allow supervised or unsupervised machine learning algorithms to analyze these data. There is also a need for use of qualitative data analytic studies as well as new methods relying, for example, on anonymous survey data to enrich our understanding of specific problem situations.

In our consideration of the wider implications of unlawful behavior, we must also consider vulnerabilities of such individuals when they come into contact with the criminal justice system as defendants, witnesses, and victims. The criminal justice system is a complex process to negotiate, and particularly so for these with social and communication vulnerabilities. As articulated in this volume, structures and supports are in place for those who are vulnerable, but unfortunately ASD is not always as obvious as, say, an intellectual disability; such individuals may not be recognized early in the criminal justice process, and the appropriate scaffolding will not, therefore, be put in place for them. It is therefore important to identify how such systems of care can be implemented. Case law does offer the opportunity to understand where such situations have been well or poorly managed, and the consequences for the individual, but ultimately a policy framework will be needed to provide more clearly defined protection. And as we reflect on these various aspects of the legal implications of ASD, it is important to think also about the wider legal frameworks by which we live, including those related to education and vocation.

Recognizing the breadth of what needs to be considered, we are faced with a number of specific dilemmas about what should be the priorities, both in terms of a research agenda moving forward, but also in regards to actual policy and practice. A principal challenge is the robustness of the research on which we rely to make judgments and decisions about risk and management. Overcoming sample size limitations will require large-scale, collaborative efforts, in a similar vein to the approach taken in genomics and other omics-focused research. It is impractical for one research group to achieve the scale necessary.

One challenge with multicenter research is methodological consistency across sites. For example, diagnosis will require expert-driven consensus, no small feat. This can be complemented with both ASD diagnostic and "diagnostic-agnostic" assessments that allow a wider pattern of strengths and difficulties to be recorded. In some ways it makes little sense to just focus specifically on diagnostic categories such as ASD, particularly if those with lesser degrees of vulnerability impacting the same traits also have similar outcomes. This ensures sample sizes are adequate for statistical power, yet at the same time still does not lose sight of the ability to think categorically in diagnostic terms.

Study design is a further consideration. For example, cross-sectional research may be useful when comparing witnesses with and without ASD or other such groups, particularly when interest is in correlated characteristics. However, to establish causality longitudinal research is needed. For large-scale projects focus groups will be needed, as will efforts to synthesize existing knowledge. In addition to the establishment of cross-disciplinary research groups, scientific advances need to be incorporated into the agenda, including those that are emerging from neuroscience and genetics. For a long time now, neuroimaging has been used as a tool to better understand brain–behavior relationships. There is a long history of neuroimaging at risk groups, particularly individuals labeled with psychopathy. Much insight has developed about patterns of brain activation during the processing of emotionally laden stimuli among such individuals, as well as structural brain differences compared to controls (Mika et al., 2020). Less is known about whether individuals with ASD with and without a history of convictions are different from a functional brain perspective, including the relationship of ASD offenders to other groups of offenders. This is critically important if we wish to view offending within a more helpful epidemiological framework.

Progress in genetics, too, will help us develop insight into those at risk of offending, particularly considering the likely contribution of common variants to ASD's heterogenic phenotype. ASD is principally a genetic disorder, but the relationship between "genes" and "behavior" is still not well understood. Similarly, studies that are examining the genetic underpinning of traits such as empathy, and mentalizing will also be relevant to our understanding of the brain basis of these same vulnerabilities among those with ASD (Woodbury-Smith et al., 2020). There are, of course, potential ethical considerations in relation to collecting genetic data, and how it may be misused.

There are certain unanswered questions that need to be prioritized. The prevalence in prisons should be calculated, as this will have immediate implications for the extent of those who may be vulnerable. Similarly, the prevalence of other neurodevelopmental disorders in the same settings and in similar jurisdictions needs to be calculated (and using identical methodology), as well as the prevalence of convictions in community samples. As mentioned above, any prevalence study will be confounded by the robustness of diagnosis, particularly among those where an existing diagnosis is not present but is instead made at the time of the study and based on screening instruments that were perhaps not designed for the prison population. Sometimes diagnoses are made without considering childhood developmental information. A more pragmatic approach would see individuals stratified according to diagnosis, including, therefore, ASD alongside social-communication disorders.

Much of what has been said above is concerned with people with ASD as perpetrators of crime, but of course they may also be victims. Even when considering involvement with terrorist organizations, it is quite likely that their vulnerability, rather than ASD per se, will have been an important factor leading to their recruitment. Other examples exist in the literature of people with ASD being drawn into criminal activity by dominant individuals whom they thought were their "friend" and with whom they believed to have developed a trusting relationship. People with ASD continue to be at risk of bullying by others throughout their lives, and this may also lead to resentment and anger. It is important not to overlook this perspective, and its impact on risk.

This book has considered these and other important questions with *knowledge translation* in mind, informing policy development, including violence prevention, alongside treatment options for clinicians. Additionally, through the accumulation of case law there is an emerging framework on how to approach difficult cases. With limited resources, such policy needs to offer options that are deliverable and that apply across cultural identities, and ideally geographic distinctions. Although law differs from one country to another, much can be learnt from other countries through comparison of the legal frameworks that exist and their evaluation.

We would be remiss to conclude this volume without discussing neurodiversity. The neurodiversity movement, defined as recognition of neurological difference as part of normal human variation, has led to shifts in how the ASD is conceptualized. In autism's 70+ year history, the emphasis has been largely disorder-focused (Baron-Cohen, 2019). The "disorder" lens identifies ASD exclusively as a problem to cure.

Key arguments against the "disorder" conceptualization come from the community of autistic self-advocates. One of the most common arguments against viewing ASD as a disorder is that considering autism as a condition that requires a cure then leads to a focus on genetic and other etiological research, which diverts resources away from improving the quality of life of autistic individuals who are already here and requiring acceptance, services, and supports. Certainly, this is a departure from the traditional view in a medical model, often espoused by parents of autistic people who are severely impacted who seek to effective therapies and amelioration of behaviors like severe self-injury or aggression. In the medical model, identifying the cause and limiting the negative impacts of ASD is a priority (Kapp et al., 2013).

Ultimately, scientists and clinicians will need to consult with multiple stakeholders in the community in order to make decisions about the most responsible way to proceed (Kapp et al., 2013). Their heterogeneity of the autism spectrum means that there may not be a single answer to the challenge of how to conceptualize autism. Understanding and using of the distinctions between disorder (a problem to be cured), disease (disorder with a known causal mechanism), disability (a person's deficits are below the norm and interfere with functioning), and difference (natural variation in a trait) (as described in Baren-Cohen, 2019) will be key to progress in both research and practice.

References

Allely, C. S. (2019). Firesetting and arson in individuals with autism spectrum disorder: A systematic PRISMA review. *Journal of Intellectual Disabilities and Offending Behaviour.*

Anderson, C., & Butt, C. (2018). Young adults on the autism spectrum: The struggle for appropriate services. *Journal of Autism and Developmental Disorders, 48*(11), 3912–3925.

Anderson, C., Lupfer, A., & Shattuck, P. (2018). Barriers to receipt of services for young adults with autism. *Pediatrics, 141*(Suppl 4), S300–S305.

Aspritiech. (2019). *Annual report.* https://www.aspiritech.org/.

Baron-Cohen, S. (2017). Editorial perspective: Neurodiversity—A revolutionary concept for autism and psychiatry. *Journal of Child Psychology and Psychiatry, 58*(6), 744–747.

Bennett, M. (2016). "What is life like in the twilight years?" A letter about the scant amount of literature on the elderly with autism spectrum disorders. *Journal of Autism and Developmental Disorders, 46*(5), 1883–1884.

Eskow, K., Chasson, G., & Summers, G. (2015). A cross-sectional cohort study of a large, statewide Medicaid home and community-based services autism waiver program. *Journal of Autism and Developmental Disorders, 45*(3), 626–635.

Freckelton Sc, I., & List, D. (2009). Asperger's disorder, criminal responsibility and criminal culpability. *Psychiatry, Psychology and Law, 16*(1), 16–40.

Grindal, T., Schifter, L. A., Schwartz, G., & Hehir, T. (2019). Racial differences in special education identification and placement: Evidence across three states. *Harvard Educational Review, 89*(4), 525–553.

Hall, I. (2000). Young offenders with a learning disability. *Advances in Psychiatric Treatment, 6,* 278–284.

Järbrink, K., & Knapp, M. (2001). The economic impact of autism in Britain. *Autism, 5*(1), 7–22.

Kapp, S. K., Gillespie-Lynch, K., Sherman, L. E., & Hutman, T. (2013). Deficit, difference, or both? Autism and neurodiversity. *Developmental Psychology, 49*(1), 59–71. https://doi.org/10.1037/a0028353.

Lindsay, S., Osten, V., Rezai, M., & Bui, S. (2019). Disclosure and workplace accommodations for people with autism: A systematic review. *Disability and Rehabilitation*, 1–14.

Maenner, M. J. (2020). Prevalence of autism spectrum disorder among children aged 8 years—Autism and developmental disabilities monitoring network, 11 sites, United States, 2016. *MMWR. Surveillance Summaries, 69.*

Mallitt, K. A., & Jorm, L. R. (2018). Diagnosis incidence of autism spectrum disorders is underestimated in Australian children, and there are inequalities in access to diagnosis and treatment services: A data linkage study of health service usage. *International Journal of Population Data Science, 3*(4).

Mazurek, M. O., Stobbe, G., Loftin, R., Malow, B. A., Agrawal, M. M., Tapia, M., Hess, A., Farmer, J., Cheak-Zamora, N., Kuhlthau, K., & Sohl, K. (2019). ECHO Autism transition: Enhancing healthcare for adolescents and young adults with autism spectrum disorder. *Autism: The International Journal of Research and Practice.* https://doi.org/10.1177/1362361319879616

Mika, J., Vaurio, O., Tiihonen J., & Lähteenvuo, M. (2020). A systematic literature review of neuroimaging of psychopathic traits. *Frontiers in Psychiatry, 10,* 1027.

Mottron, L. (2011). The power of autism. *Nature (London), 479*(7371), 33–35. https://doi.org/10.1038/479033a.

Mouridsen, S. E., Rich, B., Isager, T., & Nedergaard, N. J. (2008). Pervasive developmental disorders and criminal behavior: A case control study. *International Journal of Offender Therapy and Comparative Criminology, 52*(2), 196–205.

O'Connor, C., Burke, J., & Rooney, B. (2019). Diagnostic disclosure and social marginalisation of adults with ASD: Is there a relationship and what mediates it? *Journal of Autism and Developmental Disorders,* 1–13.

Odom, S. L., Parrish, T. B., & Hikido, C. (2001). The costs of inclusive and traditional special education preschool services. *Journal of Special Education Leadership, 14*(1), 33–41.

Rivard, M., Magnan, M., & Boulé, M. (2019). Snakes and ladders: Barriers and facilitators experienced by immigrant families when accessing an autism spectrum disorder diagnosis. *Journal of Developmental and Physical Disabilities, 31*(4), 519–539.

Solomon, C. (2020). Autism and employment: Implications for employers and adults with ASD. *Journal of Autism and Developmental Disorders.* https://doi.org/10.1007/s10803-020-04537-w.

Trevisan, D., & Birmingham, E. (2016). Examining the relationship between autistic traits and college adjustment. *Autism, 20*(6), 719–729.

Woodbury-Smith M., Paterson, A. D., Szatmari, P., & Scherer, S. W. (2020). Genome-wide association study of emotional empathy in children. *Scientific Reports, 10,* 7469.

Wright, S. D., Wright, C. A., D'Astous, V., & Wadsworth, A. M. (2019). Autism aging. *Gerontology & Geriatrics Education, 40*(3), 322–338.

Yell, M. L., & Bateman, D. F. (2017). Endrew F. v. Douglas County School District (2017) FAPE and the US Supreme Court. *TEACHING Exceptional Children, 50*(1), 7–15.

Index

F. R. Volkmar et al. (eds.), *Handbook of Autism Spectrum Disorder and the Law*,
https://doi.org/10.1007/978-3-030-70913-6

CPSIA information can be obtained
at www.ICGtesting.com
Printed in the USA
BVHW012023240921
617509BV00002B/7